ADVANCES IN THE DIAGNOSIS AND TREATMENT OF VASCULITIS

Edited by **Luis M. Amezcua-Guerra**

Advances in the Diagnosis and Treatment of Vasculitis
Edited by Luis M. Amezcua-Guerra

Published by InTech
Janeza Trdine 9, 51000 Rijeka, Croatia

Publishing Process Manager Dragana Manestar

Technical Editor Teodora Smiljanic

Cover Designer InTech Design Team

Additional hard copies can be obtained from orders@intechopen.com

Advances in the Diagnosis and Treatment of Vasculitis,
Edited by Luis M. Amezcua-Guerra
p. cm.
ISBN 978-953-307-786-4

For EU product safety concerns:
IN TECH d.o.o., Prolaz Marije Krucifikse Kozulić 3, 51000 Rijeka, Croatia,
info@intechopen.com or visit our website at intechopen.com.

Meet the editor

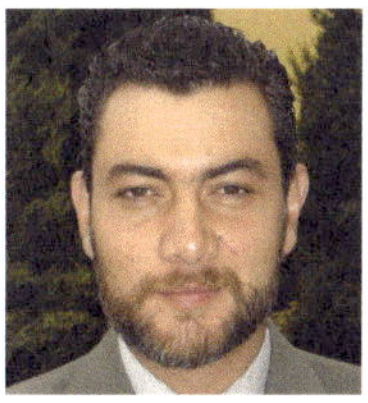

Dr. Luis M. Amezcua-Guerra is a Professor of Rheumatology and Immunology at the Instituto Nacional de Cardiología in Mexico City, Mexico. He is a postgraduate in Rheumatology and Internal Medicine at the School of Medicine, Universidad Nacional Autónoma de México. His work has been seminal to identify and characterize the immune mechanisms that underlie erosive arthritis in systemic lupus erythematosus, especially those related to the abnormal behavior of citrulline and C-reactive protein. He has also been involved in the study of kidney damage in Takayasu's arteritis as well as in the existence of subclinical tissue damage in patients with asymptomatic hyperuricemia. Dr. Amezcua-Guerra teaches immunology to postgraduate students in Rheumatology at the Universidad Nacional Autónoma de México and to undergraduate students at the School of Medicine, La Salle University.

Contents

Preface

"But there were also other fevers, as will be described. Many had their mouths affected with aphthous ulcerations. There were also many defluxions about the genital parts, and ulcerations, boils (phymata), externally and internally, about the groins. Watery ophthalmies of a chronic character, with pains; fungous excrescences of the eyelids, externally and internally, called fig, which destroyed the sight of many persons. There were fungous growths, in many other instances, on ulcers, especially on those seated on the genital organs".

This archetypal description of the Adamantiades-Behçet´s disease remains as valid today as when it was detailed by Hippokrates of Kos (460-377 BC) in his *Epidemion*, book III, part 7 (Hipp. Epid. 3.3.7).

Nevertheless, in these last 2500 years we have advanced a lot in the knowledge of vasculitis, a fascinating array of life-threatening and minor diseases caused by inflammatory conditions that affect the blood vessels. Indeed, research in immunology has invigorated the entire field of vasculitis, shaping a rational approach to its etiology, pathogenesis, diagnosis and treatment, which is the matter of the present book.

This is not a textbook on vasculitis, since it was never intended as a compilation of comprehensive reviews. Rather, it represents the view of each author on selected topics related to vasculitis, verifying the scientific evidence with their own expertise. In other words, this book represents the amalgam between an evidence-based medicine to one based on eminence. Only outstanding experts within defined scientific fields of research in vasculitis from all over the world were invited to participate in this publication. This resulted in an exciting combination of original contributions, structured reviews, overviews, state-of the-art articles, and even the proposal of novel etiopathogenetic models of disease.

Organizing this diversity of manuscripts has not been easy, and I am not certain how long will take readers to cover this *Vasculitis* book from beginning to end, but all the authors have endeavored to draw them into this volume by keeping both the text and the accompanying figures and tables lucid and memorable. This book has been intended to provide a broad base upon which one can build additional knowledge acquired from other sources.

I invite you to read both consecutive but separable books on *Vasculitis* to better understand these fascinating but complex diseases.

"*Advances in the Diagnosis and Treatment of Vasculitis*" contains a section that provides practical information about the screening approach to vasculitis by laboratory analysis, histopathology and advanced image techniques. The part "Advances in the treatment of vasculitis" provides the current standard treatment as well as new and more specific interventions including biologic agents, reparative surgery, and experimental therapies. Finally, miscellaneous issues such as the extra temporal manifestations of "temporal arteritis" or the diffuse alveolar hemorrhage syndrome are covered.

I am thankful to all the contributing authors. Their expert knowledge and experience has guaranteed a thoughtful and innovative approach for rheumatologists, nephrologists and other specialists interested in the fascinating field of vasculitis. Each author must be certain that their efforts will benefit to all patients suffering from these serious diseases.

I am also grateful to Aleksandar Lazinica for this kind invitation to edit the present book; thank you for your confidence. Off note, this book could not have been edited without the dedicated technical assistance of the publishing process managers, Petra Zobic and Dragana Manestar; thank you for your patience and willingness.

What began for Celsus as *Rubor et tumor cum calore et dolore* and led to Virchow's *Functio laesa* has grown beyond the therapeutic targeting of cytokines. As editor, I hope that some of the enthusiasm and excitement of the contributing authors may be shared by each reader of this book.

Dr. Luis M. Amezcua-Guerra, MD
Department of Immunology
The National Institute of Cardiology "Ignacio Chávez"
Mexico City
Mexico

Part 1

Diagnostic Approaches in Vasculitis

1

ANCA Diagnostics in Clinical Practice: New Developments

Jan Damoiseaux, Jos Austen and Jan Willem Cohen Tervaert
Maastricht University Medical Center
The Netherlands

1. Introduction

Anti-neutrophil cytoplasmic antibodies (ANCA) are the hallmark of the so-called ANCA-associated vasculitides (AAV) (Jennette & Falk, 1997). These primary small-vessel vasculitides comprise granulomatosis with polyangiitis (GPA, previously referred to as Wegener's granulomatosis) (Falk et al, 2011), the Churg-Straus syndrome (CSS), microscopic polyangiitis (MPA), and renal-limited necrotizing crescentic glomerulonephritis (NCGN). These disease entities can be discriminated based on systemic symptoms of disease (GPA, CSS, and MPA) versus clinical manifestations that are restricted to the kidneys (NCGN). The systemic diseases can further be subdivided by the presence (GPA and CSS) or absence (MPA) of granulomatous lesions in the airways, while GPA and CSS can be distinguished based on the presence of asthmatic manifestations and/or eosinophilia in CSS, but not in GPA. Classification criteria for these diseases have been defined by the American college of rheumatology (ACR; Fries et al, 1990) and the Chapel Hill consensus conference (Jennette, 1994). The presence of ANCA, however, is not part of these criteria which are primarily based on clinical manifestations and histopathology as observed in biopsies obtained from the affected tissues. More recently a novel consensus methodology for the classification of AAV was developed and validated for epidemiological studies (Watts et al, 2007). Importantly, the latter classification criteria incorporated the ANCA status of the patient.

By definition ANCA are directed to the cytoplasmic components of neutrophilic granulocytes. In particular the constituents of the granules appear to be the antigenic targets. With respect to AAV the serine protease (PR)3 and myeloperoxidase (MPO) are the most important autoantigens. ANCA were originally detected by indirect immunofluorescence (IIF) on ethanol-fixed neutrophils. According to the international consensus on ANCA detection four patterns have to be distinguished (Savige et al, 1999). First, the *classical* (C-)ANCA is characterized by a granular, cytoplasmic fluorescence with central or interlobular accentuation; second, a diffuse flat cytoplasmic fluorescence without interlobular accentuation may be referred to as atypical C-ANCA. In clinical practice, however, this pattern is not distinguished by many clinical laboratories. Third, the *perinuclear* (P-)ANCA is characterized by perinuclear staining, with or without nuclear extension. Reading of the P-ANCA pattern may be hampered by the presence of interfering antinuclear antibodies (ANA). Finally, if a combination of cytoplasmic and perinuclear staining occurs, this is called atypical ANCA. The perinuclear staining pattern actually is an artefact, since formalin-fixation produces a cytoplasmic staining pattern, indistinguishable

from C-ANCA on ethanol-fixed neutrophils. Recently, we reviewed the history of ANCA detection (Cohen Tervaert & Damoiseaux, 2009). It is more than 50 years ago that ANCA were first described in relation with chronic, inflammatory diseases, like rheumatoid arthritis, ulcerative colitis and chronic autoimmune hepatitis. Only in 1985 the association with vasculitis, in particular GPA, was noticed. In these patients IIF revealed a C-ANCA and the antigen recognized proved to be PR3. In a number of GPA cases, however, the sera revealed a P-ANCA and this staining pattern appeared to be more prevalent in MPA and CSS. The antigen recognized in the AAV patients with P-ANCA proved to be MPO. The autoantibodies reactive to these two catalytic enzymes are referred to as PR3-ANCA and MPO-ANCA, respectively. The relation between C-ANCA and PR3-ANCA, and especially between P-ANCA and MPO-ANCA is far from perfect. In particular in chronic, inflammatory diseases other than AAV, the ANCA are directed to multiple other constituents of the neutrophilic granules (like cathepsin G, catalase, α-enolase, elastase, lysozyme, lactoferrin, azurocidin, and bactericidal permeability-increasing protein) and in these cases the P-ANCA is not the result of reactivity with MPO. Hence, the consensus on ANCA detection is to screen sera with IIF and to identify the antigen-specificity with assays specific for PR3 and MPO (Savige et al, 1999). Preferentially, all sera should even be analysed by both IIF and antigen-specific assays.
In this chapter we will first discuss the technologies used for detection of ANCA, including IIF and antigen-specific assays. Next, the international consensus on ANCA testing will be discussed in light of the new technical developments. Finally, we will discuss novel ways of reporting results to the clinic to facilitate the interpretation. These issues will all be dealt with only in terms of the diagnostic phase of AAV; ANCA detection in relation to follow-up of AAV or in light of other disease entities, will not be discussed.

2. Methods for ANCA detection

As mentioned above, ANCA are traditionally detected by IIF. For detection of autoantibodies by IIF serum samples are diluted and incubated with antigen substrate to allow specific binding of autoantibodies (Fig. 1) (Damoiseaux & Cohen Tervaert, 2005). The antigen substrate consists of neutrophilic granulocytes on glass slides that are prepared with a fixative to enable autoantibody binding. In stead of neutrophils it is advocated to be better to use total white blood cells in order to identify true neutrophil specific autoantibodies (Wiik, 1980). In most assays the serum is diluted ~20 times, but one should be aware that the test result of an IIF assay is not only dependent on the serum dilution, but also on the quality of the substrate, the conjugate, and the fluorescence microscope. The latter, however, is more standardized since the introduction of LED-technology as light source. After washing to remove non-specific antibodies, the substrate is incubated with an anti-human IgG antibody reagent conjugated to fluorescein isothiocyanate (FITC). The final three-part complex, consisting of fluorescent secondary antibody, human autoantibody, and antigen can be visualized with the aid of fluorescent microscopy enabling the distinction of different patterns, for instance C-ANCA or P-ANCA. Typical for ANCA detection by IIF is that the substrate, i.e. neutrophilic granulocytes, is fixed with ethanol. This results in (partial) destruction of the lipid bilayer of the cytoplasmic granules enabling the constituents to freely diffuse in the cytoplasm. The strongly cationic enzymes, including MPO, then bind to the negatively charged nuclear membrane, while less cationic enzymes, like PR3 (pI 9.1) remain within the cytoplasm. The artifactual P-ANCA pattern is best illustrated upon fixation of the neutrophils with formalin. In that case the different constituents of the neutrophils are cross-linked and therefore remain within the cytoplasmic granules revealing a C-ANCA pattern. This holds at least for MPO, but other constituents in the granules may be sensitive to formalin-fixation and therefore loose reactivity. Reading of ANCA slides is subjective, labour intensive, and requires expertise of the technicians involved. Thus far, automation of reading ANCA slides is limited. We applied a method of image analyses as a novel approach for the quantification of ANCA levels during follow-up of AAV patients (Boomsma et al, 2003). This technique enabled ANCA quantification by IIF in a single serum dilution. No major differences were observed between image analysis and other techniques in their capacity to predict relapses of disease activity. Therefore, automated ANCA quantification by IIF should also be possible in the diagnostic stage. One step beyond quantification, however, is appropriate recognition of ANCA patterns. Several diagnostic companies have developed software for automated pattern recognition (Hiemann et al, 2009). The software may be fixed, or ready to include pattern information acquired during application of the device in clinical practice. The latter, self-learning device is, however, at risk of a gradual shift in the pattern recognition. Thus far, no studies have been published on automated ANCA pattern recognition.

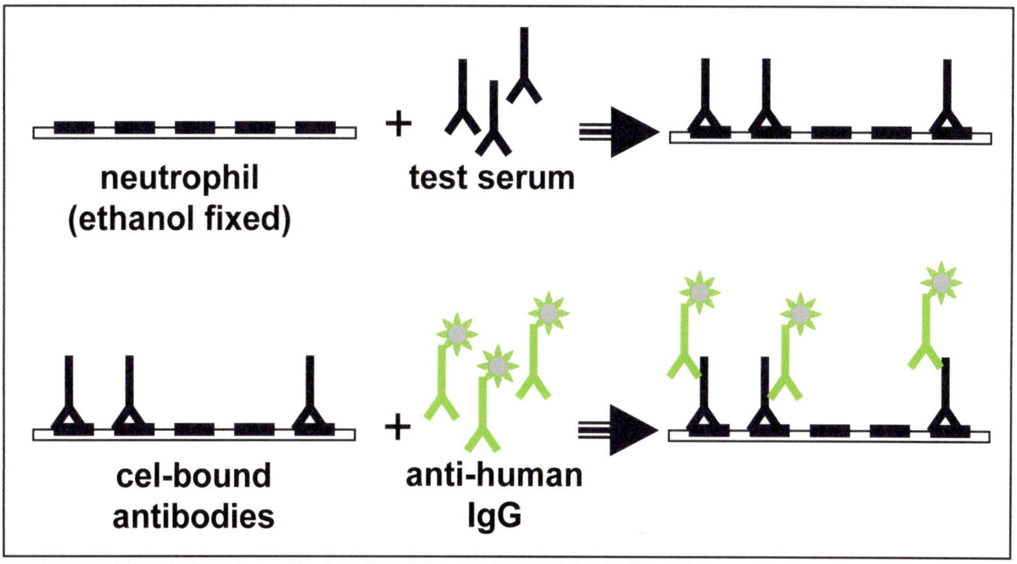

Antineutrophil cytoplasmic antibodies (ANCA) are detected by indirect immunofluorescence (IIF). Slides of ethanol-fixed neutrophils are incubated with patient serum and visualized by FITC-labelled anti-human immunoglobulin G. Fluorescent microscopy may reveal distinct staining patterns.

Fig. 1. ANCA detection by IIF.

Antigen-specificity of ANCA is generally determined by enzyme-linked immunosorbent assays (ELISA). In most cases a direct, non-competitive ELISA is the method of choice for detection of antigen-specific antibodies (Fig. 2a) (Damoiseaux & Cohen Tervaert, 2005). In this assay the antigen is solid-phase bound to the microtiter plates and unoccupied protein-binding sites on the carrier are blocked to prevent non-specific binding of antibodies. Since the antigen is directly coated to the solid-phase, this type of ELISA is referred to as direct ELISA. After coating of the antigen, patient serum is diluted and incubated to enable antigen-specific binding of autoantibodies as present in the serum sample. After washing to remove non-specific antibodies, the anti-human IgG reagent, conjugated with an enzyme like horseradish peroxidase or alkaline phosphatase, is added. Binding of the anti-human IgG conjugate with the antigen-antibody complex, leads to the formation of an enzyme-labelled three-part complex that converts the finally added substrate to form a coloured solution. The rate of colour formation is a function of the amount of autoantibody present in the serum sample. Therefore, the ELISA is considered a true quantitative assay when a reference standard is available, which happens to be the case for both PR3-ANCA as well as MPO-ANCA (IUIS-CDC reference preparations). These standards enable to report the results in international units, an important step forward in standardisation of ANCA diagnostics. During the last decade, multiple variants of the direct ELISA have become available. These assays may differ in terms of the carrier, for instance a membrane in dot-blot assays (Rutgers et al, 2004) and line-immuno-assays (LIA) or beads in multiplex flow cytometry (Nifli et al, 2006; Damoiseaux et al, 2007; Kaul et al, 2009), or by replacement of the enzyme by a fluorochrome, like in fluorescent-enzyme immuno-assays (FEIA) (Damoiseaux et al, 2005) as well as the Luminex-based technology (Nifli et al, 2006; Damoiseaux et al, 2007; Kaul et al, 2009). More recently, also assays based on chemiluminesence technology have become available. Some of the novel assays have the advantage that they simultaneously measure PR3- and MPO-ANCA, and often include anti-GBM antibodies as well. On the other hand, the dot-blot assays and LIA only reveal qualitative results and may be subjective in their read-out. Optimally, the dot-blot assays and LIA are scanned and analysed by appropriate software that takes into account the signal of a cut-off control integrated in the system.

The second generation antigen-specific assays for ANCA detection is based on the so-called capture technology (Fig. 2b). In these ELISA-based tests a monoclonal antibody, specific for either PR3 or MPO, is coated to the carrier and, next, the antigen preparation, either as a crude neutrophil extract (Cohen Tervaert et al, 1990) or as purified antigens (Westman et al, 1998; Boomsma et al, 2001) is added. The antigen is now captured by the monoclonal antibody, hence the name, and the assay is continued with subsequent incubations with patient serum, anti-human IgG conjugate, and, finally, the substrate, similar as in the direct ELISA described above. Theoretically, the advantage of the capture technology is twofold: 1. because of the better consolidation of the three dimensional structure of the antigen the sensitivity will be increased, and 2. because of the additional purification of the antigen by the use of the capturing monoclonal antibody the specificity will be increased. For detection of PR3-ANCA, indeed, both the sensitivity and the specificity are increased in the capture ELISA as compared to the direct ELISA (Csernok et al, 2004). However, capture ELISA's for MPO-ANCA only have increased specificity, but not sensitivity (Boomsma et al, 2001).

Quite recently, third generation ANCA assays were introduced which are referred to as anchor ELISA (Fig. 2c). In these assays the antigen is conjugated to a peptide linker which is used for coating to the carrier. Like in the capture ELISA the three dimensional configuration of the antigen is better maintained and this may result in improved sensitivity. Indeed, an increase in sensitivity for PR3-ANCA was observed in particular in patients with limited disease manifestations (Hellmich et al, 2007; Roggenbuck et al, 2009). These assays were first developed for PR3-ANCA only, but are now also available for MPO-ANCA, although for the latter assay no data are available yet.

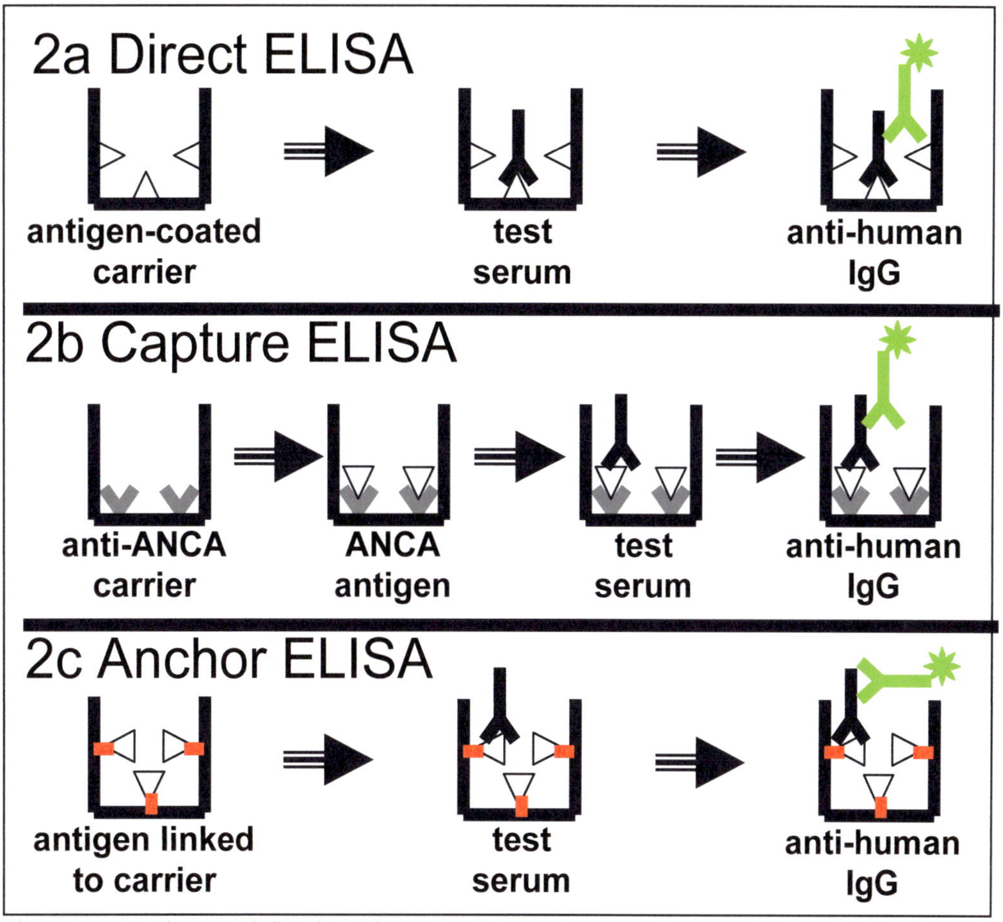

The antigen is either coated directly to the carrier (2a), or via a capturing monoclonal antibody (2b), or via a peptide linker (2c). Incubation with the patient serum and the final detection reagent is similar in these assays.

Fig. 2. PR3- and MPO-ANCA detection by antigen-specific assays.

Interestingly, in almost all antigen-specific assays native antigen, purified from human neutrophils, is used. Assays based on recombinant antigen have appeared difficult to develop (Jenne & Kuhl, 2006). There is, however, one direct ELISA based on a mixture of native and recombinant PR3 on the market. The performance of this assay is very similar to the anchor ELISA's (Damoiseaux et al, 2009a). It is speculated that the HIS-tag, which is normally genetically attached to a recombinant protein for purification purposes, functions as a linker peptide for anchoring the antigen to the carrier.

Finally, there is a novel technology that combines IIF and antigen specificity within a single assay. This biochip technology is a composite substrate of ethanol- and formalin-fixed granulocytes, Hep-2 cells and monkey liver (both for detecting potential interference of ANA), and microdots consisting of the PR3 and MPO antigens. This method has a very high concordance with a multi-test reference method based on IIF, direct ELISA, and capture ELISA (Damoiseaux et al, 2009b). More recently the biochip has even been extended by the inclusion of microdots consisting of the Goodpasture antigen, i.e. the non-collagenous part of the alpha 3 chain of type IV collagen. Although the biochip technology is qualitative in nature, it is very useful in screening new patients suspected of AAV and, in the extended version, of the Goodpasture's syndrome.

3. Guidelines for ANCA detection

In 1999 an international consensus statement on testing and reporting of ANCA has been published (Savige et al, 1999). This is a consensus based on expert opinion. Importantly, this consensus has defined clinical indications for ANCA testing (Table 1). These indications are relevant as far as there is no other obvious cause for the clinical manifestations and they are restricted to the diseases that are associated with small vessel vasculitis. Other diseases that may be associated with ANCA (not MPO- or PR3-ANCA) are included in an addendum (Savige et al, 2003). The clinical indications as defined in table 1 are validated in a retrospective study (Mandl et al, 2002). When the guidelines for requesting ANCA would have been followed, there would have been a decrease of 23% in ANCA requests, while none of the vasculitis patients would have been missed. Due to the retrospective approach, there might have been a bias in potential misclassification. However, none of the ANCA-negative patients developed AAV within 8 to 12 months follow-up. This is somewhat surprising since AAV patients may also present with (epi)scleritis and/or other symptoms that are not included in table 1 (Cohen Tervaert et al, 1987). More recently, an extended gating policy for requesting ANCA has been evaluated (Arnold et al, 2010). Besides clinical manifestations that have a significant pre-test probability of small vessel vasculitis (grossly similar as indicated in table 1), ANCA testing was also granted for the following specialties: rheumatology, nephrology,

- Glomerulonephritis, especially rapidly progressive glomerulonephritis
- Pulmonary hemorrhage, especially pulmonary renal syndrome
- Cutaneous vasculitis with systemic features
- Multiple lung nodules
- Chronic destructive disease of the upper airways
- Long-standing sinusitis or otitis
- Subglottic tracheal stenosis
- Mononeuritis multiplex or other peripheral neuropathy
- Retro-orbital mass

Table 1. Clinical indications for antineutrophil cytoplasmic antibody testing (Savige et al, 1999).

chest medicine, medical ophthalmology and ENT surgery. Additionally, a close liaison was ensured between the laboratory and referring clinician in order to offer requesters the option of further discussion. This approach resulted in a 50% decrease in ANCA requests and obviously in a concomitant reduction in false-positive results. Importantly, the gating policy did not result in either a missed or delayed diagnosis of small vessel vasculitis belonging to the spectrum of AAV.

According to the international consensus statement ANCA testing should start with screening the samples by IIF on ethanol-fixed neutrophils; titration may be useful but is optional. At least the IIF positive samples, irrespective of the pattern, should be tested in a quantitative way by ELISA for both PR3- and MPO-ANCA. Although the consensus states that antigen specificity should be determined by ELISA, it is obvious that other novel assays, nowadays available, may also be applied for detection of PR3- and MPO-ANCA. The consensus is somewhat diffuse with respect to the interpretation of the results. Basically, one expects that only the combination C-ANCA/PR3-ANCA or P-ANCA/MPO-ANCA is relevant for the diagnosis of AAV (atypical ANCA or interfering ANA may replace the respective fluorescence patterns). However, the consensus allows the interpretation of results that reveal positivity only by IIF as being relevant for the diagnosis of AAV. This was merely based on the finding that ~10% of ANCA positive serum samples in patients with GPA or MPA were positive by IIF but negative by direct ELISA. As mentioned, by using capture and/or anchor ELISA's only few samples of AAV patients that are positive by IIF are negative by antigen specific assays. Furthermore, it is obvious that the specificity of this approach (IIF positive only) is strongly reduced. If it concerns a C-ANCA, the IIF result may only be relevant when there is a strong clinical suspicion of AAV, i.e., a high pre-test probability. However, the gap between P-ANCA reactivity and MPO-ANCA will not be closed, because autoantibodies to many other antigens, that are probably irrelevant for AAV give rise to this pattern.

As mentioned above, the international consensus is based on expert opinion. A systematic review of the literature on the role of ANCA testing for AAV is hampered by several issues:

- Standardization of assays is poor: only recently an international standard preparation (IUIS-CDC reference preparations) has become available for PR3- and MPO-ANCA, and the cut-off value in different assays is often not optimal (Holle et al, 2006),
- Serum dilutions for IIF are variable: the consensus does not decide for a 1:20 or a 1:40 dilution and correctly states that the cut-off for IIF not only depends on the serum dilution, but also on the substrate, the conjugate and the microscope,
- Many studies do not use diagnostic samples for testing the utility of novel assays. This is mandatory because, due to epitope spreading and affinity maturation, the autoantibody composite may change during ongoing disease,
- Characteristics of ANCA tests are often expressed in the context of the total AAV population. However, when including the total AAV population, test characteristics will depend on the mixture of the distinct diseases since they differ in the prevalence of PR3- and MPO-ANCA (Wiik, 2002). Also the geographical area may influence test characteristics because the prevalence of MPO-ANCA decreases, while the prevalence of PR3-ANCA increases, when more remote from the equator (Watts et al, 2005).

Altogether, there is one meta-analysis available that evaluates the value of ANCA testing, i.e., the combination C-ANCA/PR3-ANCA or P-ANCA/MPO-ANCA, in the whole spectrum of AAV (Choi et al, 2001). This meta-analysis is based on only 5 studies that fulfilled the stringent inclusion criteria. The study showed that the consensus approach for testing in combination with the strict interpretation revealed a sensitivity of 84.7% and a specificity of 98,6%. Although the specificity is high, one should be aware that the prevalence of AAV is only 15/100.000 (Mohammad et al, 2007 and references herein). The positive predictive value, therefore, will be very low if the selection of patients to be tested for ANCA is not based on appropriate clinical manifestations (Table 1).

Although the current consensus states that screening should be performed with IIF because 10% of the AAV patients may be only positive by IIF, they also advise to assess all samples for both PR3- and MPO-ANCA because 5% of the AAV patients may be positive by ELISA but negative by IIF. When strict criteria are used for interpretation of ANCA results, i.e., the combination C-ANCA/PR3-ANCA or P-ANCA/MPO-ANCA, it does not matter which test is being used as screening assay. There are, however, several arguments that plead for IIF as the best choice. First, depending on the amount of ANCA requests in a laboratory and the

degree of automation, it may be more cost effective to screen with a single assay (IIF) versus two assays (PR3- and MPO-ANCA). The advent of multiplex testing, and in particular the biochip method, neutralizes this argument. Second, ANCA IIF results, but not antigen specific assays, may also be important for other chronic inflammatory diseases like inflammatory bowel disease, primary biliary sclerosis, primary sclerosing cholangitis, and chronic, active autoimmune hepatitis (Kallenberg et al, 1992). The way of testing and reporting ANCA in these chronic inflammatory diseases is described in the addendum to the international consensus (Savige et al, 2003). Third, it is often argued that the utility of the IIF technology is hampered by the requirement of expertise of reading the results. This is a relevant point, but if only PR3- and MPO-ANCA positive samples are tested by IIF, the expertise will be more difficult to maintain because the number of samples tested by IIF will be strongly reduced. On the other hand, the continuous improvement of the antigen specific assays, in particular the capture- and anchor-assays, may have resulted in the IIF being redundant. Indeed, decision tree analysis of different testing strategies revealed that a strategy based on screening for ANCA with ELISA or FEIA and confirmation by IIF is a valuable alternative to screening with IIF and confirming with ELISA or FEIA (Vermeersch et al, 2008).
Finally, the current international consensus does not discuss the need for rapid ANCA testing being available. Especially renal and pulmonary manifestations may have a rapidly progressive onset which requires early diagnosis and treatment in order to prevent organ failure or even death of the patient. In these patients it is important to have results available within 24 hours. Because rapidly progressive glomerulonephritis and alveolar haemorrhage have a high pre-test probability for the diagnosis AAV, it may be sufficient to test only with antigen specific assays, i.e., PR3- and MPO-ANCA, and not IIF. Since the Goodpasture syndrome is also within the differential diagnoses of the renal-pulmonary syndrome, it is advised to include additional testing for anti-GBM antibodies. Although nowadays most automates for autoantibody testing have random access and thereby enable rapid testing in the routine setting, there are also several rapid test assays available for laboratories that have not yet automated their ANCA diagnostics (Westman et al, 1997; Rutgers et al, 2004). Interestingly, capture technology has recently been introduced in these rapid tests. Results obtained in the rapid tests are often qualitative only and should eventually be confirmed and quantified by the assays being in use for routine testing.

4. Interpretation of ANCA results

According to the international consensus positive ANCA IIF results should be reported by the pattern (C-ANCA, atypical C-ANCA, P-ANCA, atypical ANCA, or not to be determined because of interfering ANA). Results of the antigen specific assays should be reported in arbitrary units in combination with the cut-off value. Assays that are calibrated on the new international standard can be expressed in international units. Preferentially, results of IIF and antigen specific assays should be released simultaneously. It is also advised that results are reported together with information regarding the interpretation. This information may include sensitivity and specificity values. It should be realized, however, that such information is of limited value for a clinician who has to decide on the diagnosis of a single patient.
An alternative way of presenting data, which is more valuable for an individual patient, is by likelihood ratios (Bossuyt, 2009). The likelihood ratio provides an estimation of whether there will be significant change in pre-test to post-test probability of a disease given the test result (American college of rheumatology, 2002). A likelihood ratio of 1 implies that the test, either positive or negative, will add nothing to the diagnosis. The higher the likelihood ratio

(>1) for a positive test result, the higher the probability that the patient will have the respective disease, while the lower the likelihood ratio (<1) for a negative test result, the lower the probability that the patient will have the respective disease. Importantly, likelihood ratios can also be determined for combinations of assays, like IIF and antigen-specific assays (Choi et al, 2001). The likelihood ratios depend on multiple independent parameters. First, the positive likelihood ratio corresponds to sensitivity / (1 - specificity) and the negative likelihood ratio to specificity / (1 - sensitivity). In clinical practice specificity is defined by the clinicians that request for ANCA: when the clinicians do not adhere strictly to the clinical manifestations defined in table 1, this may result in an increase in the number of false positive results and thus a reduced specificity. Similarly, if the final diagnosis of AAV is incorrect, this will affect the sensitivity. Altogether, this implies that the likelihood ratios of a certain test depend on the local settings, i.e., the clinicians involved. Second, the test system used for ANCA detection will influence the likelihood ratios. It is obvious that, as compared to antigen-specific assays, the likelihood ratio's for ANCA detection by IIF are less useful for the diagnosis of AAV, but also between distinct antigen-specific assays there may exist huge differences, especially when the cut-offs are not optimal. Finally, the level of the positive test result is associated with distinct likelihood ratios. The likelihood ratios have been defined as a function of ANCA concentration for different assays and from this study it is concluded that likelihood ratios can be best presented for different test-result intervals (Vermeersch et al, 2009). Since the patient population that requires ANCA testing and test system used for ANCA testing will be different between hospitals, this might imply that the likelihood ratios have to be determined locally based on consecutive, diagnostic samples that are sent to the laboratory for ANCA testing. Obviously, standardization of the clinical manifestations that warrant ANCA testing, together with standardization of the assays, for instance by the introduction of the international standards, will add to the generic use of likelihood ratios.

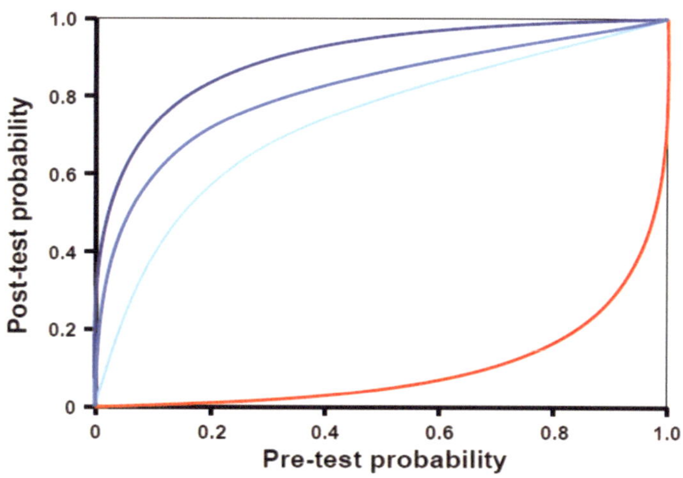

The red curve represents a negative test-result, the light-blue curve a low-positive test result, the medium-blue curve an intermediate-positive test result, and the dark-blue curve a high-positive test result. This is an imaginary example; the curves depend on multiple parameters, like the assay of choice and the patient population that is tested.

Fig. 3. The function between pre-test probability and post-test probability representing test-result intervals.

Although in the diagnostic process of AAV likelihood ratios are of increased value, as compared to sensitivity and specificity, they still require transformation of pre-test probability to post-test probability. Likelihood ratios can be used to calculate post-test probabilities by application of Bayes' rule (Bossuyt, 2009). As depicted in figure 3, this will reveal the function between pre-test probability and post-test probability for both a positive, as well as a negative test result. Most optimal would be the report of results in relation to such pre-test versus post-test diagrams, ideally representing test-result intervals.

5. Discussion

ANCA are associated with distinct forms of primary small vessel vasculitides, collectively referred to as ANCA-associated vasculitis (AAV) (Jennette & Falk, 1997). ANCA were originally identified by IIF. Importantly, however, only ANCA directed to PR3 (PR3-ANCA) or MPO (MPO-ANCA) are relevant for the diagnosis AAV. Therefore there is international consensus that ANCA should be detected by a combination of IIF and antigen-specific assays, i.e. detection of PR3- and MPO-ANCA (Savige et al, 1999). In recent years multiple new developments have influenced detection and interpretation of ANCA. Several novel technologies have become available for antigen-specific ANCA detection. Most of these technologies apply direct binding of the antigen to a carrier and these developments have enabled automation as well as multiplex testing of antigen-specificities. New generations of ANCA tests are based on indirect binding of the antigen to the carrier, either via a monoclonal antibody (second generation capture technology) or via a peptide linker (third generation anchor technology). Although data on the third generation ANCA tests is still scarce, second generation tests have proven to be superior to traditional ELISA(-like) technologies. These second and, possibly, third generation technologies even challenge the dogma of the need for performing IIF as screening assay. The wish to abandon IIF is primarily instigated by the fact that this technology has several disadvantages. Especially the subjective reading of the slides is a serious drawback of this technique. The advent of microscope devices that have integrated software for pattern recognition might overcome this problem (Hiemann et al, 2009). Also for this development there is insufficient data if this approach is going to work in the near future for ANCA IIF. In the end, decision tree analyses have to give the ultimate answer on the role of IIF in ANCA diagnostics (Vermeersch et al, 2008). Finally, with respect to interpretation of ANCA results it is suggested that the data should be interpreted in the light of likelihood ratios for test result intervals (Bossuyt, 2009). This implies that the likelihood ratio increases with increasing ANCA levels. It is evident that these likelihood ratios are different for distinct assays, but it remains to be determined whether such likelihood ratios can be generalized and are applicable in different centres. Ideally, results are reported together with graphics for pre- versus post-test probabilities because this greatly facilitates interpretation by the clinicians. However, this requires adaptation of most hospital information systems to enable a link to the relevant graphics instead of providing only reference values.

Altogether, the new developments in ANCA diagnostics of the last decade are such that revision of the current international consensus on ANCA is required. Importantly, the most recent developments, like third generation assays and automated pattern recognition software, need further evaluation to obtain objective data to be included. This might enable the development of evidence based guidelines instead of a consensus based on expert opinion. Issues that should be considered to be included in a novel consensus are summarized in Table 2. Besides the issues dealt with in this chapter, it is also relevant to define other issues, like the role of formalin-fixed neutrophils as a substrate in IIF and the usefulness of testing for other ANCA specificities. Formalin fixation of neutrophils destroys the antigenicity of multiple (irrelevant) antigens, including interfering ANA as well as multiple antigens other than PR3 or MPO, and reveals the shift in staining pattern from P-ANCA on ethanol-fixed neutrophils to C-ANCA on formalin-fixed neutrophils. As mentioned, the biochip technology enables to combine both substrates in a single incubation (Damoiseaux et al, 2009b). The usefulness of formalin-fixation is already a longstanding discussion (Bird, 1999). If eventually the role of IIF is considered to be redundant, the role of formalin-fixed neutrophils will be finished as well. With respect to other antigen-specificities of ANCA, there are at least three interesting candidates. First, anti-human elastase (HLE)-ANCA seems to be specific for midline destructive disease and/or vasculitis (Cohen Tervaert et al, 1993). Importantly, HLE-ANCA is relevant to identify drug-induced vasculitis (Merkel, 2001). In case of necrotizing lesions of the midline, i.e., nasal septum or palatum, detection of HLE-ANCA may discriminate between GPA and cocaine abuse (Trimarchi et al, 2001). However, thus far the assay is not standardized and data are limited. A second antigen of use might be the bactericidal-permeability increasing protein (BPI). BPI-ANCA have been associated with cystic fibrosis, but may also occur in other chronic inflammatory diseases. In terms of AAV detection, BPI-ANCA may be relevant to explain a C-ANCA result by IIF that can not be confirmed by specific assays for PR3-ANCA. In such a situation the likelihood for AAV is strongly decreased. Finally, human LAMP-2 has been described as a valuable ANCA subtype (Kain et al, 2008). In neutrophils, LAMP-2 is integrated into the membranes of MPO- and PR3-containing vesicles, and thus autoantibodies to LAMP-2 give positive results in ANCA IIF. These antibodies are typically associated with pauci-immune focal necrotizing glomerulonephritis and often co-occur with MPO- or PR3-ANCA. Altogether, more data is required before these different ANCA specificities can be included in routine ANCA diagnostics.

1. Is it possible to screen by antigen-specific assays instead of IIF?
2. Are second (and perhaps third) generation antigen-specific assays mandatory for the diagnosis of ANCA-associated vasculitis?
3. Are antigen-specific assays to be calibrated on the international standard preparations for MPO- and PR3-ANCA?
4. Is there a place for antigen-specific assays other than MPO and PR3?
5. Is there still a role for indirect immunofluorescence (IIF)?
6. Are formalin-fixed (next to ethanol-fixed) neutrophils to be used in IIF?
7. Should rapid-testing be available in every routine laboratory that offers ANCA tests?
8. Is it manageable to present results as likelihood ratios for test result intervals?

Table 2. Issues to be incorporated in a novel international consensus on ANCA diagnostics.

6. Conclusion

Laboratory diagnostics of ANCA has evolved in fifty years with respect to assay technology and automation. The number of ANCA requests has increased simultaneously and this inevitably results in an increase in false-positive results. Altogether, these changes ask for a novel international consensus statement as well as a change in the way of reporting results.

7. References

American college of rheumatology ad hoc committee on immunologic testing guidelines. (2002). Guidelines for immunologic laboratory testing in the rheumatic diseases: an introduction. *Arthritis & Rheumatism (Arthritis Care & Research)*, 27, 429-433.

Arnold, D.F., Timms, A., Luqmani, R. & Misbah, S.A. (2010). Does a gating policy for ANCA overlook patients with ANCA associated vasculitis? An audit of 263 patients. *Journal of Clinical Pathology*, 63, 678-680.

Bird, A.G. (1999). Is there life in the formalin fixed neutrophil for ANCA testing? No! *Journal of Clinical Pathology*, 52, 403-404.

Boomsma, M.M., Stegeman, C.A., Oost-Kort, W.W., Kallenberg, C.G., Moguilevsky, N., Limburg, P.C. & Cohen Tervaert, J.W. (2001). Native and recombinant proteins to analyze auto-antibodies to myeloperoxidase in pauci-immune crescentic glomerulonephritis. *Journal of Immunological Methods*, 254, 47-58.

Boomsma, M.M., Damoiseaux, J.G.M.C., Stegeman, C.A., Kallenberg, C.G.M., Patnaik, M, Peter, J.B. & Cohen Tervaert, J.W. (2003). Image analysis: a novel approach for the quantification of antineutrophil cytoplasmic antibody levels in patients with Wegener's granulomatosis. *Journal of Immunological Methods*, 274, 27-35.

Bossuyt, X. (2009). Clinical characteristics of a laboratory test. A practical approach in the autoimmune laboratory. *Autoimmunity Reviews*, 8, 543-548.

Choi, H.K., Liu, S., Merkel, P.A., Colditz, G.A. & Niles, J.L. (2001). Diagnostic performance of antineutrophil cytoplasmic antibody tests for idiopathic vasculitides: metaanalysis with a focus on antimyeloperoxidase antibodies. *Journal of Rheumatology*, 28, 1584-1590.

Cohen Tervaert, J.W., Van der Woude, F.J. & Kallenberg, C.G. (1987). Analysis of symptoms preceding the diagnosis of Wegener's disease. *Nederlands Tijdschrift voor Geneeskunde*, 131, 1391-1394.

Cohen Tervaert, J.W., Goldschmeding, R., Elema, J.D., Van der Giessen, M., Huitema, M.G., Van der Hem, G.K., The, T.H., Von dem Borne, A.E. & Kallenberg, C.G. (1990). Autoantibodies against myeloid lysosomal enzymes in crescentic glomerulonephritis. *Kidney International*, 37, 799-806.

Cohen Tervaert, J.W., Mulder, L., Stegeman, C.A., Elema, J., Huitema, M., The, H. & Kallenberg, C.G. (1993). Occurrence of autoantibodies to human leucocyte elastase in Wegener's granulomatosis and other inflammatory disorders. *Annals of the Rheumatic Diseases*, 52, 115-120.

Cohen Tervaert, J.W. & Damoiseaux, J. (2009). Fifty years of antineutrophil cytoplasmic antibodies (ANCA) testing: do we need to revise the international consensus statement on testing and reporting on ANCA? *Acta Pathologica, Microbiologica et Immunologica Scandinavica*, 117 (S127), 55-59.

Csernok, E., Holle, J., Hellmich, B., Cohen Tervaert, J.W., Kallenberg, C.G., Limburg, P.C., Niles, J., Pan, G., Specks, U., Westman, K., Wieslander, J., De Groot, K. & Gross, W.L. (2004). Evaluation of capture ELISA for detection of antineutrophil cytoplasmic antibodies directed against proteinase 3 in Wegener's granulomatosis: first results from a multicentre study. *Rheumatology*, 43, 174-180.

Damoiseaux, J. & Cohen Tervaert, J.W. (2005). Tests for autoantibodies, In: *Encyclopedic reference of immunotoxicology*, Ed. H. Vohr, 68-72, Springer-Verlag, Heidelberg.

Damoiseaux, J.G., Slot, M.C., Vaessen, M., Stegeman, C.A., Van Paassen, P. & Cohen Tervaert, J.W. (2005). Evaluation of a new fluorescent-enzyme immuno-assay for diagnosis and follow-up of ANCA-associated vasculitis. *Journal of Clinical Immunology*, 25, 202-208.

Damoiseaux, J., Vaessen, M., Knapen, Y., Csernok, E., Stegeman, C.A., Van Paassen, P. & Cohen Tervaert, J.W. (2007). Evaluation of the FIDIS vasculitis multiplex immunoassay for diagnosis and follow-up of ANCA-associated vasculitis and Goodpasture's disease. Annals of the New York Academy of Sciences, 1109, 454-463.

Damoiseaux, J., Dähnrich, C., Rosemann, A., Probst, C., Komorowski, L., Stegeman, C.A., Egerer, K., Hiepe, F., Van Paassen, P., Stöcker, W., Schlumberger, W. & Cohen Tervaert, J.W. (2009a). A novel enzyme-linked immunosorbent assay using a mixture of human native and recombinant proteinase-3 significantly improves the diagnostic potential for antineutrophil cytoplasmic antibody-associated vasculitis. *Annals of the Rheumatic Diseases*, 68, 228-233.

Damoiseaux, J., Steller, U., Buschtez, M., Vaessen, M., Rosemann, A., Van Paassen, P., Stöcker, W., Fechner, K. & Cohen Tervaert, J.W. (2009b). EUROPLUS™ ANCA BIOCHIP mosaic: PR3 and MPO antigen microdot simprove the laboratory diagnostics of ANCA-associated vasculitis. *Journal of Immunological Methods*, 348, 67-73.

Falk, R.J., Gross, W.L., Guillevin, L., Hoffman, G., Jayne, D.R., Jennette, J.C., Kallenberg, C.G., Luqmani, R., Mahr, A.D., Matteson, E.L., Merkel, P.A., Specks, U.& Watts, R. (2011). Granulomatosis with polyangiitis (Wegener's): an alternative name for Wegener's granulomatosis. Annals of the Rheumatic Diseases, 70, 704.

Fries, J.F., Hunder, G.G., Bloch, D.A., Michel, B.A., Arend, W.P., Calabrese, L.H., Fauci, A.S., Leavitt, R.Y., Lie, J.T., Lightfoot, R.W., Masi, A.T., McShane, D.J., Mills, J.A., Stevens, M.B., Wallace, S.L. & Zvaifler, N.J. (1990). The American College of Rheumatology 1990 criteria for the classification of vasculitis: summary. *Arthritis & Rheumatism*, 33, 1135-1136.

Hellmich, B., Csernok, E., Fredenhagen, G. & Gross, W.L. (2007). A novel high sensitivity ELISA for detection of anti-neutrophil cytoplasm antibodies against proteinase-3. *Clinical and Experimental Rheumatology*, 25 (S44), S1-S5.

Hiemann, R., Büttner, T., Krieger, T., Roggenbuck, D., Sack, U. & Conrad, K. (2009). Challenges of automated screening and differentiation of non-organ specific autoantibodies on HEp-2 cells. *Autoimmunity Reviews*, 9, 17-22.

Holle, J.U., Hellmich, B., Backes, M., Gross, W.L. & Csernok, E. (2006). Variations in performance characteristics of commercial enzyme immunoassay kits for detection of antineutrophil cytoplasmic antibodies: what is the optimal cut off? *Annals of the Rheumatic Diseases*, 64, 1773-1779.

Jenne, D.E. & Kuhl, A. (2006). Production and applications of recombinant proteinase 3, Wegener's autoantigen: problems and perspectives. Clinical Nephrology, 66, 153-159.

Jennete, J.C., Falk, R.J., Andrassy, K., Bacon, P.A., Churg, J., Gross, W.L., Hagen, E.C., Hoffman, G.S., Hunder, G.G., Kallenberg, C.G., Mccluskey, R., Sinico, R.A., Rees, A.J., Van Es, L.A., Waldherr, R. & Wiik, A. (1994). Nomenclature of systemic vasculitides. Proposal of an international consensus conference. *Arthritis & Rheumatism*, 37, 187-192.

Jennette, J.C. & Falk, R.J. (1997). Small-vessel vasculitis. *New England Journal of Medicine*, 337, 1512-1523.

Kain, R., Exner, M., Brandes, R., Ziebermayr, R., Cunningham, D., Alderson, C.A., Davidovits, A., Raab, I., Jahn, R., Ashour, O., Spitzauer, S., Sunder-Plassmann, G. Fukuda, M., Klemm, P., Rees, A.J. & Kerjaschki, D. (2008). Molecular mimicry in pauci-immune focal necrotizing glomerulonephritis. Nature Medicine, 14, 1088-1096.

Kallenberg, C.G., Mulder, A.H. & Cohen Tervaert, J.W. (1992). Antineutrophil cytoplasmic antibodies: a still growing class of autoantibodies in inflammatory disorders. *American Journal of Medicine*, 93, 675-682.

Kaul, R., Johnson, K., Scholz, H. & Marr, G. (2009). Performance of the BioPlex™ 2200 autoimmune vasculitis kit. *Autoimmunity Reviews*, 8, 224-227.

Mandl, L.A., Solomon, D.H., Smith, E.L,. Lew, R.A., Katz, J.N. & Shmerling, R.H. (2002). Using antineutrophil cytoplasmic antibody testing to diagnose vasculitis: can test-ordering guidelines improve diagnostic accuracy? *Archives Internal Medicine* 162, 1509-1514.

Merkel, P.A. (2001). Drug-induced vasculitis. *Rheumatic Disease Clinics North America*, 27, 849-862.

Mohammad, A.J., Jacobsson, L.T.H., Mahr, A.D., Sturfelt, G. & Segelmark, M. (2007). Prevalence of Wegener's granulomatosis, microsopic polyangiitis, polyarteritis nodosa and Churg-Strauss syndrome within a defined population in southern Sweden. *Rheumatology*, 46, 1329-1337.

Nifli, A.-P., Notas, G., Mamoulaki, M., Niniraki, M., Ampartzaki, V., Theodoropoulos, P.A., Kopnitsky, M. & Castanas, E. (2006). Comparison of a multiplex, bead-based fluorescent assay and immunofluorescence methods for the detection of ANA and ANCA autoantibodies in human serum. *Journal of Immunological Methods*, 311, 189-197.

Roggenbuck, D., Buettner, T., Hoffmann, L., Schmechta, H., Reinhold, D. & Conrad, K. (2009). High-sensitivity detection of autoantibodies against proteinase-3 by a novel third-generation enzyme-linked immunosorbent assay. *Annals of the New York Academy of Sciences*, 1173, 41-46.

Rutgers, A., Damoiseaux, J.G., Roozendaal, C., Limburg, P.C., Stegeman, C.A. & Cohen Tervaert, J.C. (2004). ANCA-GBM dot-blot: evaluation of an assay in the differential diagnosis of patients presenting with rapidly progressive glomerulonephritis. *Journal of Clinical Immunology*, 24, 435-404.

Savige, J., Gillis, D., Benson, E., Davies, D., Esnault, V., Falk, R.J., Hagen, E.C., Jayne, D., Jennette, J.C., Paspaliaris, B., Pollock, W., Pusey, C., Savage, C.O.S., Silvestrini, R., Van der Woude, F., Wieslander, J. & Wiik, A. (1999). International consensus statement on testing and reporting of antineutrophil cytoplasmic antibodies (ANCA). American Journal of Clinical Pathology, 111, 507-513.

Savige, J., Dimech, W., Fritzler, M., Goeken, J., Hagen, E.C., Jennette, J.C., McEvoy, R., Pusey, C., Pollock, W., Trevisin, M., Wiik, A. & Wong, R. (2003). Addendum to the international consensus statement on testing and reporting of antineutrophil cytoplasmic antibodies. American Journal of Clinical Pathology, 120, 312-318.

Trimarchi, M., Gregorini, G., Facchetti, F., Morassi, M.L., Manfredini, C., Maroldi, R., Nicolai, P., Russell, K.A., McDonald, T.J. & Specks, U. (2001). Cocaine-induced midline destructive lesions. Clinical, radiographic, histopathologic, and serologic features and their differentiation from Wegener granulomatosis. *Medicine*, 80, 391-404.

Vermeersch, P., Vervaeke, S., Blockmans, D., Van Hoovels, L., Mariën, G., Vanmaele, H. & Bossuyt, X. (2008). Determination of anti-neutrophil cytoplasmic antibodies in small vessel vasculitis: comparative analysis of different strategies. *Clinica Chimica Acta*, 397, 77-81.

Vermeersch, P., Blockmans, D. & Bossuyt, X. (2009). Use of likelihood ratio scan improve the clinical usefulness of enzyme immunoassays for the diagnosis of small-vessel vasculitis. *Clinical Chemistry*, 55, 1886-1888.

Watts, R., Lane, S., Hanslik, T., Hauser, T., Hellmich, B., Koldingsnes, W., Mahr, A., Segelmark, M., Cohen Tervaert, JW. & Scott, D. (2007). Development and validation of a consensus methodology for the classification of the ANCA-associated vasculitides and polyarteritis nodosa for epidemiological studies. *Annals of the Rheumatic Diseases*, 66, 222-227.

Westman, K.W., Bygren, P.G., Eilert, I., Wiik, A. & Wieslander, J. (1997). Rapid screening assay for anti-GBM antibody and ANCAs: an important tool for the differential diagnosis of pulmonary renal syndromes. *Nephrology Dialysis and Transplantation*, 12, 1863-1868.

Westman, K.W., Selga, D., Bygren, P., Segelmark, M., Baslund, B., Wiik, A. & Wieslander, J. (1998). Clinical evaluation of a capture ELISA for detection of proteinase-3 antineutrophil cytoplasmic antibody. *Kidney International*, 53, 1230-1236.

Wiik, A. (1980). Granulocyte-specific antinuclear antibodies. Possible significance for the pathogenesis, clinical features and diagnosis of rheumatoid arthritis. *Allergy*, 35, 263-289.

Wiik, A. (2002). Rational use of ANCA in the diagnosis of vasculitis. *Rheumatology*, 41, 481-483.

2

Histopathology of Cutaneous Vasculitis

Ko-Ron Chen
Head of Department of Dermatology, Saiseikai Central Hospital Tokyo, Japan

1. Introduction

Vasculitis is an inflammatory process occurring primarily on the vessel wall. It results in vessel wall destruction and subsequent hemorrhagic and ischemic events. Skin is the most common target organ for vasculitis.[1,2,3,4]

Cutaneous vasculitis includes vasculitis of the dermal small vessels[5] and subcutaneous small muscular vessels.[6] It can be a self-limited benign disease restricted to the skin or be a significant component of many systemic vasculitic syndromes such as collagen disease-associated vasculitis or anti-neutrophil cytoplasmic antibody (ANCA)-associated primary vasculitic syndromes.

Cutaneous vasculitis most frequently manifests as palpable purpura or infiltrated erythema (indicating dermal small vessel vasculitis), and less frequently as nodular erythema, livedo racemosa, deep ulcers, or digital gangrene (indicating deep dermal vasculitis or subcutaneous muscular-vessel vasculitis). Cutaneous vasculitis presents as a constellation of clinical and histopathologic findings since the size of vessel involved correlates with the clinical findings.[1,2,3,4]

A diagnosis of cutaneous vasculitis is best determined by the histopathologic findings of the vessel size involved and the principal inflammatory response. Histopathologic findings are also crucial for distinguishing authentic cutaneous vasculitis from cutaneous pseudovasculitis[7] (a heterogeneous collection of disorders that clinically produce hemorrhages [i.e., petechiae, purpura, and ecchymoses] or vessel occlusion [which results in livedo, cyanosis, ulcers, digital necrosis, and/or gangrene] and simulate cutaneous vasculitis but without the histopathologic evidence of vasculitis).[7]

This chapter will describe the morphological approach to cutaneous vasculitis, including:

1. The diagnostic criteria for small vessel vasculitis and for subcutaneous muscular vessel vasculitis (e.g., arteritis and phlebitis);
2. The details of the inflammatory stages of muscular vessel vasculitis (based on morphological changes during the inflammatory process, which strongly affect the treatment for vasculitis);
3. The histopathologic classification of cutaneous vasculitis (based on the size of the affected vessel [e.g., small vessels or muscular vessels] and the predominant inflammatory cell types [e.g., neutrophils, eosinophils, lymphocytes, histiocytes]) and their related disorders.

Distinguishing between subcutaneous muscular arteritis and phlebitis will be also discussed since the morphological features of the subcutaneous veins in the lower legs, such as a compact concentric smooth muscle pattern with a round lumen and no obvious bundled formation, mimic features that are characteristic of arteries. This may lead to phlebitis or thrombophlebitis being misdiagnosed as arteritis and result in unnecessary overtreatment.

2. Morphology and distribution of cutaneous vessels

Types of vessels

Small artery
Small vein
Arteriole
Venule and capillary

Small arteries are defined as arteries having a caliber of 100 μm to 1000 μm

Where a skin biopsy reaches into the subcutis, the arterial caliber level is less than 1000μm. Therefore, histopathologically proven arteritis identified from skin lesions should involve small-sized arteries, rather than medium-sized arteries (which have calibers larger than 1000 μm). The distribution of small arteries is from the lower dermis (where the arterial size ranges from 100 μm to 200 μm) to the subcutis (where the arterial size ranges from 100 μm to 1000 μm). Small arteries usually have a tunica intima (containing an endothelial cell layer with an underlying layer of a sharp internal elastic lamina) and a tunica media (containing two to 10 concentric compact continuous smooth muscular layers with very few elastic fibers in the muscular layer). These are characteristic of small arteries. The tunica adventitia - the outer layer of small arteries - is generally unidentifiable, having few perivascular collagen fibers and identifiable elastic fibers (Figures 1 and 2).

Small veins are defined as veins having a caliber between 100 μm and 1000 μm.

Small veins are distributed from the lower dermis to the subcutis. The lack of an internal elastic lamina and discontinuous bundles of muscle in the elastic fiber-rich muscular medial layer are characteristic of small veins (Figures1 and 2).

Arterioles are defined as arteries having a caliber of less than 100 μm.

The tunica intima in arterioles is characterized by a layer consisting only of endothelial cells with an underlying internal elastic lamina, as seen in small arteries. The tunica media in arterioles is characterized by approximately one to two concentric smooth muscular layers. The tunica adventitia in arterioles is usually unidentifiable (Figure 3).

Venules are defined as veins having a caliber of less than 100 μm.

Venules contain one to two muscular layers in the tunica media and may have a perivascular fibrotic layer in the tunica adventitia. The lack of the internal elastic lamina is a feature that distinguishes venules from arterioles (Figures 3 and 4).
All small vessels in the superficial to mid-dermis are arterioles, venules, and capillaries since the vessels are smaller than 100 μm (Figure 3). All of the small vessels in the dermis are less than 200 μm, including capillaries, venules, arterioles, small veins and small arteries. (The small arteries and veins in the dermis range from 100 μm to 200 μm.). The size of the small arteries at the dermo-subcutaneous junction ranges from 200 μm to 400 μm (Figures 2, 22D, and 22F). These arteries are commonly involved in cutaneous polyarteritis nodosa.

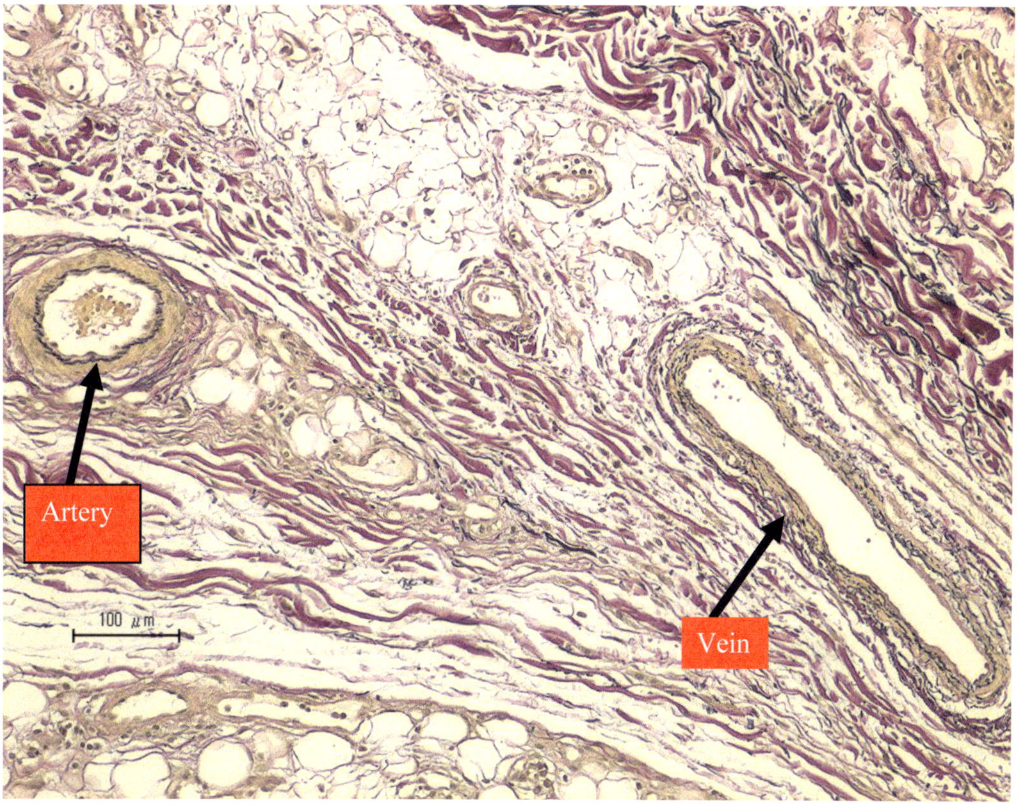

Fig. 1. (elastic tissue stain) The distinction between a deep dermal small artery and vein.

Note the characteristic sharp internal elastic fiber encircling the lumen but the absence of elastic fiber in the muscular medial layer of the artery. By contrast, there is an absence of an internal elastic lamina and there are multiple layers of elastic fibers in the medial muscular layer of the vein.

3. Points and pitfalls of distinguishing between arterial and venous vessels

1) Dermal arterioles vs. dermal venules

Points:

- Arterioles have an internal elastic lamina adhering to the outside of the endothelial cell layer (Figure 3).
- Venules lack an internal elastic lamina (Figure 3).

Pitfalls:

- The presence of a perivascular layer of elastic fiber in venules may mimic the internal elastic lamina in arterioles (Figure 3), especially if the outline of the vessel wall in venules has become unclear because of inflammation (Figure 4).

2) Subcutaneous arteries vs. subcutaneous veins[8]

Points:

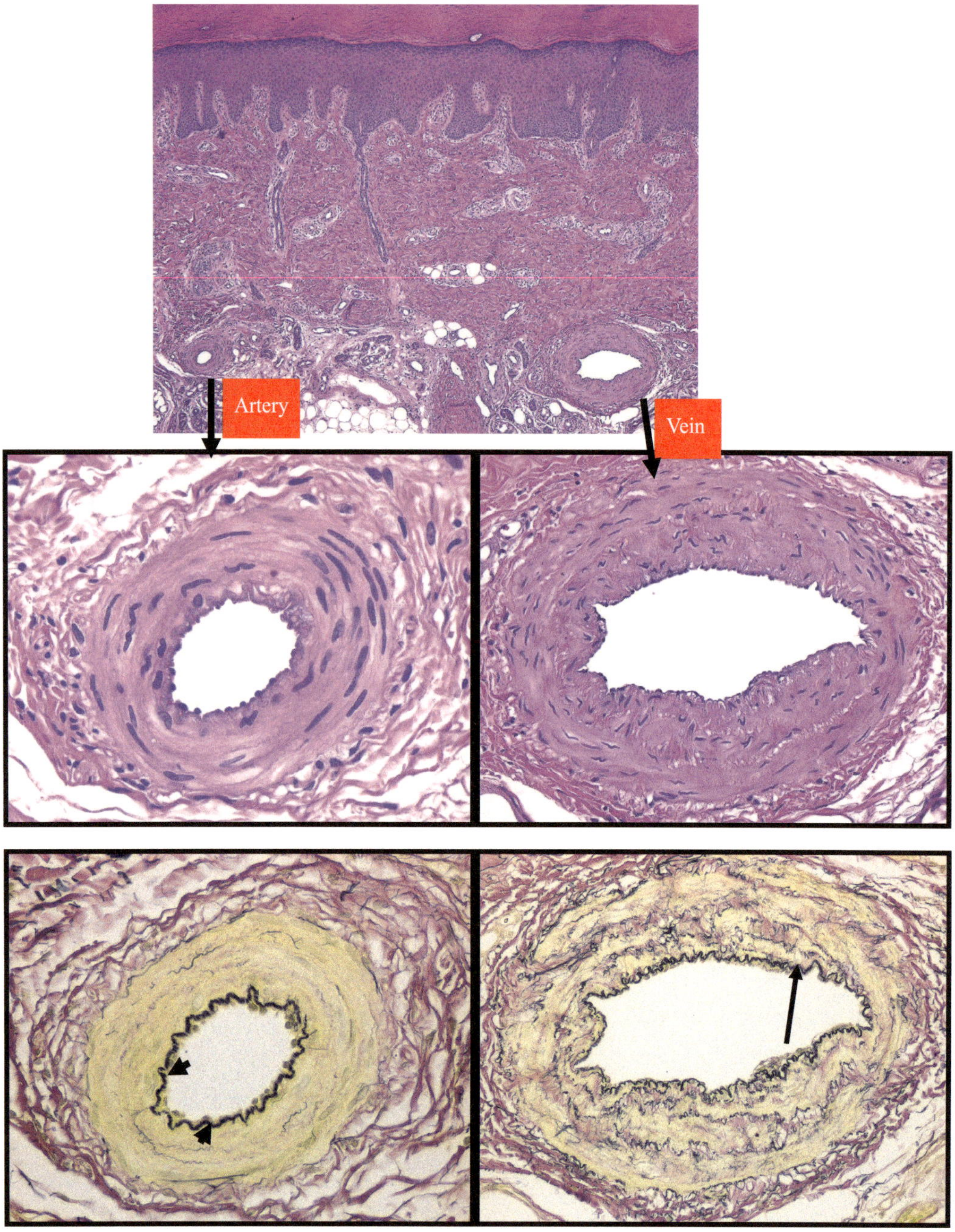

Fig. 2. The distinction between a small muscular artery and vein at the dermo-subcutaneous junction.

These vessels are from an infiltrated erythematous lesion on the inner sole. The compact concentric muscular layers and the internal elastic lamina-like elastic fiber in the intima (arrow at bottom right: [elastic tissue stain]) in the vein resemble the features of an artery.

However, the concentric continuous wreath-like smooth muscular pattern with the lack of elastic fibers in the medial muscular layer in an artery (bottom left: [elastic tissue stain]) is distinguishable from the discontinuous bundled smooth muscular layers separated by abundant elastic fibers in the medial muscular layer in the vein (bottom right). Moreover, the sharp even thickness of the internal elastic lamina (arrow heads) in the artery is dissimilar to the uneven feature of the internal elastic lamina-like elastic fiber (arrow) in the vein.

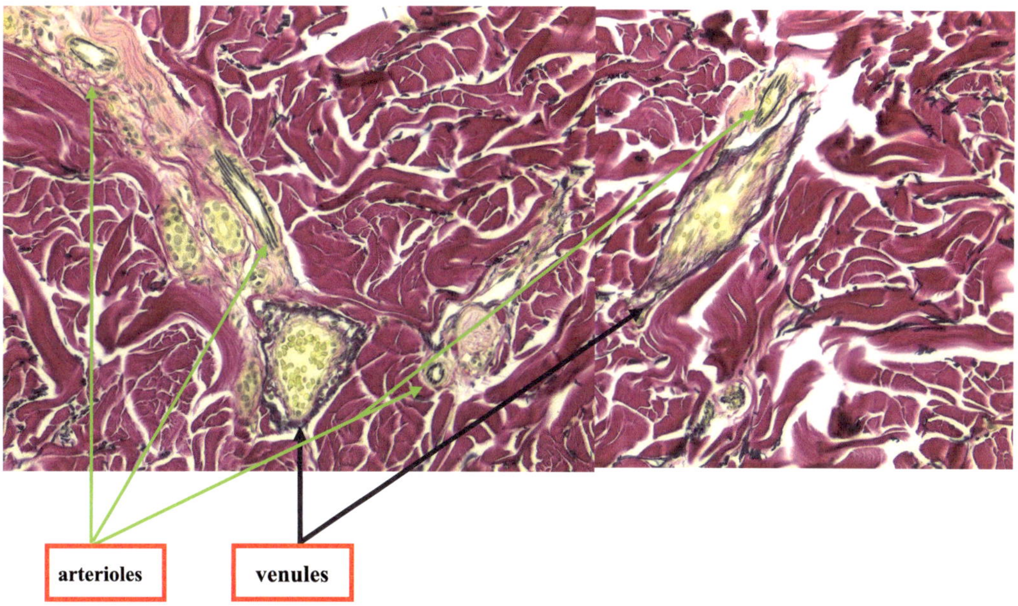

Fig. 3. Dermal arterioles and venules. (elastic tissue stain)

Arterioles contain one to two medial muscular layers with a sharp layer of internal elastic lamina (green arrows) adhering to the outside of the endothelial cell layer (which faces the lumen). By contrast, the venules lack an internal elastic lamina but have a layer of perivascular elastic fiber that may be mistaken for the authentic internal elastic lamina of arterioles.

Arterial wall (Figures 1 and 2)

- The smooth muscle layers in the media have a compact concentric and continuous distribution.
- A lack of elastic fibers in the medial layer.
- A sharp, evenly thick internal elastic lamina is present.

Venous wall (Figures 1 and 2)

- Smooth muscle layers in the media have a discontinuous bundled distribution.
- Prominent elastic fibers in the medial layer are present.
- Absence of an authentic internal elastic lamina.
- Venous valves may be present.

Pitfalls: (Figure 2)

- The presence of the intimal elastic fibers in veins (arrow at the bottom right of Figure 2) may mimic the internal elastic lamina in arteries (arrow heads at bottom left of Figure 2), while the uneven thickness and partial multilayer of the intimal elastic fibers in veins are distinguishable.
- Morphological features of the veins obtained from skin lesions of the dorsal or plantar feet may show a thick compact and continuous smooth muscle layer distribution similar to arteries.[8] The bundled smooth muscular layers, separated by abundant elastic fibers in the media of veins (bottom right of Figure 2), is distinguishable from the concentric and continuous smooth muscular layers with a lack of elastic fibers in the arterial media (bottom left of Figure 2).

4. Concept of cutaneous vasculitis

Vasculitis is an inflammatory process occurring primarily on the vessel wall, leading to vessel wall destruction and subsequent hemorrhagic and ischemic events. Cutaneous vasculitis comprises vasculitis of the dermal small vessels and the subcutaneous small muscular vessels. Basic principle of histopathologic diagnosis for cutaneous vasculitis is the morphological evidence of both (1) angiocentric infiltration of inflammatory cells and (2) damage of vessel wall. Therefore the following vasculitis-like conditions, which are different from the process of vessel damage in vasculitis, should not be interpreted as cutaneous vasculitis:

1. Vessel damage that is not caused by inflammatory cells, but is caused by a direct invasion of tumor cells or organisms, including fungi, bacteria, and viruses.
2. Vessel damage as a secondary event (i.e., innocent bystanders) caused by primary necrosis or by destruction of the connective tissue. The adjacent innocent vessels are secondarily involved in the resultant vessel destruction. This phenomenon of innocent bystanders-like secondary vessel damage is most often found in lesions of pyoderma gangrenosum, overlying ulcerative lesions, dermal/subcutaneous abscesses, and dermal/subcutaneous caseous necrosis.

5. Histopathologic diagnosis of cutaneous vasculitis

1) Biopsy: Timing, technique, and choice of lesions

An appropriate skin biopsy is the key to obtaining a significant result for cutaneous vasculitis.

Timing of biopsy:

- The pathologic features of vasculitis may be absent if the biopsy is poorly timed. A skin biopsy should not be performed for purpuric or infiltrated lesions after 48 hours, and a skin biopsy should not be performed for deep nodular erythematous lesions after 72 hours.

Choice of lesions and biopsy technique:

- A biopsy extending to the subcutis should be taken from the most palpable purpuric lesions or the most tender, reddish nodular or infiltrated lesions.
- For purpuric lesions or infiltrated erythematous lesions smaller than 5 mm, a 3 to 4 mm large punch biopsy extending to the subcutis will enable histopathologic confirmation..

- For nodular erythema lesions or infiltrated erythema larger than 5 mm, a spindle-shaped incisional biopsy extending to the subcutis with a 5 to 6 mm large tissue sample should be performed on the central lesions.
- It is better to perform two biopsies. The first, a biopsy of the most palpable and tender lesions for light microscopy examination; the second, a punch biopsy of an early erythematous or purpuric lesion for a direct immunofluorescence (DIF) examination.

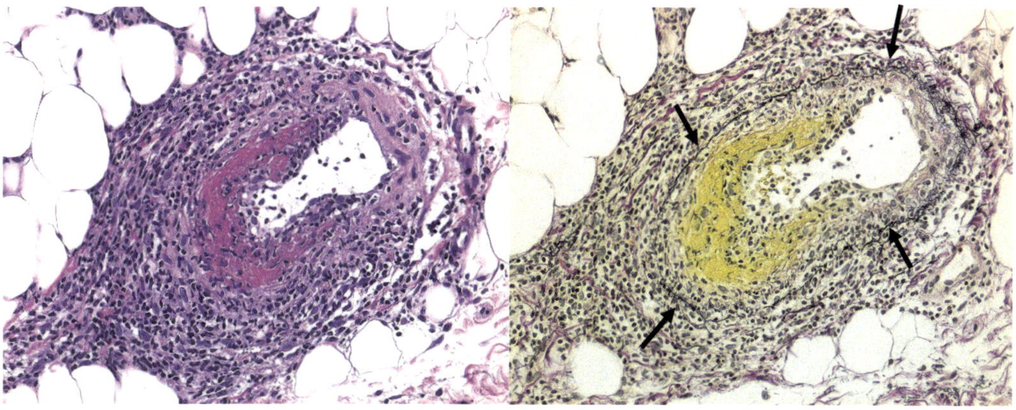

Fig. 4. Diagnostic pitfall of the internal elastic lamina-like perivascular elastic fiber (arrows) in a venule with necrotizing vasculitis. (Right): elastic tissue stain

2) Significance of direct immunofluorescence examination

A DIF examination is a crucial component of diagnosis.[1] Palpable purpura on the lower legs with a histopathologic feature of leukocytoclastic vasculitis is the most common finding in vasculitis disorders with dermal small vessel involved, which can be found in ANCA-related vasculitis (e.g., Churg-Strauss syndrome, Wegener's granulomatosis and microscopic polyangiitis); cryoglobulinemic purpura; collagen disease-associated vasculitis (e.g., rheumatoid arthritis, systemic lupus erythematosus, Sjögren disease); and Henoch-Schönlein purpura. It is therefore difficult to make a distinction just based on the cutaneous manifestations and histopathologic findings. However, the absence of immune complexes, the so-called pauci-immune vasculitis, is an expected finding in Churg-Strauss syndrome, Wegener's granulomatosis, and microscopic polyangiitis. By contrast, deposition of IgM, and/or C3 in or around the vessels characterizes immune complex-mediated vasculitis, as found in cryoglobulinemic vasculitis, rheumatoid vasculitis,[9] and systemic lupus erythematosus. Vascular deposition of IgA, rather than IgG or IgM, is required for the diagnosis of Henoch-Schönlein purpura (Figure 5). Similar to hematoxylin and eosin evaluation, the presence of diagnostic immunofluorescence patterns is inversely related to the age of the lesion biopsied. Nearly 100% of biopsies will identify immunoglobulins within the first 48 hours, followed by 70% positive results at 48-72 hours; immunoglobulins will not be detected in the lesions after 72 hours.[1]

3) Diagnostic criteria for small vessel vasculitis and muscular vessel vasculitis

1. Diagnostic criteria for small vessel vasculitis[9]

Essential findings:

i. **Perivascular infiltration of inflammatory cells**

ii. **Fibrinoid necrosis of the small vessel wall**

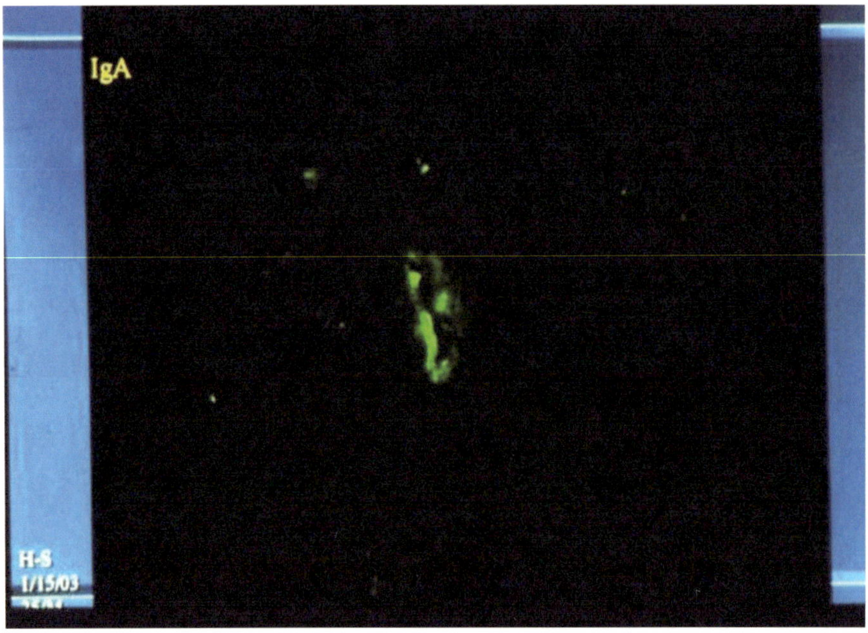

Fig. 5. The presence of an IgA vascular deposit in the papillary dermis is required for a diagnosis of Henoch-Schönlein purpura.

A histopathologic diagnosis for small vessel vasculitis should fulfill both criteria I and II above.

Other minor features, including erythrocyte extravasation and nuclear dust, are not the crucial findings for a diagnosis of small vessel vasculitis.

Q: Why is a perivascular infiltration of inflammatory cells indispensible for a diagnosis?

A: Vasculitis is an inflammatory process occurring primarily at the vessel walls. A perivascular infiltration of inflammatory cells is indispensible for a diagnosis and to avoid the diagnostic pitfalls of:

1. Vessel damage caused by direct vessel invasion by bacteria, fungi (Figure 16), or tumor cells (Figure 20), rather than by inflammatory cells; and
2. Secondary vessel wall damage (i.e., innocent bystander damage) caused by adjacent primary necrotic connective tissue, as found in lesions of dermal or subcutaneous abscess (Figures 17 and 18).

Q: Why is fibrinoid necrosis of the vessel wall indispensible for a diagnosis of small vessel vasculitis?

A: On light microscopy examination, the morphology of vessel wall fibrinoid necrosis is the sole finding of small vessel damage and is accepted as crucial in distinguishing small vessel vasculitis from vasculitis-like disorders with a perivascular infiltration of inflammatory cells (which would occur without evidence of fibrinoid necrosis of the vessel wall).

Components of small vessels in the dermis mainly comprise one to two muscular layers with an inner endothelial cell layer facing the lumen (Figure 3). The inflammatory cells can pass from the lumen through the small vessel wall without damaging the vessel wall.

Therefore, the finding of perivascular inflammatory cells infiltrating into the vessel wall is not convincing evidence of vessel wall damage. Endothelial cells, the main component of the small vessel wall, play a key role in preventing blood from coagulation. Once inflammatory cells such as neutrophils damage the endothelial cells, the endothelial cells lose their anti-coagulation function (Figure 6), resulting in the formation of fibrin thrombi at the luminal side of the damaged endothelial cell (Figures 6 and 7). A zone of a homogeneous eosinophilic deposit, (i.e., fibrinoid necrosis) - mainly containing fibrin mixed with cellular debris, including necrotic or apoptotic endothelial cells and, most often, degenerated neutrophils, and serologic proteins such as immunoglobulins and complements - eventually forms at the affected vessel wall and discharges outward to the perivascular area[3,10] (Figures 6 and 8).

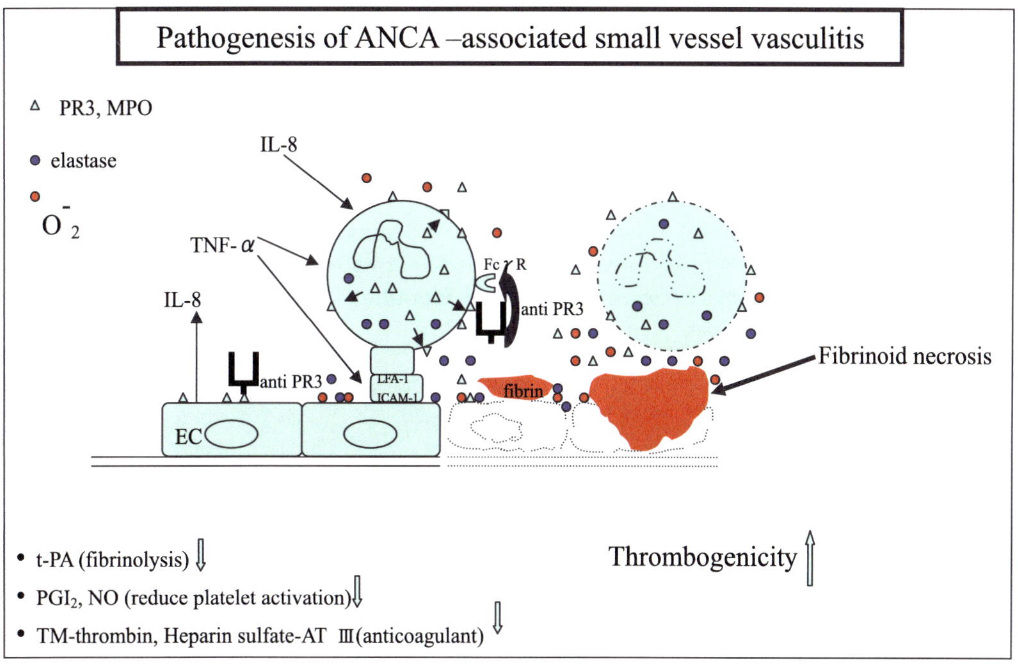

Fig. 6. Pathogenesis of ANCA –associated small vessel vasculitis

Endothelial cells damaged by inflammatory cells (e.g., neutrophils) in vasculitis will lose their anti-coagulation function, including fibrinolysis and the reduction of platelet activation, resulting in the formation of fibrin thrombi at the luminal side of the damaged endothelial cell and eventually formation of fibrinoid necrosis at the damaged vessel wall.

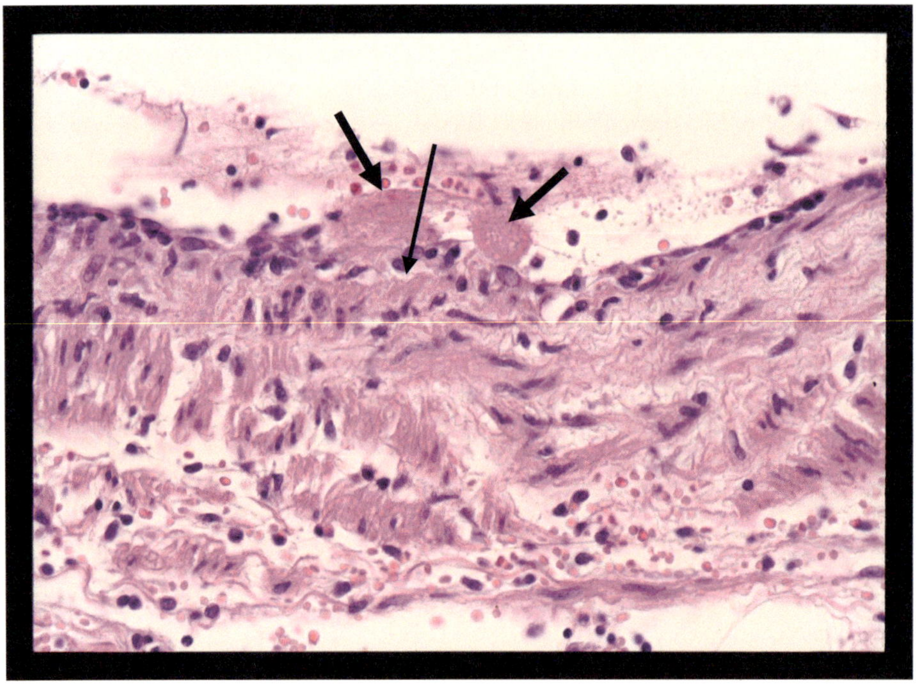

Fig. 7. Formation of fibrin thrombi at the very early stage of vasculitis.

Fibrin thrombi (thick arrows) mixed with a few inflammatory cells are adhered to the affected intima, where loss of endothelial cells can be appreciated (long arrow). By contrast, no evidence of fibrin thrombi formation can be identified at the adjacent intima where endothelial cells remain intact.

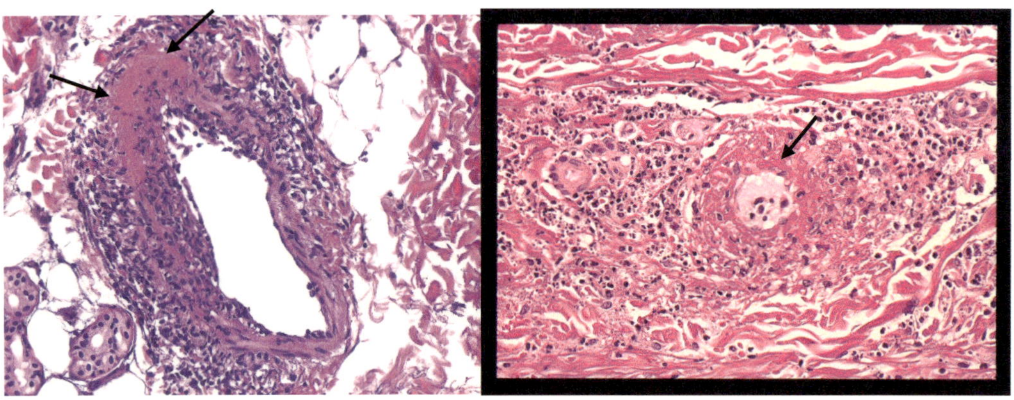

Fig. 8. Fully developed vasculitis with features of marked vessel wall fibrinoid necrosis.

The affected vessel wall (arrows) of fully developed vasculitis is characterized by a zone of a homogeneous eosinophilic deposit (i.e., fibrinoid necrosis) which mainly contains fibrin mixed with cellular debris (including degenerated neutrophils and necrotic or apoptotic endothelial cells) and serologic proteins such as immunoreactants. This subsequently discharges outwardly into the perivascular area.

2. Diagnostic criteria for muscular vessel vasculitis[9]

Essential findings:

I) Perivascular and intravascular wall infiltration of inflammatory cells

In the normal condition, the muscular vessels do not allow inflammatory cells to infiltrate into the compact muscular vessel wall. When there are inflammatory cells in the muscular vessel wall, there will always be destruction of the vessel wall, which manifests as edema of the medial layer and disruption of the muscular layers (Figures.9, 10, 11, Figure13B, Figures31B and 32C). The crucial feature of vessel wall fibrinoid necrosis, which is used for the diagnosis of small vessel vasculitis, is not essential for the diagnosis of muscular vessel vasculitis. Muscular vessel vasculitis with vessel wall fibrinoid necrosis will certainly be diagnosed as necrotizing arteritis or necrotizing phlebitis.

II) Morphological evidence of internal elastic lamina destruction, confirmed by elastic fiber staining, is needed to diagnose arteritis at the healed stage.

A feature of arteritis at the end stage (i.e., healed stage) is minimal inflammation in and around the affected artery. At this stage, it is impossible to determine, just based on hematoxylin eosin stain, if there had ever been vasculitic inflammation of the suspected artery. Disruption of the internal elastic lamina is evidence of arteritis at the healed stage (Figure 14A).

A histopathologic diagnosis for muscular vessel vasculitis should fulfill either criteria I or criteria II above.

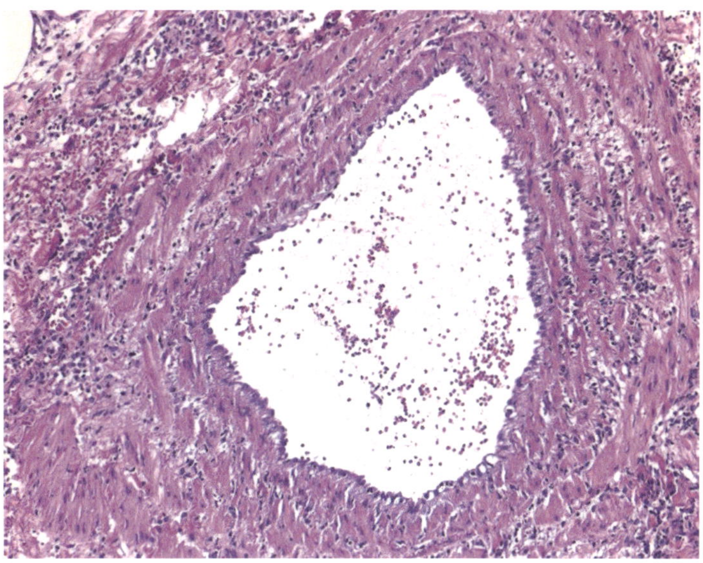

Fig. 9. Subcutaneous phlebitis with inflammatory cells in and around the muscular vessel wall is characterized by edema of the medial layers and disruption of the muscular layers with erythroctye extravasation in and around the muscular vessel wall. Note no vessel wall fibrinoid necrosis can be identified.

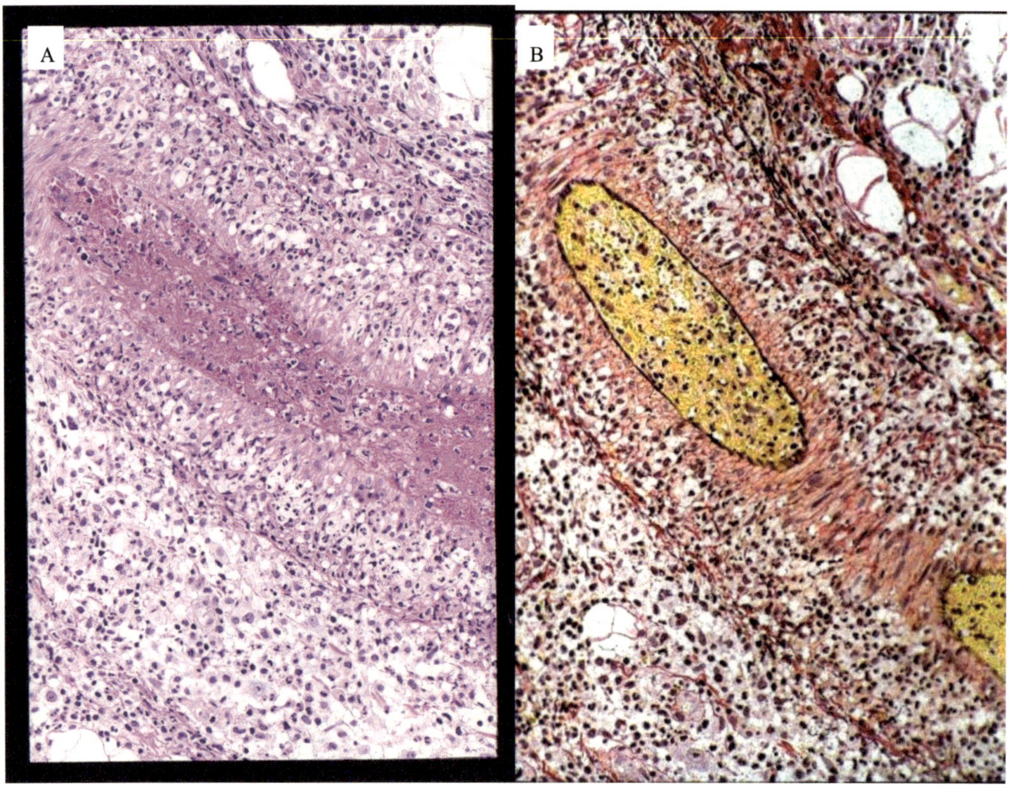

Fig. 10. Arteritis at the acute stage.

(A) A predominate infiltrate of neutrophils, with marked nuclear dust in and around the affected artery with fibrin thrombi, results in luminal occlusion. No fibrous or vascular proliferation can be found in and around the affected artery.
(B) Note that the internal elastic lamina remains intact and no fibrinoid necrosis can be identified in the vessel wall.

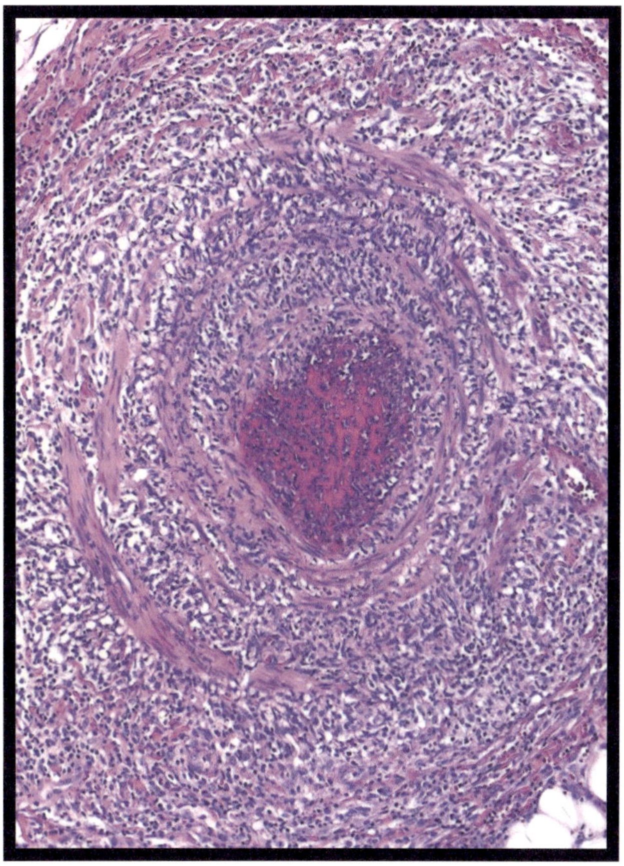

Fig. 11. Phlebitis at the acute stage.

A predominate infiltrate of neutrophils with nuclear dust in and around the affected muscular vein but without fibrous proliferation or neovascularization.

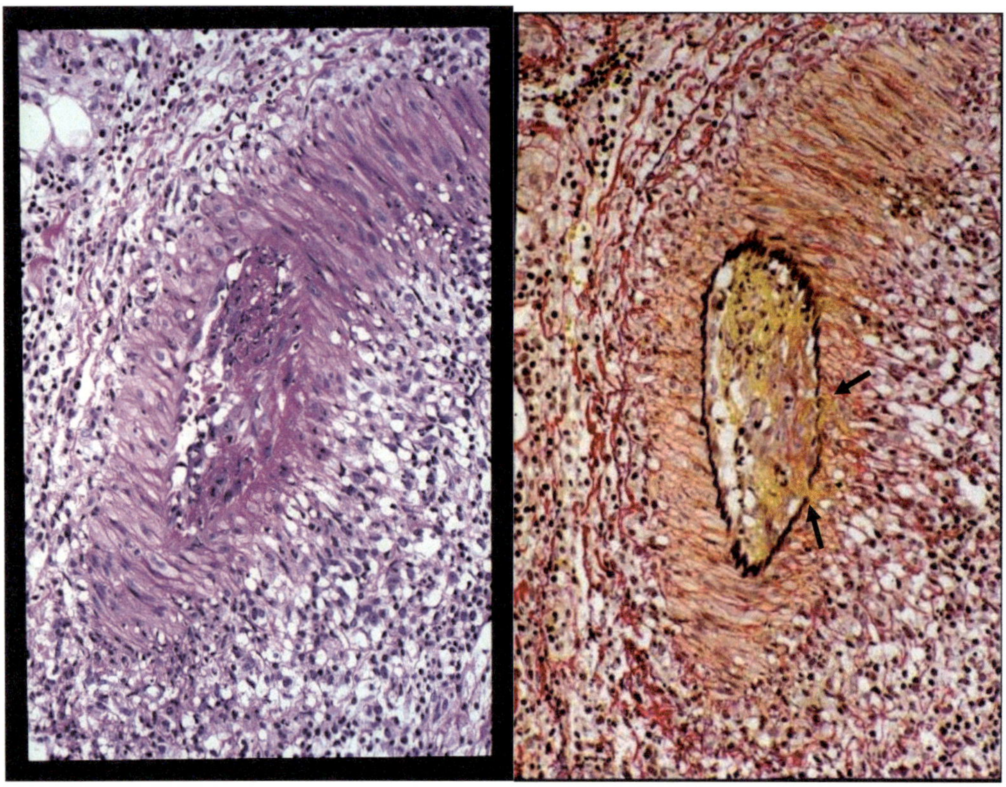

Fig. 12. A. Arteritis at the subacute stage.

(Left) The inflammatory cells comprise a mixed infiltrate of neutrophils, lymphocytes, and histiocytes; however, there is no formation of fibrous proliferation and no neovascularization in and around the vessel wall.
(Right) [elastic tissue stain] The fibrinous exudates can be seen discharging into the medial muscular layers throughout the disrupted internal elastic lamina (arrows).

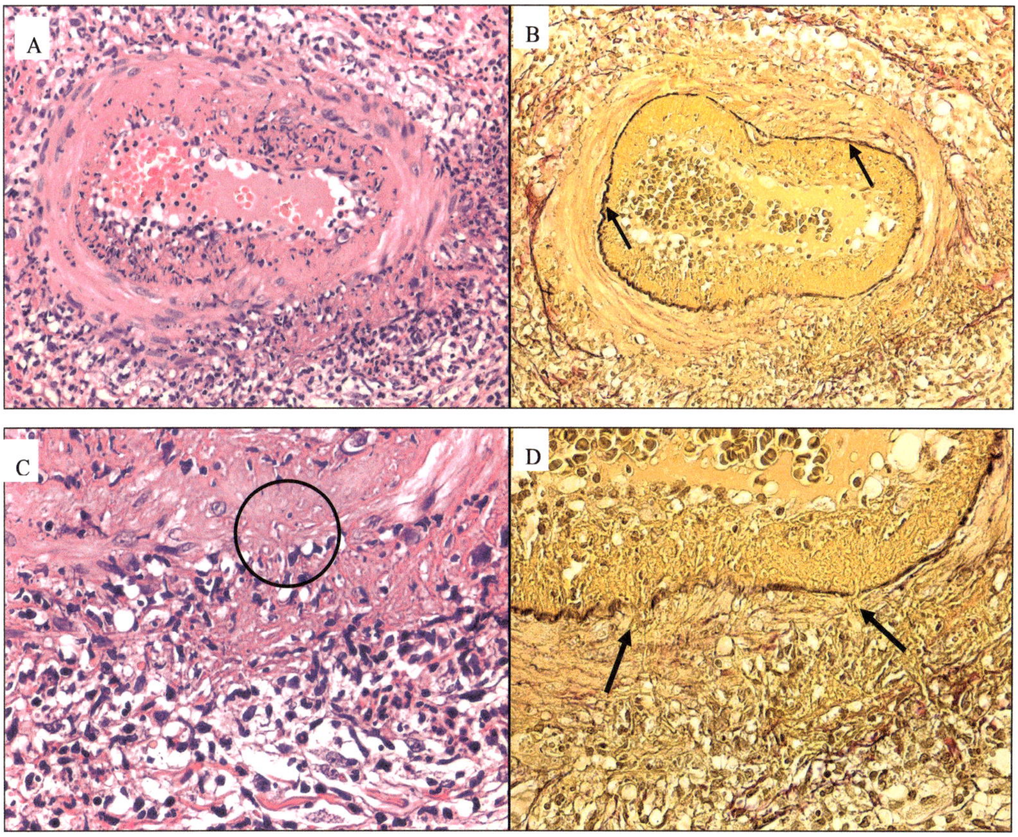

Fig. 12. B. Another arteritis at the subacute stage

(A) Arteritis at the subacute stage showing intimal concentric fibrinoid necrosis. At gross appearance, the internal elastic lamina (arrows in B: [elastic tissue stain]) remains intact, but the discharge of the fibrinoid deposit from the disrupted sites in the internal elastic lamina (spreading outward to the medial layer and perivascular area) can be appreciated at higher magnification (circle in C, arrows in D: [elastic tissue stain]).

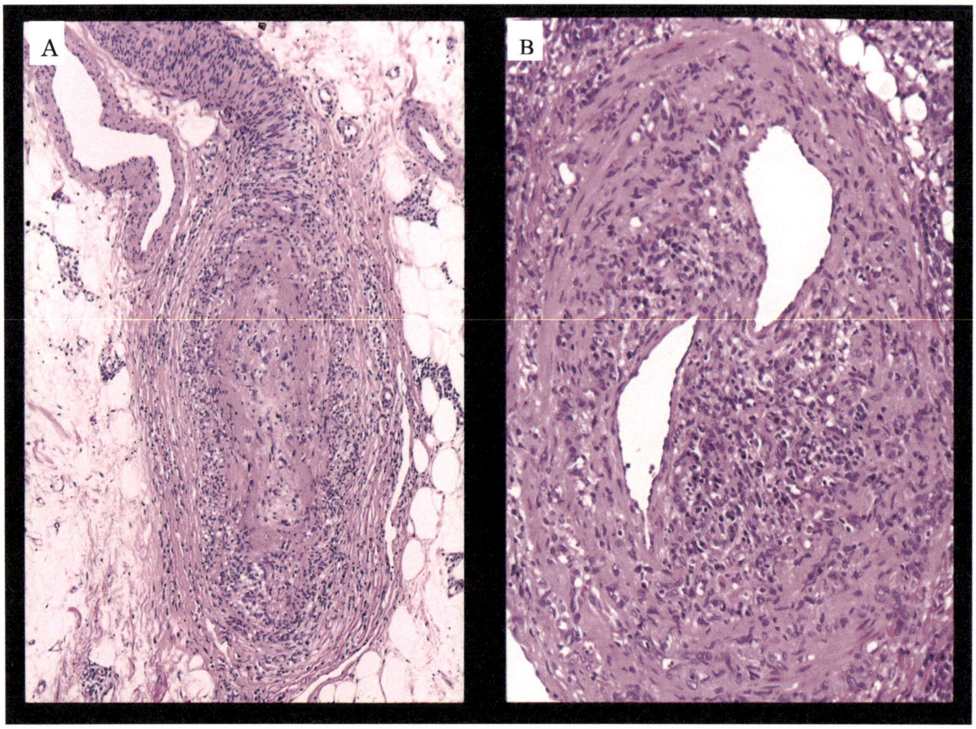

Fig. 13. (A) Arteritis at the reparative stage.(B) Phlebitis at the reparative stage.

Note the predominate infiltrate of lymphocytes and histiocytes; the neovascularization in and around the vessels; and luminal fibrous occlusion.

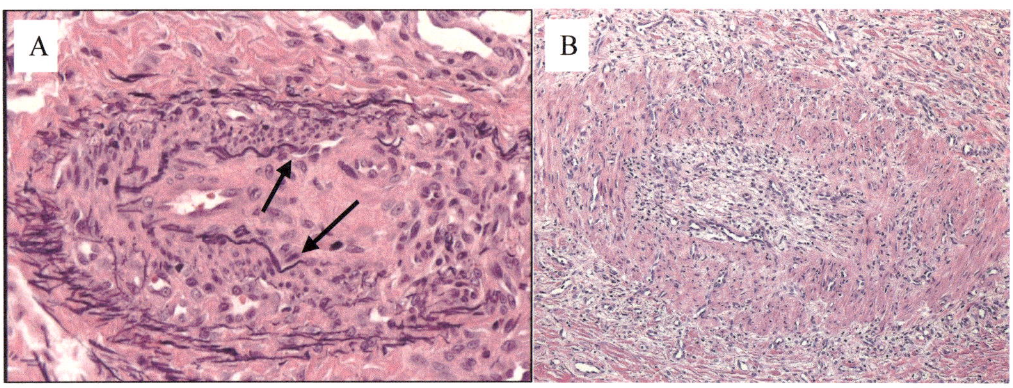

Fig. 14. (A) Arteritis at the healed stage. (B) phlebitis at the healed stage.

There is scant inflammation with marked fibrous proliferation and neovascularization in and around the affected artery and vein, with the resultant luminal occlusion.
(A) Note the marked disruption of the internal elastic lamina (arrows) at the healed stage of arteritis (elastic hematoxylin and eosin stain).
(B) The discontinuous bundled muscular layers of the vessel wall indicates that the affected vessel is a vein.

Definition of necrotizing vasculitis and its relation to small vessel vasculitis and muscular vessel vasculitis

- Necrotizing vasculitis is defined as vasculitis with vessel wall fibrinoid necrosis.
- Since vessel wall fibrinoid necrosis is the crucial finding for the diagnosis of small vessel vasculitis, all small vessel vasculitis is necrotizing vasculitis.
- Muscular vessel vasculitis is not necessarily identical to necrotizing vasculitis since vessel wall fibrinoid necrosis is not the crucial finding for muscular vessel vasculitis (Figures 9, 10, and 14).

4) Inflammatory stages of vasculitis (morphological evolution of vasculitis)

For muscular vessel vasculitis, morphological changes in the vessel wall and in the luminal and perivascular areas during the dynamic inflammatory process are diagnostically important and influence the mode of treatment. For example, patients with ulcerative lesions (caused by arteritis at the healed stage with intimal fibrous thickening resulting from luminal occlusion) should be administered anticoagulation agents and vessel dilating medications, rather than systemic steroid treatment. By contrast, for patients with lesions at either the acute or subacute stage of arteritis, initiating of systemic steroid treatment should be considered as early as possible to suppress and cease the ongoing inflammation occurring on the vessel wall; this prevents further destruction of the affected vessels .

Vasculitis of the dermal small vessels (e.g., arterioles and venules) does not have these proliferative changes as characterized by either fibrous proliferation or neovascularization of the lumen and vessel wall. However, the formation of perivascular fibrosis may be found in old lesions of certain small vessel vasculitis disorders such as erythema elevatum diutinum.

Inflammatory stages of muscular vessel vasculitis start as an acute stage, followed by a subacute stage, a reparative stage, and a healed stage.[11, 12]

Acute stage: Characterized by a predominate infiltrate of neutrophils (or eosinophils in cases of Churg-Strauss syndrome[12]) in and around the vessel wall and the lumen, but without evidence of new capillary formation (i.e., neovascularization) and fibrous proliferation in and around the vessel (Figures 10 and 11). Another feature is that the internal elastic lamina remains intact (Figure 10).

Subacute stage: Characterized by a mixed infiltrate of neutrophils, lymphocytes and histiocytes with the formation of a fibrinoid deposit (i.e., fibrinoid necrosis) in the intima of the affected arteries. This is subsequently accompanied by its discharge into the muscular medial layer and outward spread to the perivascular area throughout the sites of disrupted internal elastic lamina (Figures 12A and 12B).

Reparative stage (i.e., granulation tissue stage): Characterized by a predominate infiltrate of lymphocytes and histiocytes and fibrous and vascular proliferation in and around the affected muscular vessels. Intimal and luminal fibrous thickening results in luminal occlusion. (Figures 13 and 15b).

Healed stage (i.e., scar stage): Characterized by scant inflammation with marked fibrous proliferation and neovascularization in and around the affected muscular vessels (Figures 14A and 14B) and marked disruption of internal elastic lamina in the affected arteries (Figure 14A).

The coexistence of different stages of arteritis or phlebitis can occasionally be identified at the same skin lesion or from different biopsied lesions (Figure 15a).

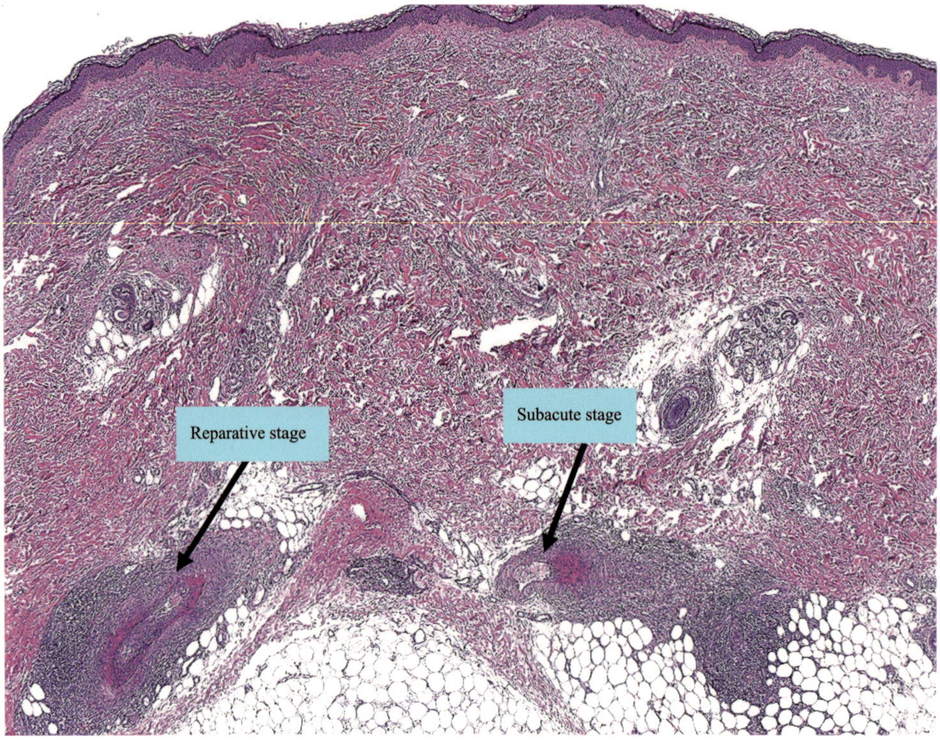

Fig. 15.a. The coexistence of different stages of arteritis from the same biopsied section.

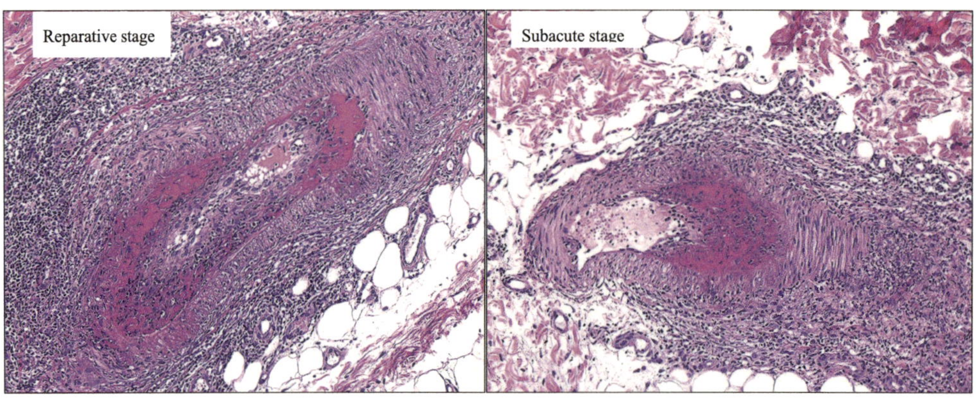

Fig. 15. b. (higher magnification of Figure 15a) (Left) The reparative stage of arteritis is characterized by a predominate infiltrate of lymphocytes and histiocytes and by intimal cellular and fibrous proliferation, resulting in luminal occlusion. (Right) The subacute stage of arteritis is characterized by a mixed infiltrate of neutrophils, lymphocytes and histiocytes with a marked intimal fibrinoid deposit. However, there is no luminal fibrous proliferation, as seen at left in Fig 15b.

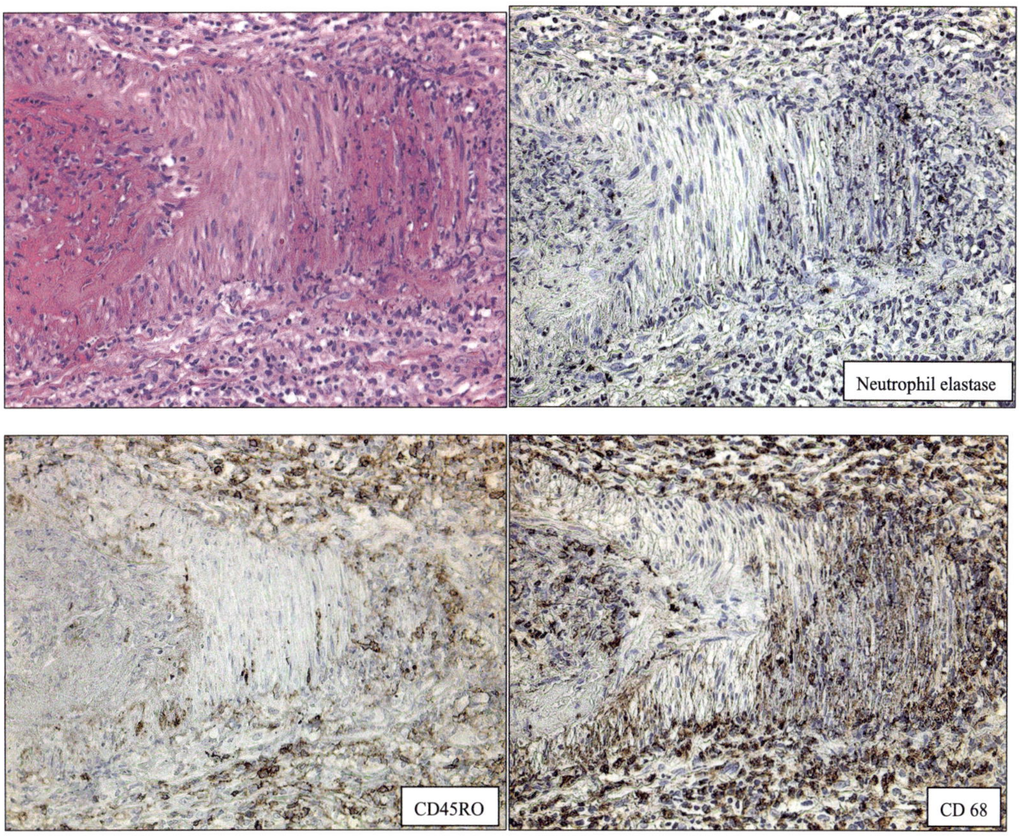

Fig. 15. c. Immunostaining of the biopsied sample of arteritis at the subacute stage in Figure 15a shows a mixed infiltrate of neutrophils (i.e., neutrophil elastase), lymphocytes (i.e., CD45RO), and histiocytes (i.e., CD68) in and around the vessel wall.

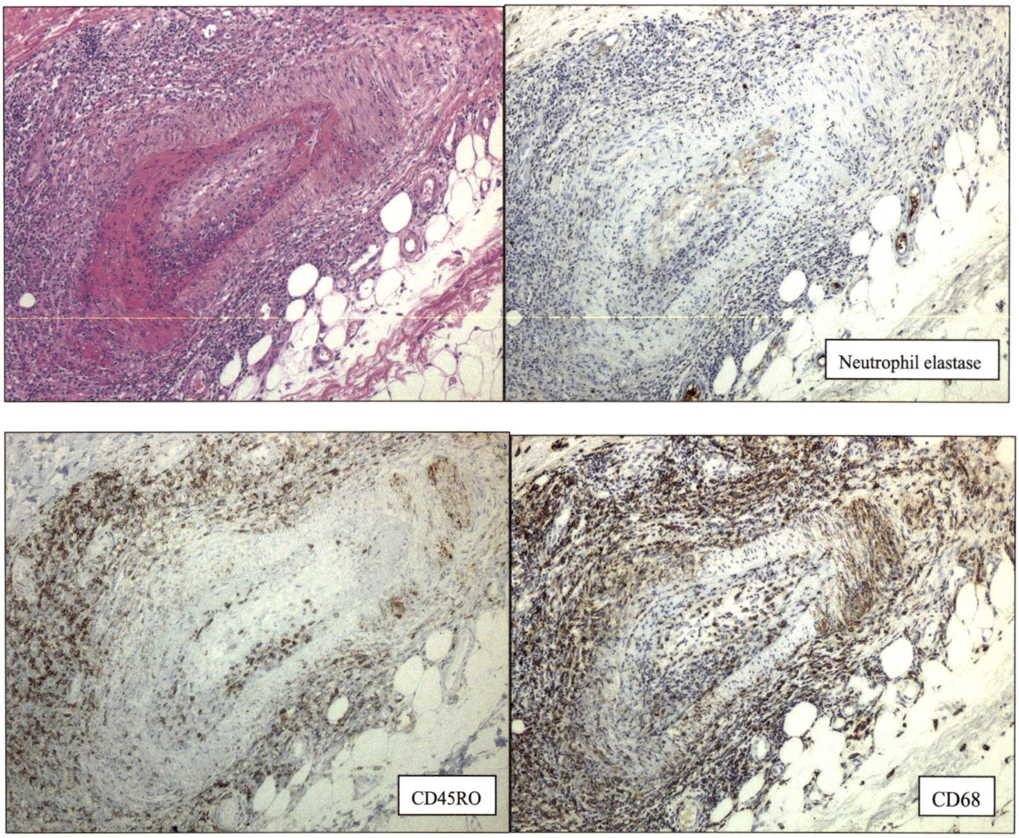

Fig. 15. d. Immunostaining of the biopsied sample of arteritis at the reparative stage in Figure 15a shows a predominate infiltrate of lymphocytes (CD45RO) and histiocytes (CD68) with virtual absence of neutrophils (i.e., neutrophil elastase) in and around the vessel wall.

5) Diagnostic pitfalls

1. **Vessel wall destruction**

Vessel destruction can be found in vasculitis-like disorders (i.e., pseudovasculitis)[7] due to direct vessel wall invasion from organisms (e.g., bacteria, fungi) (Figure 16) or tumors cells (Figure 20), rather than inflammatory cells.

2. **Fibrinoid necrosis of the vessel wall**

This crucial pathological feature of vasculitis can also be found in pseudovasculitis as a result of secondary vessel wall destruction due to lesions of a dermal/subcutaneous abscess or necrosis (Figures 17 and 18); or due to overlying ulcerative lesions (Figure 19); or due to a direct vessel wall invasion by tumor cells (Figure 20).

3. **Overlooking the main vasculitis lesion**

A vasculitic lesion presents as a segmental lesion. Therefore, features of vasculitis may be missed on the initial hematoxylin-eosin-stained section for patients with clinically suspected vasculitis. Serial sections are often required to identify the main vasculitis lesion (Figure 21).

4. **Misdiagnosis of thrombophlebitis as cutaneous polyarteritis nodosa**

Concentric compact muscular layers and internal elastic lamina are diagnostic pitfalls.[8]

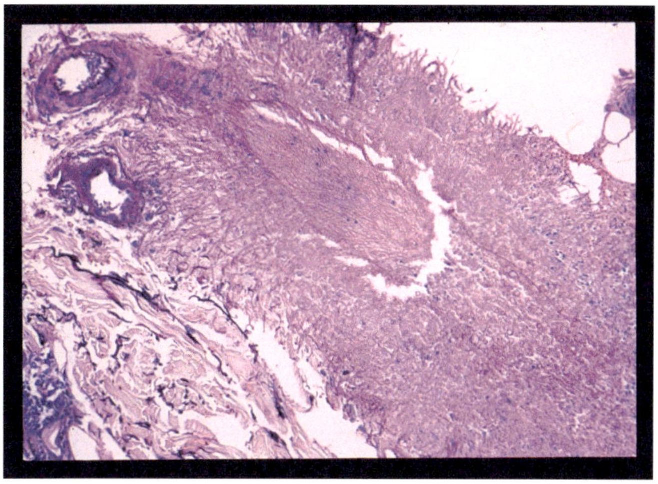

Fig. 16. Destruction of the small artery, caused by a direct vessel wall invasion from embolic *Aspergillus*.

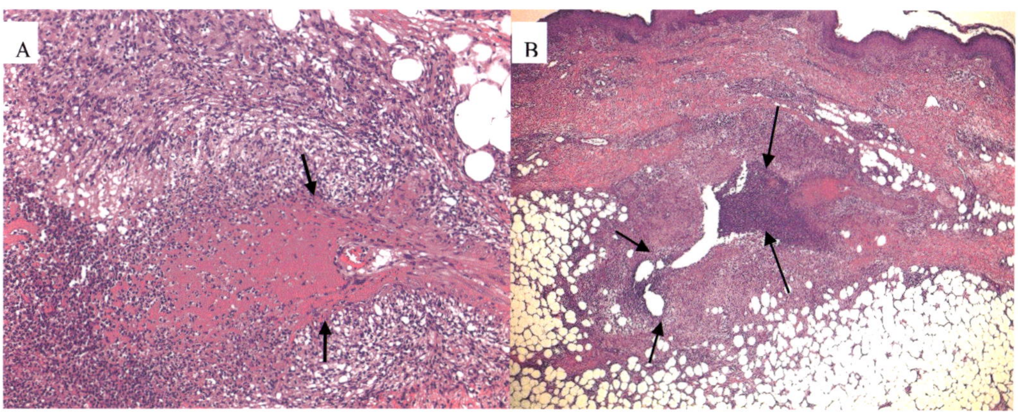

Fig. 17. Fibrinoid necrosis of the arterial vessel wall (arrows in A), resembling arteritis, is caused by secondary involvement (i.e., innocent bystanders) from an adjacent subcutaneous abscess (arrows in B).

The persistent hydrostatic pressure occurring in the lower legs usually results in hypertrophy of the medial muscular layer of the superficial subcutaneous veins, especially those located in the dorsal or plantar parts of the feet. (Figure 2) The medial muscular layer in the vein is often thicker than its muscular layer counterpart in the artery and may show a compact smooth muscular pattern with an intimal internal elastic lamina-like feature resembling the charaterisrtic features of artery. Moreover, the clinical similarities features between superficial thrombophlebitis and cutaneous polyarteritis nodosa account for the difficulty in the differential diagnosis between these two disorders. (Figures 22A-E)
An understanding of the morphologic characteristics of the veins of the lower legs (Figures 1, 2) is indispensible for a correct histopathologic diagnosis and is indispensible in avoiding the misdiagnosis of cutaneous polyarteritis nodosa and overtreatment for superficial thrombophlebitis. (Figures 22A-E).

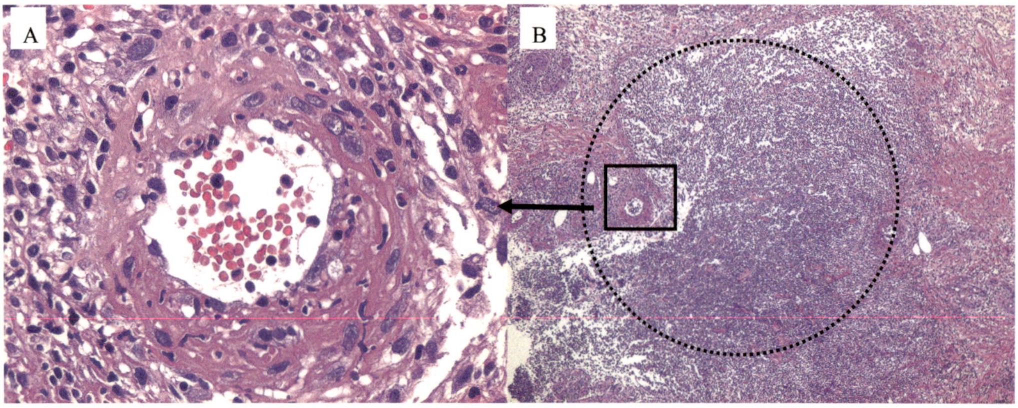

Fig. 18. (A) Vessel wall fibrinoid necrosis with infiltration of inflammatory cells is apt to be misinterpreted as necrotizing vasculitis on high magnification. However, the vessel wall destruction is caused by secondary destruction where the innocent vessel is involved in a dermal abscess (circle, in B) from a lesion of pyoderma gangrenosum.

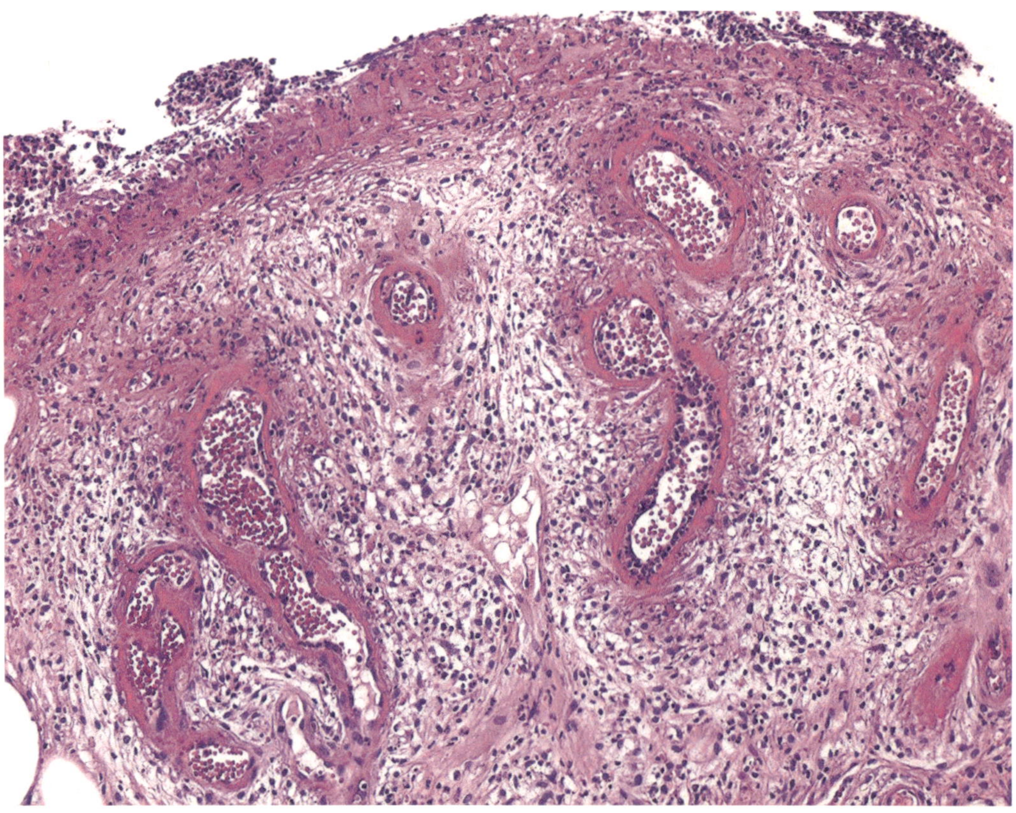

Fig. 19. Marked fibrinoid necrosis of vessel walls may be identified at sites with an overlying ulcerative lesion.

Small vessel vasculitis

Neutrophilic

Immune-complex mediated (DIF +)

Cutaneous (idiopathic) leukocytoclastic angiitis (CLA) (IgM/IgG)

(also known as: hypersensitivity vasculitis, cutaneous allergic vasculitis)

Henoch-Schonlein purpura (IgA)

Acute infantile hemorrhagic edema (IgA)

Urticarial vasculitis (IgM/IgG)

Infective endocarditis (IgM/IgG/IgA)

Chronic localized fibrosing vasculitis: Erythema elevatum diutinum (IgA)

Eosinophilic

Idiopathic cutaneous eosinophilic vasculitis

Connective tissue disease (e.g. lupus, rheumatoid arthritis, Sjögren's syndrome)

Some cases of Churg Strauss Syndrome

Granulomatous Sarcoidosis

Lymphocytic

Rickettsial & viral infections

Lichenoid dermatitides, some cases, e.g. pityriasis lichenoides, graft vs. host disease, perniosis

Rare drug reactions and arthropod assaults

Mixed, predominately small and medium vessel vasculitis

Neutrophilic

Immune-complex mediated (DIF+)

Cryoglobulinemic vasculitis (IgM/IgG)

Hepatisis B and C related vasculitis (IgM/IgG)

Connective tissue disease vasculitis (e.g. lupus, rheumatoid arthritis, Sjögren's syndrome) (IgM/IgG)

ANCA associated/pauci-immune (DIF-)

Wegener's granulomatosis

Microscopic polyangiitis

Churg-Strauss syndrome

Drug-induced ANCA vasculitis

Miscellaneous/other

Behçet's disease

Inflammatory bowel disease(Crohn's disease, ulcerative colitis)

Malignancy associated vasculitis

Eosinophilic Churg-Strauss syndrome

Lymphocytic

Degos' disease

Rickettsial & viral infections

Collagen tissue disease vasculitis (e.g. Sjögren's syndrome, lupus vasculitis)

Behçet's disease
Granulomatous
Churg-Strauss syndrome
Connective tissue disease vasculitis (e.g. lupus, rheumatoid arthritis, Sjögren's syndrome)
Inflammatory bowel disease (Crohn's disease, ulcerative colitis)
Post-herpetic eruptions
Muscular (Medium) vessel vasculitis
Neutrophilic
Polyarteritis nodosa (classic and cutaneous)
Idiopathic superficial thrombophlebitis
Eosinophilic Juvenile temporal arteritis
Granulomatous
Giant cell (temporal) arteritis
Nodular vasculitis (erythema induratum)
Lymphocytic
Sneddon's syndrome
Beurger's disease (thromboangiitis obliterans)

ANCA: antineutrophil cytoplasmic antibody. DIF +: direct immunfluorescence examination of skin lesions shows vessel wall immune-complexes and/or complement deposition. Modified from 1) Chen and Carlson. Am J Clin Dermatol 9:71-92.2008.

Table 1. Classification of cutaneous vasculitis, based on the size of the affected vessels, the predominate inflammatory cells, and the DIF studies

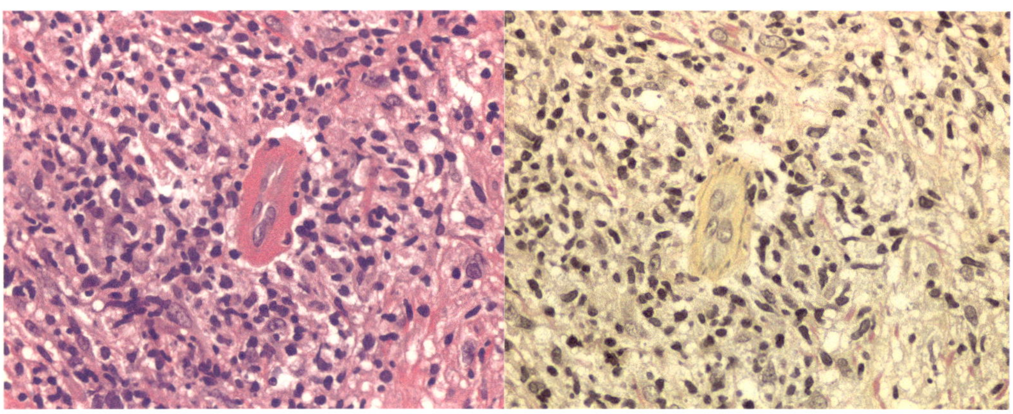

Fig. 20. Fibrinoid necrosis of the vessel wall due to a direct vessel wall invasion by tumor cells can be identified in neoplastic lesions, as seen here in a case of NK/T cell lymphoma. (Right: elastic tissue stain)

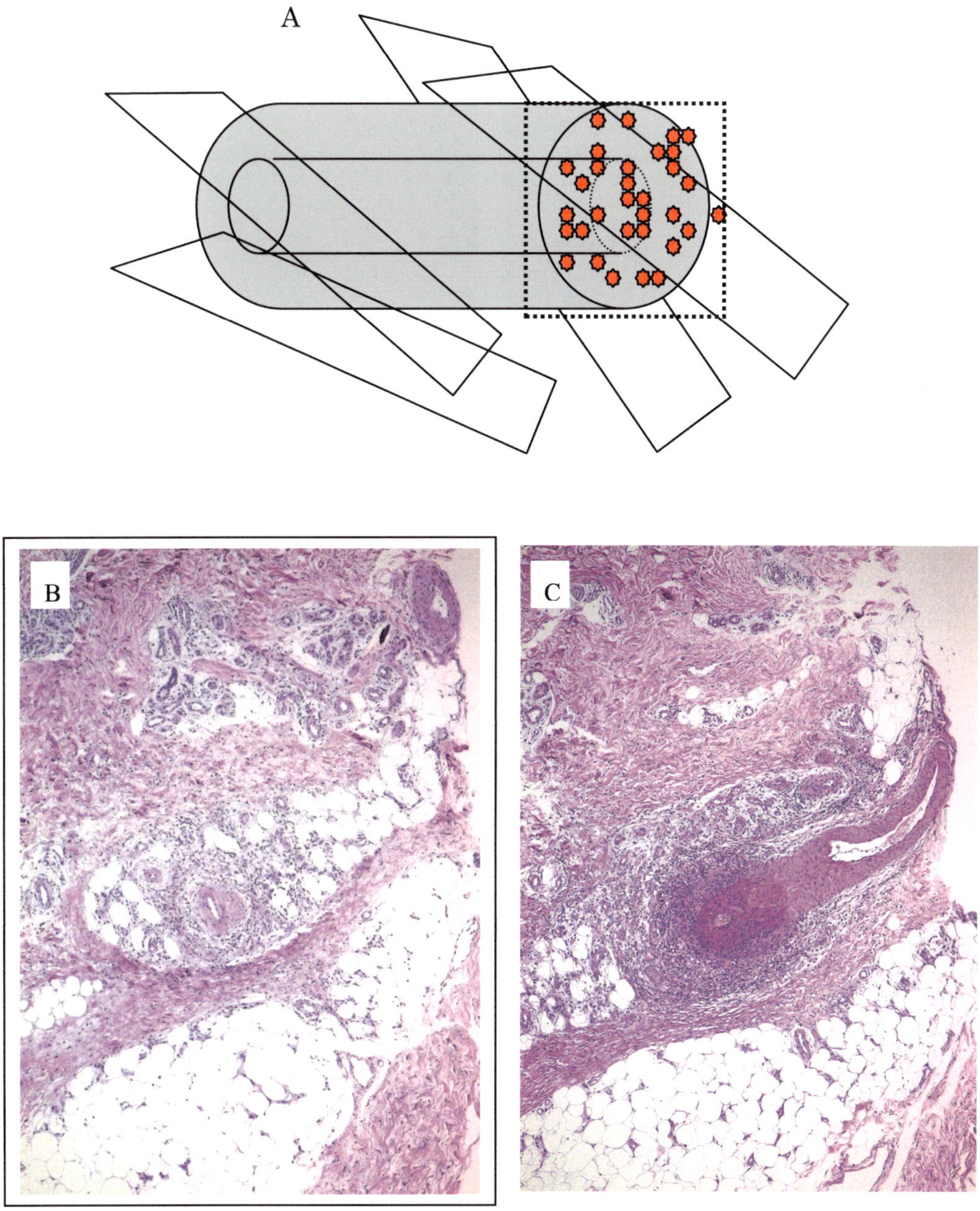

Fig. 21. (A) A pitfall in overlooking vasculitis because of an inappropriate section cut in the wrong direction. Vasculitis occurs as a segmental lesion along the affected vessels. (B) If the lesion is cut in the wrong direction, the initial section may show no evidence of vasculitis. (C) Serial sections are often required to identify the main vasculitis lesion.

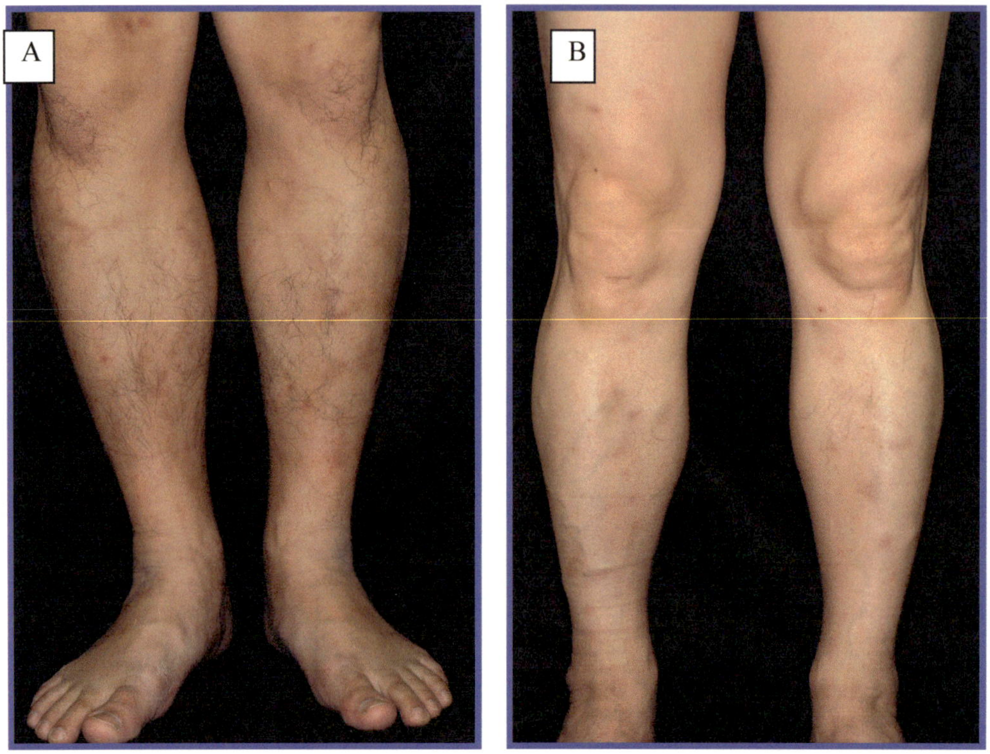

Fig. 22. (A) Superficial thrombophlebitis and (B) cutaneous polyarteritis nodosa are clinically similar.

Both show widespread nodular erythema with livedo racemosa.

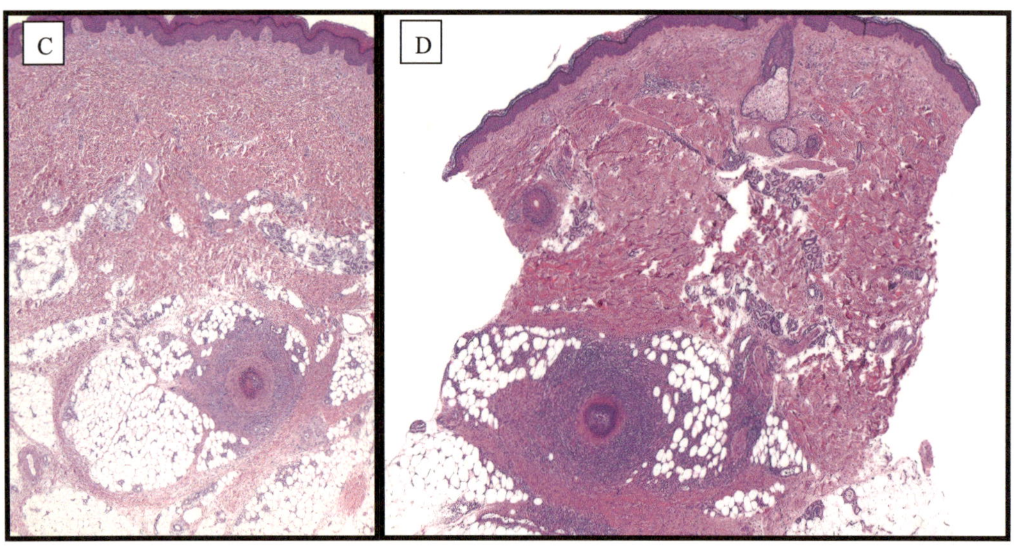

Fig. 22. (C) Superficial thrombophlebitis in figure 22A and (D) Cutaneous polyarteritis nodosa in figure 22B

They are also histopathologically similar. Both show a subcutaneous muscular vessel lesion with a compact concentric vessel wall and perivascular panniculitis.

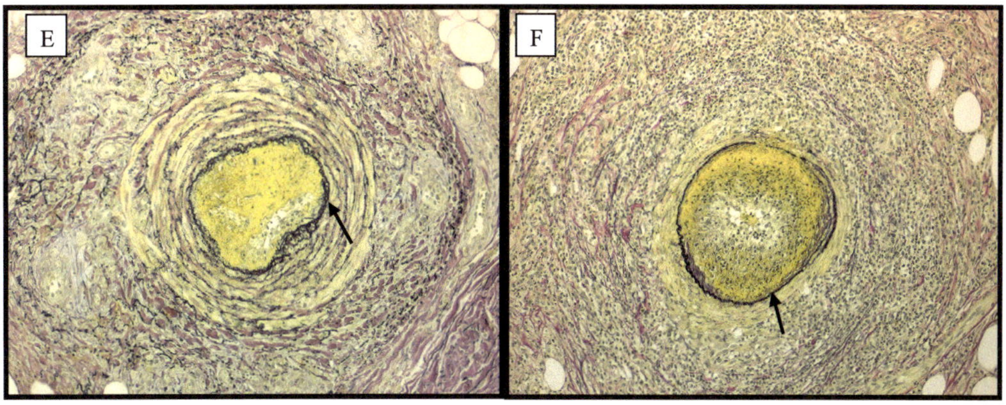

Fig. 22. (E) Thrombophlebitis (F) Cutaneous polyarteritis nodosa (elastic tissue stain)

Discontinuous bundled muscular layers separated by the rich elastic fibers in (E) thrombophlebitis is very distinguishable from the scant elastic fibers in muscular vessel wall in (F) cutaneous polyarteritis nodosa. The intimal elastic fiber in thrombophlebitis (arrow, in E) may be misinterpreted as the authentic internal elastic lamina of an artery. However, the uneven thickness and partial multilayer figures are distinguishable from the even thickness of the authentic internal elastic lamina (arrow, in F).

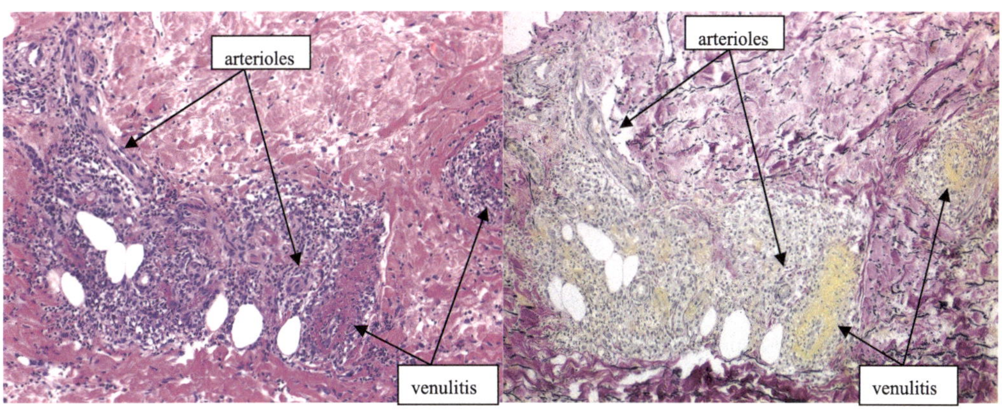

Fig. 23. The predominant vessels affected in dermal small vessel vasculitis are the venules, while their counterpart, the arterioles, are not involved. (Right: elastic tissue stain)

6. Histopathologic classifications of cutaneous vasculitis and their related disorders (Table 1)

1) Classification based on the size of the affected vessel (i.e., dermal small vessels or muscular vessels)

Dermal small vessel vasculitis and their related disorders

Dermal small vessel vasculitis predominately affecting venules (i.e., venulitis) (Figure 23) is the most common histopathologic feature of cutaneous vasculitis. However, in systemic vasculitis (such as ANCA-related vasculitis), venules and arterioles may both be affected (Figure 24). Palpable purpura on the lower legs is the most common clinical feature; other manifestations, such as infiltrated or elevated erythema, occur less often. Because many vasculitic disorders (including primary and secondary vasculitic disorders such as drug-induced vasculitis) share the histopathologic feature of dermal small vessel vasculitis and have similar cutaneous manifestations, the combination of clinical and laboratory evaluation is often needed to make the final diagnosis.

Muscular vessel vasculitis and their related disorders

Muscular vessels of the lower dermis to the subcutis are small or medium-sized arteries and veins having a caliber larger than 100 um. Small arteries or veins ranging from 200 um to 400 um at the dermo-subcutaneous junction are the vessels commonly affected in either cutaneous polyarteritis nodosa[1,6,8] (Figures 22D and 22F), in idiopathic superficial thrombophlebitis (Figures 22C and 22E), or in Behçet's disease[13] (Figure 26).

Disorders with coexistent small vessel vasculitis and muscular vessel vasculitis

Coexistent small vessel vasculitis and muscular vessel vasculitis is a feature of systemic vasculitis such as
ANCA-related vasculitis,[17,18] collagen disease,[9] and Behçet's disease,[13] or infection, inflammatory bowel disease, drug and neoplasm- related vasculitis (Figures. 25, 26, and 27).

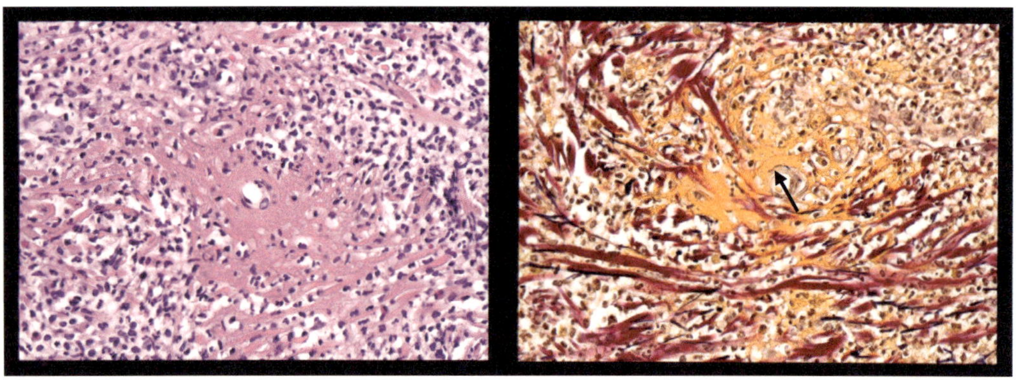

Fig. 24. Necrotizing dermal arteriolitis with a mixed infiltrate of neutrophils and eosinophils from a lesion of palpable purpura in Churg-Strauss syndrome. Note the remaining disrupted internal elastic lamina of the affected arteriole (arrow at right figure: elastic tissue stain).

2) Classification based on the predominate inflammatory cell[1,2,3,5,6]

- Neutrophilic (i.e., leukocytoclastic) vasculitis (Figures. 8, 9, 10, 11, and 26C).
- Eosinophilic vasculitis (Figure 27C). [15,16,17,18,19]
- Lymphocytic vasculitis (Figure 28) . [13,14]
- Histiocytic (i.e., granulomatous vasculitis) (Figures 29 and 30). [12,18,20,21]

Nuclear dust found in and around the affected vessels is a feature of neutrophilic vasculitis (also known as leukocytoclastic vasculitis). Eosinophilic and lymphocytic vascuiltis are both characterized by a predominate eosinophilic or lymphocytic infiltrate without nuclear dust (Figures. 27C and 28).

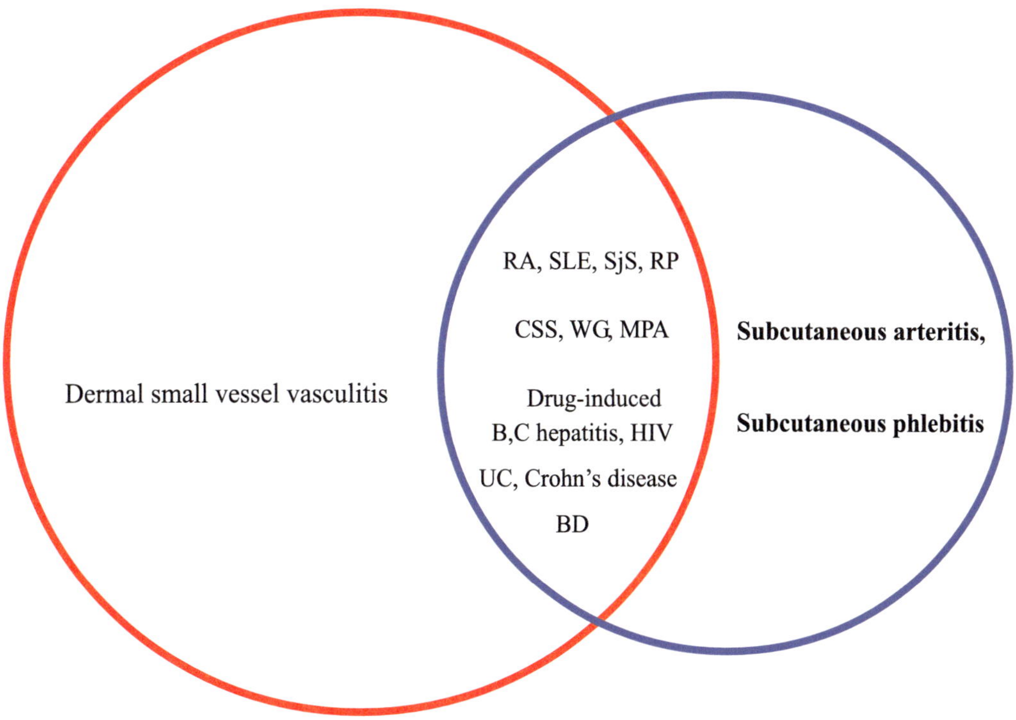

Fig. 25. Disorders with coexistent dermal small vessel vasculitis and subcutaneous arteritis or phlebitis. RP: relapsing polychondritis, CSS: Churg-Strauss syndrome, WG: Wegener's granulomatosis, MPA: microscopic polyangiitis, UC:ulcerative colitis, BD: Behçet's disease

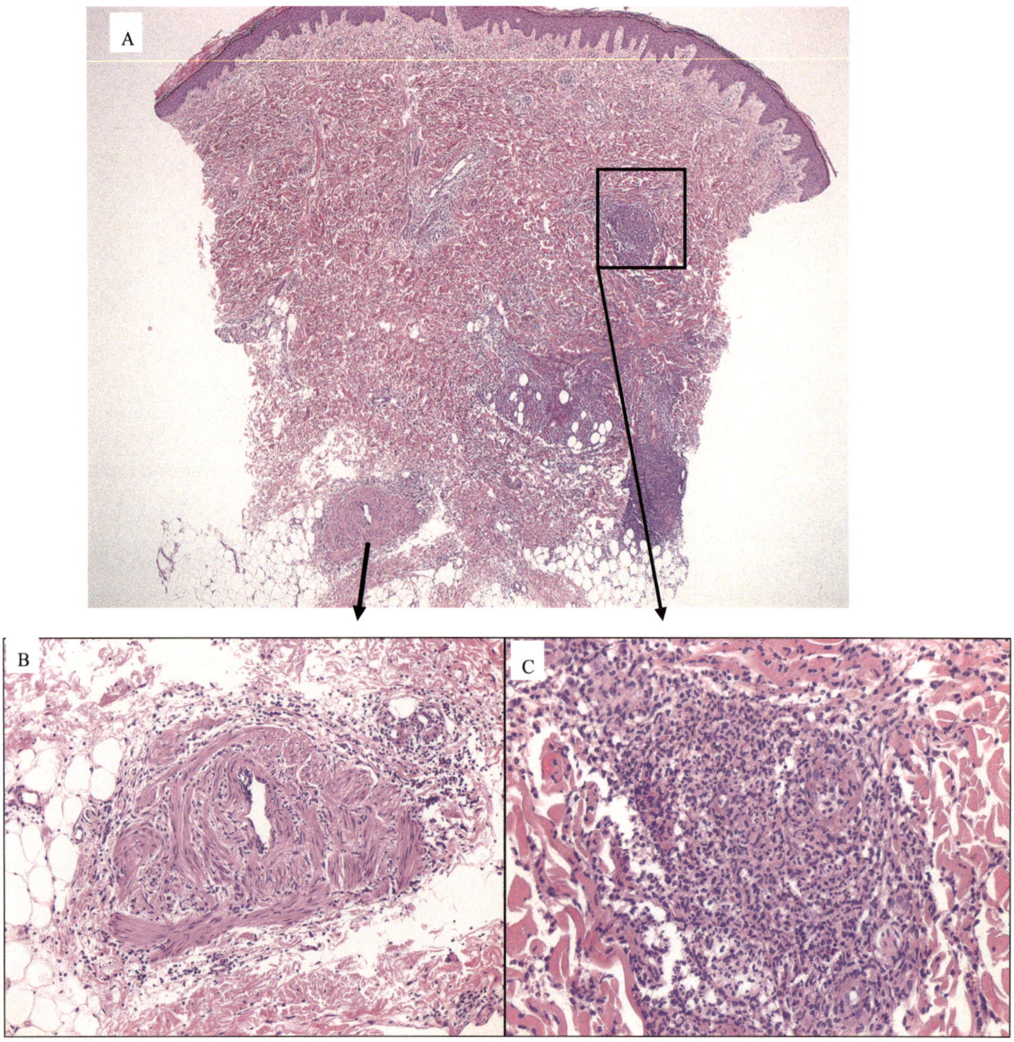

Fig. 26. (A) A unique histopathologic feature of erythema-nodosum-like lesions in Behçet's disease is the coexistence of dermo-subcutaneous phlebitis (high magnification shown in (B)) and overlying dermal small vessel vasculitis (high magnification shown in (C)) coupled with the lobular neutrophilic panniculitis.

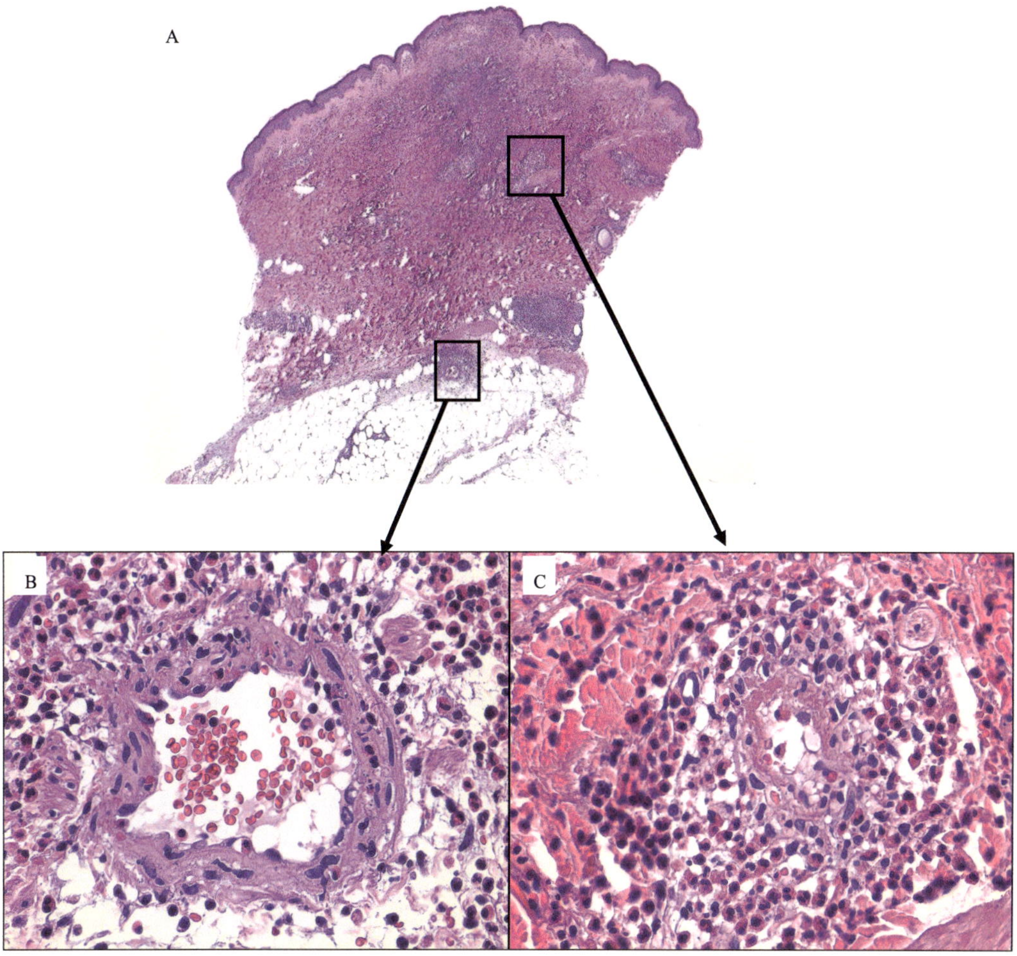

Fig. 27. (A) A unique feature of Churg-Strauss syndrome is the coexistence of dermal small vessel vasculitis (i.e., eosinophilic venulitis; (high magnification shown in (C)) and underlying granulomatous phlebitis (high magnification shown in (B)), surrounded by a marked infiltrate of eosinophils. In contrast to neutrophilic vasculitis in Figure 26C, in which nuclear dust is markedly present, eosinophilic vasculitis virtually lacks nuclear dust, as seen in (C).

3) Diagnostic clues to the correspondent vasculitis disorders

A diagnosis of vasculitis, based on the infiltrate of the predominate inflammatory cells, is a histopathologic diagnosis and generally is not the final diagnosis since most vasculitis disorders such as ANCA-related and collagen disease-related vasculitis share histopathologic features. The histopathologic features of most small vessel vasculitis are also shared by neutrophilic vasculitis. The clinical and laboratory information are generally both needed to make the final diagnosis. However, the following unique histopathologic features are the diagnostic clues to the correspondent vasculitis disorders (Table 1):

1. A mixed infiltrate rich in neutrophils and eosinophils suggests Churg-Strauss syndrome (Figure 24) or drug-induced vasculitis.

2. Subcutaneous granulomatous arteritis or phlebitis surrounded by a marked infiltrate of eosinophils is diagnostic of Churg-Strauss syndrome (Figures 27B and 29). [12,18]
3. Subcutaneous eosinophilic arteritis is diagnostic of juvenile temporal arteritis[19] and Churg-Strauss syndrome.[17]
4. Phlebitis and/or neutrophilic panniculitis with overlying dermal venulitis is a unique feature of Behçet's disease (Figure 26). [13]
5. Dermal eosinophilic vasculitis is a very rare finding. It is usually found in idiopathic cutaneous eosinophilic vasculitis,[15] collagen disease,[16] and Churg-Strauss syndrome (Figure27C). [18]
6. Dermal granulomatous vasculitis is a unique finding. It is usually found in sarcoidosis (Figure 30), postherpetic eruption, and collagen disease.
7. Subcutaneous granulomatous muscular vessel vasculitis is a unique finding. It is usually found in classic temporal arteritis (Figure 31) and nodular vasculitis also known as erythema induratum characterized by indurated erythematous lesions in the lower legs with a subcutaneous vein predominately affected (i.e., granulomatous phlebitis) in conjunction with lobular granulomatous panniculitis. It may be occasionally be found in Churg-Strauss syndrome,[12,18] collagen disease (e.g., rheumatoid arthritis); inflammatory bowel disease (e.g., ulcerative colitis, Crohn's disease); and postherpetic eruption with nodular lesions.
8. The coexistence of dermal neutrophilic vasculitis and palisaded granuloma with central basophilic degenerated collagen fibers suggests Churg-Strauss syndrome (Figure 32), Wegener's granulomatosis, and collagen disease (e.g., rheumatoid arthritis or systemic lupus erythematosus [SLE]).
9. The coexistence of dermal small vasculitis and subcutaneous arteritis should suggest a systemic vasculitis disorder such as ANCA-related vasculitis (Figure 33), collagen disease,[9] or infection-related vasculitis (e.g., hepatitis C virus-induced cryoglobulinemic purpura, inflammatory bowel disease).

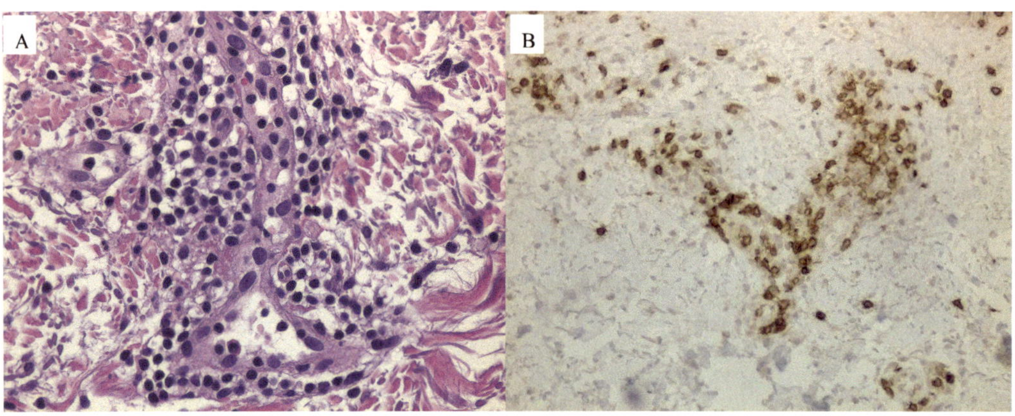

Fig. 28. Lymphocytic vasculitis. Characteristics of lymphocytic vasculitis are a predominate infiltrate of lymphocytes in (A) characterized by CD8 positive T lymphocytes in (B) with virtual absence of nuclear dust.

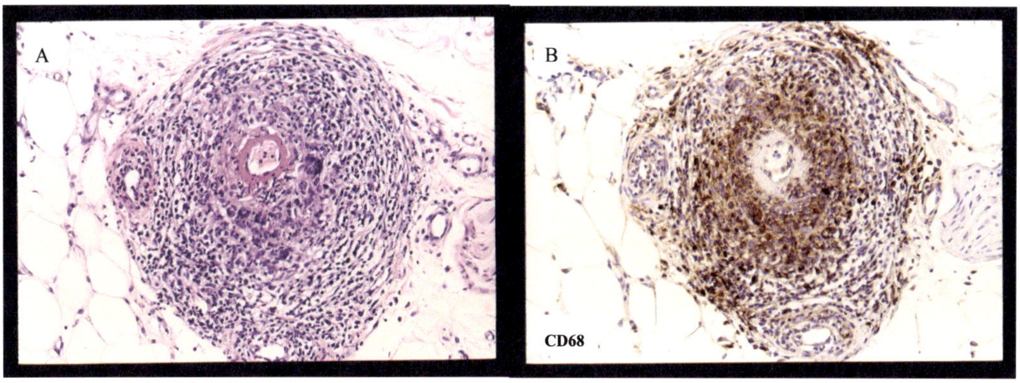

Fig. 29. (A) Subcutaneous granulomatous arteritis in Churg-Strauss syndrome. A marked angiocentric infiltrate of CD68 positive histiocytes mixed with multi-nucleated giant cells and an eosinophilic infiltrate at the periphery are diagnostic of Churg-Strauss syndrome. (B) CD68 immunostaining of the specimen.

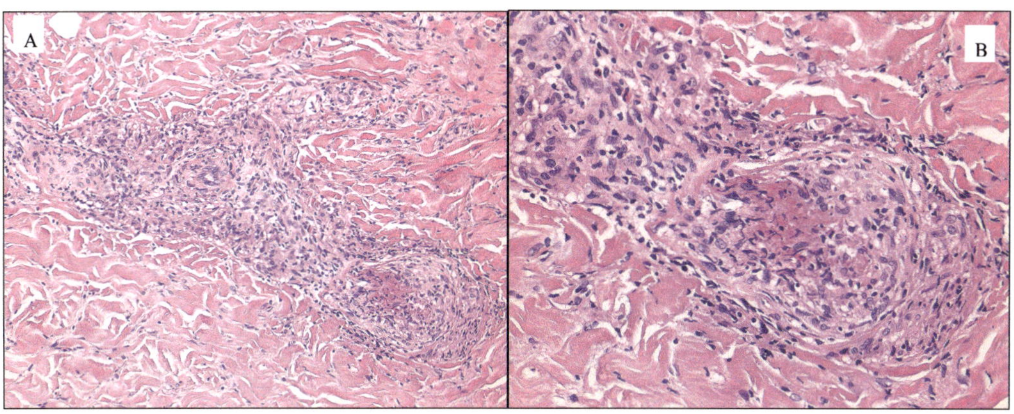

Fig. 30. (A) Dermal granulomatous vasculitis with a predominate perivascular infiltrate of histiocytes in sarcoidosis. (B) The spccimen at high magnification.

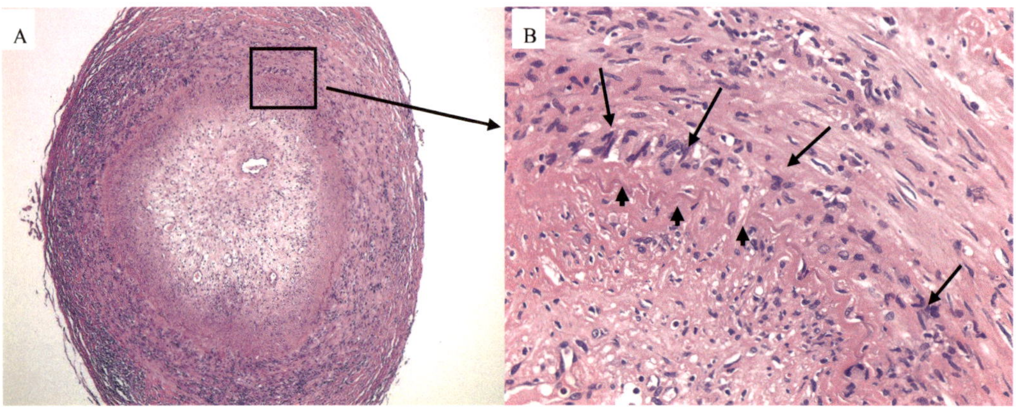

Fig. 31. (A) Subcutaneous granulomatous arteritis in temporal arteritis shows luminal occlusion by fibrous proliferation and neovascularization. (B) Note the multi-nucleated giant cells (arrows) and histiocytes in the medial layer have a palisaded arrangement along the inner disrupted internal elastic lamina (arrow heads).

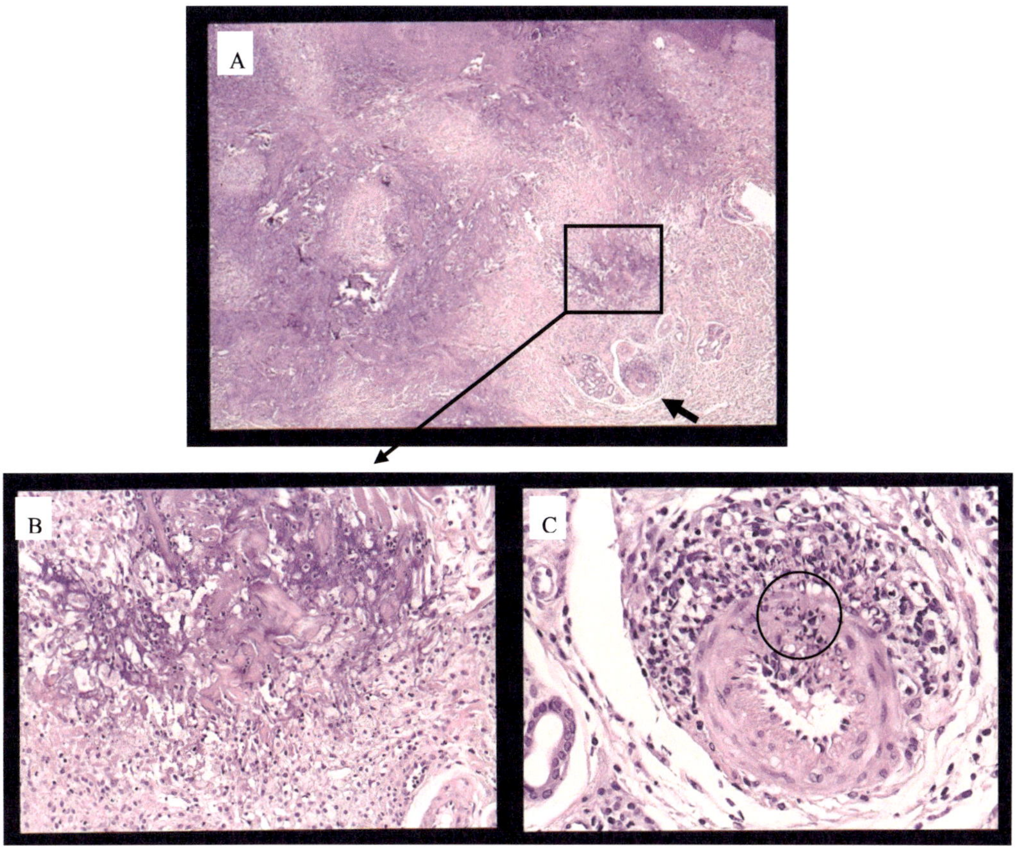

Fig. 32. (A) The coexistence of deep dermal neutrophilic arteritis (thick arrow) and foci of basophilic palisaded granulomas in a nodular lesion of Churg-Strauss syndrome.(B) A higher magnification of the palisaded granuloma. Note the central basophilic degenerated collagen fibers mixed with neutrophils and nuclear dust, and the underlying palisaded arrangement of histiocytes. (C) Arteritis at high magnification. Note the affected artery is infiltrated by neutrophils with nuclear dust in and around the disrupted muscular vessel wall (circle), and note the infiltrate of histiocytes at the periphery.

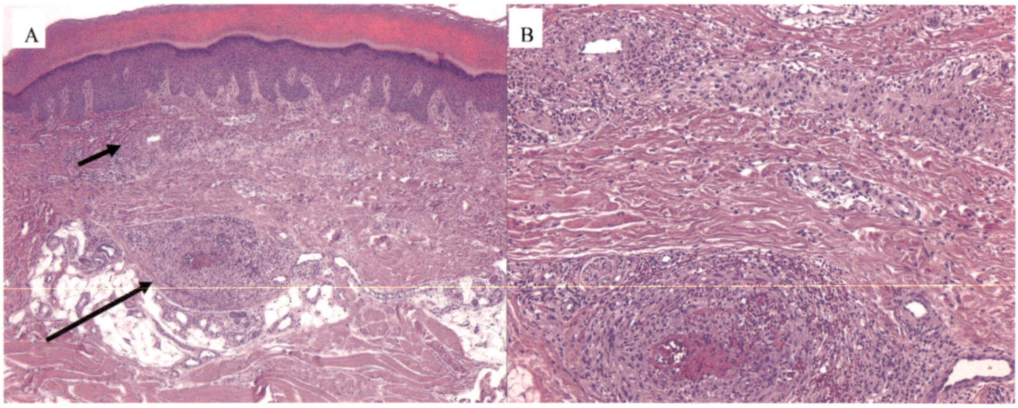

Fig. 33. (A) The coexistence of dermal small vasculitis (short arrow) and underlying arteritis (long arrow) in microscopic polyangiitis. (B) The specimen at high magnification.

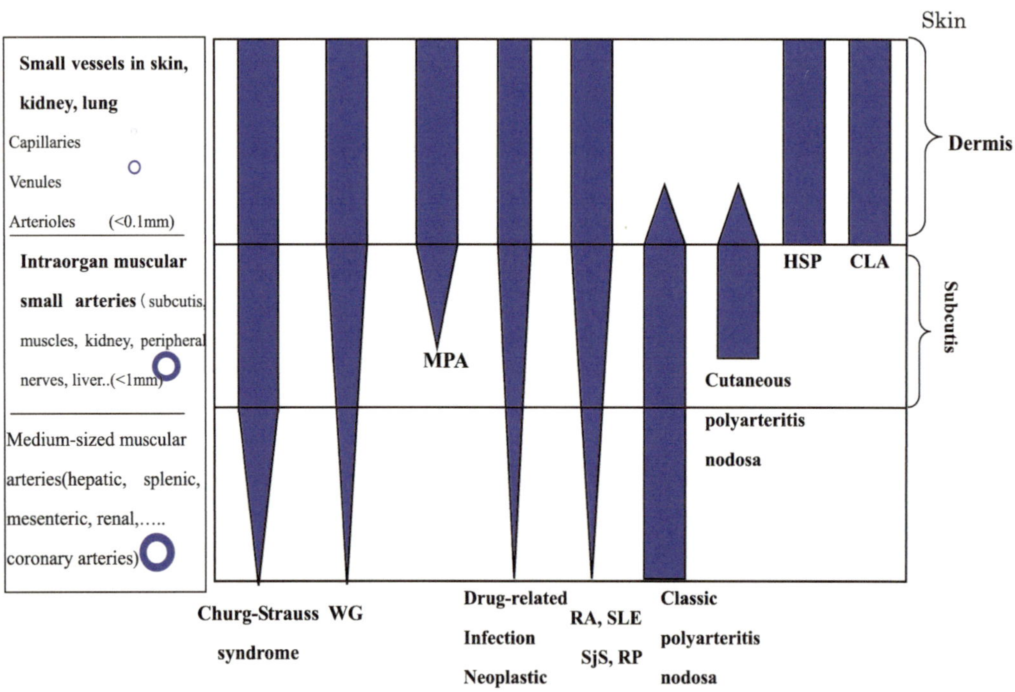

CLA:Cutaneous leukocytoclastic angiitis (also known as:idiopathic cutaneous small vessel vasculitis, cutaneous allergic vasculitis) WG: Wegener's granulomatosis, MPA: microscopic polyangiitis, HSP: Henoch-Schönlein purpura,
RP: relapsing polychondritis. Adapted from 3)Chen KR. Jpn J Dermatol, 120:2379-2391, 2010.

Fig. 34. The distribution of affected vessels in selected primary and secondary vasculitis syndromes.

7. Summary

Skin is the most common target organ for vasculitis (Figure 34). A diagnosis of cutaneous vasculitis is best determined by the histopathologic findings. However, the diagnosis may be difficult because of the constellation of clinical and histopathologic findings. The above described contents are the best approach to the complicated histopathology of cutaneous vasculitis, including the morphology of cutaneous vessels; the diagnostic criteria; the diagnostic pitfalls; and the classification, based on the size of the involved vessels and the principal inflammatory response.

8. References

[1] Chen KR, Carlson JA. Clinical approach to cutaneous vasculitis. Am J Clin Dermatol, 9:71-92, 2008.
[2] Carlson JA, Eng BT, Chen KR. Cutaneous Vasculitis Update: Diagnostic Criteria, Classification, Epidemiology, Etiology, Pathogenesis, Evaluation and Prognosis. Am J Dermatopathol, 27:504-528, 2005.
[3] Chen KR. Pathogenesis and histopathologic diagnosis of cutaneous vasculitis · Jpn J Dermatol, 120:2379-2391, 2010. (in Japanese)
[4] Sunderkotter C, Sindrilaru A. Clinical classification of vasculitis. Eur J Dermatol. 16:114-24, 2006.
[5] Carlson JA, Chen KR: Cutaneous Vasculitis Update: Small Vessel Neutrophilic Vasculitis Syndromes. Am J Dermatopathol. 28:486-506, 2006.
[6] Carlson JA, Chen KR: Cutaneous Vasculitis Update: Neutrophilic Muscular Vessel and Eosinophilic, Granulomatous, and Lymphocytic Vasculitis Syndromes. Am J Dermatopathol. 29:32-43, 2007.
[7] Carlson JA, Chen KR: Cutaneous pseudovasculitis. Am J Dermatopathol. 29:44-55, 2007.
[8] Chen KR. The misdiagnosis of superficial thrombophlebitis as cutaneous polyarteritis nodosa: Features of the internal elastic lamina and the compact concentric muscular layer as diagnostic pitfalls. Am J Dermatopathol 32:688-693, 2010.
[9] Chen KR, Toyohara A, Suzuki A, Miyakawa S: Clinical and histopathological spectrum of cutaneous vasculitis in rheumatoid arthritis. Br J Dermatol, 147:905-913, 2002.
[10] Bajema IM, Bruijn JA.. What stuff is this! A historical perspective on fibrinoid necrosis. J Pathol, 191:235-238, 2000.
[11] Ishibashi M, Chen KR: A morphological study of evolution of cutaneous polyarteritis nodosa. Am J Dermatopathol 30(4):319-26, 2008.
[12] Chen KR, Sakamoto M, Ikemoto K, et al: Granulomatous arteritis in cutaneous lesions of Churg-Strauss syndrome. J Cutan Pathol 34(4):330-7, 2007.
[13] Chen KR, Kawahara Y, Miyakawa S, Nishikawa T: Cutaneous vasculitis in Behçet's disease: a clinical and histopathologic study of 20 patients. J Am Acad Dermatol 36:689-96, 1997.
[14] Carlson JA, Mihm MC, Jr., LeBoit PE. Cutaneous lymphocytic vasculitis: a definition, a review, and a proposed classification. Semin Diagn Pathol. 13(1):72-90, 1996.
[15] Chen KR, Pittelkow MR, Su WPD, Gleich GJ, Newman W, Leiferman KM: Recurrent cutaneous eosinophilic necrotizing vasculitis: A novel eosinophil-mediated syndrome. Arch Dermatol 130:1159-1166, 1994.

[16] Chen KR, Su WPD, Pittelkow MR, Conn DL, George T, Leiferman KM: Eosinophilic vasculitis in connective tissue disease. J Am Acad Dermatol 35:173-182, 1996.

[17] Chen KR, Ohata Y, Sakurai M, Nakayama H: Churg-Strauss syndrome: Report of a case without pre-existing asthma. J Dermatol 19:40-47, 1992.

[18] Ishibashi M, Kudo S, Yamamoto K, Shimai N, Chen KR:Churg-Strauss syndrome with coexistence of eosinophilic vasculitis, granulomatous phlebitis and granulomatous dermatitis in bullous pemphigoid-like blisters. J Cutan Pathol. 38:290-294. 2011.

[19] Lie JT, Gordon LP, Titus JL. Jevenile temporal arteritis. Biopsy study of four cases. JAMA, 234;496-499, 1975.

[20] Nordborg E, Nordberg C. The inflammatory reaction in giant cell arteritis: an immunohistochemical investigation. Clin Exp Rheumatol, 16:165-8, 1998.

[21] Mambo NC. Temporal (granulomatous) arteritis: A histopathological study of 32 cases. Histopathology. 3:209-221, 1979.[

3

FDG-PET in Large Vessel Vasculitis

Quinn K.T. Ng[1], Bernd Klaeser[1], Ulrich A. Walker[2] and Martin A. Walter[1]
[1]Institute of Nuclear Medicine University Hospital Haller Building Freiburgstrasse 4 CH-3010 Bern
[2]Department of Rheumatology Felix-Platter Spital Burgfelderstr. 101 CH-4012 Basel Switzerland

1. Introduction

[18F]FDG-PET, a non-invasive metabolic imaging technique, is based on the regional distribution of fluorine-18-fluorodeoxyglucose ([18F]FDG) reflecting increased glucose consumption of tissues. This technique has become increasingly important over the years in the management of patients with malignancies, as many malignant tumors show an enhanced glucose metabolism[1]. [18F]FDG uptake in infections and other inflammatory changes seen during oncologic imaging showed indications for the versatility of [18F]FDG-PET. Activated leukocytes also overexpress glucose transporters and avidly accumulate glucose and [18F]FDG [2,3], providing an important rationale for its use in vasculitis. Remarkable images of patients with active vasculitis have been generated through [18F]FDG-PET scans[4-12]. Such images demonstrate the potential of [18F]FDG-PET for a variety of applications which implies that it may also be useful in the future for the routine evaluation of patients with several forms of vasculitis, particularly for large vessel vasculitis.

The family of vasculitides is categorized with reference to the size of vessels involved into large, medium, and small vessel vasculitis (**Table 1**). Of interest with respect to [18F]FDG-PET imaging is the group of large vessel vasculitides (giant cell arteritis and Takayasu's arteritis), other causes of aortitis and potentially also chronic periaortitis. Patients of both of these diseases regularly present a set of non-specific symptoms and laboratory tests which make their diagnosis and follow-up quite challenging. Consequently, patients may receive delays or even unsuccessful diagnostic work-up regarding their condition. The use of whole-body scanning via [18F]FDG-PET may provide a sensitive metabolic imaging modality that could lead to a more successful and shorter diagnostic workup.

The total amount of available data on [18F]FDG-PET in large vessel vasculitis is however still limited **(Table 2)**. In addition, no standardized guidelines are in place for the placement of [18F]FDG-PET imaging in the sequence of the diagnostic workup, its performance, interpretation and description. This chapter summarizes current clinical data in order to assist nuclear medicine and rheumatology practitioners in recommending, performing and interpreting the results of [18F]FDG-PET in patients with suspected large vessel vasculitis.

2. Giant cell arteritis

Giant cell arteritis was first described by Hutchinson in 1890 as a granulomatous vasculitis of large and medium sized arteries [13]. Giant cell arteritis usually affects the cranial branches of the arteries originating from the aortic arch, particularly the superficial temporal artery; however, involvement of the entire aorta and of its main branches also occurs in about 15% [14]. Giant cell arteritis is common in the Caucasian population, with an incidence of about 18 per 100,000 over 50 years of age [15-17]and affects women twice as often as men [15-17]. Autopsy studies however suggest that it may be much more common than is clinically apparent [18].

Size of vessels	Type of vasculitis	Classification Criteria*
Large	Giant cell arteritis	Age at onset of disease ≥50 yr New headache Temporal artery abnormality Elevated erythrocyte sedimentation rate Abnormal findings on biopsy of temporal artery
	Takayasu's arteritis	Age at onset of disease ≤40 yr Claudication of an extremity Decreased brachial artery pulse Difference in systolic blood pressure between arms A bruit over the subclavian arteries or the aorta Narrowing or occlusion of the entire aorta at angiography
Medium	Peri-arteritis nodosa Kawasaki's arteritis Primary CNS vasculitis Buerger's disease	
Small	Wegener's disease Churg-Strauss syndrome Microscopic polyangiitis Henoch-Schonlein purpura Essential cryoglobulinaemic vasculitis Cutaneous leukocytoclastic angiitis	

*Diagnosis of giant cell arteritis: at least 3/5 criteria; Sensitivity =93.5%, Specificity =90.5%
*Diagnosis of Takayasu's arteritis: at least 3/6 criteria; Sensitivity =91.2%, Specificity =97.8%

Table 1. Classification of vasculitis

Currently, the etiology of giant cell arteritis still remains unknown. Classic histological pictures of giant cell arteritis show granulomatous inflammation wherein giant cells are usually located at the connection between the intima and media. However, panarteritides with mixed-cell inflammatory infiltrates of lymphomononuclear cells, occasional neutrophils and eosinophils, but without giant cells are also found [19]. The focal arteritic lesions cause ischemia which subsequently leads to the sudden or gradual onset of symptoms and a variety of systemic manifestations. A variety of systemic symptoms may be present [20,21], and include myalgia, neck pain, scalp tenderness, jaw claudication, fever, tenderness of the temporal arteries, transient ischemic attacks, general malaise, fatigue, anorexia, weight loss, depression, and night sweats [20,22,23]. Headache is probably the most frequent symptom which occurs in two thirds of patients [21].

Authors	Year	Takayasu arteritis (number of patients)	Giant cell arteritis (number of patients)	Follow-up PETs	Reference
Blockmans et al.	1999	-	11*	-	63
Blockmans et al.	2000	-	25*	-	64
Belhocine et al.	2002	-	3	3	65
Meller et al.	2003	5	-	-	52
Meller et al.	2003	1	14	7	48
Bleeker-Rovers et al.	2003	1	7*	1	45
Webb et al.	2004	18	-	8	44
Brodman et al.	2004	-	22	-	46
Moosig et al.	2004	-	12*	8	47
Andrews et al.	2004	6	-	6	43
Scheel et al.	2004	-	8	8	53
Kobayashi et al.	2005	14	-	7	50
Walter et al.	2005	6	20	4	49
Blockmans et al.	2006	-	35*	22	66
Blockmans et al.	2008	-	46	25	67
Both et al.	2008	-	25	9	68
Hautzel et al.	2008	-	18	-	69
Henes et al.	2008	3	10	-	70
Janssen et al.	2008	-	11	-	71
Arnaud et al.	2009	28	-	8	72
Lee et al.	2009	32	-	-	73
Vista et al.	2010	4	-	-	74
Lehmann et al.	2011	3	17	-	75

*Giant cell arteritis and polymyalgia rheumatica patients

Table 2. Clinical studies on PET in the detection of large vessel inflammation: the present literature

3. Takayasu's arteritis

Takayasu's arteritis is named after Mikito Takayasu, who in 1908 had reported the peculiar wreath-like arteriovenous anastomoses around the papillae in a young woman with pulseless disease [24]. This large vessel vasculitis primarily affects the aorta, its main branches, and the coronary and pulmonary arteries. The incidence rate of the disease is about 2 per 1,000,000 with its onset at a mean of 35 years of age [25-27]. Takayasu's arteritis occurs worldwide, although it is considered to be more common in the Orient [28] and is 10 times more prevalent in females than in males. The etiology of Takayasu's arteritis also remains unresolved, while the clinical course includes both an early and a late phase. Pathology studies in the early phase reveal granulomatous or diffuse productive inflammation in the media and adventitia, with secondary thickening of the intima and occasional perivascular inflammation [29]. In the clinic, it is commonly the setting of fever of unknown origin with non-specific systemic symptoms. Contrary to the early phase, pathology studies in the late phase show marked thinning of the media, with disruption of elastic fibers, fibrotic thickening of the adventitia, and marked intimal proliferation[29]. The resulting variable ischemic symptoms secondary to arterial stenosis, occlusion, or arterial dilatation and aneurysmal formation cause various clinical conditions, such as arm claudication, decreased arterial pulses, carotodynia, visual loss, stroke, aortic regurgitation and arterial hypertension[30]. Topological classification of Takayasu's arteritis is based on the vascular provinces that are affected [31], with either affection of the branches of the aortic arch (Type I), the ascending aorta, aortic arch and its branches (Type IIa), the ascending aorta, aortic arch and its branches and the thoracic descending aorta (Type IIb), the thoracic descending aorta, abdominal aorta, and/or renal arteries (Type III), the abdominal aorta and/or renal arteries (Type IV) or combined features of types IIb and IV.

4. Diagnostic work-up in large vessel vasculitis

Giant cell arteritis and Takayasu's arteritis are both usually present with a wide clinical spectrum with no specific laboratory finding. The American College of Rheumatology has established a set of clinical, radiological and histological criteria to classify cases of biopsy-proven arteritis (**Table 1**) [32,33]. The presence of at least three of the described criteria is required for classifying a patient as having either Takayasu's arteritis or giant cell arteritis. These criteria provide a sensitivity of 93.5% with a specificity of 90.5% for diagnosing giant cell arteritis and a sensitivity of 91.2% with a specificity of 97.8% for diagnosing Takayasu's arteritis in biopsy-positive patients.

Although these criteria were originally designed for research purposes to help distinguish between different types of vasculitis; they are in clinical practice also frequently used for diagnosing an individual patient [34]. Nevertheless, the fact that frequent symptoms of giant cell arteritis such as jaw claudication, diplopia, neck pain, and elevated C-reactive protein are not included in the criteria, limits their widespread clinical application. Criteria that are included, such as headache and scalp tenderness can also be due to various other diseases. A normal erythrocyte sedimentation rate does not rule out giant cell arteritis, as it has been found in up to 30% of patients with biopsy-proven giant cell arteritis [35,36]. Furthermore, several patients with giant cell arteritis do only display nonspecific symptoms that does not apply to any set of criteria. Systemic giant cell arteritis symptoms such as fever, anorexia, weight loss and malaise may focus the diagnostic work-up towards a suspected malignancy, especially in older patients [37].

Frequent clinical features of Takayasu's arteritis such as fever, postural dizziness, arthralgias, weight loss, headache, hypertension, elevated erythrocytes sedimentation rate and anemia were also not included in the classification criteria of the American College of Rheumatology. In contrast, angiographic findings and non-congruent blood pressure measurements between both arms are included as part of the diagnostic criteria although they may be false negative in early vasculitis [38,39] , or when the arteritis is restricted to the abdominal aorta, its branches, or to the pulmonary artery.

The wide clinical spectrum and the diagnostic limitations of giant cell arteritis and Takayasu's arteritis frequently cause delay in their diagnosis and subsequent treatment.

5. [^{18}F]FDG-PET and [^{18}F]FDG-PET/CT

[^{18}F]FDG-PET is an operator-independent, non-invasive imaging modality which examines the regional distribution of fluorine-18-fluorodeoxyglucose. Deoxyglucose is labeled with the positron emitting radionuclide, ^{18}Fluorine, and is intravenously administered to patients. [^{18}F]FDG initially distributes in proportion to the perfusion of the organs, where it follows the same route of uptake as glucose. After entering cells through specific carriers, [^{18}F]FDG is phosphorylated to [^{18}F]FDG-6-phosphate, trapped intracellularly, but not metabolized further. The emitted positrons can be detected by a scanner and are displayed as a bright signal in the [^{18}F]FDG-PET scan, reflecting an increased glucose requirement.

Heightened glucose metabolism is a property of many malignancies, a fact which has fostered the use of [^{18}F]FDG-PET studies in the staging and follow-up in various types of cancers [1].

Modern PET-CT scanners combine PET scanners with a computed tomography scanner in a single gantry system. With these scanners, images are taken sequentially with both devices in the same session and the reading can be done with the single co-registered image. As a consequence, the functional image obtained by PET, can be correlated more precisely with the anatomic structures. PET/CT has shown an incremental diagnostic value over CT and PET alone and there is emerging evidence of a substantial impact of PET/CT imaging on patient management [40].

6. [^{18}F]FDG-PET scanning protocols for large vessel vasculitis

The American and the European Association of Nuclear Medicine have both established procedure guidelines for tumor imaging with [^{18}F]FDG-PET [41,42]. The guidelines of the American Association of Nuclear Medicine from 1998 recommend fasting at least 4 hours prior to the scan. Low blood glucose levels are recommended, the injected activity should total 350 to 750 MBq [^{18}F]FDG, and image acquisition should start 30 to 40 minutes after injection. In contrast, the guidelines of the European Association of Nuclear Medicine from the year 2003 advocate fasting at least 6 hours prior to the scan. Blood glucose level should not exceed 130mg/dl, the injected [^{18}F]FDG activity should be 6 MBq/kg body weight, and acquisition should be started 60 minutes after injection.

Both professional associations however, have not established guidelines for the PET imaging of inflammation and consequently, the present studies **(Table 2)** have used several different protocols. Pre-scan fasting intervals of 4 hours [43,44], 6 hours [45-47], and overnight fasts [48-50] were applied. Body-weight adapted protocols for the applied [^{18}F]FDG dose with 5 [49], 6 [50] or 6.5 MBq [46,51] [^{18}F]FDG per kilogram bodyweight were used. However, fixed doses of 296 MBq [52], 370 MBq [48], and 450 MBq [47] were also employed. To accelerate renal [^{18}F]FDG elimination, one group also routinely administered additional furosemide [45]. Most studies on [^{18}F]FDG-PET in large vessel vasculitis did not restrict scanning by maximal glucose levels and only three studies tolerated maximum serum glucose levels of 100mg/dl [48,52] and 180mg/dl [49]. Large differences in the time interval between [^{18}F]FDG application and image acquisition were also shown as [^{18}F]FDG-uptake periods of 45 minutes [49,50], 60 minutes [45,46,48,51,52], or 90 minutes [43,44,47] were reported. Dedicated PET scanners with full-ring detectors were generally used; nevertheless, hybrid cameras have also been successfully employed [48,52,53]. Reports on the use of combined [^{18}F]FDG-PET-CT scanners in large vessel vasculitis are available [50,54,55].

The average radiation dose from the [^{18}F]FDG-PET scan is 7mSv, the average dose from the CT scan is 18mSv. The CT dose, however, can be lowered by the use of low-dose acquisition protocols.
This summary indicates that despite a lack of standardization, [^{18}F]FDG-PET is a reliable imaging modality of large vessel vasculitis.

7. [^{18}F]FDG-PET and atherosclerosis

The accumulation of glucose analogues has not only been demonstrated in vasculitic vessels, but also in atherosclerotic plaques **(Figure 1)** [56]. Consequently, a modest large vessel [^{18}F]FDG accumulation at the level of the major vessels occurs in about 50% of all PET-scans, with increased prevalence in older people [57]. This vascular uptake might be explained by smooth muscle metabolism in the media, subendothelial smooth muscle proliferation from senescence, and the presence of macrophages within the atherosclerotic plaque. Therefore, vascular uptake found in the [^{18}F]FDG-PET scan is not specific for vasculitis.

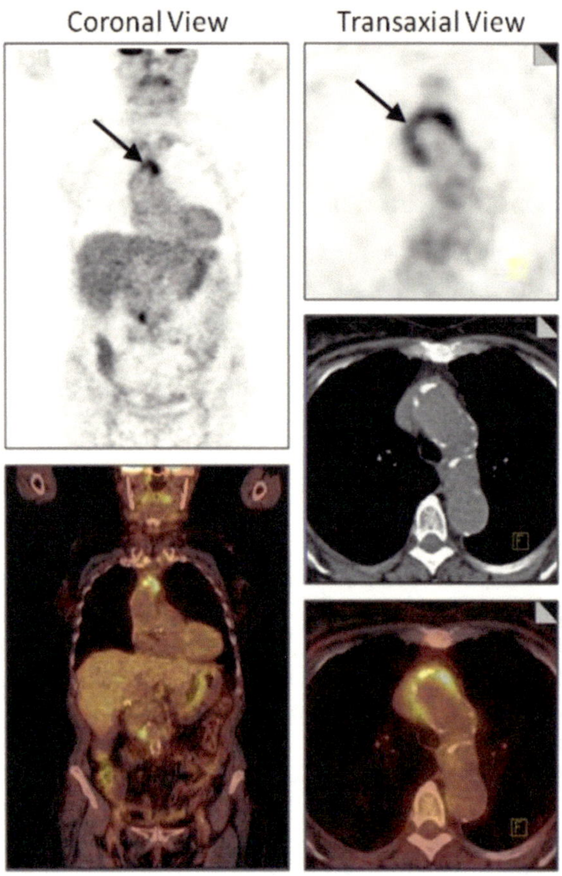

Fig. 1. 71-year-old female patient that underwent FDG-PET/CT to evaluate a suspicious lung nodule. Focal FDG uptake was found in the thoracic and abdominal aorta corresponding to circumscribed artherosclerotic and aneurysmatic wall changes (arrow; from the Institute of Nuclear Medicine, University Hosptial, Bern, CH)

Nevertheless, atherosclerotic lesions can be differentiated from vasculitic lesions by taking into account the vascular distribution, [^{18}F]FDG uptake pattern, and the intensity of the [^{18}F]FDG accumulation. For example, the internal carotid artery demonstrates atherosclerotic changes more frequently, while the external carotid artery more often reveals inflammatory changes. The uptake pattern of atherosclerotic mediastinal great vessels sometimes can be identified as ring-shaped structures, while contrary to this, the uptake pattern in the arteries of the abdomen and lower extremities are often linear and continuous [58]. Most discriminatingly, atherosclerotic lesions rarely demonstrate intense uptake of FDG [48,49].

To distinguish vasculitis from atherosclerosis, a visual scoring of vascular [^{18}F]FDG-uptake compared to the liver [^{18}F]FDG-accumulation has been established. Three grades of large vessel [^{18}F]FDG-uptake are differentiated **(Figure 2)**: a) Grade I: uptake present but lower than liver uptake, b) Grade II: similar to liver uptake, and c) Grade III: uptake higher than liver uptake. Proposed by Meller et al. [48], this scale was subsequently validated to represent the severity of inflammation [49].

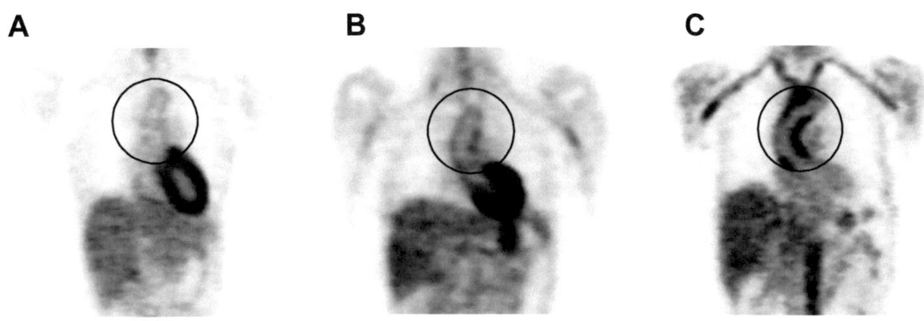

Fig. 2. The visual arteritis score as proposed by Meller et al. [48]. The severity of large vessel [18F]FDG-uptake is visually graded: **A)** Grade 1: uptake present but lower than liver uptake; **B)** Grade 2: similar to liver uptake; **C)** Grade 3: uptake higher than liver uptake (images derived from reference [49]).

So far, this score has been employed in two reference collectives without clinical symptoms or laboratory signs of large vessel inflammation in order to determine the uptake in non-vasculitic vessels [48,49]. Grade I vessel uptake was frequently found in the thoracic part of the aorta which was most likely due to atherosclerosis. Accordingly, only Grade II or III [^{18}F]FDG-uptake in the thoracic aorta and any visible uptake in other segments should routinely be judged as active large vessel inflammation. In this manner, the majority of lesions can be ruled out as due to atherosclerosis. On the other hand, computed quantification of [^{18}F]FDG-uptake using the [^{18}F]FDG *standardized uptake value* (SUV) has not shown to be useful in discriminating atherosclerosis from vasculitis yet.

8. [^{18}F]FDG-PET for diagnosing giant cell arteritis

The diagnosis of giant cell arteritis is currently based mainly on clinical evaluation, laboratory results, and temporal biopsy, but a gold standard is lacking. Despite recent advances, no imaging modality has been included in the American College of Rheumatology diagnostic criteria for giant cell arteritis **(Table 1)**. Nevertheless, [^{18}F]FDG-

PET has indicated its usefulness clinically for a number of studies through better evidence, as compared to Takayasu's arteritis, due to the higher frequency of the disease **(Table 2)**.
The uptake pattern in large vessels affected by giant cell arteritis was linear, continuous, and was predominantly of Grade II. The thoracic vessels were most frequently affected, followed by the abdominal vessels [48,49]. In the published studies, the ability of [^{18}F]FDG-PET to detect large vessel inflammation differed considerably. In studies employing patients with polymyalgia rheumatica and giant cell arteritis, sensitivities between 56% and 100% were reported [45,46,51,53], with a specificity between 77% and 98% [51]. The large differences seen between the studies can partially be explained by dissimilar disease activity; as suggested by one study demonstrating that the sensitivity depends on the degree of inflammation **(Figure 4)**. C-reactive protein has shown to be a better predictor for the sensitivity of [^{18}F]FDG-PET in giant cell arteritis than the erythrocyte sedimentation rate [49].
Studies employing [^{18}F]FDG-PET and Magnetic Resonance Imaging (MRI) revealed comparable sensitivities for both methods. [^{18}F]FDG-PET may have the advantage that it simultaneously identifies more affected vessels [48,53], possibly reflecting the fact that metabolic changes normally precede morphologic changes in giant cell arteritis. Additionally, [^{18}F]FDG-PET might also allow new insights into the pathology of giant cell arteritis and polymyalgia rheumatica. A study demonstrated inflammation of the aorta or its major branches in 92% of patients with polymyalgia rheumatica. Tracer uptake was strongly correlated with the erythrocyte sedimentation rate and the C-reactive protein. These data underline that polymyalgia rheumatica frequently may be accompanied by subclinical vasculitis [47].
[^{18}F]FDG-PET also offers the possibility of whole-body screening in one procedure which may become helpful in the follow-up of patients with giant cell arteritis. The results of computed quantification of vascular [^{18}F]FDG accumulation correlate well and better than Magnetic Resonance Imaging with the clinical course also at longitudinal follow up [47,48].
The value of [^{18}F]FDG-PET for diagnosing temporal arteritis has however been questioned in a study of 22 patients, 17 of which had involvement of the temporal arteries which was not detected by [^{18}F]FDG-PET [46]. The high [^{18}F]FDG uptake of the brain and the small diameter of the temporal arteries limited its sensitivity in the detection of cranial vessel involvement with the whole-body PET technique used. Newer generation PET/CT scanners offer an image resolution corresponding to a three-fold improvement compared to the technology used in the aforementioned study (2mm vs. 7mm), potentially allowing to image even smaller arteries as the temporal arteries. Further clinical studies must are warranted to clarify the potential role of PET in the non-invasive work-up of temporal vasculitis.

9. [^{18}F]FDG-PET for diagnosing Takayasu's arteritis

The diagnosis of Takayasu's arteritis frequently integrates imaging and angiographic **(Table 1)**. However, angiographic alterations usually occur in the late phase of Takayasu's arteritis while metabolic changes are already present in the early phases. The data on the use of [^{18}F]FDG-PET in Takayasu's arteritis are less robust compared to those in giant cell arteritis **(Table 2)**, accounting for the different prevalences of both vasculitides.
During the early phase of Takayasu's arteritis, the [^{18}F]FDG uptake pattern is linear and continuous **(Figure 3A)**, while in the late phase the pattern can become patchier rather than continuous but still remains in a linear distribution [44]. Three studies reported sensitivities of [^{18}F]FDG-PET between 83% and 100% [43,44,52], which is comparable to Magnetic Resonance

Imaging. Additionally, metabolic imaging using [^{18}F]FDG-PET for Takayasu's arteritis has identified more affected vascular regions than morphologic imaging using Magnetic Resonance Imaging [52]. However, unlike Magnetic Resonance Imaging, [^{18}F]FDG-PET does not give any information about the wall structure or the lumen of affected vessels.

Similarly to giant cell arteritis, there is a clear correlation between the activity of vessel inflammation and the sensitivity of [^{18}F]FDG-PET. [^{18}F]FDG-PET positive patients have shown significantly higher erythrocyte sedimentation rates and C-reactive protein levels as compared to [^{18}F]FDG-PET negative patients, with the C-reactive protein being the superior marker [44].

Follow-ups in Takayasu's arteritis only based on clinical symptoms alone have shown to be of limited accuracy. In a previous report, biopsies showed active inflammation in 44% of patients thought to be in clinical remission [59]. However, [^{18}F]FDG-PET is able to detect more sites than just those that were clinically active [44]. This makes [^{18}F]FDG-PET a promising candidate to be regularly employed in the follow-up of Takayasu's arteritis **(Figure 3)** due its high sensitivity and the good correlation with the outcome [43,44,49].

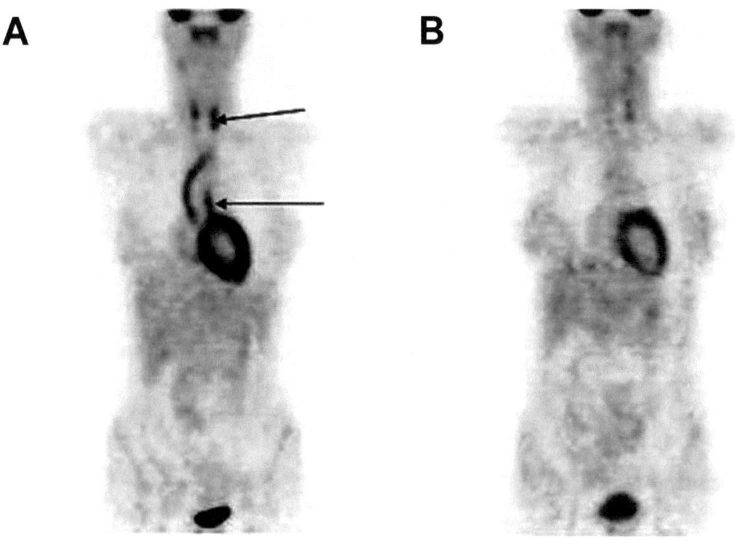

Fig. 3. **A)** [^{18}F]FDG-PET of a patient with Takayasu's arteritis with markedly abnormal uptake of [^{18}F]FDG in the aortic arch and carotide arteries (arrows). **B)** [^{18}F]FDG-PET scan of the same patient in clinical remission after treatment with prednisone and intravenous cyclophosphamide (from reference [43])

10. [^{18}F]FDG-PET-CT in large vessel vasculitis

The combination of [^{18}F]FDG-PET scanners with Computed Tomography (CT) has gained importance in the management of patients with malignancies [60-62] by allowing the integration of morphologic and metabolic information for detection, staging, and therapy control. Rapidly increasing availability of [^{18}F]FDG-PET-CT scanners are also opening new opportunities for its application in rheumatology by allowing the investigation of both morphologic and metabolic activity while significantly improving the localization of affected vessels. Two case reports have already indicated the value of [^{18}F]FDG-PET-CT

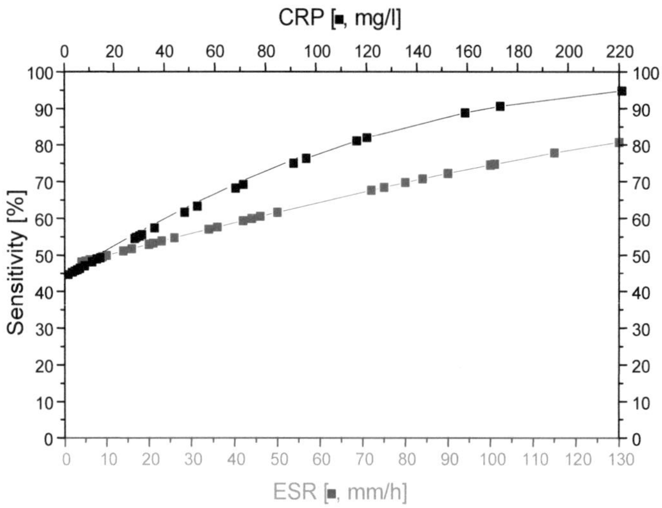

Fig. 4. Sensitivity of Large Vessel Vasculitis [18F]FDG-PET as a function of C-reactive protein (CRP)levels and erythrocyte sedimentation rate (ES§) , respectively. High sensitivity for detection of large vessel vasculitis is reached at high CRP and ESR levels (from reference [49]).

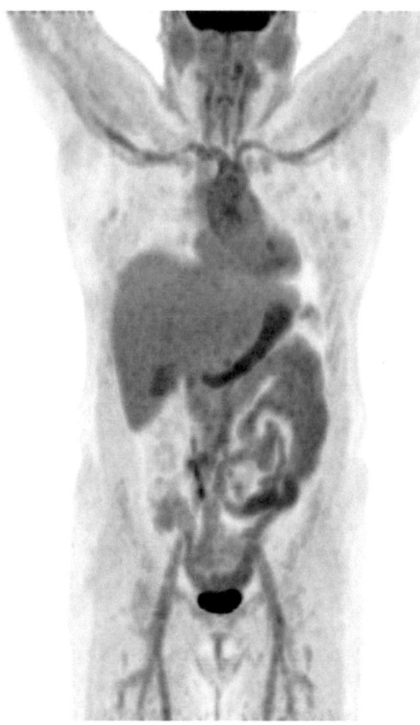

Fig. 5. 52 year-old female patient with clinical suspision of a large vessel vasculitis. The FDG-PET/CT shows intense tracer uptake along the aortic arch, the supraaortic branches and the supraclavicular arteries. There is also uptake along the abdominal aorta and femoral arteries and branches.

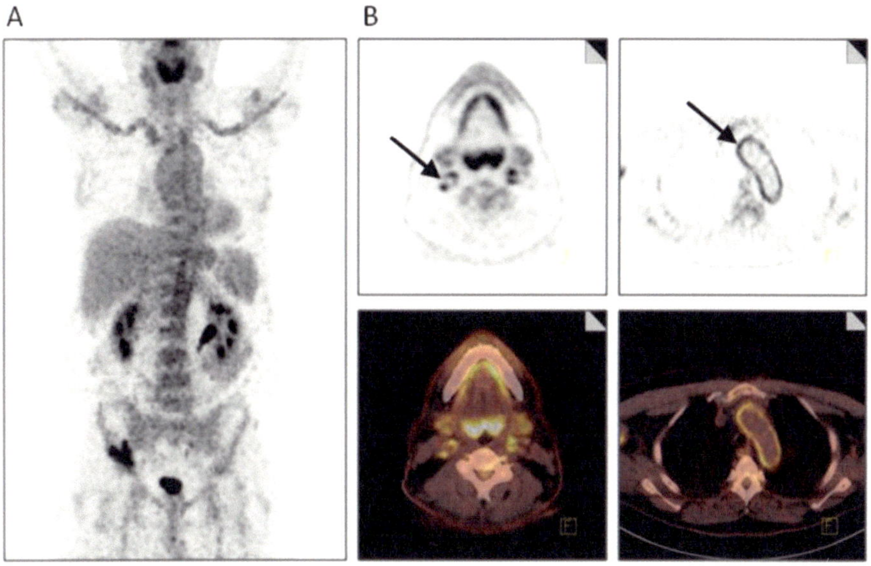

Fig. 6. FDG-PET/CT of a 67-year-old male patient with recent loss of weight and continious deterioration of his general condition. The PET/CT performed did not support the clinical suspicion of a malignant tumor but showed intense vessel uptake (**A**). Additional high-resolution PET images of the chest and neck illustrate the ability of state-of-the-art PET machines to visualize circumscribed wall inflammation even in medium sized arteries as the carotic sinus and the vessel wall of the aortic arch (**B**)

scanners in large vessel vasculitis [53,54] and one clinical trial has investigated its value in 14 patients [50]. The co-registered CT scan was most useful for the anatomic identification of vascular [^{18}F]FDG-uptake, especially in case of rather moderate [^{18}F]FDG-accumulation. Furthermore, the anatomic identification of mediastinal [^{18}F]FDG uptake, particularly in the pulmonary arteries was significantly improved **(Figure 5)**. The coregistered CT scan allows for a sensitive detection of calcified plaques to discriminate vasculitis from inflammatory arteriosclerotic changes.

11. Conclusions

In conclusion, whole-body imaging with [^{18}F]FDG-PET is highly effective in assessing the extent of giant cell arteritis and Takayasu's arteritis, respectively.
[^{18}F]FDG-PET has shown to have identified more affected vascular regions than morphologic imaging with Magnetic Resonance Imaging in both diseases.
A unique feature and strength of FDG-PET is the opportunity to monitor disease activity non-invasively. In contrast to other imaging modalities PET allows for an immediate assessment of response to anti-inflammatory treatment and is suitable to guide therapy.
Recent developments in PET technology such as integrated PET/CT machines and increased image resolution of the PET submodality imply significant improvements for vaculitis imaging with FDG.
Further studies are warranted to evaluate the diagnostic benefit of these newer technical developments.

[^{18}F]FDG-PET has the clear potential to develop into a valuable tool in the diagnostic work-up of both giant cell arteritis and Takayasu's arteritis, and may become a first-line investigation technique for non-invasive therapy monitoring. However, consensus regarding the imaging procedures as well as further clinical evidence is urgently needed.

12. References

[1] Been LB, Suurmeijer AJ, Cobben DC, Jager PL, Hoekstra HJ, Elsinga PH. [18F]FLT-PET in oncology: current status and opportunities. Eur J Nucl Med Mol Imaging 2004;31(12):1659-72.

[2] Ishimori T, Saga T, Mamede M, Kobayashi H, Higashi T, Nakamoto Y, Sato N, Konishi J. Increased (18)F-FDG uptake in a model of inflammation: concanavalin A-mediated lymphocyte activation. J Nucl Med 2002;43(5):658-63.

[3] Jones HA, Cadwallader KA, White JF, Uddin M, Peters AM, Chilvers ER. Dissociation between respiratory burst activity and deoxyglucose uptake in human neutrophil granulocytes: implications for interpretation of (18)F-FDG PET images. J Nucl Med 2002;43(5):652-7.

[4] Turlakow A, Yeung HW, Pui J, Macapinlac H, Liebovitz E, Rusch V, Goy A, Larson SM. Fludeoxyglucose positron emission tomography in the diagnosis of giant cell arteritis. Arch Intern Med 2001;161(7):1003-7.

[5] Blockmans D, Van Moer E, Dehem J, Feys C, Mortelmans L. Positron emission tomography can reveal abdominal periaortitis. Clin Nucl Med 2002;27(3):211-2.

[6] Wenger M, Gasser R, Donnemiller E, Erler H, Glossmann H, Patsch JR, Moncayo R, Schirmer M. Images in cardiovascular medicine. Generalized large vessel arteritis visualized by 18fluorodeoxyglucose-positron emission tomography. Circulation 2003;107(6):923.

[7] Brodmann M, Lipp RW, Aigner R, Pilger E. Positron emission tomography reveals extended thoracic and abdominal peri-aortitis. Vasc Med 2003;8(2):127-8.

[8] Wiest R, Gluck T, Schonberger J, Scholmerich J, Eilles C, Muller-Ladner U. Clinical image: occult large vessel vasculitis diagnosed by PET imaging. Rheumatol Int 2001;20(6):250.

[9] De Winter F, Petrovic M, Van de Wiele C, Vogelaers D, Afschrift M, Dierckx RA. Imaging of giant cell arteritis: evidence of splenic involvement using FDG positron emission tomography. Clin Nucl Med 2000;25(8):633-4.

[10] Hara M, Goodman PC, Leder RA. FDG-PET finding in early-phase Takayasu arteritis. J Comput Assist Tomogr 1999;23(1):16-8.

[11] Malik IS, Harare O, A AL-N, Beatt K, Mason J. Takayasu's arteritis: management of left main stem stenosis. Heart 2003;89(3):e9.

[12] Walter MA, Melzer RA, Graf M, Tyndall A, Muller-Brand J, Nitzsche EU. [18F]FDG-PET of giant-cell aortitis. Rheumatology (Oxford) 2005;44(5):690-1.

[13] Hutchinson J. On a peculiar form of thrombotic arteritis of the aged which is sometimes productive or gangrene. Arch Surg 1890;1:323-329.

[14] Klein RG, Hunder GG, Stanson AW, Sheps SG. Large artery involvement in giant cell (temporal) arteritis. Ann Intern Med 1975;83(6):806-12.

[15] Salvarani C, Gabriel SE, O'Fallon WM, Hunder GG. The incidence of giant cell arteritis in Olmsted County, Minnesota: apparent fluctuations in a cyclic pattern. Ann Intern Med 1995;123(3):192-4.

[16] Franzen P, Sutinen S, von Knorring J. Giant cell arteritis and polymyalgia rheumatica in a region of Finland: an epidemiologic, clinical and pathologic study, 1984-1988. J Rheumatol 1992;19(2):273-6.
[17] Gonzalez-Gay MA, Alonso MD, Aguero JJ, Bal M, Fernandez-Camblor B, Sanchez-Andrade A. Giant cell arteritis in Mediterranean countries: comment on the article by Salvarani et al. Arthritis Rheum 1992;35(10):1249-50.
[18] Ostberg G. An arteritis with special reference to polymyalgia arteritica. Acta Pathol Microbiol Scand [A] 1973;237:Suppl 237:1-59.
[19] Lie JT. Illustrated histopathologic classification criteria for selected vasculitis syndromes. American College of Rheumatology Subcommittee on Classification of Vasculitis. Arthritis Rheum 1990;33(8):1074-87.
[20] Weyand CM. The Dunlop-Dottridge Lecture: The pathogenesis of giant cell arteritis. J Rheumatol 2000;27(2):517-22.
[21] Salvarani C, Macchioni PL, Tartoni PL, Rossi F, Baricchi R, Castri C, Chiaravalloti F, Portioli I. Polymyalgia rheumatica and giant cell arteritis: a 5-year epidemiologic and clinical study in Reggio Emilia, Italy. Clin Exp Rheumatol 1987;5(3):205-15.
[22] Huston KA, Hunder GG. Giant cell (cranial) arteritis: a clinical review. Am Heart J 1980;100(1):99-105.
[23] Calamia KT, Hunder GG. Giant cell arteritis (temporal arteritis) presenting as fever of undetermined origin. Arthritis Rheum 1981;24(11):1414-8.
[24] Takayasu M. Case with unusual changes of the central vessels in the retina. Acta Soc Ophthal Jpn 1908;12:554-5.
[25] Waern AU, Andersson P, Hemmingsson A. Takayasu's arteritis: a hospital-region based study on occurrence, treatment and prognosis. Angiology 1983;34(5):311-20.
[26] Hall S, Barr W, Lie JT, Stanson AW, Kazmier FJ, Hunder GG. Takayasu arteritis. A study of 32 North American patients. Medicine (Baltimore) 1985;64(2):89-99.
[27] el-Reshaid K, Varro J, al-Duwairi Q, Anim JT. Takayasu's arteritis in Kuwait. J Trop Med Hyg 1995;98(5):299-305.
[28] Lande A. Abdominal Takayasu's aortitis, the middle aortic syndrome and atherosclerosis. A critical review. Int Angiol 1998;17(1):1-9.
[29] Nasu T. Pathology of pulseless disease. A systematic study and critical review of twenty-one autopsy cases reported in Japan. Angiology 1963;14:225-42.
[30] Matsunaga N, Hayashi K, Sakamoto I, Ogawa Y, Matsumoto T. Takayasu arteritis: protean radiologic manifestations and diagnosis. Radiographics 1997;17(3):579-94.
[31] Moriwaki R, Noda M, Yajima M, Sharma BK, Numano F. Clinical manifestations of Takayasu arteritis in India and Japan--new classification of angiographic findings. Angiology 1997;48(5):369-79.
[32] Hunder GG, Bloch DA, Michel BA, Stevens MB, Arend WP, Calabrese LH, Edworthy SM, Fauci AS, Leavitt RY, Lie JT and others. The American College of Rheumatology 1990 criteria for the classification of giant cell arteritis. Arthritis Rheum 1990;33(8):1122-8.
[33] Arend WP, Michel BA, Bloch DA, Hunder GG, Calabrese LH, Edworthy SM, Fauci AS, Leavitt RY, Lie JT, Lightfoot RW, Jr. and others. The American College of Rheumatology 1990 criteria for the classification of Takayasu arteritis. Arthritis Rheum 1990;33(8):1129-34.

[34] Rao JK, Allen NB, Pincus T. Limitations of the 1990 American College of Rheumatology classification criteria in the diagnosis of vasculitis. Ann Intern Med 1998;129(5):345-52.
[35] Salvarani C, Hunder GG. Giant cell arteritis with low erythrocyte sedimentation rate: frequency of occurence in a population-based study. Arthritis Rheum 2001;45(2):140-5.
[36] Hayreh SS, Zimmerman B. Management of giant cell arteritis. Our 27-year clinical study: new light on old controversies. Ophthalmologica 2003;217(4):239-59.
[37] Gonzalez-Gay MA, Garcia-Porrua C, Salvarani C, Olivieri I, Hunder GG. The spectrum of conditions mimicking polymyalgia rheumatica in Northwestern Spain. J Rheumatol 2000;27(9):2179-84.
[38] Lambert M, Hachulla E, Hatron PY, Perez-Cousin M, Beregi JP, Warembourg H, Devulder B. [Takayasu's arteritis: vascular investigations and therapeutic management. Experience with 16 patients]. Rev Med Interne 1998;19(12):878-84.
[39] Lambert M, Hatron PY, Hachulla E, Warembourg H, Devulder B. Takayasu's arteritis diagnosed at the early systemic phase: diagnosis with noninvasive investigation despite normal findings on angiography. J Rheumatol 1998;25(2):376-7.
[40] Czernin J, Benz MR, Allen-Auerbach MS. PET/CT imaging: The incremental value of assessing the glucose metabolic phenotype and the structure of cancers in a single examination. Eur J Radiol;73(3):470-80.
[41] Schelbert HR, Hoh CK, Royal HD, Brown M, Dahlbom MN, Dehdashti F, Wahl RL. Procedure guideline for tumor imaging using fluorine-18-FDG. Society of Nuclear Medicine. J Nucl Med 1998;39(7):1302-5.
[42] Bombardieri E, Aktolun C, Baum RP, Bishof-Delaloye A, Buscombe J, Chatal JF, Maffioli L, Moncayo R, Mortelmans L, Reske SN. FDG-PET: procedure guidelines for tumour imaging. Eur J Nucl Med Mol Imaging 2003;30(12):BP115-24.
[43] Andrews J, Al-Nahhas A, Pennell DJ, Hossain MS, Davies KA, Haskard DO, Mason JC. Non-invasive imaging in the diagnosis and management of Takayasu's arteritis. Ann Rheum Dis 2004;63(8):995-1000.
[44] Webb M, Chambers A, A AL-N, Mason JC, Maudlin L, Rahman L, Frank J. The role of 18F-FDG PET in characterising disease activity in Takayasu arteritis. Eur J Nucl Med Mol Imaging 2004;31(5):627-34.
[45] Bleeker-Rovers CP, Bredie SJ, van der Meer JW, Corstens FH, Oyen WJ. F-18-fluorodeoxyglucose positron emission tomography in diagnosis and follow-up of patients with different types of vasculitis. Neth J Med 2003;61(10):323-9.
[46] Brodmann M, Lipp RW, Passath A, Seinost G, Pabst E, Pilger E. The role of 2-18F-fluoro-2-deoxy-D-glucose positron emission tomography in the diagnosis of giant cell arteritis of the temporal arteries. Rheumatology (Oxford) 2004;43(2):241-2.
[47] Moosig F, Czech N, Mehl C, Henze E, Zeuner RA, Kneba M, Schroder JO. Correlation between 18-fluorodeoxyglucose accumulation in large vessels and serological markers of inflammation in polymyalgia rheumatica: a quantitative PET study. Ann Rheum Dis 2004;63(7):870-3.
[48] Meller J, Strutz F, Siefker U, Scheel A, Sahlmann CO, Lehmann K, Conrad M, Vosshenrich R. Early diagnosis and follow-up of aortitis with [(18)F]FDG PET and MRI. Eur J Nucl Med Mol Imaging 2003;30(5):730-6.

[49] Walter MA, Melzer RA, Schindler C, Muller-Brand J, Tyndall A, Nitzsche EU. The value of [18F]FDG-PET in the diagnosis of large-vessel vasculitis and the assessment of activity and extent of disease. Eur J Nucl Med Mol Imaging 2005;32(6):674-81.
[50] Kobayashi Y, Ishii K, Oda K, Nariai T, Tanaka Y, Ishiwata K, Numano F. Aortic wall inflammation due to Takayasu arteritis imaged with 18F-FDG PET coregistered with enhanced CT. J Nucl Med 2005;46(6):917-22.
[51] Blockmans D, Stroobants S, Maes A, Mortelmans L. Positron emission tomography in giant cell arteritis and polymyalgia rheumatica: evidence for inflammation of the aortic arch. Am J Med 2000;108(3):246-9.
[52] Meller J, Grabbe E, Becker W, Vosshenrich R. Value of F-18 FDG hybrid camera PET and MRI in early takayasu aortitis. Eur Radiol 2003;13(2):400-5.
[53] Scheel AK, Meller J, Vosshenrich R, Kohlhoff E, Siefker U, Muller GA, Strutz F. Diagnosis and follow up of aortitis in the elderly. Ann Rheum Dis 2004;63(11):1507-10.
[54] Kroger K, Antoch G, Goyen M, Freudenberg LS, Veit P, Janicke I, Bockisch A, Forsting M. Positron emission tomography/computed tomography improves diagnostics of inflammatory arteritis. Heart Vessels 2005;20(4):179-83.
[55] Antoch G, Freudenberg LS, Debatin JF, Kroger K. Images in vascular medicine. Diagnosis of giant cell arteritis with PET/CT. Vasc Med 2003;8(4):281-2.
[56] Rudd JH, Warburton EA, Fryer TD, Jones HA, Clark JC, Antoun N, Johnstrom P, Davenport AP, Kirkpatrick PJ, Arch BN and others. Imaging atherosclerotic plaque inflammation with [18F]-fluorodeoxyglucose positron emission tomography. Circulation 2002;105(23):2708-11.
[57] Yun M, Jang S, Cucchiara A, Newberg AB, Alavi A. 18F FDG uptake in the large arteries: a correlation study with the atherogenic risk factors. Semin Nucl Med 2002;32(1):70-6.
[58] Yun M, Yeh D, Araujo LI, Jang S, Newberg A, Alavi A. F-18 FDG uptake in the large arteries: a new observation. Clin Nucl Med 2001;26(4):314-9.
[59] Kerr GS, Hallahan CW, Giordano J, Leavitt RY, Fauci AS, Rottem M, Hoffman GS. Takayasu arteritis. Ann Intern Med 1994;120(11):919-29.
[60] Sachelarie I, Kerr K, Ghesani M, Blum RH. Integrated PET-CT: evidence-based review of oncology indications. Oncology (Williston Park) 2005;19(4):481-90; discussion 490-2, 495-6.
[61] Macapinlac HA. FDG PET and PET/CT imaging in lymphoma and melanoma. Cancer J 2004;10(4):262-70.
[62] Frank SJ, Chao KS, Schwartz DL, Weber RS, Apisarnthanarax S, Macapinlac HA. Technology insight: PET and PET/CT in head and neck tumor staging and radiation therapy planning. Nat Clin Pract Oncol 2005;2(10):526-33.
[63] Blockmans D, Maes A, Stroobants S, Nuyts J, Bormans G, Knockaert D, Bobbaers H, Mortelmans L. New arguments for a vasculitic nature of polymyalgia rheumatica using positron emission tomography. Rheumatology (Oxford) 1999;38(5):444-7.
[64] Blockmans D, Baeyens H, Van Loon R, Lauwers G, Bobbaers H. Periaortitis and aortic dissection due to Wegener's granulomatosis. Clin Rheumatol 2000;19(2):161-4.
[65] Belhocine T, Kaye O, Delanaye P, Corman V, Baghaie M, Deprez M, Daenen F, De Barsy C, Beckers C, Gomez P and others. [Horton's disease and extra-temporal vessel

locations: role of 18FDG PET scan. Report of 3 cases and review of the literature]. Rev Med Interne 2002;23(7):584-91.

[66] Blockmans D, Ceuninck Ld, Vanderschueren S, Knockaert D, Mortelmans L, Bobbaers H. Repetitive 18F-fluorodeoxyglucose positron emission tomography in giant cell arteritis: A prospective study of 35 patients. Arthritis Care & Research 2006;55(1):131-137.

[67] Blockmans D, Coudyzer W, Vanderschueren S, Stroobants S, Loeckx D, Heye S, De Ceuninck L, Marchal G, Bobbaers H. Relationship between fluorodeoxyglucose uptake in the large vessels and late aortic diameter in giant cell arteritis. Rheumatology 2008;47(8):1179-1184.

[68] Both M, Ahmadi-Simab K, Reuter M, Dourvos O, Fritzer E, Ullrich S, Gross WL, Heller M, BÃ¤hre M. MRI and FDG-PET in the assessment of inflammatory aortic arch syndrome in complicated courses of giant cell arteritis. Annals of the Rheumatic Diseases 2008;67(7):1030-1033.

[69] Hautzel H, Sander O, Heinzel A, Schneider M, Muller H-W. Assessment of Large-Vessel Involvement in Giant Cell Arteritis with 18F-FDG PET: Introducing an ROC-Analysis-Based Cutoff Ratio. J Nucl Med 2008;49(7):1107-1113.

[70] Henes J, Müller M, Krieger J, Balletshofer B, Pfannenberg A, Kanz L, Kötter I. [18F] FDG-PET/CT as a new and sensitive imaging method for the diagnosis of large-vessel vasculitis. Clinical and experimental rheumatology 2008;26(3).

[71] Janssen SP, Comans EH, Voskuyl AE, Wisselink W, Smulders YM. Giant cell arteritis: Heterogeneity in clinical presentation and imaging results. Journal of Vascular Surgery 2008;48(4):1025-1031.

[72] Arnaud L, Haroche J, Malek Z, Archambaud F, Gambotti L, Grimon G, Kas A, Costedoat-Chalumeau N, Cacoub P, Toledano D and others. Is 18F-fluorodeoxyglucose positron emission tomography scanning a reliable way to assess disease activity in takayasu arteritis? Arthritis & Rheumatism 2009;60(4):1193-1200.

[73] Lee SG, Ryu JS, Kim HO, Oh JS, Kim YG, Lee CK, Yoo B. Evaluation of disease activity using F-18 FDG PET-CT in patients with Takayasu arteritis. Clinical nuclear medicine 2009;34(11):749.

[74] Vista EGS, Santos Estrella PV, Lichauco JJT. Flourine-18 flourodeoxyglucose Positron Emission Tomography as a non-invasive test of disease activity in Takayasu's arteritis -- A report of four cases. Autoimmunity Reviews 2010;9(7):503-506.

[75] Lehmann P, Buchtala S, Achajew N, Haerle P, Ehrenstein B, Lighvani H, Fleck M, Marienhagen J. 18F-FDG PET as a diagnostic procedure in large vessel vasculitis—a controlled, blinded re-examination of routine PET scans. Clinical Rheumatology 2011;30(1):37-42.[

Part 2

Advances in the Treatment of Vasculitis

4

Treatment of Different Types of Vasculitis

Hisayoshi Imanishi[1,3] and Daisuke Tsuruta[2,3]
[1]*The Department of Dermatology, Saiseikai Tondabayashi Hospital, Osaka,*
[2]*The Department of Dermatology, Kurume University School of Medicine, and Kurume Institute of Cutaneous Cell Biology, Fukuoka,*
[3]*The Department of Dermatology, Osaka City University Graduate School of Medicine, Osaka,*
Japan

1. Introduction

Vasculitis is classified by the size of the blood vessels affected by inflammatory reactions. In vasculitis of skin, many patients show obvious purpura and ulceration. Because many vasculitides can be noticed by these skin manifestations, dermatologists should be well informed about vasculitis. It is difficult to manage vasculitis after the diagnosis has been performed, and it is particularly difficult to treat systemic vasculitides, because they are potentially life threatening. The purpose of this chapter is to provide treatment guidelines for the primary vasculitic diseases.

2. Giant cell arteritis

Giant cell arteritis is an inflammation of medium- and large-sized arteries that characteristically affects one or more branches of the carotid artery, particularly the temporal artery (Salvarani C et al., 2002), but it is a systemic disease that can affect arteries in multiple locations, particularly the aorta and its main branches. Polymyalgia rheumatica, which is characterized by stiffness, aching, and pain in the muscles of the neck, shoulders, lower back, hips, and thighs, can occur with giant cell arteritis (Langford CA, 2010).

It is very important for patients who are strongly suspected of having giant cell arteritis to be treated immediately in order to protect their vision. When patients show ischemic symptoms, treatment should be started before checking the results of a temporal artery biopsy. A temporal artery biopsy after treatment has begun is exceedingly useful for making a diagnosis (Langford CA, 2010).

The aim of treatment is to improve the symptoms such as headache, jaw claudication, tenderness of scalp, and polymyalgia rheumatica and to prevent complications occurring as a result of vascular occlusion causing tissue infarction.

Glucocorticoids rapidly improve cranial and systemic symptoms and prevent visual complications in patients with giant cell arteritis rapidly. Aiello et al. reported that the probability of loss of vision developing after initiating oral glucocorticoid treatment was determined to be 1% (Aiello PD et al., 1993). The initial dose of prednisone is usually 40 to 60 mg/day (Langford CA, 2010), but the other report has stated that a dose under

40 mg/day is effective in more than 90% of patients (Hashimoto et al., 1999). After an initial dose of 60 mg/day, the dose can usually be decreased to 50 mg/day after 2 weeks and to 40 mg/day after 4 weeks (Langford CA, 2010). After clinical symptoms and laboratory data improve, the dose of prednisone was decreased by approximately 10% of the total daily dose every 1 to 2 weeks (Salvarani C et al., 2002).

Patients with recent or impending visual loss may be treated with initial pulsed intravenous doses of methylprednisolone (1,000 mg every day for three days) (Salvarani C et al., 2002). Corticosteroids may prevent but usually do not reverse visual loss.

Polymyalgia rheumatica can occur in 40% to 60% of patients with giant cell arteritis as a complication. Treatment with 10 to 20 mg/day prednisone can be effective in isolated polymyalgia rheumatica.

If the treatment does not result in improvement of symptoms, giant cell arteritis is suggested as an underlying disease (Langford CA, 2010).

To reduce significant steroid side effects or relapse on tapering the steroid dose, methotrexate is often added to the steroid (Hoffman GS et al., 2002; Jover JA et al., 2001; Mahr AD et al., 2007). A dose of 81 mg/day of aspirin has been reported to decrease the risk of cranial ischemic complications and all patients without a contraindication should be treated by aspirin together with prednisone (Lee MS et al., 2006; Nesher G et al., 2004).

Other drugs, such as cyclophosphamide, azathioprine, and etanercept, have been applied with variable success, although the success rates were generally less than hoped for success.

3. Takayasu arteritis

Takayasu arteritis, which has also been known as the *aortic arch syndrome*, is an inflammatory and stenotic disease of medium- and large-sized arteries characterized by a strong predilection for the aortic arch and its branches (Langford CA & Fauci AS, 2008).

For the first 1 to 3 months, patients are treated with 1 mg/kg/day prednisone as an initial dose. After that, the dose is tapered to withdrawal over a 6- to 12-month period (Langford CA, 2010).

If the disease activity persists in spite of treatment with glucocorticoids or the dose of glucocorticoids cannot be tapered, cytotoxic therapy is primarily administrated (Langford CA, 2010). Doses of 15 to 25 mg/week methotrexate in combination with glucocorticoids may induce remission and minimize glucocorticoid therapy and toxicity in most of these patients (Hoffman GS et al., 1994). Azathioprine is used for the patients who are steroid-resistant or have severe side effects by glucocorticoids. Cyclophosphamide has been used in patients with Takayasu arteritis refractory to glucocorticoids (Shelhamer JH et al., 1985). In the patients with intractable Takayasu arteritis, anti-TNF therapy may lead to durable remission in a majority of patients and facilitate dose reduction or discontinuation of prednisone and other immunosuppressive therapy (Molloy ES et al., 2008).

Vascular reconstructive surgery or angioplasty are adjunctive therapeautic options in some patients (Gota CE & Mandell BF, 2008).

4. Polyarteritis nodosa

Polyarteritis nodosa constitutes a necrotizing inflammation of medium-sized or small arteries (Cox NH et al., 2010; Jennette JC et al., 1994). Polyarteritis nodosa does not show

glomerulonephritis or vasculitis in arterioles, capillaries or venules (Cox NH et al., 2010). Affected patients may have several signs and symptons involving multiple organ systems (Cox NH et al., 2010). Ischaemia, infarcts and haemorrhage result from the vasculitis and lead to end-organ damage in patient with polyarteritis nodosa (Cox NH et al., 2010).
Therapy for polyarteritis nodosa is still somewhat empiric. If patients have critical organ involvement, such as renal insufficiency, gastrointestinal ischemia, cardiomyopathy, dense peripheral neuropathy, or central nervous system involvement, they should be treated with 2 mg/kg/day cyclophosphamide and glucocorticoids (Gayraud M et al., 2001). In patients who do not have immediate critical organ involvement, glucocorticoids alone may be sufficient therapy. Patients who cannot taper glucocorticoids and are unresponsive to other therapy may be treated by cyclophosphamide with glucocorticoids (Langford CA, 2010).
In patients whose disease is strongly suspected to be caused by streptococcal infection and repeat recurrence, penicillin antibiotics may be given as preventive treatment. But it has not been reported that penicillin antibiotics alone are effective and the efficacy of this therapy has not been proved in randomized trials (Katsuoka K et al., 2008).
Nonsteroidal anti-inflammatory drugs may be administratered to polyarteritis nodosa patients with little or no evidence of systemic disease (Katsuoka K et al., 2008).
Vasodilator and antithrombotic agents may be used together with other drugs and have been especially promoted to be used in patients with skin ulcers and necrosis (Choi SW et al., 2006; Gonzalez-Fernandez MA & Garcia-Consuegra J, 2007; Lim MJ et al., 2006; Zulian F et al., 2004; Zulian F et al., 1998).
Dapsone and colchicines may be given to patients who are refractory to other therapy (Guillevin L, 1986; Thompson DM et al., 1976; Vignes S et al., 2005).
When active hepatitis B or C infection is present, an antiviral agent should be part of the treatment regimen, with the goal of containing viral replication and cause seroconversion (Langford CA, 2010).
Glucocorticoids, alone or combined with cyclophosphamide, might be given to patients in combination with apheresis (Guillevin L et al., 2005).
The possibility of drug-induced polyarteritis nodosa syndromes should always be considered. Propylthiouracil, hydralazine, leukotriene inhibitors, sulfasalazine, minocycline, D-penicillamine, ciprofloxacin, phenytoin, and allopurinol are included among the drugs that may cause these symptoms (Gota CE & Mandell BF, 2008).

5. Wegener granulomatosis

Wegener granulomatosis is a relatively uncommon, potentially lethal, and multisystem disease characterized by clinical disease involving the upper and lower respiratory tracts and kidneys with histological evidence of granulomatous inflammation, vasculitis of the small- to medium-sized vessels, and a pauci-immune glomerulonephritis (Hoffman GS et al., 1992).
Active Wegener granulomatosis is potentially life-threatening, therefore glucocorticoids combined with a cytotoxic agent are required as initial treatment. Patients with active severe Wegener granulomatosis should initially be treated with 2 mg/kg/day cyclophosphamide and simultaneously with prednisone at 1 mg/kg/day (Langford CA, 2010). After 4 weeks of

treatment, the prednisone is tapered and withdrawn by 6 to 12 months, if the treatment improves the patient's condition. Cyclophosphamide treatment for 3 to 6 months is performed, and then, cyclophosphamide is discontinued and the treatment is switched to a less toxic medication for remission maintenance (Langford CA, 2010). If patients have active but non-severe disease, the treatment by prednisone together with 20 to 25 mg/week methotrexate is effective at inducing and then maintaining remission (De Groot K et al., 2005).

It has been reported that the withdrawal of cyclophosphamide and the substitution of azathioprine after remission did not increase the rate of relapse (Jayne D et al., 2003).

Treatment with trimethoprim–sulfamethoxazole (co-trimoxazole) reduces the incidence of relapse in patients with Wegener's granulomatosis in remission (Stegeman CA et al., 1996).

Plasma exchange increased the rate of renal recovery in patients that presented with renal failure (Jayne DR et al., 2007).

6. Microscopic polyangiitis

Microscopic polyangiitis was originally considered to be a branch of polyarteritis nodosa; it includes glomerulonephritis and occasionally pulmonary hemorrhage. According to the Chapel Hill Consensus Conference in 1994, the definition of primary systemic vasculitis (PSV) has become clear, and the disease group included microscopic polyangiitis. Microscopic polyangiitis is a systemic necrotizing vasculitis affecting the small blood vessels or small- to medium-sized arteries.

2 mg/kg/day cyclophosphamide and 1 mg/kg/day prednisone should be given as initial therapy to patients who have life-threatening disease including lung, kidney, and nerve involvement (Langford CA, 2010). The therapy follows the schedule outlined for Wegener granulomatosis. It was reported that the combination therapy with cyclophosphamide and prednisone decreased the frequency of renal failure and recurrence (Hogan SL et al., 1996), and improved survival rates (Gayraud M et al., 2001). However, infectious events were strongly associated with the combination of corticosteroid and cyclophosphamide, and were more frequent in patients older than 65 years (Gayraud M et al., 2001). Moreover, cyclophosphamide increases the incidence rate of bladder cancer and induces gonadal failure dose-dependently. Therefore the remission induction should be followed by azathioprine or methotrexate administration for remission maintenance. Patients with active non-severe disease may be treated with methotrexate for remission and maintenance.

Mychophenolate mofetil (Villiger PM & Guillevin L, 2010), rituximab (Villiger PM & Guillevin L, 2010), trimethoprim-sulfamethoxazole (Jennette JC et al., 2001), plasma exchanges (Villiger PM & Guillevin L, 2010), intravenous immunoglobulins (Villiger PM & Guillevin L, 2010) can also be effective in microscopic polyangiitis, and etanercept has been recommended as well (Keogh KA et al., 2005).

7. Churg-strauss syndrome

Churg-Strauss syndrome is a rare systemic necrotizing vasculitis of small- to medium-sized vessels that was first described in the early 1950s. In patients with late-onset asthma it is characterized by vasculitic manifestations, such as fever, cutaneous purpura and mononeuritis multiplex (Pagnoux C, 2010). In ANCA-associated vasculitides, the prognosis of Churg-Strauss syndrome is better than those of Wegener granulomatosis and microscopic polyangiitis (Guillevin L et al., 1999; Keogh KA & Specks U, 2006).

Systemic administration of steroids is effective in Churg-Strauss syndrome, and many cases show remission by this therapy. Patients are treated by administration of 1 intravenous pulse of methylprednisolone (15 mg/kg) at the start of treatment (Ribi C et al., 2008). Oral prednisone (1 mg/kg/day) is given to patients for 3 weeks. After that, the dose is tapered slowly as the symptoms and laboratory data, especially the eosinophil count, are improving.

Cases that are steroid-resistant or relapse repeatedly by steroid treatment alone are additionally given 2 mg/kg/day cyclophosphamide or 50 to 100 mg/day azathioprine (Gayraud M et al., 2001). However, cyclophosphamide with glucocorticoids should be given early to patients with life-threatening disease (Gayraud M et al., 1997; Guillevin L et al., 1999; Guillevin L & Pagnoux C, 2003; Keogh KA & Specks U, 2006; Noth I et al., 2003; Solans R et al., 2001). To decrease the side effect of cyclophosphamide, cyclophosphamide pulse therapy is recommended (Cohen P et al., 2007; Gayraud M et al., 1997; Guillevin L & Pagnoux C, 2003).

8. Cutaneous vasculitis

Cutaneous vasculitis is a frequent and often significant component of many systemic vasculitic syndromes such as lupus or rheumatoid vasculitis and ANCA-associated primary vasculitic syndromes (Carlson JA et al., 2006). It is manifested as urticaria, purpura, hemorrhagic vesicles, ulcers, nodules, livedo, infarcts, or digital gangrene. In most instances, cutaneous vasculitis shows the features of a self-limiting, single-episode phenomenon.

If the primary diseases or exposures are clarified, those are treated first.

If the patients have idiopathic cutaneous vasculitis, glucocorticoids are frequently used.

Other drugs, such a nonsteroidal anti-inflammatory agents, antihistamines, dapsone, hydroxychloroquine, colchicines, and cyclophosphamide, may also be given to the patients. But there is no optimal dosage schedule.

9. Cryoglobulinemic vasculitis

Cryoglobulins are cold-precipitable monoclonal or polyclonal immunoglobulins in serum. In the majority of cases of cryoglobulinaemia, the disease remains asymptomatic but immune complexes can form and be deposited in tissues, causing cryoglobulinemic vasculitis (Braun GS et al., 2007; Lamprecht P et al., 1999).

Asymptomatic cryoglobulinemia does not need to be treated. In symptomatic cryoglobulinemia, the treatment of the underlying disease can then proceed. If the underlying disease cannot be determined, it is idiopathic and symptomatic treatment is performed. It is important to determine the particular type of cryoglobulinemia, because the underlying disease may be associated with a particular type.

Because type I cryoglobulins usually are associated with haematological disorders, these disorders are treated preferentially.

Types II and III (mixed) cryoglobulinemias have strong connection with HCV infection (Braun GS et al., 2007). Aggressive antiviral therapy with Peg-IFNα and ribavirin provide

the best opportunity for improvement of HCV-associated cryoglobulinemic vasculitis (Langford CA, 2010; Saadoun D et al., 2008).
Plasmapheresis is performed together with administration of corticosteroids and immunosuppressive drugs in order to prevent production of abnormal protein or to treat primary disease. But it is impractical for long-term treatment (Langford CA, 2010; Siami GA & Siami FS, 1999).
Rituximab, a chimeric monoclonal anti-CD20 antibody, is suitable as a rescue therapy in resistant cryoglobulinemia associated with HCV (Ahmed MS & Wong CF, 2007). Immunosuppressive agents are typically applied in patients with severe disease symptoms such as membranoproliferative glomerulonephritis, severe peripheral or central nervous system neuropathy, severe cutaneous disease, and vasculitis involving vital organs such as the heart or gastrointestinal tract (Vassilopoulos D & Calabrese LH, 2002). Immunosuppressive agents such as cyclophosphamide, azathioprine, cyclosporine, melphalan, chlorambucil, and fludarabine are usually used together with corticosteroids (Vassilopoulos D & Calabrese LH, 2002).

10. Henoch-schönlein purpura

Henoch-Schönlein purpura is an acute, self-limited, systemic, small-vessel vasculitis. It predominantly affects children. Clinical presentation of Henoch-Schönlein purpura nephritis in adults is severe and the prognosis is relatively poor, worse than in children (Blanco R et al., 1997; Narchi H, 2005; Pillebout E et al., 2002). Therefore, more active treatment and careful follow up are needed in adults.
The treatment is not required in many cases of Henoch-Schönlein purpura because Henoch-Schönlein purpura is typically characterized by its self-limiting condition (Langford CA, 2010). Treatment with systemic application of glucocorticoids to patients with severe gastrointestinal symptoms is strongly recommended (Gunasekaran TS et al., 2000; Leung SP, 2001; Reinehr T et al., 2000; Ronkainen J et al., 2006). Prednisone does not prevent the development of renal symptoms but treats them effectively (Ronkainen J et al. reported that renal symptoms resolved in 61% of the prednisone-treated patients 80-100 mg/kg/day, compared with 34% of the placebo-receiving patients) (Ronkainen J et al., 2006). Moreover, methylprednisolone pulse therapy is effective in patients at risk of progression of nephropathy, particularly in the cases that started therapy early during the course of the disease before the crescents became fibrous (Niaudet P & Habib R, 1998).
The efficacy of immunosuppressive agents (e.g. cyclophosphamide, cyclosporin A), plasmapheresis, anticoagulant agents and antiplatelet agents is controversial.
Glucocorticoids in combination with each of these treatments can be effective in patients with severe nephritis (Flynn JT et al., 2001; Hattori M et al., 1999; Kawasaki Y et al., 2004; Ronkainen J et al., 2003; Scharer K et al., 1999; Someya T et al., 2004; Tanaka H et al., 2003; Tarshish P et al., 2004; Wyatt RJ & Hogg RJ, 2001; Zaffanello M et al., 2007).
Administration of Factor XIII, tonsillectomy, and dapsone may be useful for the patients with Henoch-Schönlein purpura, but the evidence concerning efficacy is insufficient. Factor XIII concentrate may contribute to abdominal pain relief in Henoch-Schönlein purpura patients (Shimomura N et al., 2005; Utani A et al., 1991).
Tonsillectomy may be useful for alleviating Henoch-Schönlein purpura nephropathy(Hotta O et al., 1996; Inoue CN et al., 2007; Sugiyama H et al., 2005; Tomioka S et al., 1996).

Dapsone therapy may be useful for improving purpura and arthritis (Hoffbrand BI, 1991; Iqbal H & Evans A, 2005; Ramelli GP & Bianchetti MG, 1997; Sarma PS, 1994; Shimomura N et al., 2005).

11. Kawasaki disease

Kawasaki disease is an acute multisystem vasculitis of infants and young children. This disease represents the primary cause of acquired heart disease(Barron KS et al., 1999).

For patients in the acute stage of the disease, a single high-dose intravenous immunoglobulin (2 g/kg) in combination with high-dose aspirin (80-100 mg/kg/day) is given (Muta H et al., 2004; Rowley AH & Shulman ST, 2010; Terai M & Shulman ST, 1997). However, patients in Asia are often treated with 80-100 mg/kg/day, because it is believed that 80-100 mg/kg/day of aspirin is excessively toxic in Asian children (Rowley AH & Shulman ST, 2010). Whether it is an advantage to add corticosteroid to this combination therapy is controversial (Inoue Y et al., 2006; Jibiki T et al., 2004; Newburger JW et al., 2007).

About 5-15% of Kawasaki disease patients do not respond to this therapy. A second 2 g/kg dose of intravenous immunoglobulin and a 3-day course of intravenous pulsed methylprednisolone (30 mg/kg/day) can be effective in nonresponders (Freeman AF & Shulman ST, 2004; Rowley AH & Shulman ST, 2010; Sundel RP et al., 1993).

Administration of infliximab to these patients has been reported, but the efficacy is unclear (Burns JC et al., 2008; Burns JC et al., 2005).

Low-dose aspirin (3-5 mg/kg/day) is given to the patients after the acute stage (Rowley AH & Shulman ST, 2010). In order to check the development of coronary aneurysms, an echocardiogram should be performed at 2, 6, and 8 weeks after illness onset (Langford CA, 2010). Close follow-up using ultrasonographic monitoring is needed for the patients with multiple aneurysms, giant aneurysms, or coronary artery obstruction.

12. Behçet disease

Behçet disease is a multisystem inflammatory disease with an unknown etiology that affects all types and sizes of blood vessels (Calamia KT & Kaklamanis PG, 2008; Langford CA, 2010; Yazici Y et al., 2010). Treatment of Behçet disease is adjusted depending on the type and severity of symptoms, sex, and age (Yazici Y et al., 2010).

Colchicine, 1.0-2.0 mg/day, can be effective for genital ulcers, erythema nodosum, and arthritis among women, although merely for arthritis in men (Yurdakul S et al., 2001).

Azathioprine, 2.5 mg/kg/day, is able to prevent the progression of Behçet disease, particularly the eye disease (Yazici H et al., 1990).

Cyclosporine is useful in treating ocular manifestations, oral aphthous ulcer, dermal lesions, and genital ulceration (Masuda K et al., 1989). Thalidomide, 100 mg/day, is effective for the oral and genital ulcers and papulopustular lesions (Hamuryudan V et al., 1998).

Interferon alpha-2a improves the duration and pain of oral ulcers and the frequency of genital ulcers and papulopustular lesions (Alpsoy E et al., 2002).

It was reported that tumor necrosis factor α (TNF α) antagonists, which are infliximab, etanercept, and adalimumab, improve symptoms in patients with eye, mucocutaneous, and gastrointestinal involvement, as well as neurological disease, and even pulmonary artery aneurysms (Sfikakis PP et al., 2007).

Corticosteroids are widely used in the treatment of Behçet disease (Yazici Y et al., 2010).

Topical therapy, including glucocorticoids and sucralfate suspension, can be effective for aphthous lesions and mucocutaneous disease (Alpsoy E et al., 1999; Hatemi G et al., 2009). For patients in the early disease stages of pulmonary and peripheral arterial aneurysms, cyclophosphamide pulse therapy and corticosteroids are especially effective (Yazici Y et al., 2010).

13. Acknowledgment

We thank for Dr. Koichi Nakagawa, MD, Dr. Yasuhiko Yoshida, MD, Dr. Masaru Kishida, MD, Dr. Aya Kumei, MD, Dr. Takashi Hashimoto, MD, Dr. Hiromi Kobayashi, MD, PhD, and Dr. Masamitsu Ishii, MD, PhD for helping with the preparation of the paper.

14. References

Ahmed, M.S. & Wong, C.F. (2007) Should rituximab be the rescue therapy for refractory mixed cryoglobulinemia associated with hepatitis C? *J Nephrol*, Vol. 20, No. 3, pp. 350-356, ISSN 1121-8428

Aiello, P.D., Trautmann, J.C., McPhee, T.J., Kunselman, A.R. & Hunder, G.G. (1993) Visual prognosis in giant cell arteritis. *Ophthalmology*, Vol. 100, No. 4, pp. 550-555, ISSN 0161-6420

Alpsoy, E., Durusoy, C., Yilmaz, E., Ozgurel, Y., Ermis, O., Yazar, S. & Basaran, E. (2002) Interferon alfa-2a in the treatment of Behcet disease: a randomized placebo-controlled and double-blind study. *Arch Dermatol*, Vol. 138, No. 4, pp. 467-471, ISSN 0003-987X

Alpsoy, E., Er, H., Durusoy, C. & Yilmaz, E. (1999) The use of sucralfate suspension in the treatment of oral and genital ulceration of Behcet disease: a randomized, placebo-controlled, double-blind study. *Arch Dermatol*, Vol. 135, No. 5, pp. 529-532, ISSN 0003-987X

Barron, K.S., Shulman, S.T., Rowley, A., Taubert, K., Myones, B.L., Meissner, H.C., Peters, J., Duffy, C.E., Silverman, E. & Sundel, R. (1999) Report of the National Institutes of Health Workshop on Kawasaki Disease. *J Rheumatol*, Vol. 26, No. 1, pp. 170-190, ISSN 0315-162X

Blanco, R., Martinez-Taboada, V.M., Rodriguez-Valverde, V., Garcia-Fuentes, M. & Gonzalez-Gay, M.A. (1997) Henoch-Schonlein purpura in adulthood and childhood: two different expressions of the same syndrome. *Arthritis Rheum*, Vol. 40, No. 5, pp. 859-864, ISSN 0004-3591

Braun, G.S., Horster, S., Wagner, K.S., Ihrler, S. & Schmid, H. (2007) Cryoglobulinaemic vasculitis: classification and clinical and therapeutic aspects. *Postgrad Med J*, Vol. 83, No. 976, pp. 87-94, ISSN 1469-0756

Burns, J.C., Best, B.M., Mejias, A., Mahony, L., Fixler, D.E., Jafri, H.S., Melish, M.E., Jackson, M.A., Asmar, B.I., Lang, D.J., Connor, J.D., Capparelli, E.V., Keen, M.L., Mamun, K., Keenan, G.F. & Ramilo, O. (2008) Infliximab treatment of intravenous immunoglobulin-resistant Kawasaki disease. *J Pediatr*, Vol. 153, No. 6, pp. 833-838, ISSN 1097-6833

Burns, J.C., Mason, W.H., Hauger, S.B., Janai, H., Bastian, J.F., Wohrley, J.D., Balfour, I., Shen, C.A., Michel, E.D., Shulman, S.T. & Melish, M.E. (2005) Infliximab treatment for refractory Kawasaki syndrome. *J Pediatr*, Vol. 146, No. 5, pp. 662-667, ISSN 0022-3476

Calamia, K.T. & Kaklamanis, P.G. (2008) Behcet's disease: recent advances in early diagnosis and effective treatment. *Curr Rheumatol Rep*, Vol. 10, No. 5, pp. 349-355, ISSN 1534-6307

Carlson, J.A., Cavaliere, L.F. & Grant-Kels, J.M. (2006) Cutaneous vasculitis: diagnosis and management. *Clin Dermatol*, Vol. 24, No. 5, pp. 414-429, ISSN 0738-081X

Choi, S.W., Lew, S., Cho, S.D., Cha, H.J., Eum, E.A., Jung, H.C. & Park, J.H. (2006) Cutaneous polyarteritis nodosa presented with digital gangrene: a case report. *J Korean Med Sci*, Vol. 21, No. 2, pp. 371-373, ISSN 1011-8934

Cohen, P., Pagnoux, C., Mahr, A., Arene, J.P., Mouthon, L., Le Guern, V., Andre, M.H., Gayraud, M., Jayne, D., Blockmans, D., Cordier, J.F. & Guillevin, L. (2007) Churg-Strauss syndrome with poor-prognosis factors: A prospective multicenter trial comparing glucocorticoids and six or twelve cyclophosphamide pulses in forty-eight patients. *Arthritis Rheum*, Vol. 57, No. 4, pp. 686-693, ISSN 0004-3591

Cox, N.H., Jorizzo, J.L., Bourke, J.F., Savage, C.O.S. (2010) Vasculitis, Neutrophilic Dermatoses and Related Disrders. In: *Rook's Textbook of Dermatology*, Tony Burns, Stephan Breathnach, Neil Cox, Christopher Griffiths, pp. 50. 1, Blackwell Publishing, ISBN 9781405161695, New Jersey

De Groot, K., Rasmussen, N., Bacon, P.A., Tervaert, J.W., Feighery, C., Gregorini, G., Gross, W.L., Luqmani, R. & Jayne, D.R. (2005) Randomized trial of cyclophosphamide versus methotrexate for induction of remission in early systemic antineutrophil cytoplasmic antibody-associated vasculitis. *Arthritis Rheum*, Vol. 52, No. 8, pp. 2461-2469, ISSN 0004-3591

Flynn, J.T., Smoyer, W.E., Bunchman, T.E., Kershaw, D.B. & Sedman, A.B. (2001) Treatment of Henoch-Schonlein Purpura glomerulonephritis in children with high-dose corticosteroids plus oral cyclophosphamide. *Am J Nephrol*, Vol. 21, No. 2, pp. 128-133, 0250-8095

Freeman, A.F. & Shulman, S.T. (2004) Refractory Kawasaki disease. *Pediatr Infect Dis J*, Vol. 23, No. 5, pp. 463-464, ISSN 0891-3668

Gayraud, M., Guillevin, L., Cohen, P., Lhote, F., Cacoub, P., Deblois, P., Godeau, B., Ruel, M., Vidal, E., Piontud, M., Ducroix, J.P., Lassoued, S., Christoforov, B. & Babinet, P. (1997) Treatment of good-prognosis polyarteritis nodosa and Churg-Strauss syndrome: comparison of steroids and oral or pulse cyclophosphamide in 25 patients. French Cooperative Study Group for Vasculitides. *Br J Rheumatol*, Vol. 36, No. 12, pp. 1290-1297, ISSN 0263-7103

Gayraud, M., Guillevin, L., le Toumelin, P., Cohen, P., Lhote, F., Casassus, P. & Jarrousse, B. (2001) Long-term followup of polyarteritis nodosa, microscopic polyangiitis, and Churg-Strauss syndrome: analysis of four prospective trials including 278 patients. *Arthritis Rheum*, Vol. 44, No. 3, pp. 666-675, ISSN 0004-3591

Gonzalez-Fernandez, M.A. & Garcia-Consuegra, J. (2007) Polyarteritis nodosa resistant to conventional treatment in a pediatric patient. *Ann Pharmacother*, Vol. 41, No. 5, pp. 885-890, ISSN 1542-6270

Gota, C.E. & Mandell, B.F. (2008) Systemic Necrotizing Vasculitis. In: *Fitzpatrick's Dermatology in General Medicine* (Wolff K., Goldsmith L., Katz S. I., Gilchrest B. A., S.Paller A. & Leffell D. J.), (Ed), Vol. 2, pp. 1606-1616. McGraw-Hill, New York.

Guillevin, L. (1986) Treatment of polyarteritis nodosa with dapsone. *Scand J Rheumatol*, Vol. 15, No. 1, pp. 95-96, ISSN 0300-9742

Guillevin, L., Cohen, P., Gayraud, M., Lhote, F., Jarrousse, B. & Casassus, P. (1999) Churg-Strauss syndrome. Clinical study and long-term follow-up of 96 patients. *Medicine (Baltimore)*, Vol. 78, No. 1, pp. 26-37, ISSN 0025-7974

Guillevin, L., Mahr, A., Callard, P., Godmer, P., Pagnoux, C., Leray, E. & Cohen, P. (2005) Hepatitis B virus-associated polyarteritis nodosa: clinical characteristics, outcome, and impact of treatment in 115 patients. *Medicine (Baltimore)*, Vol. 84, No. 5, pp. 313-322, ISSN 0025-7974

Guillevin, L. & Pagnoux, C. (2003) When should immunosuppressants be prescribed to treat systemic vasculitides? *Intern Med*, Vol. 42, No. 4, pp. 313-317, ISSN 0918-2918

Gunasekaran, T.S., Berman, J. & Gonzalez, M. (2000) Duodenojejunitis: is it idiopathic or is it Henoch-Schonlein purpura without the purpura? *J Pediatr Gastroenterol Nutr*, Vol. 30, No. 1, pp. 22-28, ISSN 0277-2116

Hamuryudan, V., Mat, C., Saip, S., Ozyazgan, Y., Siva, A., Yurdakul, S., Zwingenberger, K. & Yazici, H. (1998) Thalidomide in the treatment of the mucocutaneous lesions of the Behcet syndrome. A randomized, double-blind, placebo-controlled trial. *Ann Intern Med*, Vol. 128, No. 6, pp. 443-450, ISSN 0003-4819

Hatemi, G., Silman, A., Bang, D., Bodaghi, B., Chamberlain, A.M., Gul, A., Houman, M.H., Kotter, I., Olivieri, I., Salvarani, C., Sfikakis, P.P., Siva, A., Stanford, M.R., Stubiger, N., Yurdakul, S. & Yazici, H. (2009) Management of Behcet disease: a systematic literature review for the European League Against Rheumatism evidence-based recommendations for the management of Behcet disease. *Ann Rheum Dis*, Vol. 68, No. 10, pp. 1528-1534, ISSN 1468-2060

Hattori, M., Ito, K., Konomoto, T., Kawaguchi, H., Yoshioka, T. & Khono, M. (1999) Plasmapheresis as the sole therapy for rapidly progressive Henoch-Schonlein purpura nephritis in children. *Am J Kidney Dis*, Vol. 33, No. 3, pp. 427-433, ISSN 0272-6386

Hoffbrand, B.I. (1991) Dapsone in Henoch-Schonlein purpura--worth a trial. *Postgrad Med J*, Vol. 67, No. 793, pp. 961-962, ISSN 0032-5473

Hoffman, G.S., Cid, M.C., Hellmann, D.B., Guillevin, L., Stone, J.H., Schousboe, J., Cohen, P., Calabrese, L.H., Dickler, H., Merkel, P.A., Fortin, P., Flynn, J.A., Locker, G.A., Easley, K.A., Schned, E., Hunder, G.G., Sneller, M.C., Tuggle, C., Swanson, H., Hernandez-Rodriguez, J., Lopez-Soto, A., Bork, D., Hoffman, D.B., Kalunian, K., Klashman, D., Wilke, W.S., Scheetz, R.J., Mandell, B.F., Fessler, B.J., Kosmorsky, G., Prayson, R., Luqmani, R.A., Nuki, G., McRorie, E., Sherrer, Y., Baca, S., Walsh, B., Ferland, D., Soubrier, M., Choi, H.K., Gross, W., Segal, A.M., Ludivico, C. & Puechal, X. (2002) A multicenter, randomized, double-blind, placebo-controlled trial of adjuvant methotrexate treatment for giant cell arteritis. *Arthritis Rheum*, Vol. 46, No. 5, pp. 1309-1318, ISSN 0004-3591

Hoffman, G.S., Kerr, G.S., Leavitt, R.Y., Hallahan, C.W., Lebovics, R.S., Travis, W.D., Rottem, M. & Fauci, A.S. (1992) Wegener granulomatosis: an analysis of 158 patients. *Ann Intern Med*, Vol. 116, No. 6, pp. 488-498, ISSN 0003-4819

Hoffman, G.S., Leavitt, R.Y., Kerr, G.S., Rottem, M., Sneller, M.C. & Fauci, A.S. (1994) Treatment of glucocorticoid-resistant or relapsing Takayasu arteritis with methotrexate. *Arthritis Rheum*, Vol. 37, No. 4, pp. 578-582, ISSN 0004-3591

Hogan, S.L., Nachman, P.H., Wilkman, A.S., Jennette, J.C. & Falk, R.J. (1996) Prognostic markers in patients with antineutrophil cytoplasmic autoantibody-associated microscopic polyangiitis and glomerulonephritis. *J Am Soc Nephrol*, Vol. 7, No. 1, pp. 23-32, ISSN 1046-6673

Hotta, O., Taguma, Y., Yoshizawa, N., Oda, T., Nishiyama, J., Yusa, N., Chiba, S., Horigome, I., Sudo, K. & Tomioka, S. (1996) Long-term effects of intensive therapy combined with tonsillectomy in patients with IgA nephropathy. *Acta Otolaryngol Suppl*, Vol. 523, No. pp. 165-168, ISSN 0365-5237

Inoue, C.N., Chiba, Y., Morimoto, T., Nishio, T., Kondo, Y., Adachi, M. & Matsutani, S. (2007) Tonsillectomy in the treatment of pediatric Henoch-Schonlein nephritis. *Clin Nephrol*, Vol. 67, No. 5, pp. 298-305, ISSN 0301-0430

Inoue, Y., Okada, Y., Shinohara, M., Kobayashi, T., Tomomasa, T., Takeuchi, K. & Morikawa, A. (2006) A multicenter prospective randomized trial of corticosteroids in primary therapy for Kawasaki disease: clinical course and coronary artery outcome. *J Pediatr*, Vol. 149, No. 3, pp. 336-341, ISSN 0022-3476

Iqbal, H. & Evans, A. (2005) Dapsone therapy for Henoch-Schonlein purpura: a case series. *Arch Dis Child*, Vol. 90, No. 9, pp. 985-986, ISSN 1468-2044

Jayne, D., Rasmussen, N., Andrassy, K., Bacon, P., Tervaert, J.W., Dadoniene, J., Ekstrand, A., Gaskin, G., Gregorini, G., de Groot, K., Gross, W., Hagen, E.C., Mirapeix, E., Pettersson, E., Siegert, C., Sinico, A., Tesar, V., Westman, K. & Pusey, C. (2003) A randomized trial of maintenance therapy for vasculitis associated with antineutrophil cytoplasmic autoantibodies. *N Engl J Med*, Vol. 349, No. 1, pp. 36-44, ISSN 1533-4406

Jayne, D.R., Gaskin, G., Rasmussen, N., Abramowicz, D., Ferrario, F., Guillevin, L., Mirapeix, E., Savage, C.O., Sinico, R.A., Stegeman, C.A., Westman, K.W., van der Woude, F.J., de Lind van Wijngaarden, R.A. & Pusey, C.D. (2007) Randomized trial of plasma exchange or high-dosage methylprednisolone as adjunctive therapy for severe renal vasculitis. *J Am Soc Nephrol*, Vol. 18, No. 7, pp. 2180-2188, ISSN 1046-6673

Jennette, J.C. Falk, R.J., Andrassy, K., Bacon, P. A., Churg, J., Gross, W. L., Hagen, E. C., Hoffman, G. S., Hunder, G. G., Kallenberg, C. G. (1994). Nomenclature of systemic vasculitides. Proposal of an international consensus conference, *Arthritis Rheum*, Vol. 37, No. 2, pp. 187-92, ISSN 0004-3591

Jennette, J.C., Thomas, D.B. & Falk, R.J. (2001) Microscopic polyangiitis (microscopic polyarteritis). *Semin Diagn Pathol*, Vol. 18, No. 1, pp. 3-13, ISSN 0740-2570

Jibiki, T., Terai, M., Kurosaki, T., Nakajima, H., Suzuki, K., Inomata, H., Terashima, I., Honda, T., Yasukawa, K., Hamada, H. & Kohno, Y. (2004) Efficacy of intravenous immune globulin therapy combined with dexamethasone for the initial treatment of acute Kawasaki disease. *Eur J Pediatr*, Vol. 163, No. 4-5, pp. 229-233, ISSN 0340-6199

Jover, J.A., Hernandez-Garcia, C., Morado, I.C., Vargas, E., Banares, A. & Fernandez-Gutierrez, B. (2001) Combined treatment of giant-cell arteritis with methotrexate and prednisone. a randomized, double-blind, placebo-controlled trial. *Ann Intern Med*, Vol. 134, No. 2, pp. 106-114, ISSN 0003-4819

Katsuoka, K., Kawakami, T., Ishiguro, N., Sawada, Y., Chen, K., Aiba, S., Kawana, S., Izaki, S., Furukawa, F., Masuzawa, M., Sato, S. & Morita, E. (2008) *The Japanese Journal of Dermatology*, Vol. 118, No. 11, pp. 2095-2187, ISSN 0021-499X.

Kawasaki, Y., Suzuki, J. & Suzuki, H. (2004) Efficacy of methylprednisolone and urokinase pulse therapy combined with or without cyclophosphamide in severe Henoch-Schoenlein nephritis: a clinical and histopathological study. *Nephrol Dial Transplant*, Vol. 19, No. 4, pp. 858-864, ISSN 0931-0509

Keogh, K.A. & Specks, U. (2006) Churg-Strauss syndrome. *Semin Respir Crit Care Med*, Vol. 27, No. 2, pp. 148-157, ISSN 1069-3424

Keogh, K.A., Wylam, M.E., Stone, J.H. & Specks, U. (2005) Induction of remission by B lymphocyte depletion in eleven patients with refractory antineutrophil cytoplasmic antibody-associated vasculitis. *Arthritis Rheum*, Vol. 52, No. 1, pp. 262-268, ISSN 0004-3591

Lamprecht, P., Gause, A. & Gross, W.L. (1999) Cryoglobulinemic vasculitis. *Arthritis Rheum*, Vol. 42, No. 12, pp. 2507-2516, ISSN 0004-3591

Langford, C.A. (2010) Vasculitis. *J Allergy Clin Immunol*, Vol. 125, No. 2 Suppl 2, pp. S216-225, ISSN 1097-6825

Langford, C.A. & Fauci, A.S. (2008) The Vasculitis Syndromes. In: *Harrison's PRINCIPLES OF INTERNAL MEDICINE Seventeenth Edition* (Fauci A. S., Braunwald E., Kasper D. L., Hauser S. L., Longo D. L., Jameson J. L. & Loscalzo J.), (Ed), Vol. 1, pp. 2119-2131. McGraw-Hill, New York.

Lee, M.S., Smith, S.D., Galor, A. & Hoffman, G.S. (2006) Antiplatelet and anticoagulant therapy in patients with giant cell arteritis. *Arthritis Rheum*, Vol. 54, No. 10, pp. 3306-3309, ISSN 0004-3591

Leung, S.P. (2001) Use of intravenous hydrocortisone in Henoch-Schonlein purpura. *J Paediatr Child Health*, Vol. 37, No. 3, pp. 309-310, ISSN 1034-4810

Lim, M.J., Kwon, S.R., Lee, S. & Park, W. (2006) Rapid improvement of distal vasculitis in PAN related to hepatitis B with alprostadil infusion: a case report. *Rheumatol Int*, Vol. 26, No. 10, pp. 928-932, ISSN 0172-8172

Mahr, A.D., Jover, J.A., Spiera, R.F., Hernandez-Garcia, C., Fernandez-Gutierrez, B., Lavalley, M.P. & Merkel, P.A. (2007) Adjunctive methotrexate for treatment of giant cell arteritis: an individual patient data meta-analysis. *Arthritis Rheum*, Vol. 56, No. 8, pp. 2789-2797, ISSN 0004-3591

Masuda, K., Nakajima, A., Urayama, A., Nakae, K., Kogure, M. & Inaba, G. (1989) Double-masked trial of cyclosporin versus colchicine and long-term open study of cyclosporin in Behcet's disease. *Lancet*, Vol. 1, No. 8647, pp. 1093-1096, ISSN 0140-6736

Molloy, E.S., Langford, C.A., Clark, T.M., Gota, C.E. & Hoffman, G.S. (2008) Anti-tumour necrosis factor therapy in patients with refractory Takayasu arteritis: long-term follow-up. *Ann Rheum Dis*, Vol. 67, No. 11, pp. 1567-1569, ISSN 1468-2060

Muta, H., Ishii, M., Egami, K., Furui, J., Sugahara, Y., Akagi, T., Nakamura, Y., Yanagawa, H. & Matsuishi, T. (2004) Early intravenous gamma-globulin treatment for Kawasaki disease: the nationwide surveys in Japan. *J Pediatr*, Vol. 144, No. 4, pp. 496-499, ISSN 0022-3476

Narchi, H. (2005) Risk of long term renal impairment and duration of follow up recommended for Henoch-Schonlein purpura with normal or minimal urinary findings: a systematic review. *Arch Dis Child*, Vol. 90, No. 9, pp. 916-920, ISSN 1468-2044

Nesher, G., Berkun, Y., Mates, M., Baras, M., Rubinow, A. & Sonnenblick, M. (2004) Low-dose aspirin and prevention of cranial ischemic complications in giant cell arteritis. *Arthritis Rheum*, Vol. 50, No. 4, pp. 1332-1337, ISSN 0004-3591

Newburger, J.W., Sleeper, L.A., McCrindle, B.W., Minich, L.L., Gersony, W., Vetter, V.L., Atz, A.M., Li, J.S., Takahashi, M., Baker, A.L., Colan, S.D., Mitchell, P.D., Klein, G.L. & Sundel, R.P. (2007) Randomized trial of pulsed corticosteroid therapy for primary treatment of Kawasaki disease. *N Engl J Med*, Vol. 356, No. 7, pp. 663-675, ISSN 1533-4406

Niaudet, P. & Habib, R. (1998) Methylprednisolone pulse therapy in the treatment of severe forms of Schonlein-Henoch purpura nephritis. *Pediatr Nephrol*, Vol. 12, No. 3, pp. 238-243, ISSN 0931-041X

Noth, I., Strek, M.E. & Leff, A.R. (2003) Churg-Strauss syndrome. *Lancet*, Vol. 361, No. 9357, pp. 587-594, ISSN 0140-6736

Pagnoux, C. (2010) Churg-Strauss syndrome: evolving concepts. *Discov Med*, Vol. 9, No. 46, pp. 243-252, ISSN 1944-7930

Pillebout, E., Thervet, E., Hill, G., Alberti, C., Vanhille, P. & Nochy, D. (2002) Henoch-Schonlein Purpura in adults: outcome and prognostic factors. *J Am Soc Nephrol*, Vol. 13, No. 5, pp. 1271-1278, ISSN 1046-6673

Ramelli, G.P. & Bianchetti, M.G. (1997) Dapsone in cutaneous Henoch-Schonlein syndrome--worth a trial. *Acta Paediatr*, Vol. 86, No. 3, pp. 337, ISSN 0803-5253

Reinehr, T., Burk, G. & Andler, W. (2000) Does steroid treatment of abdominal pain prevent renal involvement in Henoch-Schonlein purpura? *J Pediatr Gastroenterol Nutr*, Vol. 31, No. 3, pp. 323-324, ISSN 0277-2116

Ribi, C., Cohen, P., Pagnoux, C., Mahr, A., Arene, J.P., Lauque, D., Puechal, X., Letellier, P., Delaval, P., Cordier, J.F. & Guillevin, L. (2008) Treatment of Churg-Strauss syndrome without poor-prognosis factors: a multicenter, prospective, randomized, open-label study of seventy-two patients. *Arthritis Rheum*, Vol. 58, No. 2, pp. 586-594, ISSN 0004-3591

Ronkainen, J., Autio-Harmainen, H. & Nuutinen, M. (2003) Cyclosporin A for the treatment of severe Henoch-Schonlein glomerulonephritis. *Pediatr Nephrol*, Vol. 18, No. 11, pp. 1138-1142, ISSN 0931-041X

Ronkainen, J., Koskimies, O., Ala-Houhala, M., Antikainen, M., Merenmies, J., Rajantie, J., Ormala, T., Turtinen, J. & Nuutinen, M. (2006) Early prednisone therapy in Henoch-Schonlein purpura: a randomized, double-blind, placebo-controlled trial. *J Pediatr*, Vol. 149, No. 2, pp. 241-247, ISSN 0022-3476

Rowley, A.H. & Shulman, S.T. (2010) Pathogenesis and management of Kawasaki disease. *Expert Rev Anti Infect Ther*, Vol. 8, No. 2, pp. 197-203, ISSN 1744-8336

Saadoun, D., Delluc, A., Piette, J.C. & Cacoub, P. (2008) Treatment of hepatitis C-associated mixed cryoglobulinemia vasculitis. *Curr Opin Rheumatol*, Vol. 20, No. 1, pp. 23-28, ISSN 1040-8711

Salvarani, C., Cantini, F., Boiardi, L. & Hunder, G.G. (2002) Polymyalgia rheumatica and giant-cell arteritis. *N Engl J Med*, Vol. 347, No. 4, pp. 261-271, ISSN 1533-4406

Sarma, P.S. (1994) Dapsone in Henoch-Schonlein purpura. *Postgrad Med J*, Vol. 70, No. 824, pp. 464-465, ISSN 0032-5473

Scharer, K., Krmar, R., Querfeld, U., Ruder, H., Waldherr, R. & Schaefer, F. (1999) Clinical outcome of Schonlein-Henoch purpura nephritis in children. *Pediatr Nephrol*, Vol. 13, No. 9, pp. 816-823, ISSN 0931-041X

Sfikakis, P.P., Markomichelakis, N., Alpsoy, E., Assaad-Khalil, S., Bodaghi, B., Gul, A., Ohno, S., Pipitone, N., Schirmer, M., Stanford, M., Wechsler, B., Zouboulis, C., Kaklamanis, P. & Yazici, H. (2007) Anti-TNF therapy in the management of Behcet's disease--review and basis for recommendations. *Rheumatology (Oxford)*, Vol. 46, No. 5, pp. 736-741, ISSN 1462-0324

Shelhamer, J.H., Volkman, D.J., Parrillo, J.E., Lawley, T.J., Johnston, M.R. & Fauci, A.S. (1985) Takayasu's arteritis and its therapy. *Ann Intern Med*, Vol. 103, No. 1, pp. 121-126, ISSN 0003-4819

Shimomura, N., Kawai, K., Watanabe, S., Katsuumi, K. & Ito, M. (2005) Adult Henoch-Schonlein purpura with severe abdominal pain treated with dapsone and factor XIII concentrate. *J Dermatol*, Vol. 32, No. 2, pp. 124-127, ISSN 0385-2407

Siami, G.A. & Siami, F.S. (1999) Plasmapheresis and paraproteinemia: cryoprotein-induced diseases, monoclonal gammopathy, Waldenstrom's macroglobulinemia, hyperviscosity syndrome, multiple myeloma, light chain disease, and amyloidosis. *Ther Apher*, Vol. 3, No. 1, pp. 8-19, ISSN 1091-6660

Solans, R., Bosch, J.A., Perez-Bocanegra, C., Selva, A., Huguet, P., Alijotas, J., Orriols, R., Armadans, L. & Vilardell, M. (2001) Churg-Strauss syndrome: outcome and long-term follow-up of 32 patients. *Rheumatology (Oxford)*, Vol. 40, No. 7, pp. 763-771, ISSN 1462-0324

Someya, T., Kaneko, K., Fujinaga, S., Ohtaki, R., Hira, M. & Yamashiro, Y. (2004) Cyclosporine A for heavy proteinuria in a child with Henoch-Schonlein purpura nephritis. *Pediatr Int*, Vol. 46, No. 1, pp. 111-113, ISSN 1328-8067

Stegeman, C.A., Tervaert, J.W., de Jong, P.E. & Kallenberg, C.G. (1996) Trimethoprim-sulfamethoxazole (co-trimoxazole) for the prevention of relapses of Wegener's granulomatosis. Dutch Co-Trimoxazole Wegener Study Group. *N Engl J Med*, Vol. 335, No. 1, pp. 16-20, ISSN 0028-4793

Sugiyama, H., Watanabe, N., Onoda, T., Kikumoto, Y., Yamamoto, M., Maeta, M., Ohara, N., Maeshima, Y., Yamasaki, Y. & Makino, H. (2005) Successful treatment of progressive Henoch-Schonlein purpura nephritis with tonsillectomy and steroid pulse therapy. *Intern Med*, Vol. 44, No. 6, pp. 611-615, ISSN 0918-2918

Sundel, R.P., Burns, J.C., Baker, A., Beiser, A.S. & Newburger, J.W. (1993) Gamma globulin re-treatment in Kawasaki disease. *J Pediatr*, Vol. 123, No. 4, pp. 657-659, ISSN 0022-3476

Tanaka, H., Suzuki, K., Nakahata, T., Ito, E. & Waga, S. (2003) Early treatment with oral immunosuppressants in severe proteinuric purpura nephritis. *Pediatr Nephrol*, Vol. 18, No. 4, pp. 347-350, ISSN 0931-041X

Tarshish, P., Bernstein, J. & Edelmann, C.M., Jr. (2004) Henoch-Schonlein purpura nephritis: course of disease and efficacy of cyclophosphamide. *Pediatr Nephrol*, Vol. 19, No. 1, pp. 51-56, ISSN 0931-041X

Terai, M. & Shulman, S.T. (1997) Prevalence of coronary artery abnormalities in Kawasaki disease is highly dependent on gamma globulin dose but independent of salicylate dose. *J Pediatr*, Vol. 131, No. 6, pp. 888-893, ISSN 0022-3476

Thompson, D.M., Heaf, P.J. & Robinsin, T.W. (1976) Australia antigen polyarteritis treated with prednisone and dapsone. *Proc R Soc Med*, Vol. 69, No. 6, pp. 389-390, ISSN 0035-9157

Tomioka, S., Miyoshi, K., Tabata, K., Hotta, O. & Taguma, Y. (1996) Clinical study of chronic tonsillitis with IgA nephropathy treated by tonsillectomy. *Acta Otolaryngol Suppl*, Vol. 523, No. pp. 175-177, ISSN 0365-5237

Utani, A., Ohta, M., Shinya, A., Ohno, S., Takakuwa, H., Yamamoto, T., Suzaki, T. & Danno, K. (1991) Successful treatment of adult Henoch-Schonlein purpura with factor XIII concentrate. *J Am Acad Dermatol*, Vol. 24, No. 3, pp. 438-442, ISSN 0190-9622

Vassilopoulos, D. & Calabrese, L.H. (2002) Hepatitis C virus infection and vasculitis: implications of antiviral and immunosuppressive therapies. *Arthritis Rheum*, Vol. 46, No. 3, pp. 585-597, ISSN 0004-3591

Vignes, S., Stoyanova, M., Vasseur, E., Haicault de la Regontais, G. & Hanslik, T. (2005) [Reversible lower limb lymphedema as the first manifestation of cutaneous periarteritis nodosa]. *Rev Med Interne*, Vol. 26, No. 1, pp. 58-60, ISSN 0248-8663

Villiger, P.M. & Guillevin, L. (2010) Microscopic polyangiitis: Clinical presentation. *Autoimmun Rev*, Vol. 9, No. 12, pp. 812-819, ISSN 1873-0183

Wyatt, R.J. & Hogg, R.J. (2001) Evidence-based assessment of treatment options for children with IgA nephropathies. *Pediatr Nephrol*, Vol. 16, No. 2, pp. 156-167, ISSN 0931-041X

Yazici, H., Pazarli, H., Barnes, C.G., Tuzun, Y., Ozyazgan, Y., Silman, A., Serdaroglu, S., Oguz, V., Yurdakul, S., Lovatt, G.E. & et al. (1990) A controlled trial of azathioprine in Behcet's syndrome. *N Engl J Med*, Vol. 322, No. 5, pp. 281-285, ISSN 0028-4793

Yazici, Y., Yurdakul, S. & Yazici, H. (2010) Behcet's syndrome. *Curr Rheumatol Rep*, Vol. 12, No. 6, pp. 429-435, ISSN 1534-6307

Yurdakul, S., Mat, C., Tuzun, Y., Ozyazgan, Y., Hamuryudan, V., Uysal, O., Senocak, M. & Yazici, H. (2001) A double-blind trial of colchicine in Behcet's syndrome. *Arthritis Rheum*, Vol. 44, No. 11, pp. 2686-2692, ISSN 0004-3591

Zaffanello, M., Brugnara, M. & Franchini, M. (2007) Therapy for children with henoch-schonlein purpura nephritis: a systematic review. *ScientificWorldJournal*, Vol. 7, No. pp. 20-30, ISSN 1537-744X

Zulian, F., Corona, F., Gerloni, V., Falcini, F., Buoncompagni, A., Scarazatti, M., Martini, G. & Zacchello, F. (2004) Safety and efficacy of iloprost for the treatment of ischaemic digits in paediatric connective tissue diseases. *Rheumatology (Oxford)*, Vol. 43, No. 2, pp. 229-233, ISSN 1462-0324

Zulian, F., Costantini, C., Montesco, M.C., Schiavon, F. & Zacchello, F. (1998) Successful treatment of gangrene in systemic necrotizing vasculitis with iloprost. *Br J Rheumatol*, Vol. 37, No. 2, pp. 228-230, ISSN 0263-7103

5

Treatment of ANCA – Associated Vasculitis

Christina G. Katsiari and Lazaros Sakkas
Department of Rheumatology, School of Medicine, University of Thessaly, Larissa, Greece

1. Introduction

ANCA - associated vasculitis (AAV) encompass Wegener granulomatosus (WG), Churg Strauss syndrome (CSS) and Microscopic Polyangiitis (MPA). Granuloma formation characterizes both WG and CSS, while necrotising inflammation of middle to small arteries, pauci-immune glomerulonephritis and production of ANCA typify all three of them. Common clinical and laboratory features point towards common pathogenetic mechanisms and thus therapeutic approach have evolved over the years from treatment of individual members of the group to unified treatment strategies. It is the presentation of the disease rather than a particular AAV that guides treatment decisions. Clinical subtypes of AAV according to the extend and the severity of the disease, have been proposed by the European Vasculitis Study (EUVAS) Group (Jayne & Rasmussen 1997) (Table 1): AAV can be presented as localized, early systemic, generalized, severe or refractory disease. This classification currently serves as the basis for the assignment of different treatment regimens.

Forty years ago AAV was a rapidly fatal disease. One-year survival was estimated to be less than 20%, mainly due to pulmonary and/or renal failure and steroids-related infection (Hoffman et al. 1992). The introduction of oral cyclophosphamide (CyP) during the '70s radically changed the prognosis of AAV. Recent data from the EUVAS Group trials show that survival at 1-year is currently almost 90%. CyP in combination with prednisone remain today the cornerstone of treatment of AAV. However, several issues have emerged: a) there are still patients that either die early in the course of the disease or display progressive disease refractory to conventional treatment, b) relapses are frequent, affecting approximately 50% of patients with AAV during extended follow-up, c) the burden of drug-related toxicity is high, as serious adverse events affect approximately 40% of the patients. In addition to glucocorticoids toxicity, CyP can acutely lead to cytopenias, hemorrhagic cystitis and infections along with late complications including gonadal insufficiency and infertility, myelodysplasias and bladder cancer.

In an effort to minimize CyP toxicity as well as to find regimens that could replace CyP in cases of non-responding, refractory, or relapsing disease, several treatment options have been considered. During the last 20 years and despite the rarity of AAV, several multi-center, multi-national randomized control trials (RCTs) were conducted largely due to the combined efforts of EUVAS Group and the VCRC (Vasculitis Clinical Research Consortium), which have altered our treatment practice as it will be discussed below. Treatment of AAV consists of an initial phase aiming at rapid induction of remission and a second phase where maintenance of remission is sought.

AAV Subtype	Description
Localized	one system, typically the upper respiratory track in WG
Early Systemic	involvement of multiple sites but without impending renal or other vital organ failure
Generalized	impending vital organ failure or renal involvement with creatinine level below 5.6 mg/dL (500μmol/L)
Severe	vital organ failure, typically renal involvement with serum creatinine over 5.6 mg/dL (500μmol/L)
Refractory	progressive disease despite conventional treatment

Table 1. Clinical Subtypes of AAV according to the extend and the severity of the disease

2. Induction of remission

The gold standard for induction of remission in most cases of AAV has been the combination of high dose prednisolone (1mg/kg/day with or without previous pulses 1g/d x 3d) with CyP either orally (2mg/kg/day) or intravenously (0.75 g/m^2 every month for 6 months) (Adu et al. 1997; Guillevin et al. 1997). In order to reduce the cumulative dose of drugs and thus adverse effects, current treatment strategies are differentiated according to the presentation of the disease (Table 1) and along with different schemes of CyP administration include several other medications such as rituximab, mycophenolate mofetil (MMF) and methotrexate (MTX).

2.1 Generalized AAV

Generalized AAV refers to patients who display imminent vital organ failure or renal involvement with creatinine level below 5.6 mg/dL (500μmol/L).

In an earlier study including 47 patients with generalized AAV and renal involvement intravenous pulses of CyP (0.75 g/m^2, monthly for 6 months) were equally effective in achieving remission as oral CyP. Moreover, fewer incidents of cytopenia and infections had been recorded in the pulse group (Haubitz & Schellong 1998).

A randomized controlled trial by EUVAS, termed CYCLOPS, compared another scheme of pulse cyclophosphamide with daily oral cyclophosphamide for the induction of remission of AAV (De Groot et al. 2009). Patients with generalized AAV (n=149) and renal involvement received prednisolone plus either pulse cyclophosphamide (15 mg/kg every 2-3 weeks; n = 76) or daily oral cyclophosphamide (2 mg/kg per day; n=73). The efficacy of both regimens was similar in inducing remission. Lower cumulative dose of CyP was achieved in the pulse group, which displayed fewer episodes of leukopenia. It should be noted though that following pulse treatment there was a tendency towards a higher rate of relapse compared to oral treatment during the 9-month follow-up of the study.

Although it is not clear whether there are significant differences regarding efficacy and safety between the 2 schemes of CyP pulses, EULAR recommendations endorse the following strategy (Mukhtyar et al. 2009): administration of 15mg/kg of CyP every 2 weeks for 3 pulses and then every 3 weeks for additional 3-6 pulses. According to the same set of recommendations prednisolone intake should start at 1mg/kg/day (or 60mg/day) for 1 month, tapered to 15mg/day at 3 months and 7.5mg/day at 12 months.

Following the paradigm of lupus nephritis, MMF has been examined whether it can replace CyP for the induction of remission in AAV. In a study including 35 patients with AAV renal vasculitis with serum creatinine <5.6 mg/dL, 18 received MMF (2g/day) and 17 monthly pulses of CyP (0.75–1.0 g/m^2) for 6 months (Hu et al. 2008). According to the study, complete remission was achieved in 78% in the MMF group compared to 47% in the CyP group. Whether MMF truly bears superiority towards CyP remains to be verified in large controlled trilas. MYCYC (http://clinicaltrials.gov/ct2/show/ NCT00414128 (2010)), a multi-center controlled trial by EUVAS comparing the efficacy of MMF and CyP has been initiated. Notably, MMF will be used at the increased dose of 3g/day.

Rituximab, an anti-CD20 chimeric monoclonal antibody that effectively depletes B cells, has recently received much attention regarding its treatment potential in AAV. The number of activated B cells in AAV is associated with disease activity and the extend of organ involvement. Moreover, B cells generate ANCA-producing plasma cells. Studies in humans and animal models support the concept that ANCA have a central role in the pathogenesis and maintenance of AAV (Xiao et al. 2002)

The efficacy of rituximab to induce remission in generalized AAV was examined in two RCTs. In RITUXVAS trial (Jones et al. 2010), 11 patients received pulses CyP plus glucocorticoids and 33 patients additionally received rituximab. The rituximab group received four infusions of rituximab 375 mg/m^2 per week plus two infusions of intravenous cyclophosphamide 15 mg/kg. The cyclophosphamide group received between six and ten infusions of cyclophosphamide 15 mg/kg. Azathioprine was used as maintenance therapy in all patients. At 12 months, remission rates were comparable between the two groups (76% for rituximab and 82% for CyP group). Rituximab (375 mg/m^2 per week for four weeks) was also compared with oral CyP (2 mg/ kg per day) in addition to glucocorticoids in the RAVE trial (Stone et al. 2010). At 6 months remission rates were 64% for the rituximab and 53% for the CyP group. These lower rates of remission compared to other studies were probably due to the aggressive tapering of corticosteroids employed.

Overall, both studies show that rituximab therapy is not inferior to CyP (oral or pulses) treatment for the induction of remission in patients with generilized AAV. It should be noted, however, that adverse effects were also comparable between rituximab and CyP receivers an issue that has to be further addressed in studies with extended follow-up. Rituximab can thus replace CyP treatment especially in patients where CyP is contraindicated and could be the drug of choice in patients with childbearing potential. In spring of 2011, rituximab became the first drug to get an FDA approval for the treatment of AAV.

2.2 Early systemic AAV

Early systemic AAV refers to patients with involvement of multiple sites but without imminent renal or other vital organ failure.

Following initial open label studies with promising results, the NORAM study (De Groot et al. 2005), a RCT initiated by EUVAS, evaluated the efficacy of MTX as a potentially less toxic than CyP alternative to induce remission in patients with early systemic AAV. In addition to corticosteroids, patients received either oral CyP (2 mg/Kg per day) or oral MTX (initial dose 15mg/week that was increased to 20-25mg/week) for 12 months. Patients' follow-up lasted 18 months, and during the last 6 months all medications were stopped. At 12 months remission rates between the two groups were comparable (89.8% for MTX and 93.5% for oral CyP). Time to remission in overall was also comparable. However, some patients with pulmonary involvement or relatively extensive disease in the MTX group had delayed onset of remission. In addition, at 18 months the relapse rate in the MTX group was 69.5%, which was significantly higher compared to that observed in the CyP group (46.5%). These high relapse rates in both treatment arms suggest that treatment of early systemic AAV should last beyond 1 year. The overall frequency of adverse events did not differ between the two groups. Leukopenia was prevalent with the use of CyP as was liver dysfunction with the use of MTX. In view of the results of the NORAM study, EULAR recommend MTX as an alternative to CyP for remission induction in non-organ-threatening or non-life threatening AAV.

2.3 Severe AAV

Severe AAV refers to patients with vital organ failure, typically renal involvement with serum creatinine over 5.6 mg/dL (500µmol/L).

Patients with life- and/or vital organ threatening manifestations, such as diffuse alveolar hemorrhage (DAH), severe rapidly progressive glomerulonephritis (serum creatinine >5.6 mg/dL), glomerulonephritis with double serum positivity for MPO-ANCA and anti-glomerular basement membrane antibodies (Rutgers et al. 2005), require urgent, aggressive treatment. Supportive measures such as blood transfusion and mechanical ventilation or hemodialysis are frequently required.

In a EUVAS trial called MEPEX (Jayne et al. 2007) the effectiveness of plasma exchange was evaluated in patients with severe AAV involving acute renal failure. All 137 patients received oral CyP and prednisolone. One group was assigned to additionally receive three infusions of 1g methylprednisolone pulse therapy (n=67) and a second to receive seven courses of plasma exchanges (n=70). At 3 months, 69% of patients who received plasma exchanges were alive and dialysis independent compared to the significantly lower 49% of patients treated with methylprednisolone pulses.

The usefulness of plasma exchange in patients already on dialysis at the time of diagnosis has also been suggested (de Lind et al. 2007). Intravenous pulses methylprednisolone as adjunctive therapy in patients with severe tubular atrophy and <18% normal glomeruli increased the chance of therapy-related death over the chance of dialysis independence. The same was true for the group receiving plasma exchange only when the proportion of normal glomeruli reached a value of <2%.

Although there are no RCT available, plasma exchanges appear to be warranted in patients with DAH. In a retrospective review of 20 patients with DAH that were presented at a single institute and were treated with plasma exchanges in addition to intravenous methylprednisolone with or without CyP, resolution of lung hemorrhage was achieved in all 20 patients after an average number of 6.4 treatments. Historical review of 11 patients hospitalized at the same centre and did not receive plasma exchanges revealed 3 deaths. (Klemmer Am J Kid Dis 2003).

2.4 Other treatments

Anti-Tumor Necrosis Factor (anti-TNF) regimens have been considered as an alternative to current treatment for over a decade. Based on the beneficial effects of TNF blockade in other chronic inflammatory disorders and the fact that several lines of evidence implicate TNF in the pathogenesis of AAV in humans and animal models of the disease, several small pilot studies evaluated the therapeutic potential of infliximab revealing promising results. However, data derived from subsequent studies were conflicting and could not corroborate any additional benefit from the use of infliximab in patients with AAV (Booth et al. 2004; Josselin et al. 2008; Morgan et al. 2010). It should be noted that there is no RCT for infliximab in AAV. On the contrary, the effect of entanercept, another anti-TNF agent, was examined in a large RCT (WGET) with patients suffering from WG (Wegener's G.E.T.W. 2005). In WGET, etanercept was used as an additional therapy to standard treatment for the induction and maintenance of remission in 180 patients with WG. At 27 months, remission rates and time-to-remission, were not significantly different between the two groups. It should be emphasized that six patients in the etanercept group developed solid cancers compared to no such malignancies in the control group (Stone et al. 2006). Hence, etanercept is considered ineffective and potentially hazardous when added to standard therapy for induction and maintenance of remission in WG. The overall experience with anti-TNF drugs in AAV is either negative or inconclusive. Skepticism has replaced initial enthusiasm and currently the use of TNF blockade in patients with AAV appears remote.

Drug	Dosage	Comments
Prednisolone	60 mg/day for 1 month tapered to 15 mg/day at 3 months	Use IV methylprednisolone 500-1,000 mg/day for 3 days in critical organ manifestations
Cyclophosphamide IV pulse	15 mg/Kg 2-weekly for 3 pulses, then 3-weekly for 3-6 pulses	Oral cyclophosphamide (2 mg/Kg/day) might be used adjusted to keep WBC >3,000/μL
Methotrexate	Starting dose 15 mg/week, increased to 20-25 mg/week at 2 months	Use in non critical organ manifestations (normal serum creatinine)
Rituximab IV	375 mg/m2/week for 4 pulses	Use in intolerance to CyP and in young patients with non-severe critical organ manifestations
Mycophenolate Mofetil	2 g/day	In patients with moderate renal involvement who cannot take cyclophosphamide
Plasmapheresis		Use in critical organ manifestations (serum creatinine >5.6 mg/dL, lung hemorrhage)

Table 2. Induction of remission in ANCA-associated vasculitis

Since ANCA may have a central role in the pathogenesis of AAV, the idea to target autoreactive T cells that drive the production of ANCA excreeting-plasma cells appears to be a logical treatment approach. Abatacept, a CTLA4—Ig molecule, blocks the co-stimulatory talk between T and B cells and has been proven efficacious in the treatment of rheumatoid arthritis. A RCT to evaluate relapse rate over a 24 month period in patients treated for 12 months with abatacept in addition to standard treatment (MTX plus prednisone) had been initiated but unfortunately was recently terminated due to slow recruitment (ABAVAS Study NCT00482066).

Recent data generated increased interest towards the role of the complement pathway in the pathogenesis of AAV, which appears to have an essential role on how ANCA can damage the vascular wall. Eculizumab is a monoclonal antibody that blocks the activation of C5, a central component of the complement cascade. Blockade of C5 activation was shown to have substantial therapeutic effect in animal models of AAV. A similar approach to treat patients with AAV will be evaluated in a pilot study with 10 patients receiving eculizumab in addition to standard treatment (study NCT01275287).

In anticipation of novel treatments, drugs currently used to induce remission in AAV are summarized in Table 2 and include corticosteroids, CyP, MTX, MMF, Rituximab and plasmapheresis.

3. Maintenance of remission

The majority of patients with AAV can achieve remission within the first 6 months of treatment. However, if no other care is undertaken over half of the patients may have a relapse within the first 2 years following remission (De Groot et al. 2005). Relapses in AAV were associated with subsequent progression to end-stage renal disease (Hogan et al. 2005). Moreover, the number of relapses for an individual patient was a strong predictor of damage during follow-up, as measured by the Vasculitis Damage Index (Koldingsnes & Nossent 2002). Therefore maintenance, once remission is achieved, is essential for the long term outcome of patients with AAV.

CyP as oral (1.5mg/kg per day) or infusion regimen (0.75/m^2, effusion every 3 months) was initially the standard regimen to maintain remission (Hoffman et al. 1992). Because of the serious adverse events related to long term exposure to CyP less toxic drugs have been proposed such as azathioprine, methotrexate, leflunomide or MMF

The CYCAZAREM study by EUVAS randomly assigned 144 patients with AAV (who achieved remission with oral CyP and prednisolone) to receive either azathioprine (2 mg/kg per day; n = 71) or CyP (1.5 mg/kg per day; n = 73) (Jayne et al. 2003). Both treatment groups continued to receive prednisolone (7.5 mg per day). At 18 months of follow-up, relapses had occurred in 15.5% and 13.7% of patients in the azathioprine and CyP group, respectively, suggesting that azathioprine is as effective as CyP for maintaining remission in AAV. Adverse events were comparable between the two treatment groups.

In a RCT by the French Vasculitis Study Group, 126 patients with WG or MPA following induction therapy, were randomly assigned to receive either oral azathioprine (2 mg/kg per day; n = 63) or methotrexate (0.3 mg/kg per week, progressively increased to 25 mg per week; n = 63) for 12 months. No significant difference was found between the two groups in terms of relapse-free survival and toxicity at a follow-up period of 29 ± 13 months (Pagnoux et al. 2008).

In another RCT, 54 patients with WG (who achieved remission after treatment with cyclophosphamide and prednisolone) were randomly assigned oral leflunomide (30 mg per day) or oral methotrexate (starting with 7.5 mg per week and reaching 20 mg per week after 8 weeks) for 2 years (Metzler et al. 2007). Leflunomide was more effective in preventing relapses than oral methotrexate (6 versus 13 relapses, respectively), but was associated with a higher rate of adverse events. However, this study was underpowered; it was initially designed for 154 patients but only 54 were enrolled.

The potential benefit of MMF treatment for maintenance of remission in AAV has been demonstrated in preliminary uncontrolled studies (Silva et al. 2010). On the basis of these studies, an RCT by EUVAS, termed IMPROVE, comparing MMF with azathioprine for maintenance of remission in renal vasculitis, has been carried out (Hiemstra et al. 2010). Among 156 patients treated either with AZA (starting at 2 mg/kg/d) or MMF (starting at 2000 mg/d) following induction of remission with CyP and prednisolone, patients on MMF experienced more relapses compared to AZA group.

Some observational studies provide preliminary data regarding the efficacy of other regimens to maintain remission in patients with AAV. Rituximab appears to be beneficial (Stasi et al. 2006; Rhee et al. 2010). A large RCT currently evaluates the efficacy of rituximab in comparison to AZA (MAINRITSAN , Study NCT00748644). On the contrary, addition of intravenous immunoglobulin (IVIg) to standard maintenance treatment (AZA plus prednisone) does not prevent relapses (Fortin et al. 2009).

In overall, treatment with low-dose prednisolone plus AZA (2 mg/Kg/day until 12 months then 1.5 mg/Kg/day) (Jayne et al. 2003; Pagnoux et al. 2008), or MTX (20-25 mg/week) (Pagnoux et al. 2008) is currently the preferred approach for maintenance of remission in AAV. The duration of maintenance is not known but should be >24 months (Lapraik et al. 2007) (Table 3).

Drug	Dosage	Comments
Prednisolone	Starting from 15 mg/day at 3 months tapered to 7.5 mg/day at 12 months	Alternate-day schemes have also been applied to minimize side effects. Should probably be avoided in generalized or severe forms of the disease
Cyclophosphamide IV pulse	0.75 mg/m^2 every 3 months	Oral cyclophosphamide (1.5 mg/Kg/day) might be used adjusted to keep WBC >3,000/μL in patients who experience frequent relapses
Azathioprine	2 mg/kg/day for 12 months then 1.5 mg/kg/day	Currently the gold standard for maintenance of remission
Methotrexate	Starting dose 0.3/kg per week, increased to 25 mg per week	At high doses is a good alternative to Azathioprine
Rituximab IV	375 mg/m^2 every 6 months	Waits to be compared with Azathiprione. Should be considered in patients where AZA or MTX is either contraindicated or ineffective.
Maintenance treatment should last > 24 months		

Table 3. Maintenance of remission in ANCA-associated vasculitis

4. Relapse

Symptoms and signs of apparent AAV relapse, especially in patients on immunosuppression, should be differentiated from infections and malignancies. Relapse can be treated with oral or IV pulses of CyP plus prednisolone (60 mg/day) (Wegener's G.E.T.W. 2005). Patients intolerant to CyP can receive MMF (Stassen et al. 2007) or rituximab. IVIg (added to maintenance treatment) can achieve remission (Martinez et al. 2008) and it is particularly useful until infection is ruled out.

5. Refractory disease

Refractory disease refers to patients who experience progressive disease despite conventional treatment.

Patients with refractory disease should be treated in specialized centers. Rituximab has been successful in CyP-refractory disease in observational studies (Smith et al. 2006; Keogh et al. 2006; Jones et al. 2009; Keogh et al. 2005). Deoxyspergualin (0.5 mg/Kg/day subcutaneously in 6 cycles of 21 days with 7-day intervals), an antiproliferative agent licensed in Japan for acute renal transplant rejection, showed promise in phase II study (Flossmann et al. 2009). Infliximab was beneficial in refractory disease in observational studies (Josselin et al. 2008) but when added to standard induction treatment did not make any difference (Morgan et al. 2010).

6. Special issues

6.1 End stage renal disease (ESRD) and renal transplantation

Relapse of ANCA-associated vasculitis is significantly less frequent (0.08 episodes/person-year) in ESRD patients compared with patients with preserved renal function (0.16-0.20 episodes/person-year), but infection, an important cause of death is almost double in frequency in ESRD (Lionaki et al. 2009). Therefore, immunosuppression in patients with ESRD may be limited to patients with active vasculitis.

Patients with ESRD can receive renal transplants. The overall survival of renal transplants is 90% at 5 years (Gera et al. 2007), and 70% at 10 years (Little et al. 2009). In one study, risk factors for renal transplant rejection was transplantation <12 months postvasculitis remission (Little et al. 2009). Therefore, renal transplantation should be considered in patients with ESRD with sustained remission of vasculitis.

6.2 Subglottic stenosis

Patients with active disease receive aggressive treatment with prednisolone and CyP, and tracheostomy, if needed. Rituximab may also be used in case of CyP inadequate response. In inactive disease, intralesional costicosteroid with dilatation is generally effective (Hernandez-Rodriguez et al. 2010).

6.3 Orbital mass

Aggressive treatment with steroids and CyP is the standard of care. Rituximab is effective in refractory cases

6.4 Precautions

CyP dose should be adjusted for renal function and age.

There should be vigilance for side effects of drugs used (CyP, rituximab, MTX, IVIg, plasmapheresis). Patients should be checked for tuberculosis with chest x-rays and PPD skin test, and patients with latent tuberculosis should receive prophylaxis with isoniazid plus vitamin B6. Patients on IV pulse CyP, receive antiemetic drug (ondesarton) immediately prior to and 8 hours after the CyP pulse. On the day of IV CyP pulse, patients receive oral or IV hydration with 2-3 liters of fluid. They also receive IV 2-mercaptoethanesulfonate (mesna) (20% of CyP dose) immediately before and at 2, 4 and 8 hours after the CyP pulse to reduce irritation of urinary bladder. The dose of next IV CyP pulse is adjusted to keep nadir WBC (12-14 days after the IV pulse) >3,000/μL. The rate of leucopenia, infections, and gonadal toxicity is reduced in the IV pulse CyP compared to oral CyP regimen (De Groot et al. 2009; Haubitz & Schellong 1998). Oral mesna is also beneficial for patients on oral CyP.

According to a recent study ever-tobacco smoking and previous episode of hemorrhagic cystitis were strong predictors for the development of cancer in the urinary tract. Thus patients with these characteristics need close surveillance.

All patients receiving CyP are advised to take prophylaxis against Pneumocystis jiroveci with trimethoprime/sulphamethoxazole (800/160 mg thrice weekly). This may also prevent relapses in patients with respiratory involvement (Zycinska et al. 2009).

Gonadal failure is a common side effect in patients treated with CyP, where the risk increases in parallel with the increase of the cumulative dose received. No standard care to preserve gonadal function has been proposed for patients with AAV under CyP. Similar issues encountered in patients with systemic lupus erythematosus (SLE) have been addressed. For women with SLE two protocols exist: administration of leuprolide acetate with or without transdermal estrogen and depo-progesterone for contraception. Leuprolide should be administered 10-14 days prior to each CyP infusion. In men with SLE, administration of intramuscular monthly injections of testosterone has been proposed. Analogous approaches should probably be established for young patients with AAV at risk.

Patients on immunosuppression should not be vaccinated with live attenuated vaccines. They can and should be vaccinated with dead pathogens. Patients with WG exhibit adequate antibody (Holvast et al. 2009) and cell-mediated (Holvast ARD2010) immune response to influenza vaccines (Holvast et al. 2010).

7. Conclusion

The treatment of ANCA-associated vasculitis (AAV) has evolved over the years from treatment of individual members of the group i.e Wegener granulomatosis(WG), Churg-Strauss syndrome (CSS), microscopic polyangiitis (MPA), to unified treatment. For years, treatment of WG was corticosteroids plus oral cyclophosphamide (CyP), which was effective but had a high frequency of severe adverse effects (Hoffman AIM1992). To reduce the adverse effects of CyP, notably, bone marrow suppression and infections, hemorrhagic cystitis, gonadal toxicity, and tumors, other regimens were sought. So, intense immunosuppression with CyP is used only for induction of remission, and then remission is maintained with drugs with fewer side effects, such as azathioprine (AZA) and methotrexate (MTX). In addition, the regimen for the induction of remission is individualized according to disease severity.

8. References

Adu, D., Pall, A., Luqmani, R.A., Richards, N.T., Howie, A.J., Emery, P., Michael, J., Savage, C.O. & Bacon, P.A. (1997) Controlled trial of pulse versus continuous prednisolone and cyclophosphamide in the treatment of systemic vasculitis. *QJM: monthly journal of the Association of Physicians*, 90, pp. 401.

Booth, A., Harper, L., Hammad, T., Bacon, P., Griffith, M., Levy, J., Savage, C., Pusey, C. & Jayne, D. (2004) Prospective study of TNFalpha blockade with infliximab in anti-neutrophil cytoplasmic antibody-associated systemic vasculitis. *Journal of the American Society of Nephrology: JASN*, 15, pp. 717.

De Groot, K., Harper, L., Jayne, D.R., Flores, S.L.F., Gregorini, G., Gross, W.L., Luqmani, R., Pusey, C.D., Rasmussen, N. & Sinico, R.A. (2009) Pulse versus daily oral cyclophosphamide for induction of remission in antineutrophil cytoplasmic antibody-associated vasculitis: a randomized trial. *Annals of internal medicine*, 150, pp. 670.

De Groot, K., Rasmussen, N., Bacon, P.A., Tervaert, J.W., Feighery, C., Gregorini, G., Gross, W.L., Luqmani, R. & Jayne, D.R. (2005) Randomized trial of cyclophosphamide versus methotrexate for induction of remission in early systemic antineutrophil cytoplasmic antibody-associated vasculitis. *Arthritis and rheumatism*, 52, pp. 2461.

De Lind, V.W.R.A., Hauer, H.A., Wolterbeek, R., Jayne, D.R., Gaskin, G. & RASMUSSEN, N. (2007) Chances of renal recovery for dialysis-dependent ANCA-associated glomerulonephritis. *Journal of the American Society of Nephrology: JASN*, 18, pp. 2189.

Flossmann, O., Baslund, B., Bruchfeld, A., Cohen, T.J.W., Hall, C., Heinzel, P., Hellmich, B., Luqmani, R.A., Nemoto, K. & Tesar, V. (2009) Deoxyspergualin in relapsing and refractory Wegener's granulomatosis. *Annals of the rheumatic diseases*, 68, pp. 1125.

Fortin, P.M., Tejani, A.M., Bassett, K. & Musini, V.M. (2009) Intravenous immunoglobulin as adjuvant therapy for Wegener's granulomatosis. *Cochrane database of systematic reviews (Online)*, pp. CD007057.

Gera, M., Griffin, M.D., Specks, U., Leung, N., Stegall, M.D. & Fervenza, F.C. (2007) Recurrence of ANCA-associated vasculitis following renal transplantation in the modern era of immunosupression. *Kidney international*, 71, pp. 1296.

Guillevin, L., Cordier, J.F., Lhote, F., Cohen, P., Jarrousse, B., Royer, I., Lesavre, P., Jacquot, C., Bindi, P. & Bielefeld, P. (1997) A prospective, multicenter, randomized trial comparing steroids and pulse cyclophosphamide versus steroids and oral cyclophosphamide in the treatment of generalized Wegener's granulomatosis. *Arthritis and rheumatism*, 40, pp. 2187.

Haubitz, M. & Schellong, S. (1998) Intravenous pulse administration of cyclophosphamide versus daily oral treatment in patients with antineutrophil cytoplasmic antibody-associated vasculitis and renal involvement: a prospective, randomized study. *Arthritis and rheumatism*, 41, pp. 1835.

Hernandez-Rodriguez, J., Hoffman, G.S. & Koening, C.L. (2010) Surgical interventions and local therapy for Wegener's granulomatosis. *Current opinion in rheumatology*, 22, pp. 29.

Hiemstra, T.F., Walsh, M., Mahr, A., Savage, C.O., DE Groot, K., Harper, L., Hauser, T., Neumann, I., Tesar, V. & Wissing, K.M. (2010) Mycophenolate Mofetil vs Azathioprine for Remission Maintenance in Antineutrophil Cytoplasmic Antibody-Associated Vasculitis: A Randomized Controlled Trial. *JAMA: the journal of the American Medical Association.*

Hoffman, G.S., Kerr, G.S., Leavitt, R.Y., Hallahan, C.W., Lebovics, R.S., Travis, W.D., Rottem, M. & Fauci, A.S. (1992) Wegener granulomatosis: an analysis of 158 patients. *Annals of internal medicine*, 116, pp. 488.

Hogan, S.L., Falk, R.J., Chin, H., Cai, J., Jennette, C.E., Jennette, J.C. & Nachman, P.H. (2005) Predictors of relapse and treatment resistance in antineutrophil cytoplasmic antibody-associated small-vessel vasculitis. *Annals of internal medicine*, 143, pp. 621.

Holvast, A., DE Haan, A., Van Assen, S., Stegeman, C.A., Huitema, M.G., Huckriede, A., Benne, C.A., Westra, J., Palache, A. & Wilschut, J. (2010) Cell-mediated immune responses to influenza vaccination in Wegener's granulomatosis. *Annals of the rheumatic diseases*, 69, pp. 924.

Holvast, A., Stegeman, C.A., Benne, C.A., Huckriede, A., Wilschut, J.C., Palache, A.M., Kallenberg, C.G. & Bijl, M. (2009) Wegener's granulomatosis patients show an adequate antibody response to influenza vaccination. *Annals of the rheumatic diseases*, 68, pp. 873.

Hu, W., Liu, C., Xie, H., Chen, H., Liu, Z. & LI, L. (2008) Mycophenolate mofetil versus cyclophosphamide for inducing remission of ANCA vasculitis with moderate renal involvement. *Nephrology, dialysis, transplantation: official publication of the European Dialysis and Transplant Association-European Renal Association*, 23, pp. 1307.

Jayne, D., Rasmussen, N., Andrassy, K., Bacon, P., Tervaert, J.W., Dadonienθ,J., Ekstrand, A., Gaskin, G., Gregorini, G. & De Groot, K. (2003) A randomized trial of maintenance therapy for vasculitis associated with antineutrophil cytoplasmic autoantibodies. *The New England journal of medicine*, 349, pp. 36.

Jayne, D.R., Gaskin, G., Rasmussen, N., Abramowicz, D., Ferrario, F., Guillevin, L., Mirapeix, E., Savage, C.O., Sinico, R.A. & Stegeman, C.A. (2007) Randomized trial of plasma exchange or high-dosage methylprednisolone as adjunctive therapy for severe renal vasculitis. *Journal of the American Society of Nephrology: JASN*, 18, pp. 2180.

Jayne, D.R. & Rasmussen, N. (1997) Treatment of antineutrophil cytoplasm autoantibody-associated systemic vasculitis: initiatives of the European Community Systemic Vasculitis Clinical Trials Study Group. *Journal of the American Society of Nephrology: JASN*, 72, pp. 737.

Jones, R.B., Cohen, T.J.W., Hauser, T., Luqmani, R., Morgan, M.D., Peh, C.A., Savage, C.O., Segelmark, M., Tesar, V. & Van Paassen, P. (2010) Rituximab versus

Cyclophosphamide in ANCA-Associated Renal Vasculitis. *The New England journal of medicine*, 363, pp. 211.

Jones, R.B., Ferraro, A.J., Chaudhry, A.N., Brogan, P., Salama, A.D., Smith, K.G., Savage, C.O. & Jayne, D.R. (2009) A multicenter survey of rituximab therapy for refractory antineutrophil cytoplasmic antibody-associated vasculitis. *Arthritis and rheumatism*, 60, pp. 2156.

Josselin, L., Mahr, A., Cohen, P., Pagnoux, C., Guaydier-Souquiφres, G., Hayem, G., Job-Deslandre, C., Liferman, F., Pourrat, J. & Guillevin, L. (2008) Infliximab efficacy and safety against refractory systemic necrotising vasculitides: long-term follow-up of 15 patients. *Annals of the rheumatic diseases*, 67, pp. 1343.

Keogh, K.A., Wylam, M.E., Stone, J.H. & Specks, U. (2005) Induction of remission by B lymphocyte depletion in eleven patients with refractory antineutrophil cytoplasmic antibody-associated vasculitis. *Arthritis and rheumatism*, 52, pp. 262.

Keogh, K.A., Ytterberg, S.R., Fervenza, F.C., Carlson, K.A., Schroeder, D.R. & Specks, U. (2006) Rituximab for Refractory Wegener's Granulomatosis: Report of a Prospective, Open-Label Pilot Trial. *American Journal of Respiratory and Critical Care Medicine*, 173, pp. 180.

Koldingsnes, W. & Nossent, H. (2002) Predictors of survival and organ damage in Wegener's granulomatosis. *Rheumatology (Oxford, England)*, 41, pp. 572.

Lapraik, C., Watts, R., Bacon, P., Carruthers, D., Chakravarty, K., D'cruz, D., Guillevin, L., Harper, L., Jayne, D. & Luqmani, R. (2007) BSR and BHPR guidelines for the management of adults with ANCA associated vasculitis. *Rheumatology (Oxford, England)*, 46, pp. 1615.

Lionaki, S., Hogan, S.L., Jennette, C.E., Hu, Y., Hamra, J.B., Jennette, J.C., Falk, R.J. & Nachman, P.H. (2009) The clinical course of ANCA small-vessel vasculitis on chronic dialysis. *Kidney international*, 76, pp. 644.

Little, M.A., Hassan, B., Jacques, S., Game, D., Salisbury, E., Courtney, A.E., Brown, C., Salama, A.D. & Harper, L. (2009) Renal transplantation in systemic vasculitis: when is it safe? *Nephrology, dialysis, transplantation: official publication of the European Dialysis and Transplant Association-European Renal Association*, 24, pp. 3219.

Martinez, V., Cohen, P., Pagnoux, C., Vinzio, S., Mahr, A., Mouthon, L., Sailler, L., Delaunay, C., Sadoun, A. & Guillevin, L. (2008) Intravenous immunoglobulins for relapses of systemic vasculitides associated with antineutrophil cytoplasmic autoantibodies: results of a multicenter, prospective, open-label study of twenty-two patients. *Arthritis and rheumatism*, 58, pp. 308.

Metzler, C., Miehle, N., Manger, K., Iking-Konert, C., DE Groot, K., Hellmich, B., Gross, W.L. & Reinhold-Keller, E. (2007) Elevated relapse rate under oral methotrexate versus leflunomide for maintenance of remission in Wegener's granulomatosis. *Rheumatology (Oxford, England)*, 46, pp. 1087.

Morgan, M.D., Drayson, M.T., Savage, C.O. & Harper, L. (2010) Addition of Infliximab to Standard Therapy for ANCA-Associated Vasculitis. *Nephron.Clinical practice*, 117, pp. c89.

Mukhtyar, C., Guillevin, L., Cid, M.C., Dasgupta, B., DE Groot, K., Gross, W., Hauser, T., Hellmich, B., Jayne, D. & Kallenberg, C.G. (2009) Eular recommendations for the management of primary small and medium vessel vasculitis. *Annals of the rheumatic diseases*, 68, pp. 310.

Pagnoux, C., Mahr, A., Hamidou, M.A., Boffa, J.J., Ruivard, M., Ducroix, J.P., Kyndt, X., Lifermann, F., Papo, T. & Lambert, M. (2008) Azathioprine or methotrexate maintenance for ANCA-associated vasculitis. *The New England journal of medicine*, 359, pp. 2790.

Rhee, E.P., Laliberte, K.A. & Niles, J.L. (2010) Rituximab as Maintenance Therapy for Anti-Neutrophil Cytoplasmic Antibody-Associated Vasculitis. *Clinical journal of the American Society of Nephrology: CJASN.*

Rutgers, A., Slot, M., Van Paassen, P., Van Breda, V.P., Heeringa, P. & Tervaert, J.W. (2005) Coexistence of anti-glomerular basement membrane antibodies and myeloperoxidase-ANCAs in crescentic glomerulonephritis. *American journal of kidney diseases: the official journal of the National Kidney Foundation*, 46, pp. 253.

Silva, F., Specks, U., Kalra, S., Hogan, M.C., Leung, N., Sethi, S. & Fervenza, F.C. (2010) Mycophenolate mofetil for induction and maintenance of remission in microscopic polyangiitis with mild to moderate renal involvement--a prospective, open-label pilot trial. *Clinical journal of the American Society of Nephrology: CJASN*, 5, pp. 445.

Smith, K.G., Jones, R.B., Burns, S.M. & Jayne, D.R. (2006) Long-term comparison of rituximab treatment for refractory systemic lupus erythematosus and vasculitis: Remission, relapse, and re-treatment. *Arthritis and rheumatism*, 54, pp. 2970.

Stasi, R., Stipa, E., Del Poeta, G., Amadori, S., Newland, A.C. & Provan, D. (2006) Long-term observation of patients with anti-neutrophil cytoplasmic antibody-associated vasculitis treated with rituximab. *Rheumatology (Oxford, England)*, 45, pp. 1432.

Stassen, P.M., Tervaert, J.W.C. & Stegeman, C.A. (2007) Induction of remission in active anti neutrophil cytoplasmic antibody associated vasculitis with mycophenolate mofetil in patients who cannot be treated with cyclophosphamide. *Annals of the rheumatic diseases*, 66, pp. 798.

Stone, J.H., Holbrook, J.T., Marriott, M.A., Tibbs, A.K., Sejismundo, L.P., Min, Y.I., SPECKS, U., MERKEL, P.A., SPIERA, R. & DAVIS, J.C. (2006) Solid malignancies among patients in the Wegener's Granulomatosis Etanercept Trial. *Arthritis and rheumatism*, 54, pp. 1608.

Stone, J.H., Merkel, P.A., Spiera, R., Seo, P., Langford, C.A., Hoffman, G.S., Kallenberg, C.G., ST Clair, E.W., Turkiewicz, A. & Tchao, N.K. (2010) Rituximab versus Cyclophosphamide for ANCA-Associated Vasculitis. *The New England journal of medicine*, 363, pp. 221.

Wegener's G.E.T.W. (2005) Etanercept plus standard therapy for Wegener's granulomatosis. *The New England journal of medicine*, 352, pp. 351.

Xiao, H., Heeringa, P., Hu, P., Liu, Z., Zhao, M., Aratani, Y., Maeda, N., Falk, R.J. & JENNETTE, J.C. (2002) Antineutrophil cytoplasmic autoantibodies specific for myeloperoxidase cause glomerulonephritis and vasculitis in mice. *The Journal of clinical investigation*, 110, pp. 955.

Zycinska, K., Wardyn, K.A., Zielonka, T.M., Krupa, R. & Lukas, W. (2009) Co-trimoxazole and prevention of relapses of PR3-ANCA positive vasculitis with pulmonary involvement. *European journal of medical research*, 14, pp. 265.

6

Biologic Agents for the Treatment of Systemic Vasculitis

P. Sfriso and F. Schiavon
Division of Rheumatology, University of Padova, Italy

1. Introduction

Vasculitis is a disorders characterized by the presence of blood vessel inflammation. It can appear in a wide range of forms: the inflammation can occur in association with an underlying disease or exposure, called secondary vasculitis, or in primary vasculitis blood inflammation occurs for unknown reasons. When this disorder strikes it can lead to blood vessels stenosis/occlusion, causing organ ischemia, or thinning of the blood vessels that results in the formation of aneurysm or hemorrhages. Every size of blood vessels can be affected by the inflammatory process and the size of the vessels involved influences the clinical manifestations. Several classification systems have been proposed but the classification that has been unanimously adopted by the scientific community is the Chapel Hill Nomenclature that classifies vasculitis into small, medium or large vessels vasculitis depending on the calibre of the vessels involved. (Jennette et al, 1994) These three types of vasculitis differ in severity, ranging from a self-limited illness to conditions that can be life-threatening in the absence of prompt treatment. Therapy originally involved treating the patients with glucocorticoids but subsequently, with the improvement of our knowledge about vasculitis pathogenesis, immunosuppressive agents such as methotrexate, azathioprine and cyclophosphamide have been introduced. These drugs have vastly improved the previously dismal prognosis associated with many of these diseases, they are widely used and represent the standard against which newer therapies should be compared. Nevertheless despite this optimal standard therapy, the diseases does not got into full remission for 20 to 30% of patients and in addition, a smaller proportion of patients develop a more severe disease (Hiemstra & Jayne, 2009) Five years post diagnosis, 50% of patients will relapse in spite of having undergone at least 2 years of therapy (Booth el al, 2003) and approximately 25% will experience a refractary course manifested by incomplete disease control or frequent relapses despite remission-manteining therapy. Moreover the toxicity that is caused by the drugs causes severe side effects. For exaples, it has reported that during prolonged treatment with cyclophosphamide, infection and malignancy are the most cause of death in the first year (Bougarit el al, 2005).The toxicity of cyclophosphamide, particularly that associated with long term and repeat use of the agent, has emerged as the principle challenge in managing patients. To minimize the side effects, current approaches include initial use of cyclophosphamide to induce remission followed by use of less toxic immunosuppressive agents for mainteinance. Although this strategy has reduced the malignancy and infection risk, they remain present. High doses of glucocorticoids can also contribute to severe infection. In the last 10 years important progress has been made on the pathogenesis of vasculitis and several factors have been identified as potential therapeutic targets. These include ANCA antibodies, whose pathogenic role in small vessel vasculitis has been demonstrated by evidence in vivo (Halbwachs-Mecarelli, 1995; Huugen, 2007; Kain, 2008; Little, 2005; Pfister, 2004; Xiao, 2002, 2005, 2007; Ruth, 2006) and in vitro tests (Kallemberg, 2008; Schreiber 2003; Van Rossum. 2004; Witko-Sarsat, 1999), tumor necrosis factor alpha (TNFα) (Huugen et al, 2005) interleukin 6 (IL-6) (Noris et al, 1999) and T and B lymphocytes (Walsh & Jayne 2007) . Therefore, targeted therapies have been introduced in the treatment of vasculitis, in order to decrease treatment toxicity as well the propensity to relapse.

1.1 Role of TNF-α in the pathogenesis of vasculitis

TNF is the prototype of a gene superfamily that is important in regulating many biologic function. Science has identified approximately 40 members of the TNF superfamily and knowledges about their function is rapidly emerging. The identification of a TNF-α dependent cytokine cascade in the cultures of synovium present in the joint of patients with rheumatoid arthritis led to the discovery of the role of this cytokine in RA. The development of anti TNF-α therapies constitute still today a major advance in the treatment of RA. There is also evidence that TNF-α plays a role in glomerular inflammation, produced not only by infiltrating macrophages but also by several intrinsic renal cell types. The production of TNF has been demostrated within glomeruli in both experimental and human glomerulonephritis including that associated with ANCA antibody (Noronha et al, 1993) and its role in the recruitment of leukocytes to inflammatory sites in rodent model of ANCA associated vasculitis (Feldmann & Pusey, 2006). In *vitro* studies suggest that the interaction of ANCA and TNF-α primed neutrophils results in the activation of neutrophils as well as degranulation, causing subsequent endothelial cell damage and amplification of the inflammatory process by means of further leukocytes recruitment (Gross, 2004). Moreover, animal models suggest that TNF-α plays a key role in granuloma formation (Noronha, 1993) and that anti TNF-α treatment attenuates manifestations in animal MPO-ANCA- induced glomerulonephritis (Huugen et al, 2005). TNF represented therefore a good therapeutic target and due to the success of blocking TNF in RA, this approach was also tested on vasculitis diseases.

Three agents directed against TNF are currently approvated for the use: Infliximab, Etanercept and Adalimimab. Infliximab is a chimeric monoclonal antibody comprised of the human IgG1 constant region fused with the murine variable region recognized TNF. Adalimumab has a similar structure but is fully humanized. Infliximab and Adalimumab can bind to circulating and membrane bound TNF. Etanercept is a fusion protein composed of 2 extracellular p75 receptors domains linked by the Fc portion of human IgG1. Infliximab and Adalimumab can induce apoptosis in cell expressing TNF, while Etanercept does not induced apoptosis in TNF-expressing cells.

1.2 B limphocytes in the pathogenesis of vasculitis

The primary role of B cells in the pathogenesis of several autoimmune diseases has been demonstrated by the presence of autoantibodies in the patient's serum. B cells are the precursor of antibody-producing cells (plasma cells). In addition to producing ANCA these cells can contribute to the pathogenesis of Wegener's granulomatosis by instigating costimulation and antigen presentation within granulomata (Voswinkel et al, 2008). B cells can interact on an antigen presentig cell (APC) to the T cells, secrete a variety of cytokines (e.g. IL-6, IL-10. TNF α), function as an (auto-) antigen-presenting cell themselves and curry out a role of regulatory cells (Pistoia, 1997; Harris, 2000; Serra, 2006). In Wegener's granulomatosis granulomas of the upper respiratory tract display features of lymphoid-like tissue neoformation and are infiltrated by cluster of B lymphocytes in vicinicity to PR3 cells, dendritic cells and plasma cells. Moreover, antigen (PR3)-driven selection within the immunoglobulin's heavy chain gene repertoire in different granuloma tissues are found (Youinou, 2007) suggesting an initial selection and affinity maturation of B cells within granuloma. B cell activating factor (BAFF) is a central cytokine in B cell development and survival (Mackay et al, 2003) and is elevated in the serum of patients with Wegener's Granulamatosis (Bader, 201; Krumboltz, 2005). BAFF is secreted by activated neutrophils, which play a central role in the pathogenesis of Wegener's granulomatosis, (Scapini et al 2005) and in turn could drive B cell expansion and subsequent ANCA production. Therefore B cells represent an optimal target for biological drugs. Rituximab is a chimeric monoclonal antibody directed against the cell surface protein CD20. This antibody is comprised of the variable regions derived from a murine anti CD-20 antibody fused to human IgG constant regions (Grillo-Lopez et al, 2000). CD 20 is a highly specific surface antigen that is expressed on pre-B and mature B cells but is not found on precursors or plasma cells. The Fab region of Rituximab recognizes the four amino acid sequence on a large extra-cellular loop of the CD 20 molecules (Gurcan et al, 2009). The binding of Rituximab to CD 20 leads to significant depletion of peripheral B cells, inducing cell death. Although the mechanisms involved are not fully understood.(Reff et al, 1994) the experimental evidences demonstrated al least 3 different mechanisms:

Complement–dependent cytotoxicity (CDC), involving the complement protein C1q, with formation of pores in the cell membrane and cell lysis

Antibody dependent cellular cytotoxicity (ADCC) which leads to membrane damage and cell lysis via the recruitment of macrophages, natural killer and cytotoxic cells

Apoptosis by the direct cross linking of CD 20 on B cell (Mease, 2008) .

Rituximab was approved by FDA to use in the treatment of low grade Not Hodgking Lymphoma in 1997 and in 2006 for the treatment of RA. Besides RA, growing experience with Rituximab therapy indicates that it may be effective in the treatment of other rheumatic diseases such as Sjogren syndrome, dermatomyositis-polymiositis, systemic lupus erythematosus and systemic vasculitis.

2. Large vessels vasculitis

2.1 Giant cells arteritis

Giant cell arteritis is a vasculitis of the large-vessel that occours excusively in patients over 50 years of age. Giant cell arteritis involves the aorta and external carotid arteries and their branches and produces intimal hyperplasia and luminal obstruction leading to ischemic manifestations. Visual loss can occour as a consequence of acute anterior ischemic optic neuritis. This represent the most severe complication. The pathophysiology of giant cell arteritis is still poorly understood but T-cells and dendritic cells play a pivotal role. Dendritic cells activate T-cells that produce TNF-α and other proinflammatory citokines contributing to the activation of macrophages and further recruitment of T cells and macrophages in the inflammatory lesion (Ly et al , 2010). Moreover TNF-α is present in high levels inside temporal artery lesions in patients with giant cell arteritis, particularly in corrispondences to the granulomatous areas (Hernandez-Rodriguez et al, 2004). Small case series and case reports present evidence that infliximab could be used as a steroid sparing agent for giant cell arteritis (Airo 2002; Andronopoulos, 2003; Cantini, 2001). A randomized, placebo controlled, double-blind multicenter trial was conducted in 2007 to determine the efficacy of infliximab in treating giant cell arteritis. Fourty-four patients with newly diagnosed of giant cell arteritis were randomly assigned to receive infliximab (5 mg/kg of body weight) or placebo in a 2:1 ratio, in addition to prednisone. Primary end points were the number of patients who did not relapse during a 22 week period nor suffered side effects. Secondary end points included time to first relapse, cumulative glucocorticoid dose and the number of patients who remained relapse-free even when the steroid dosage was tapered to 10 mg/day. Infliximab therapy did not increase the proportion of patients without relapse (43% vs 50% respectively P = 0.65), nor did it increase the proportion of patients whose glucocorticoid dosages were tapered to 10 mg/day without suffering a relapse (61% vs 75% respectively P = 0.31). The incidence of infection was 71% with infliximab and 56% with placebo (difference of 15%, 95% confidence interval (CI) 14-45% (Hoffman et al, 2007). The authors concluded that infliximab was unlikely to be effective in the treatment of giant cell arteritis. The data about the role that Etanercept and Adalimumab play in treating giant cell arteritis are inconclusive: A double blind placebo controlled trial was conducted in 2008 with Etanercept .Seventeen patients partecipated in the study. The primary outcome was that the patients were able to stop the corticosteroid therapy and still keep the disease under control for over one year. After 12 months 50% of the patients in the Etanercept group and 22,2% in the placebo group were able to keep the disease under control without corticosteroid therapy (p value not significant) (Martinez-Toboada et al, 2008). Adalimumab, a fully humanized monoclonal antibody directed against TNF, was successfully used only in one case of giant cell arteritis refractory to steroid therapy (Ahmed et al, 2007) . There are also two isolated reports of new-onset giant cell arteritis in patients receiving etanercept and adalimumab associated with methotrexate for rheumatoid arthritis (Leydet-Quilici 2007; Seton, 2004). Finally a single report has described successful in treating giant cell arteritis with Rituximab combined with cyclophosphamide (Bhatia et al, 2005).

2.2 Takayasu's arteritis

Takayasu's arteritis is an idiopathic systemic granulomatosis disease of the large and medium-sized vessels that may lead to segmental stenosis, occlusion, dilatation and/or aneurysm formation in the aorta and/or its main branches. Coronary and polmonary arteries may also be affected. Takayasu's arteritis is characterized by the formation of granuloma on vessel walls and several proinflammatory cytokines, including TNF are associated with the development of granuloma (Park et al, 20). It is therefore reasonable to consider that TNF inhibition might be useful in the therapy of Takayasu's arteritis. The first case series were conducted by Hoffman in 2004. Fifteen patients with active relapsing Takayasu's arteritis were selected. Seven received etanercept, (later the medication was changed to infliximab for 3 patients) and eight received infliximab. Ten of the 15 patients went into complete remission that was sustained for 1 to 3.3 years without steroid therapy. Four patients achieved partial remission with a reduction in the glucocorticoid therapy > 50%, whereas therapy failed for only 1 patient. For 9 of the 14 respondents,an increase in the anti TNF dosage (up to 10 mg/Kg for infliximab and 50 mg 2/weekly for etanercept) was required to sustain remission. Two relapse occurred during periods when the therapy was interrupted (both with etanercept) but the patients re established full remission upon re introduction of the therapy. (Hoffman et al 2004). Since the first initial studies of the use of antiTNF therapy in the treatment of Takayasu's arteritis, the successful use of this therapy has been reported by multiple investigators (Calderon, 2010; Della Rossa, 2005; Jolly, 2005; Karageorgaki, 2007; Maffei, 2009; Tanaka, 2006; Tato, 2005) . The largest sample of studies examined 25 patients with active relapsing Takayasu' s arteritis treated with infliximab (21 pts) or etanercept (9 pts, later therapy was changed to infliximab for 5 pts) and followed them for a median of 28 months. Four of the 9 patients initially treated with etanercept enjoyed a complete remission and 2 experienced partial remission. Of the 6 patients who achieved remission 3 relapsed. Of the 21 patients treated with infliximab (including the 5 previously treated with etanercept) 12 achieved complete remission and 6 patients went into partial remission. Three patient discontinued infliximab; 12 of the remaining 18 patients relapsed and required treatment with a higher dose of infliximab administered at shorter intervals (Molloy et al, 2008). These studies suggest that anti TNF therapy may provide long term remission for patients with refractory Takayasu's arteritis and thus justify a randomized controlled clinical trial. Lastly it was also reported that treatment using Tocilizumab, a humanized anti interleukin-6-receptor antibody in a patient with refractory Takayasu's arteritis was successful (Nishimoto et al, 2008)

3. Medium vessel arteritis

3.1 Polyarteritis nodosa

Polyarteritis nodosa is a necrotizing vasculitis that affects small and medium-size arteries and affects patients of all ages. Standard treatment with corticosteroids and cyclophosphamide has drammatically improved the prognosis but medication induced morbidity is frequent. The successful use of anti TNF therapy in treating adult and chilhood systemic or cutaneous PAN has been reported in several papers (Al-Bishri J et al, 2005; Brik R et al, 2007; de Kort AWK et al, 2006; Feinstein J et al,2005; Garcia-Porrua et al, 2003; Vega Gutierrez J et al, 2007; Wahezi DM et al, 2010; Wu K et al, 2006**)** The largest study sample was conducted over three years and examined 11 young patients treated with TNF α inhibitors, 8 with Infliximab, (2 later changed the therapy to Adalimumab and Rituximab) and 3 patients were treated with Etanercept The dosage of Infliximab given to patients varied from 3 to 6 mg/Kg and a dose of 0.8 mg/Kg for Etanercept. Side effects appeared in three patients: a *staphylococcus epidermidis* sepsis and cerebral abscesses following Infliximab therapy and a bowel perforation a month after starting Etanercept. There was a significant reduction in the median daily prednisolone requirement and a reduction of ESR and PCR (Eleftheriou D et al, 2009). Therefore, biologic therapy represents an effective treatment option for patients with Polyarteritis nodosa-resistant vasculitis. Lastly, in 2008 a case of cutaneous corticosteroid and immunosuppressive-resistant Polyarteritis nodosa in a 47 year old man was successfully treated by Rituximab (Sonomoto K et al, 2008).

4. Small vessels arteritis

4.1 ANCA-associated vasculitis

The antineutrophil cytoplasmic antibody (ANCA) associated systemic vasculitis is a group of multisystemic diseases predominantly characterized by small vessel vasculitis and the occurrence of ANCA in most but not all cases. These diseases include Wegener's granulomatosis, microscopic polyangiitis, renal-limited vasculitis and Churg-Strauss angiitis. Despite significant progress in managing these diseases there are no satisfactory treatment options for patients suffering either refractory or frequently relapsing disease. These patients moreover are a high risk of cumulative toxicity from the medications. Recent advances in biological therapy has helped to establish new options for patients that are resistant to conventional treatment

4.1.1 Anti TNFα inhibitors

Little is know regarding the efficacy of anti TNF therapy in treating microscopic polyangiitis and Churg-Strauss Syndrome (Arbach et al 2002, Josselin L et al 2008) A TNF blocker was tested specifically on patients with Wegener's granulomatosis. In the Wegener's granulomatosis etanercept trial (WGET), a multi-center, placebo controlled trial, 180 patients were randomized to receive adjunctive therapy with etanercept versus placebo, in addition to standard care immunosuppression (with cyclophosphamide or methotrexate). There were no differences in remission rates and time to remission at the end of follow-up (after 27 months) between the two groups (69.7 vs 75.3% p=0.39). In addition,there were no observed differences in the relative risk of disease flares up between the two groups (p= 0.54). Six solid tumors developed in patients in the etanercept group, whereas none were observed in the placebo group (p=0.01) with a standardized incidence ratio (SIR) of 3.12 (95% CI 1.15-6.80) (Wegener's granulomatosis etanercept trial, 2005) Additional follow-up of 140 partecipants in the WGET showed that this increased risk of developing solid tumor malignancies in the etanercept group persisted 3.5 years following the conclusion of the study (SIR 4.4 p= 0.01) (Chung S & Seo, 2009). A potential explanation of these surprising negative results might be that Etanercept is not effective in inflammatory granulomatosis diseases. In fact, Etanercept is not effective in treating Crohn disease and sarcoidosis which are both characterized by granulomatous inflammation (Sandborn et al, 2001). Four case series and a prospective open-label trial have been published describing the use of Infliximab in Wegener's granulomatosis (Table I). Infliximab use has been reported in 51 patients with Wegener's granulomatosis. All patients were treated with doses between 3 mg/Kg and 5 mg/Kg at a frequency of one to two monthly i.v injections. Except for 1 trial, all the patients continued standard therapy for systemic vasculitis. The Bartolucci group stopped all immunosuppressants (apart from steroids) when they commenced infliximab and the drugs were reintroduced on day 42. The cohort of patient partecipating in the study was mixed and included new cases, relapse and persistent disease cases. In the Booth's group, patients were divided into two groups, new patients and persistent disease patients. The patients with persistent disease who benefited from infliximab continued on the medication for a total of one year. All others, including all patients in the new arm received infliximab for only 10 weeks. In the other trials Infliximab was administered for three to six month Fourty-five out of 51 patients (88.23%) experienced remission, partial or complete. Relapse occurred in 7 patients (13.72%), 4 out of these 7 patients were still receiving anti TNFα blocker drugs. Side effects were reported in 9 patients (17,64%): 2 patients died one for diffuse pulmonary hemorrhage attribuited to pulmonary vasculitis and the other from bronchopneumonia However, these two patients had MPO-ANCA related renal vasculitis rather than Wegener's granulomatosis. Seven patients had severe infections, 1 suffering from *Haemophilis influenzae* pneumonia, 1 with recurrent *Klebsiella* urinary tract infections, 2 patients with recurrent *St. aureus* skin abscesses, 1 has an uncharacterized diarrheal illness and 1 had *Nocardia* endophtalmitis requiring evisceration of the eye. All the patients also received prednisolone and immunosuppressive therapy (Bartolucci 2002; Booth 2002, 2004; Josselin, 2008; Lamprecht P 2002). These studies suggest that Infliximab, in conjunction with steroid and immunosuppressive agents, appears to be effective for inducing remission in ANCA associated vasculitis or in the treatment of refractory forms. Careful attention must be given concerning the increased risk of serious infection. Nevertheless the use of Infliximab in treating vasculitis must await until corroboration from larger controlled studies and should not be used as first line therapy, but after a review of the risk and benefits of the therapy, considered in the treatment of refractory disease.

4.1.2 Rituximab

Use of Rituximab in treating refractory or relapsing ANCA-associated vasculitis has been tested via case reports, case series and also prospective open-label trials, retrospective study and open label randomized trial. In case series study of refractory/relapsing Wegener's granulomatosis patients, Rituximab therapy was introduced adjunct to ongoing therapy and within a 7 to 36 month follow-up, there a complete remission. Eight case series with 110 patients were reported (87 affected by WG, 14 affected by MPA, 5 by CSS and 4 by unclassified vasculitis). Ninety-five patients were ANCA PR3 or MPO positive (86,36%). The Rituximab regimen varied from 375 mg/m^2 i.v weekly x 4 weeks to 500 mg i.v weekly x 4 weeks to 1000 mg i.v given each 2 or 3 weeks or 2 infusions of 750 mg/m^2 given 2 weeks or 1 infusion of 3.2 gm). Tab 1

Study type	Study authors	N° patients	Rituximab regimen	Patients outcomes
8 case series	Omdal, Gottemborg, Keogh Eriksson, Tamura, Brihave, Jones	45	Mainly 375 mg/m^2 Weekly x 4 weeks	CR= 30-100% PR= 10-30% R=10-60% (6-18 months)
4 prospective open label trials	Keogh, Aries, Stasi, Smith	38	Mainly 375 mg/m^2 Weekly x 4 weeks With or without Immunosuppression	CR=25-100% PR=9-25% R=10-50% (9-24 months)
2 open label randomized trial	Jones, Stone	142	375 mg/m^2 weekly X 4 weeks	CR= 63-91% R=3-6% (median 12 months)

CR= complete remission; PR= partial remission; R= relapse

Table 1. Rituximab use in ANCA associated vasculitis

Seventy-six out 110 patients went into full remission (69.09%), 18 patients went into partial remission (16,36%), and no response occurred for 4 patients (3,63%). Of the 76 patients who went into full remission, 38 of these (50%) experienced relapse, not always associated with ANCA positivity or a rise in ANCA levels. Fifty-seven serious side effects were observed and 1 patient died for adenoviral pneumonitis; the lung infection developed after several immunosuppressive therapy were administered before Rituximab treatment and after the addition of anti TNF-α drug (Adalimumab). (Brihaye, 2007; Eriksson, 2005; Gottemberg, 2005, Keogh, 2005; Jones, 2009; Omdal; 2005 Seo, 2008; Tamura, 2006). In 2006, four prospective open-label trial were published. The treatment protocol included administering Rituximab in doses of 375 mg/m^2 i.v. every 4 weeks x 4 doses. In two of four trials, Rituximab was used alone without the introduction of other immunosuppressive drugs (Keogh et al, 2006, Stasi et al, 2006). Thirty out of 39 patients went into complete remission (76.92% of total patients), partial remission were observed in 3 of the 39 patients (7.69%) and complete failure of treatment was measured in 6 out of 31 (15.38%). Ten patients relapsed between 9 to 24 months and all of these were re-treated with rituximab risulting in a new sustained response in all the patients. (Aries, 2006; Keogh, 2006; Smith, 2006; Stasi, 2006). Circulating B-cells were monitored and it was noted that they rapidly became undetectable after the treatment. However, in the majority of patients, B-cells gradually returned after 6 to 9 months, although some patients maintained very low levels of the cells for a long time. A relationship between relapse and re-appearance of the B cell population has been put forth, but clinical data shows that relapses are not always associated with the return of circulating B cells and in turn, B-cell re-appearance is not always followed by a relapse. Finally, two pivotal studies, whose results have been recently published in NEJM, were carried out in order to determine the real efficacy of anti B-lymphocyte therapy compared with cyclophosphamide in the induction phase of treatment of ANCA-associated vasculitis. Jones et al reported on the results of a open-label, two group, parallel design, multi-center randomized trial of Rituximab versus Cyclophosphamide treatment involving 44 patients affected by ANCA-associated renal vasculitis. (RITUXIVAS). Patients who were randomly assigned to the Rituximab group also received at least two doses of intravenous cyclophosphamide at a dose of 15 mg per kilogram along with the first and the third Rituximab infusion and not receive azathioprine to maintain remission. Patients in the control group received a validated regimen of intravenous cyclophosphamide for 3 to 6 months followed by azathioprine. Sustained remission was achieved in 25 of 33 patients in the Rituximab group (76%) and 9 of 11 patients in the control group (82%). Six patients in the rituximab group and 1 patient in the control group died within the first 12 months. Three patients did not achieve a sustained remission. The median time it took for remission of symtoms was 90 days in the rituximab group and 94 days in the control group (P= 0.87). A total of 31 severe side effects occurred in 14 of the 33 patients in the Rituximab group (42%) and 12 severe side effects occurred in 4 of the 11 patients in the control group (36%). Incidence rates for severe side effects were 1.00 per patient-year in the Rituximab group (95% CI. 069 to 1.44) and 1.10 per patient-year in the control group (95% CI, 0.61 to 1.99 P=0.77). The frequency of infections was 36% in the Rituximab group and 27% in the control group (Jones et al, 2010). A second multi-center randomized, duoble blind trial of Rituximab treatment compared with cyclophosphamide was reported by Stone (RAVE). One hundred and ninety-seven ANCA-positive patients with Wegener's granulomatosis or micropolyangiitis were enrolled in the study. Patients assigned to the Rituximab group did not receive any cyclophosphamide treatment while patients in the control group received oral cyclophosphamide (2 mg per Kilogram of body weight adjusted for renal insufficiency). When they went into remission, usually between 3 to 6 months later, they were eligible to switch from cyclophosphamide to azathioprine (2 mg per Kilogram per day). Sixty-three of the 99 patients in the Rituximab group (64%) and 52 the 98 patients in the control group (53%) achieved remission and stopped steroid therapy (P=0.09). Among patients with relapsing disease at baseline Rituximab was more efficacious than cyclophosphamide (respectively 67% and 42% achieved remission). Fourteen patients in the Rituximab group (14%) and 17 in the control group (17%) had side effects that lead to a discontinuation of the treatment. Two patients in the control group and 1 patient in the Rituximab group died. During the first 6 months of the trial, a malignant tumor was diagnosed in one patient in each group; but after 6 months 5 malignant tumour developed in the patients, four in the Rituximab group and one receiving cyclophosphamide treatment (Stone et al, 2010). Therefore similar conclusion are reached in the two studies. Both trial showed that rituximab was effective in inducing remission but unfortunately the rate of side effects was the same for the Rituximab and cyclophosphamide groups (RAVE trial). Similarly in the RITUXIVAS study, 6 of the 33 patients in the Rituximab group died as well as 2 of 11 patients in the control group. Moreover the RAVE trial also demonstrated an un-expected elevated number of malignant tumour appearing over a relatively short treatment period. Therefore Rituximab might be considered as an option for first-line therapy and the induction of remission of ANCA-associated vasculitis. It is still unclear if anti-B-cell therapy might alter the immunopathogenetic process, permitting the discontinuation or reduction of therapy (steroids and immunosuppressants) to maintain remission

5. Cryoglobulinemic vasculitis

Cryoglobulins are cold-precipitable monoclonal or polyclonal immunoglobulins that can occur in conjunction with a variety of other diseases, including plasmacell or lymphoid neoplasms, chronic infection and inflammatory disease. Three subtypes of crioglobulins can be identified using immunochemical analysi. Type I crioglobulins are single monoclonal immunoglobulins (most commonly monoclonal IgM) ad are almost exclusively associated with malignant hematologic disorder. Type 2 cryoglobulins consist of polyclonal IgG with monoclonal IgM with rheumatoid factor activity.Type 3 are polyclonal IgG and polyclonal IgM with rheumatoid factor activity. Since the discovery of the hepatitis C virus (HCV) it has been demonstrated that the majority of cases of cryoglobulinemia are related to HCV infection (Cacoub & Saadoun, 2008). In mixed cryoglobulin HCV- related vasculitis, a combined therapy of interferon-alpha (IFN-α) and ribavirin provide the best opportunity for improvement but long term resolution of symptoms is limited to patients who have a sustained virologic response (Saadoun et al, 2008). In addition, the therapy is often not tolerated or controindicated. Plasmapheresis is not applicable for long term management and immunosuppressant agents (Cyclophosphamide, Azathioprine, Methotrexate) have been used but, mostly type 2 cryoglobulinemia vasculitis treated with Rituximab. No randomized controlled trials have been carried out. Nine uncontrolled studies with patients samples ranging from 5 to 23 patients have been reported while the other patients came from case reports (Bryce,2006; Cavallo, 2009; Quartuccio, 2006; Roccatello, 2008; Saadoum, 2008; Sansonno, 2003; Sene, 2009; Terrier, 2010; Visenti, 2007; Zaja, 2003). In most of the studies, Rituximab was administered at the dose of 375 mg/m^2 weekly for 4 weeks, sometimes followed by two extra infusion at 1 and 2 months, but also in higher amounts (two 1,000 mg-Rituximab infusion at days 1 and 15) and a lower dose (250 mg/m^2 at days 1 and 8). As reported by Sen, the higher dose seems to be correlated with a higher risk of side effects. Three patients developed severe systemic reactions after the first infusion of 1,000 mg. Two patients developed a typical serum sickness syndrome with accompanying fever, arthralgia, purpura and increased of serum parameters of inflammation 7 and 9 days after the infusion. The final outcome was a spontaneous resolution in one patient and the other developed cardiac and kidney problems that required steroid treatment. In vitro immunochemical assays showed that Rituximab formed a complex with the cryoprecipitating IgMκ that had rheumatoid factor activity and the in vitro addition of Rituximab to serum containig rheumatoid factor-positive IgMκ tipe II mixed cryoglobulin was associated with visibly accelerated cryoprecipitation. The author suggested that Rituximab should be administrated with caution in patients with cryoglobulinemic type II vasculitis with high levels of cryoglobulins and low C4 levels and that the 375 mg protocol is preferred (Sene, 2009). The most reported clinical manifestation of vasculitis is neuropathy and skin involvement. A complete remission from symtoms was seen in 87 patients (53%); a total of 31 (18.90%) had partially responded to treatment and 20 (12.19%) did not respond to treatment at all. A significant reduction in levels of rheumatoid factor, cryoglobulins and IgM was reported after Rituximab therapy. Overall, 38 (23.17%) out of 164 patients treated with Rituximab reported side effects. In addition to serum sickness and severe flares of vasculitis, the other side effects reported included a thrombosis of the retinal artery, the development of cold agglutinin disease and serious infectious complications. After the treatment with Rituximab, death was reported in 9 cases, 3 from liver carcinoma, one patient died of cirrhosis, one had a vasculitis relapse, one died of multiple organ failure due to cold agglutinin disease, another patient died from *Cryptococcus neoformans* menigoencephalitis, one patient died of septic shock after an intestinal perforation and the last died of an unknown cause. Skin manifestations and arthralgias frequently responded well to treatment with Rituximab, whereas symptoms of neuropathy and renal involvement were more resistant to treatment. Clinical relapse occurred in 20% to 50% of the patients, 12 to 14 months following the Rituximab administration. Most of the patients responded well to a 2nd course of the drug therapy (Terrier et al, 2010). As demonstrated by Saadoun in a prospective cohort study of 38 patients who received a combination of Rituximab (375 mg/m^2) once a week for 1 month, followed by Peg-IFN-α (180 μg/week or 1.5 μg/Kg/week) plus ribavirin (600-1200 mg) daily, as compared with 55 patients treated by Peg-IFN-α/ribavirin with the same modalities the combination of Rituximab plus Peg-interferon-α/ribavirin seems to be more effective than Peg-IFN/ribavirin in treating HCV-associated cryoglobulinemic vasculitis. Out of the entire patients population, a complete clinical response was achieved in 73.1% of patients, cryoglobulin clearance in 52.7% of patients and a sustained virologic response in 59.1% of patients. Compared with Peg-IFN-α/ribavirin Rituximab plus Peg-IFN-α/ribavirin-treated patients had a shorter clinical response time, better renal response rates and a higher rates of cryoglobulin clearance. Seventeen patients (18.3%) experienced relapse, including 10 patients treated with Peg-IFN-α/ribavirin and 7 with Rituximab with Peg-IFN-α/ribavirin. Treatment was well tolerated with 11% of patients (distribuited equally bertween the two group) discontinuing therapy and no worsenig of HCV RNA under Rituximab was observed (Saadoun, et al, 2010) Finally the efficacy of Rituximab therapy in treating 19 patients with HCV-associated mixed cryoglobulinemi and severe liver disease was reported. Fifteen of 19 patients had liver cirrhosis with ascitic decompensation in 6 cases. Rituximab was administered at a dose of 375 mg/m2 body surface area once a week over a 1 month period. A complete relief from the symptoms of mixed cryoglobulinemia (purpura, arthralgia, leg ulcers, paresthesias) was observed in 12 patients and partial relief in 7 patients. Complete cryocrit negativization was observed in 9 patients, a cryocrit decrease greater than 50% was evaluated in 2 patients, and in 3 patients there was a decrease of cryocrit between 25% and 50%, whereas in 5 patients no consistent cryocrit reduction was shown. An improvement of hepatic function and an impressive reduction in the degree of ascites in patients with liver cirrhosis was observed in most patients with advances disease. A transient increase of viremia was also observed (Petrarca et al, 2010) As a single agent, Rituximab seems to be a safe and effective therapy for treating patients with cryoglobulinemic vasculitis. However it is not a curative treatment. The combination therapy with Peg-IFN-α/ribavirin seems to be more effective than Peg-IFN-α/ribavirin since this combination synergizes the immunologic effect of antiviral therapy.

6. Behçet disease

Behçet disease is a multisystemic chronic-relapsing inflammatory disorders classified among the vasculitis that presents clinical features of mucocutaneous lesions and ocular, vascular, articular, gastrointestinal, urogenital, pulmonary and neurologic involvement. Some evidences suggests that TNF-α plays a critical role in the pathogenesis of the disease. In seven open label, prospective self controlled studies patients with ocular manifestations that were unresponsive to standard immunosuppressive treatment were given infliximab i.v. infusion. Infliximab was given alone or in addition to the previous treatment (mostly prednisone, azathioprine and cyclosporin) at a dose of 5 mg/Kg. Time of treatment varied: a single infusion (Skikakis et al, 2004) , 2 infusions (Al- Rayes et al, 2008), at time 0, 2 and 4 and then every 6-8 weeks (Tognon, et al, 2007) at time 0, 2, 6, 10 weeks (Ohno et al, 2004), 0, 2, 6, 14 weeks (Tugal-Tutkun et al 2005) , 0, 2, and 6 weeks and monthly for ad additional 4-6 months and every 8 weeks thereafter (El-Asrar 2005; Accorinti, 2007) The follow-up period was from 1 month to 36 months. Complete remission of uveitis was achieved in 59 out of 78 patients (75.64%). Adalimumab it also reported to be an effective drug alternative that improved visual acuity in a case series of 11 male patients (Bawazeer & Raffa, 2010).In addition to the aforementioned studies, many small case series and case reports suggest that patients with mucocutaneous lesions, gastrointestinal symptoms and arthritis exhibit a rapid and sustained responses to infliximab therapy (Sfikakis et al, 2007). Recently a case series of 6 patients with intestinal involvement was reported by Naganuma. All patient were steroid-dependent and refractory to immunosuppressants. The drug infusion schedule was 5 mg/kg body weight at 0,2 and 6 weeks and every 8 weeks thereafter. Four patients went into remission and all of the aforementioned mantained this state for up to 3 years. Two patients with ileal ulceration required surgery. Infliximab has also been utilized to treat parenchymal central nervous system involvement.with a favorably outcome (Pipitone et al, 2008). The first controlled study of anti TNF-α treatment was conducted with etanercept. In a double-blind, placebo-controlled study of 40 male patients, the authors reported that etanercept, administered at a dose of 25 mg twice a week for 4 week is effective in suppressing oral ulcers and nodular and papulopustular lesions. No differences was observed in regards to pathergy test, genital ulcers and arthritis (Melikoglu et al, 2005). A recent position paper concluded that infliximab is recommended as first line treatment option for patients with bilateral posterior uveitis or with unilateral involvement with visual acuity < 0.2 because the fast onset of response is critical in preventing fixed retinal lesions and permanent visual loss. In patients with SNC, intestinal, mucocutaneous manifestations or arthritis infliximab can be used as an add-on therapy for severe manifestations or refractory illness or used in treating patients that are intolerant to traditional immunosuppressive regimens (Sfikakis et al, 2007) Tab 2

Subset	TNF inhibitors type	Efficacy
Posterior segment Intraocular inflammation	Infliximab 5 mg/Kg Etanercept 25 mg x 2 weekly Adalimumab 40 mg every 2 weeks	+ + +
Mucocutaneous manifestations - Oral ulcers	Infliximab 3 or 5 mg/Kg Etanercept 25 mg x 2 weeky	+ +
- Genital ulcers	Infliximab 3 or 5 mg/Kg Etanercept 25 mg x 2 weekly	+ -
-Nodular lesions or psudofollicolitis	Infliximab 3 or 5 mg/Kg Etanercept 25 mg x 2 weekly	+ +
- Skin pathergy	Etanercept 25 mg x 2 weekly	-
Arthritis	Infliximab 3 or 5 mg/Kg Etanercept 25 mg x 2 weekly	+ +/-
Intestinal inflammation	Infliximab 5 mg/Kg	+
Parenchimal CNS involvement	Infliximab 5 mg/Kg	+
Major vessel involvement	Not enough data	

Table 2. Anti TNF agents in Behçet disease

7. Conclusion

The advent of biologic drug therapy to treat systemic vasculitis is the beginning of a new era in which highly toxic immunosuppressive therapy may be replaced by a more sophisticated and targeted approach. However, data from the national arthritis registries demonstrate a higher risk of opportunistic infections in patients treated with these biologic drugs. Moreover, we don't have experiences with the long term consequences of these agents, particularly about the increased risk of malignancy in patients affected by vasculitis. Given the rarity of these diseases, international collaboration will be crucial in defining the future role of these agents in the treatment of vasculitis..

8. References

Accorinti M, Pirraglia MP, Paroli MP, Priori R, Conti F, Pivetti-Pezzi P Infliximab treatment for ocular and extraocular manifestations of Behcet disease. JPN. J. Ophthamol. 2007; 51: 191-96

Ahmed MM, Mubashir E, Hayat S, Fowler M, Berney SM Treatment of recractory temporal arteritis with adalimumab Clin Rheumatol. 2007; 26: 1353-55

Airo P, Antonioli CM, Vianelli M, Toniati P. Antitumor necrosis factor treatment with infliximab in a case of giant cell arteritis resistant to steroid and immunosuppressive drugs. Rheumatology (Oxford) 2002; 41: 347-49

Al Bishri J, Le Riche N, Pope JE. Refractory polyarteritis nodosa successfully treated with infliximab J. Rheumatol 2005; 32: 1371-3

Al-Rayes H, Al-Swailem R, Al-Balawi M, Al-Dohayan N, Al-Zaidi S, Tariq M Safety and efficacy of infliximab therapy in active Behcet's uveitis: an open-label trial. Rheumatol. Int. 2008; 29: 53-57

Andronopoulos AP, Meimaris N, Daoussis D, Bounas A, Giannopoulos G. Experience with infliximab (anti TNF alpha monoclonal antibody) as monotherapy for giant cell arteritis. Ann Rheum Dis 2003; 62: 1116

Arbach O, Gross WL, Gause A. Treatment of refractory Churg-Strauss Syndrome (CSS) by TNF apha blockade. Immunobiology 2002; 206: 496-501

Aries PM, Hellmich B, Voswinkel J, Both M, Nölle B, Holl-Ulrich K, Lamprecht P, Gross WL Lack of efficacy of rituximab in Wegener's granulomatosis with refractory granulomatous manifestations. Ann Rheum Dis. 2006; 65: 853-8

Bader L, Koldingsnes W, Nossent J. B-lymphocyte activating factor levels are increased in patients with Wegener's granulomatosis and inversely correlated with ANCA titer. Clin Rheumatol 2010; 29: 1031-35

Bartolucci P, Ramoelina J, Cohen P, Mahr A, Godmer P, Le Hello C, Guillevin L Efficacy of the anti TNF-α antibody infliximab against refractory systemic vasculitides: an open pilot study on 10 patients. Rheumatology. 2002; 41: 1126-1132

Bawazeer A, Raffa LH. Clinical experience with adalimumab in the treatment of ocular Behcet disease. Ocul. Immunol. Inflamm. 2010; 18: 226-32

Bhatia A, Eli PJ, Edwards JC. Anti CD-20 monoclonal antibody (rituximab) as an adjunct in the treatment of giant cell arteritis Ann Rheum Dis. 2005; 64: 1099-1100

Booth AD, Jefferson HJ, Ayliffe W, Andrews PA; Jayne DR. Safety and efficacy of TNF- α blockade in relapsing vasculitis Ann Rheum Dis. 2002; 61: 559

Booth AD, Almond MK, Burns A, Ellis P, Gaskin G, Neild GH, Plaisance M, Pusey CD, Jayne DR; Pan-Thames Renal Research Group. Outcome of ANCA-associated renal vasculitis: a 5-year retrospective study. Am J Kidney Dis. 2003 Apr;41(4):776-84.

Booth A, Harper L, Hammad T, Bacon P, Griffith M, Levy J, Savage C, Pusey C, Jayne D. Prospective study of TNF- α blockade with infliximab in anti-neutrophil cytoplasmic antibody-associated systemic vasculitis J. AM. Soc. Nephrol. 2004; 15: 717-12

Bougarit A, Le Toumelin P, Pagnoux C, Cohen P, Mahr A, Le Guern V, Mouthon L, Guillevin L Deaths occuring during the first year after treatment onset for Polyarterityis Nodosa, Microscopic Polyangitiis and Churg- Strauss Syndrome. Medicine 2005; 84: 323-30

Brihaye B, Aouba A, Pagnoux C, Cohen P, Lacassin F, Guillevin L. Adjunction of rituximab to steroids and immunosuppressants for refractory/relapsing Wegener's granulomatosis: a study on 8 patients. Clin Exp. Rheumatol. 2007; 25 (1 suppl 44): S23-S27

Brik R, Gepstein V, Shahar E, Goldsher D, Berkowitz D Tumor necrosis factor blockade in the management of children with orphan diseases. Clin Rheumatol 2007; 26: 1783-85

Bryce AH, Dispenzieri A, Kyle RA, Lacy MQ, Rajkumar SV Response to rituximab in patients with type II cryoglobulinemia Clin. Lymphoma Myeloma 2006; 7: 140-44

Cacoub P, Saadoun D Hepatitis C virus infection induced vasculitis. Clin Rev Allergy Immunol 2008; 35: 30-9

Calderon R, Estrada S, Ramirez del la Piscina P, Salvador M, Zabaleta S, Enciso C, Delgado E, Garcia-Campos F Infliximab therapy in a patient with refractory ileocolic Crohn' s disease and Takayasu arteritis Rev Esp Enferm Dig. 2010; 102: 145-6

Cantini F, Niccoli L, Salvarani C, Padula A, Olivieri I. Treatment of longstanding active giant cell arteritis with infliximab: report of four cases. Arthritis Rheum 2001; 44: 2933-2935

Cavallo R, Roccatello D, Menegatti E, Naretto C, Napoli F, Baldovino S. Rituximab in cryoglobulinemic peripheral neuropathy J. Neurol 2009; 256: 1076-82

Chung SA, Seo P. Advances in the use of biologic agents for the treatment of systemic vasculitis. Curr. Opin. Rheumatol 2009; 21: 3-9

De Kort SWK, van Rossum MAJ, Ten Cate R. Infliximab in a child with therapy resistant systemic vasculitis Clin Rheumatol 2006; 25: 769-771

Della Rossa A, Tavoni A, Merlini G, Baldini C, Sebastiani M, Lombardi M, Neglia D, Bombardieri S. Two Takayasu arteritis patients successfully treated with infliximab: a potential disease-modifyng agent? Rheumatology. 2005; 44: 1074-75

El Asrar, AMA, Abboud EB, Aldihbni H, Al-Arfaj A. Long-term safety and efficicacy of infliximab therapy in refractory uveitis due to Behcet disease. Int. Ophthamol. 2005; 26: 83-92

Eleftheroiou D, Melo M, Marks SD, Tullus K, Sills J, Cleary G, Dolezalova P, Ozen S, Plikington C, Woo P, Klein N, Dillon MJ Brogan PA Biologic therapy in primary systemic vasculitis of the young. Rheumatology 2009; 48: 978-86

Eriksson P. Nine patients with antineutrophil cytoplasmic antobody-positive vasculitis successfully treated with rituximab J Int. Med. 2005; 257: 540-8

Feinstein J, Arroyo R. Successful treatment of chilhood onset refractory polyarteritis nodosa with tumor necrosis factor alpha blockade. J Clin Rheumatol. 2005; 11: 219-22

Feldmann M, Pusey CD. Is there a role for TNF-α in anti-neutrophil cytoplasmic antibody-associated vasculitis?. Lessons from other chronic inflammatory diseases. J Am Soc. Nephrol. 2006; 17: 1243-52

Garcia-Porrua C, Gonzalez-Gay MA. Successfull treatment to infliximab in a patient with undifferentiated spondyloarthropathy coexisting with polyarteritis nodosa-like cutaneous vasculitis. Clin. Exp. Rheumatol. 2003; 21: S138

Grillo-Lopez AJ, White CA, Dallaire BK, Varns CL, Shen CD, Wei A, Leonard JE, McClure A, Weaver R, Cairelli S, Rosenberg J.Rituximab: the first monoclonal antibody approved for the treatment of lymphoma. Curr. Pharm Biotechonol 2000; 1: 1-9

Gross WL Immunopathology and new therapeutic considerations in ANCA- associated vasculitis. Autoimmun. Rev. 2004; 3: S47-S48

Gottemberg JE, Guillevin L, Lambotte O, Combe B, Allanore Y, Cantagrel A, Larroche C, Soubrier M, Bouillet L, Dougados M, Fain O, Farge D, Kyndt X, Lortholary O, Masson C, Moura B, Thomas T, Wendling D, Anaya JM, Sibilia J, Mariette X. Tolerance and short term efficacy of rituximab in 43 patients with systemic autoimmune diseases. Ann Rheum Dis. 2005; 64: 913-20

Gurcan HM, Keskin DB, Stern JNH, Nitzberg MA, Shekani H, Ahmed AR A review of the current use of rituximab in autoimmune diseases. Intern immunopharm. 2009; 9: 10-25

Halbwachs-Mecarelli L, Bessou G, Lesavre P, Lopez S, Witko-Sarsat V Bimodal distribution of proteinase 3 (PR3) surface expression reflects a costitutive heterogeneity in the polimorphonuclear neutrophil pool FEBS letter 1995; 374: 29-33

Harris DP, Haynes L, Sayles PC, Duso DK, Eaton SM, Lepak NM, Johnson LL, Swain SL, Lund FE. .Reciprocal regulation of polarized cytokine production by effector B and T cells. Nat. Immunol. 2000; 1: 475-82

Hernandez-Rodriguez J, Segarra M, Vilardell C, Sanchez M, Garcia-Martinez A, Esteban MJ, Queralt C, Grau JM, Urbano-Marquez A, Palacin A, Colomer D, Cid M.C. Tissue production of pro-inflammatory cytokines (IL-1b, TNF α and IL-6) correlates with the intensity of the systemic inflammatory response and with corticosteroid requirements in giant-cell arteritis Rheumatology 2004;43:294–301

Hiemstra TF, Jayne DR. Newer therapies for vasculitis Best Pract. Res Clin Rheumatol. 2009; 23: 379-389

Huugen D, Xiao H, van Esch A, Falk RJ, Peutz-Kootstra CJ, Buurman WA, Tervaert JW, Jennette JC, Heeringa P. Aggravation of antimyeloperoxidase antibody-induced glomerulonephritis by bacterial lipopolysaccharide: role of tumor necrosis factor-α Am J Pathol 2005; 167:47-58

Huugen D, van Esch A, Xiao H, Peutz,- Koostra CJ, Buurman WA, Tervaert JW, Jennette JC, Heeringa P. Inhibition of complement factor C3 protects against antimyeloperoxidase antibody-induced glomerulonephritis in mice Kidney Int. 2007;71: 646-654

Hoffman GS, Merkel PA, Brasington RD, Lenschow DJ, Liang P. Anti-tumor necrosis factor therapy in patients with difficult to treat Takayasu arteritis. Arthiritis Rheum. 2004; 50: 2296-2304

Hoffman GS, Cid MC, Rendt-Zagar K, Merkel PA, Weyand CM, Stone JH, Salvarani C, Xu W, Visvanathan S, Rahman MU. Infliximab for mainenance of glucocorticoid-induced remission of giant cell arteritis. Ann Int Med. 2007; 146: 621-630

Jennette JC, Falk RJ, Andrassy K, Bacon PA, Churg J, Gross WL, Hagen EC, Hoffman GS, Hunder GG, Kallenberg CG, et al Nomenclature of systemic vasculitides. Proposal of an international consensus conference. Arthritis Rheum 1994; 37: 310-392

Jones RB, Ferraro AJ, Chaudhry AN, Brogan P, Salama AD, Smith KGC, Savage COS, Jayne DRW. A multicenter survey of rituximab therapy for refractory antineutrophil cytoplasmic antibody-associated vasculitis. Arthritis. Rheum.. 2009; 60: 2156-68

Jones RB, Tervaert JWC, Hauser T, Luqmani R, Morgan MD, Peh CA, Savage CO, Segelmark M, Tesar V, van Passen P, Walsh D, Walsh M, Westman K, Jayne DRW. Rituximab versus cyclophosphamide in ANCA-associated renal vasculitis. NEJM 2010; 363: 211-20

Jolly M, Curran JJ Infliximab responsive uveitis and vasculitis in a patient with Takayasu arteritis. J. Clin. Rheumatol. 2005; 11: 213-5

Josselin L, Mahr A, Cohen P, Pagnoux C, Guaydler-Souquieres G, Hayem G, Job-Deslandre C, Liferman F, Pourrat J, Guillevin L. Infliximab efficacy and safety against refractory systemic necrotising vasculitides: long-term follow-up of 15 patients. Ann Rheum Dis. 2008; 67: 1434-6

Kain R, Exner M, Ziebermayr R, Cunningham D, Alderson CA, Davidovits A, Raab I, Jahn R, Ashour O, Spitzauer S, Sunder-Plassmann G, Fukuda M, Klemm P, Rees AJ, Kerjasiski D. Molecular mimicry in pauci-immune focal necrotizing glomerulonephritis Nat Med 2008; 14: 1088-1096

Kallemberg CGM Pathogenesis of PR3 ANCA-associated vasculitis J Autoimmun. 2008; 30: 29-36

Karageorgaki ZT, Mavragani CP, Papathanasiou MA, Skopouli FN Infliximab in Takayasu arteritis. A safe alternative? Clin Rheumatol 2007; 26: 984-7

Keogh KA, Wylam ME, Stone JH, Specks U. Induction of remission by B lymphocyte depletion in eleven patients with refractory antineutrophil cytoplasmic antibody-associated vasculitis. Arthritis Rheum. 2005; 52: 262-8

Keogh KA, Yttemberg SR, Fervenza FC, Carlson KA, Schroeder DR, Specks U. Rituximab for refractory Wegener's granulomatosis. Am J Respir Crit Care Med. 2006; 173: 180-7

Krumboltz M, Specks U, Wick M, Kalled SL, Jenne D, Meinl E. BAFF is elevated in serum of patients with Wegener's granulomatosis. J. Autoimmun. 2005; 25: 298-302

Lamprecht P, Voswinkel J, Lilienthal T, Nolle B, Heller M, Gross WL, Gause A. Effectiveness of TNF-α blockade with infliximab in refractory Wegener's granulomatosis. Rheumatology 2002; 41: 1303-07

Leydet-Quilici H, Luc M, Armingeat T, Pham T, Lafforgue P. Giant cell arteritis during adalimumab treatment for rheumatoid arthritis. Joint Bone Spain 2007; 74: 303-4

Little MA, Smyth CL, Yadav R, Ambrose L, Cook HT, Nourshargh S, Pusey CD. Antineutrophil cytoplasm antibodies directed against myeloperoxidase augment leucocyte-microvascular interactions in vivo. Blood 2005; 106: 2050-58

Ly K-H, Regent A, Tamby MC, Mouthon L. Pathogenesis of giant cell arteritis: more than just an inflammatory conditions? Autoimmunity Rev. 2010; 9: 635-45

Mackay F, Schneider P, Rennert P, Browing J. BAFF and APRIL: a tutorial on B cell survival. Ann Rev Immunol. 2003; 21: 231-264

Maffei S, Di Rienzo M, Santoro S, Puccetti L, Pasqui AL. Refractory Takayasu arteritis successfully treated with infliximab. Eur. Rev Med Pharmacol. Sci. 2009; 13: 63-65

Martinez-Toboada VM, Rodriguez-Valverde V, Carreño L, Lopez-Longo J, Figueroa M, Belzunegui J, Mola EM, Bonilla G A double-blind placebo controlled trial of etanercept in patients with giant cell arteritis and corticosteroid side effects. Ann. Rheum Dis. 2008; 67: 625-30

Mease PJ B-cell-targeted therapy in autoimmune disease: rationale, mechanisms and clinical application. J Rheumatol. 2008; 35: 1245-55

Melikoglu M, Fresko I, Mat C, Ozyagan Y, Gogus F, Yurdakul S, Hamuryudan V, Yacizi H. Short term of etanercept in Behcet disease: a double-blind, placebo controlled study. J. Rheumatol. 2005; 32: 98-105

Molloy ES, Langford CA, Clark TM, Gota CE, Hoffmann GS Anti tumor necrosis factor therapy in patients with refractory Takayasu arteritis: long term follow-up. Ann Rheum Dis. 2008; 67: 1567-9

Naganuma M, Sakuraba A, Hisamatsu T, Ochiai H, Hasegawa H, Ogata H, Iwao Y, Hibi T. Efficacy of Infliximab for reduction and manteinance of remission in intestinal Behcet disease. Inflamm Bowel Dis. 2008; 14: 1259-64

Nishimoto N, Nakahara H, Yoshio-Hoshino N, Mima T. Successfull treatment of a patient with Takayasu arteritis using a humanized anti-interleukin 6-receptor antibody Arthritis Rheum 2008; 58: 1197-1200

Noris M, Daina E, Gamba S, Bonazzola S, Remuzzi G Interleukin-6 and RANTES in Takayasu arteritis: a guide for therapeutic decisions?. Circulation 1999; 100: 55-60

Noronha IL, Kruger C, Andrassy K, Ritz E, Waldherr R. In situ production of TNF-α IL-1b, and IL-2R in ANCA positive glomerulonephritis. Kidney Int. 1993; 43: 682-692

Omdal R, Wildhagen K, Hansen T, Gunnarsson R, Kristoffersen G. Anti CD-20 therapy of treatment-resistant Wegener's granulomatosis: favourable but temporary response Scand J Rheumatol. 2005; 34: 229-32

Ohno S, Nakamura S, Hori S, Shimakawa M, Kawashima H, Mochizuki M, Sugita S, Ueno S, Yoshizaki K, Inaba G. Efficacy, safety and pharmacokinetics of multiple administration of infliximab in Behcet disease with refractory uveoretinitis. J. Rheumatol. 2004; 31: 1362-68

Park MC, Lee SW, Park YB, Lee SK: Serum citokines profiles and their correlations with disease activity in Takayasu's arteritis Rheumatology 2006; 45: 545-8

Petrarca A, Rigacci L, Caini P, Colagrande S, Romagnoli P, Vizzuti F, Arena U, Giannini C, Monti M, Montalto P, Matucci-Cerinic M, Bosi A, Laffi G, Zignego AL Safety and efficacy of rituximab in patients with hepatitis C-virus related mixed cryoglobulinemia and severe liver disease. Blood. 2010; 116: 335-34

Pfister H, Ollert M, Frohlich LF, Quintanilla-Martinez L, Colby TV, Specks U, Jenne D. Antineutrophil cytoplasmic autoantibodies against the murine homolog of proteinase 3 (Wegener autoantigen) are pathogenetic in vivo Blood 2004; 104: 1411-18

Pipitone N, Olivieri I, Padula A, D'Angelo S, Nigro A, Zuccoli G, Boiardi L, Salvarani C. Infliximab for the treatment of neuro-Behcet's disease: a case series and review of the literature. Arthritis Rheum. 2008; 59: 285-290

Pistoia V. Production of cytokines by B cell in health and disease. Immunol. Today 1997; 18: 343-50

Quartuccio L, Soardo G, Romano G, Zaja F, Scott, CA, De Marchi G, Fabris M, Ferraccioli G, De Vita S. Rituximab treatment for glomerulonephritis in HCV-associated mixed cryoglobulinemia: efficacy and safety in the absence of steroid. Rheumatology 2006; 45: 842-46

Reff ME, Carner K, Chambers KS, Chinn PC, Leonard JE, Raab R, Newman RA, Hanna N, Anderson DR. Depletion of B cells in vivo by a chimeric mouse human monoclonal antibody to CD 20. Blood 1994; 82: 435-45

Roccatello D, Baldovino S, Rossi D, Giachino O, Mansouri M Rituximab as a therapeutic tool in severe mixed cryoglobulinemia Clin Rev Allergy Immunol. 2008; 34: 111-117

Ruth AJ, Kitching AR, Kwan RY, Odobasic D, Ooi JD, Timoshanko JR, Hickey MJ, Holdsworth SR: Anti-neutrophil cytoplasmic antibodies and effector CD4+ cells play non-redundant roles in anti-myelopexidase crescentic glomerulonephritis J Am Soc. Nephrol. 2006; 17: 1940-9

Saadoun D, Delluc A, Piette JC Cacoub P. Treatment of hepatitis C-associated mixed cryoglobulinemia vasculitis. Curr. Opin. Rheumatol. 2008; 20: 23-8

Saadoun D, Resche-Rigon M, Sene D, Perard L, Piette JC, Cacoub P Rituximab combined with peg-interferon-ribavirin in refractory HCV-associated cryoglobulinemia vasculitis Ann. Rheum Dis. 2008: 67: 1431-1436

Saadoun D, Resche Rigon M, Sene D, Terrier B, Karras A, Perard L, Schoindre Y, Coppere B, Blanc F, Musset L, Piette JC, Rosenzwaig M Cacoub P. Rituximab plus Peg-interferon-α ribavirin compared with Peg-interferon-α/ribavirin in hepatitis C-related mixed cryoglobulinemia Blood 2010; 116: 326-34

Sandborn WJ, Hanauer SB, Katz S, Safdi M, Wolf DG, Baerg RD,Tremaine DJ,Johnson T, Diehl NN, Zinmeister AR. Etanercept for active Crohn disease: a randomized, double blind, placebo controlled trial Gastroenterology 2001; 121: 1088-94

Sansonno D, De Re V, Lauletta G, Tucci FA, Boiocchi M, Dammacco F. Monoclonal antibody treatment of mixed cryoglobulinemia resistant to interferon α with an anti CD20 Blood 2003; 101: 3818-3826

Scapini P, Carletto A, Nardelli B, Calzetti F, Roschle V, Merigo F, Tamassia N, Pieropan S, Biasi D, Sbarbati A, Sozzani S, Bambara L, Cassatella MA.. Proinflammatory mediators elicit secretion of the intracellular B-lymphocytes stimulate pool (BlyS) that is stored in activated neutrophils: implication for inflammatory diseases Blood 2005; 2: 830-837

Schreiber A, Busjahn A, Luft FC, Kettritz R Membrane expression of proteinase 3 is genetically determined. J. Am. Soc. Nephrol. 2003; 14: 69-75

Sfikakis PP, Kaklamanis PH, Elezoglu A, Katsilambros N, Theodossiadis PG, Papafthimiou S, Markomichelakis N. Infliximab for recurrent, sight-threatening ocular inflammation in Adamantiades-Behcet disease. Ann Int. Med. 2004; 140: 404-6

Sfikakis PP, Markomichelakis N, Alpsoy E, Assad-Kahil S, Bodaghi B, Gul A, Ohno S, Pipitone N, Schirmer M, Stanford M, Wechsler B, Zouboulis C, Kaklamanis P, Yacizi H. Anti TNF therapy in the management of Behcet disease-review and basis for reccomendations. Rheumatology 2007; 46: 736-741

Sene D, Ghillani-Dalbin P, Amoura Z, Musset L, Cacoub P Rituximab may form a complex IgMκ mixed cryoglobulin and induce severe systemic reactions in patients with hepatitis C virus-induced vasculitis Arthritis Rheum 2009; 60: 3848-55

Seo P, Specks U, Keogh K. Efficacy of rituximab in limited Wegener's granulomatosis with refractory granulomatous manifestations. J. Rheumatol. 2008; 35: 2017-23

Serra P, Santamaria P To B regulated: B cells as members of the regulatory workforce. Trend Immunol. 2006; 27: 7-10

Seton M. Giant cell arteritis in a patient taking etanercept and methotrexate. J. Rheumatol. 2004; 31: 1467

Smith KG, Jones RB, Burms SM, Jayne DR. Long term comparison of rituximab treatment for refractory systemic lupus erythematosus and vasculitis. Remission, relapse and re-treatment. Arthritis. Rheum. 2006; 54: 2970-82

Sonomoto K, Watanabe MT, Takahama S, Nakamura M, Ando H, Minami R, Yamamoto M, Saito T, Imayama S, Hosokawa C, Suematsu E. A case of polyarteritis nodosa successfully treated by rituximab Nihon Rinsho Meneki Gakkai Kaishi 2008; 31: 119-23

Stasi R, Stipa E, Del Poeta G, Amadori S, Newland AC, Provan D. Long term observation of patients with anti-neutrophil cytoplasmic antibody-associated vasculitis treated with rituximab. Rheumatology. 2006; 45: 1432-6

Stone JH, Merkel PA, Spiera R, Seo P, Langford CA, Hoffman GS, Kallemberg CGM, St Cliar EW, Turkiewicz A, Tchao N, Webber L, Ding L, Seijsmundo LP, Mieras K, Weitzenkamp D, Ilke D, Seyfert-Margolis V, Mueller M, Brunetta P, Allen NB, Fervenza FC; Geetha D, Keogh KA, Kissin EY, Monach PA, Peikert T, Stegeman C, Yttemberg SY, Specks U. Rituximab versus cyclophosphamide in ANCA-associated renal vasculitis. NEJM 2010; 363: 221-32

Tamura N, Matsudaira R, Hirashima M, Ikeda M, Tajima M, Nawata M, Morimoto S, Kaneda K, Kobayashi S, Hashimoto H, Takasaki Y. Two cases of refractory Wegener's granulomatosis successfully treated witn rituximab. Intern. Med.2007; 46: 409-14

Tanaka F, Kawakami A, Iwanaga N, Tamai M, Izumi Y, Aratake K, Arima K, Kamachi M, Nakamura H, Huang M, Ida H, Origuchi T, Eguchi K Infliximab is effective for Takayasu arteritis refractory to glucocorticoid and methotrexate. Intern Med 2006; 45: 313-6

Tatò F, Rieger J, Hoffman U. Refractory Takayasu's arteritis successfully treated with the human monoclonal anti-tumor necrosis factor antibody adalimumab Int Angiol 2005; 24: 304-7

Terrier B, Launay D, Kaplanski G, Hot A, Larroche C, Cathebras P, Cfombe B, De Jaurreguiberry J.P, Meyer O, Schaeverbeke T, Somogy A, Tricot L, Zenone T, Ravaud P, Gottemberg JE, Mariette X, Cacoub P. Safety and efficacy of rituximab in nonviral cryoglobulinemia vasculitis: data from the French autoimmunity and rutuximab registry. Arthritis Care and Res. 2010; 62: 1787-95

Tognon S, Graziani G, Marcolongo R. Anti TNF-α therapy in seven patients with Behcet disease Ann. N.Y. Acad. Sci. 2007; 1110: 474-84

Tugal-Tutkun I, Mudun A, Urgancioglu M, Kamali S, Kasapoglu E, Inanc M, Gul A. Efficacy of infliximab in the treatment of uveitis that is resistant to treatment with the combination of Azathioprine, Cyclosporin and corticosteroids in Behcet disease. Arhtritis Rheum 2005; 52: 2478-2484

Utz JP, Limper AH, Kalra S, Specks U, Scott JP, Vuk-Pavlovic Z, Schroeder D. Etanercept for the treatment of stage II and III progressive pulmonary sarcoidosis. Chest 2003; 124: 177-85

Van Rossum AP, Rarok AA, Huitema MG, Fassina G, Limburg PC, Kallemberg CGM Costitutive membrane expression of proteinase 3 (PR3) and neutrophil activation by antiPR3 antibodies.J. Leukoc Biol 2004; 76: 1162-70

Vega-Gutierrez J, Rodriguez Prieto MA, Garcia Riuz JM Successfull treatment of childhood cutaneous polyarteritis nodosa with infliximab. JEADV 2007; 536: 570-71

Visenti M, Granata M, Veneziano ML, Borghese F, Carlesino M, Pimpinelli F, Fiorilli M, Casato M Efficacy of low dose rituximab for mixed cryoglobulinemia Clin. Immunol. 2007; 125: 30-33

Voswinkel J, Assmann G, Held G, Pitann S, Gross WL, Holl-Ulrich K, Herlyn K, A. Mueller. Sigle cells analysis of B lymphocytes from Wegener's granulomatosis: B cells receptor display affinity maturation within the granulomatous lesions. Clin Exp. Immunol. 2008; 154: 339-345

Wahezi DM, Gomes WA, Illowite NT. Cranial nerve involvement with juvenile polyarteritis nodosa: clinical manifestations and treatment. Pediatrics 2010; 126: 719-22

Walsh M, Jayne DR Rituximab in the treatment of antineutrophil cytoplasm antibody associated vasculitis and systemic lupus erythematosus. Kidney Int. 2007; 27: 676-82

Wegener's granulomatosis etanercept trial (WGET) research group- Etanercept plus standard therapy for Wegener's granulomatosis N Engl. J. Med. 2005; 352: 351-61

Witko-Sarsat V, Lesavre P, Lopez S, Bessou G, Hieblot C, Prum B, Noël LH, Guillevin L, Ravaud P, Sermet-Gaudelus I, Timsit J, Grünfeld JP, Halbwachs-Mecarelli L. A large subset of neutrophils expressing membrane proteinase 3 is a risk factor for vasculitis and rheumatoid arthritis J. AM. Soc. Nephrol. 1999; 10: 1224-33

Wu K, Throssell D A new treatment for polyarteritis nodosa Nephrol. Dial Transplant 2006; 21: 1710-1712

Xiao H, Heeringa P, Hu P, Liu Z, Zaho M, Aratani Y, Maeda N, Falk RJ, Jennette JC Antineutrophil cytoplasmic autoantibodies specific for myeloperoxidase cause glomerulonephritis and vasculitis in mice J. Clin. Invest.2002 110; 955-963

Xiao H, Schreiber P, Liu Z, Huugen D, Maeda N, Falk RJ, Jennette JC The role of neutrophils in the induction of glomerulonephritis by anti mieloperoxydase antibodies. Am. J. Pathol. 2005; 167: 39-45

Xiao, H, Schreiber A, Heeringa P, Falk RJ, Jennette JC Alternative complement pathway in the pathogenesis of disease mediated by antineutrophil cytoplasmic autoantibodies Am J Pathol. 2007; 170: 52-64

Youinou P. B cell conduct the lymphocyte orchestra. J. Autoimmun. 2007; 28: 143-151

Zaja F, De Vita S, Mazzaro C, Sacco S, Damiani D. Efficacy and safety of rituximab in type II mixed cryoglobulinemia Blood 2003; 101: 3827-3834

7

The Role of Biological Therapies in the Management of Systemic Vasculitis

Paloma Vela and Mariano Andrés
Sección de Reumatología, Hospital General Universitario de Alicante
Spain

1. Introduction

Systemic vasculitides are multisystem disorders with an autoimmune basis leading to blood vessel inflammation. Vasculitis present a wide spectrum, being classified regarding different aspects on pathogenesis, histopathology or laboratory findings. The most common used classification considers size of the vessel predominantly affected, established at Chapel Hill Consensus Conference (Jennete et al, 1994): large-sized vessels (giant-cell arteritis, Takayasu's arteritis), medium-sized vessels (polyarteritis nodosa, Kawasaki's disease) and small-sized vessels (Wegener granulomatosis, microscopic polyangiitis, Churg-Strauss syndrome, cryoglobulinemia, Henoch-Schönlein purpura, and cutaneous leukocytoclastic angiitis). Behçet's disease affects small and large vessels of the arterial and venous systems. Systemic vasculitis predominantly associated with the presence of serum anti-neutrophil cytoplasmic antibodies (ANCA) are known as ANCA-associated vasculitis, in spite of about 10-20% of this vasculitis present with classical clinical picture but ANCA negative.

Systemic vasculitis are rare diseases with wide and heterogenic range of manifestations, so leading prospective controlled clinical trials in pathogenesis and management of these diseases is difficult. Despite these limitations, first descriptions about vasculitis in mid-20th century ascertained that some forms of vasculitis are severe and potentially fatal in a short-term period (weeks-months) with no treatment. These are mainly Wegener disease and microscopic polyangiits with critical organ involvement (kidney, lung, gastrointestinal system or central nervous system), but they are not the only ones. Introduction of glucocorticoids and, later, immunosuppressive agents (cyclophosphamide, methotrexate, azathioprine, etc.) contributed to achieve remission of these diseases and prevent further organ damage, former potentially fatal.

But nowadays many questions are still unsolved. In ANCA-associated vasculitis, high rate of remission (about 80-90% patients) is followed by an unacceptable rate of relapses, which is especially important in Wegener granulomatosis, reaching up to 50% of patients within 2 years after the diagnosis (Hoffman et al, 1992), with further morbidity and mortality. Another concern is about cytotoxic regimens for induction of remission on these diseases: although current schemes are less toxic, severe infections and bone marrow toxicity still are major problems, so serious adverse events and mortality in early stages are not related to disease activity, but to therapy in a significant proportion of cases (Little MA et al, 2010).

In last decade, the advent of target-defined drugs, known as biological agents, became a substantial advance for the management of several diseases in different medical areas, as

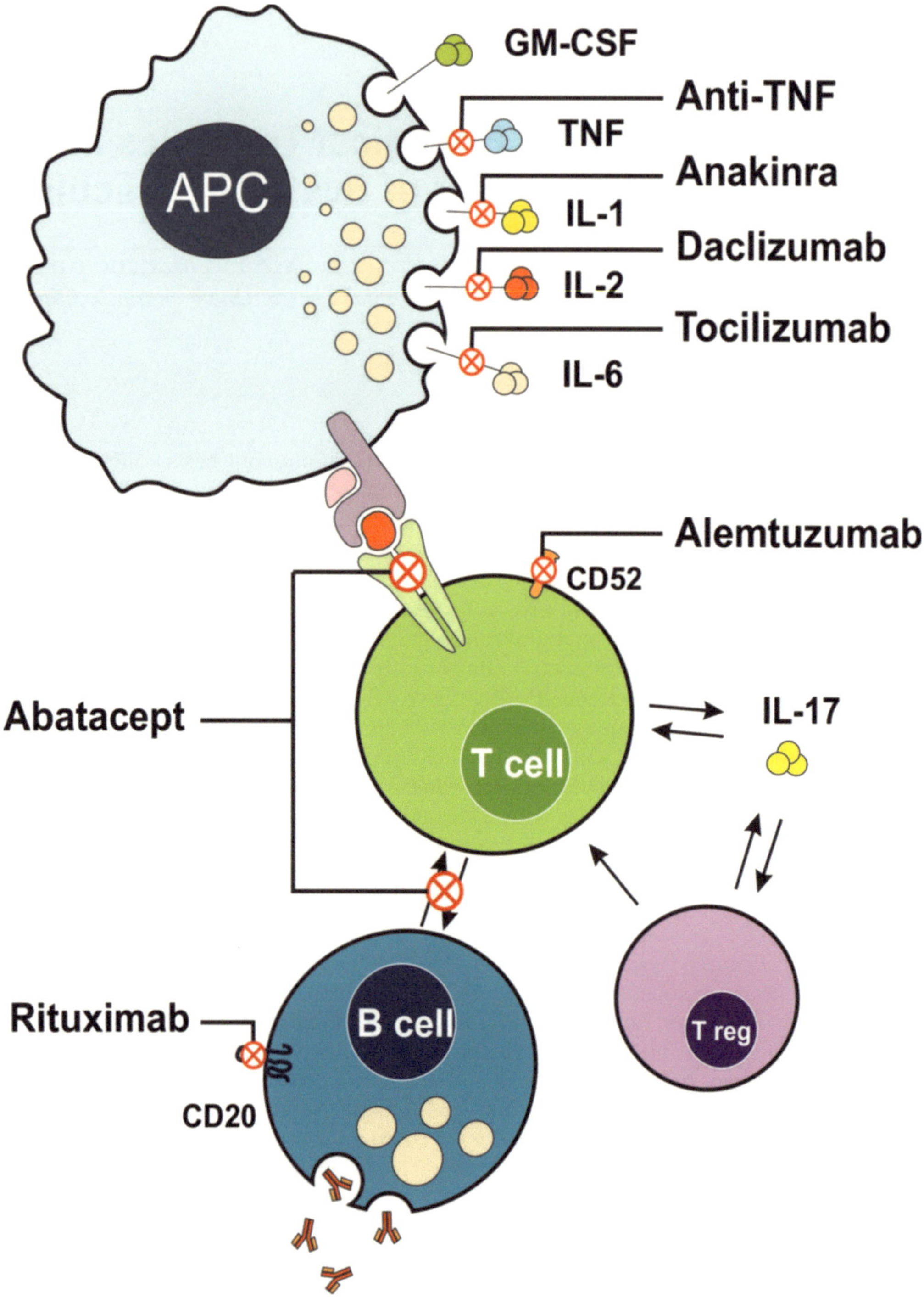

Fig. 1. Common biological agents and their targets on immune system cells and molecules. APC: antigen-presenting cell; GM-CSF: granulocyte-monocyte colonial stimulating factor; TNF: tumour necrosis factor; IL: interleukin. [*Figure by Enrique Sillero MD*].

rheumatology, nephrology, haematology, oncology, dermatology or digestive medicine. They are immunological agents, monoclonal antibodies or recombinant soluble receptors, designed against simple targets on serum (for example, tumor necrosis factor-α, interleukin-1 or interleukin-6) or cell surface (for example, CD20, CD3 or epidermical growing factor receptor) (Figure 1). In autoimmune disorders, biological agents proved to be highly effective in rheumatoid arthritis, inflammatory bowel disease, psoriasis or autoimmune haemolytic anaemia, also in refractory forms. As any other agents, biological therapies carry some adverse events, as increased risk of infections, hypersensitivity or infusion-related reactions and skin disorders. An increased risk of further malignancies is not clear. But overall benefit-risk ratio is very high.

In systemic vasculitis, the introduction of biological therapy in last decade has provided the hope of a more targeted treatment with greater efficacy, fewer side effects and longer-lasting remissions. They may also be a promising solution for refractory cases. In this chapter, the current evidence about the use of biological agents in systemic vasculitis will be reviewed.

2. ANCA-associated vasculitis

2.1 Introduction

Wegener's granulomatosis, Churg-Strauss syndrome and microscopic polyangiitis are types of systemic vasculitis associated to the presence of detectable serum anti-neutrophil cytoplasmic antibodies (ANCA). Less than 10% of cases of polyarteritis nodosa show positive ANCA. As previously described, ANCA vasculitis are severe conditions with a fatal outcome with no treatment. Former high mortality rates became lower after the introduction of an intensive management with immunosuppressive agents as cyclophosphamide. Despite this improvement, unacceptable rates of relapses and drug-related adverse events made the search of more effective and more safety agents highly desirable, and biological agents have been used and tested with this purpose. Their results will be discussed in this section.

2.2 TNF blockade

Anti-tumour necrosis factor (TNF) agents have been widely used in ANCA-associated vasculitis. TNFα is a prominent cytokine involved in the formation of granuloma in infectious and inflammatory diseases, and many other evidence support TNF blockade in ANCA-associated vasculitis: TNF gene expression and cytokine production by lymphocytes is increased in patients with Wegener (Deguchi et al, 1990; Ludviksson et al, 1998); TNF soluble receptor levels seemed to correlate with disease activity (Nassonov at al, 1997) and TNF-positive cells predominate in inflammatory infiltrates found in renal biopsies from patients with ANCA vasculitis (Noronha I et al, 1993).

Uncontrolled studies where anti-TNF drugs were used in patients with refractory ANCA vasculitis showed promising results in efficacy and safety. Chimeric monoclonal antibody infliximab was tried in six patients with refractory Wegener granulomatosis - one persistent and five relapsing diseases - in a preliminary study (Lamprecht et al, 2002). In different dosage (3mg/kg in 2 patients and 5 mg/kg in 4 patients), the addition of infliximab to standard therapy achieved remission in five out six patients, being discontinued in the remaining one due to a non-confirmed infection. In another study (Booth et al, 2004), an open-labelled multicenter non-controlled trial, infliximab was associated with a high rate of remission (88% patients in about 6 weeks) in 28 patients with Wegener granulomatosis and microscopic polyangiitis. Disease activity scores, inflammatory markers and prednisolone doses were significantly reduced all throughout the study. These promising data with infliximab carried on some queries: discontinuation of the drug followed by high rate of relapses in a short period - about 20%patients in 16 months of follow-up; there were no control group; patients presented a significant rate of severe adverse events, with 2 deaths, 6 severe infections and one malignancy. The pattern of organ involvement and detected microorganism were consistent with recognized events in other infliximab-treated disorders.

In an exploratory study (Stone et al, 2001), fusion protein etanercept - a combination of p75 soluble TNFα receptor and Fc portion of human IgG1 – were added to standard therapy for patients with refractory Wegener granulomatosis, persistently active or relapsing forms. Twenty patients received etanercept 25mg subcutaneous twice a week for 6 months. The study endpoint was safety and there was no control group. After 6 months of follow up, the most common adverse event was related to injection site reactions, and no serious adverse events were detected. Though no study endpoint, good results were noted in efficacy; the authors found a reduction in disease activity, even remissions in 80% of patients, with reductions in prednisolone doses.

These promising results in safety and efficacy led to further randomized controlled trial (WGET Research Group, 2005). In this multicenter, randomized, double-blind, placebo-controlled trial, 181 patients with active Wegener disease – not other forms of ANCA vasculitis were included – were randomized to receive etanercept 25mg subcutaneously twice a week or placebo, along with standard therapy, in order to evaluate the maintenance of remission. Surprisingly, no significant differences were found in the rate of sustained remission – 69% patients in etanercept group versus 75% patients in control group – and results did not depend on severity or duration of the disease. But the most astonishing finding was related to safety: both groups presented a similar rate of severe adverse events; in etanercept group, however, 6 malignancies were detected, with none in placebo group. It is a standardised incidence rate over 300% compared to expected rate in this group matching per age and sex. It is noteworthy that relapsing disease, what means more previous exposure to immunosuppressive agents, was higher in etanercept group.

Recently, fully humanised TNFα monoclonal antibody adalimumab has been tested in ANCA-associated vasculitis (Laurino et al, 2010). An open-label, prospective uncontrolled trial was underwent to study adalimumab (40mg subcutaneously every 2 weeks) as an adjuvant to standard therapy in flares of Wegener granulomatosis and microscopic polyangiits. Results were comparable to infliximab: a high rate of remission followed by frequent relapses (6 out 14 patients in less than 2 years after remission) and 2 cases of severe infections, one fatal.

Data about TNFα blockade in other forms of necrotising systemic vasculitis are scarce. Churg-Strauss syndrome is often mild and controlled with glucocorticoids. But data suggest that small portion of patients will present a severe disease requiring intensive treatment. Anti-TNF agents might be an effective option for these patients (Arbach et al, 2002). Currently very rare after widespread hepatitis B vaccination, polyarteritis nodosa is a systemic necrotising vasculitis affecting medium-sized vessels and seldom associated to ANCA (less than 10% of cases). A case of refractory and severe polyarteritis nodosa successfully treated with infliximab has been reported (Al-Bishri et al, 2005).

In summary, huge evidence about TNFα blockade in ANCA-associated vasculitis is lacking. High rates of remission in refractory cases were found, especially in uncontrolled studies;

but high rate of relapses after discontinuation and intolerable severe adverse events (especially infections and increased risk of malignancies - found with etanercept) make anti-TNF agents not formally recommended for the management of ANCA-associated vasculitis.

2.3 B-cell targeted therapies

B-lymphocytes are one of the cornerstone cells in immune system, with pleiotropic effects: antibody production, antigen presentation, cytokine secretion or T-lymphocytes regulation. As previously mentioned, systemic necrotising vasculitis are largely related to ANCA autoantibodies against neutrophil proteins, mainly proteinase-3 and myeloperoxidase. B-lymphocytes are responsible of ANCA production, and plasma activated B-cell titre is related to disease activity (Popa et al, 1999). So B-cells are a logical target for the management of ANCA-associated vasculitis.

Rituximab is a chimeric monoclonal antibody against CD20; CD20 is a surface marker found almost exclusively in B-lymphocytes (immature and mature cells), except of plasma cells. Rituximab is an effective agent for B-cell non-Hodgkin lymphoma and several autoimmune disorders, as rheumatoid arthritis. Several case reports and small series found rituximab as a potential agent for patients with refractory ANCA vasculitis (Specs et al, 2001; Omdal et al, 2005; Stasi et al, 2006; Tektonidou & Skopouli, 2006; Tamura et al, 2007; Ferraro et al, 2008; Sanchez-Cano et al, 2008; Seo et al, 2008). Encouraged by previous reports, a prospective open-label pilot trial with rituximab in refractory Wegener granulomatosis was underwent (Keogh et al, 2006). In this trial, ten patients with refractory disease - three with persistent and seven with relapsing disease - were treated with rituximab 4 weekly infusions of 375mg/m^2, along with glucocorticoids. All of these patients achieved complete remission in less than 5 months after last infusion, and 9 out ten continued with remission at the end of the study (12months); only one patient relapsed, at 9 months. In this trial, clinical response appeared to be related to successful B-cell depletion. Another trial (Jones et al, 2009), larger (65 patient) but retrospective, supported this results: rituximab induced remission in 75% of patients with relapsing or persistent ANCA-associated vasculitis, in this case also including microscopic polyangiitis and Churg-Strauss syndrome. Relapse occurred in 57% of patients, but subsequent courses also achieved remission.

These very promising data from uncontrolled studies warranted confirmation in randomised controlled trials. Two were recently published. RITUXVAS trial (Jones et al, 2010) was a non-inferiority open-label trial about rituximab as an induction of remission agent in ANCA-associated vasculitis with renal involvement, compared to standard regime (cyclophosphamide and steroids). Patients in treatment group received rituximab using lymphoma scheme (375mg/m2 weekly 4 weeks) along with cyclophosphamide (15mg/kg 2 i.v. pulses with the first and third rituximab infusions) and glucocorticoids. Patients with new Wegener disease, microscopic polyangiitis and renal-limited vasculitis were enrolled and randomised to each group in a 3:1 ratio. No differences in sustained remission were found between both groups (76% in rituximab group versus 82% in control group, p=0.68), time to remission was similar (about 90 days) and safety data was comparable. Fifteen percent of patients in rituximab group and 10% patients in control group relapsed after 12 months of follow-up. Stone et al (2010) conducted the RAVE trial, a double-blind, randomised control trial where rituximab was tested as non-inferior to cyclophosphamide for induction of remission in ANCA-associated vasculitis. Investigators recruited patients with active disease, newly diagnosed or relapsed. In this trial, rituximab (lymphoma scheme) plus placebo was compared to daily oral cyclophosphamide plus placebo.

Remission rate was similar in both groups - 64% rituximab versus 53% control - being noteworthy that was lower than usual remission rates, about 80-90% (Hoffman et al, 1992). In relapsing subgroup rituximab was superior to cyclophosphamide; a possible explanation might be that patients with relapsing disease were initially treated with cyclophosphamide and are less likely to respond to new cyclophosphamide rather than those with new-onset disease. Relapses were low and did not differ between groups. Safety data was again comparable, with more leukopenia in cyclophosphamide group.

If B-cell repopulation or ANCA levels should guide further courses of rituximab in order to prevent relapse is still to be determined. In trial by Keogh et al (2006), B-cells depleted in all patients after rituximab, and further ANCA levels augments (previously decreased in all patients) coincided or followed B-cell reconstitution; in this trial only one patient relapsed, preceded by B-cell repopulation and ANCA increase. But this association was not found in other studies (Jones et al, 2009).

Churg-Strauss syndrome was seldom included in above studies, but successful outcome in refractory cases using rituximab has been reported as well (Kaushik et al, 2006; Koukoulaki et al, 2006; Pepper et al, 2008]. We found no data about rituximab in polyangiitis nodosa.

In summary, B-cells are a very promising target as a part of the management of ANCA-associated vasculitis. Presented data support the use of rituximab as an induction of remission agent, especially in persistent or relapsing disease. Due to randomised controlled trial results, rituximab should be even consider as a first-line agent, though is not licensed for this employ. One grey area of ANCA-associated vasculitis remains unanswered with rituximab: while successful results in remission have been reported, patients still present an unacceptable rate of relapses. RITUXVAS and RAVE trials did not explore rituximab as a maintenance agent, and follow-up was too short (12 and 6 months respectively) to assess it. Further studies are warranted and desirable.

2.4 T-cell targeted therapies

Along with B cells, autoreactive T lymphocytes have a major role in pathogenesis of ANCA-associated vasculitis (Popa et al, 2002). So T-cell depletion might have a role in the management of these conditions. Alemtuzumab (CAMPATH-1H) is a humanised monoclonal antibody against CD52, present in T lymphocytes and macrophages, leading to T cell depletion. Tested in other immune disorders - like rheumatoid arthritis, multiple sclerosis or renal transplantation - alemtuzumab was used in refractory cases of ANCA-associated vasculitis, especially Wegener disease. Walsh et al (2008) reported long-term results of 71 patients with refractory or relapsing disease treated with alemtuzumab. Use of alemtuzumab achieved high remission rates (85% of patients) but high relapsing rate as well (60%), and patients developed an unacceptable rate of severe adverse events, in particular infections. Infections are probably due to deep immune suppression by alemtuzumab, but it is noteworthy that several patients had other risk factors for severe infections: 23% showed undetectable CD4+ cells before alemtuzumab probably related to prior intensive immunosuppressive agents, 8% were hemodyalisis-dependent and 18% presented a life-threatening disease requiring intensive unit care. Data with anti-thymocyte globulin, which also leads to lymphocyte depletion, is quite similar (Lukas & Keller, 1998; Hagen et al, 1995]. No further controlled trials have been undertaken.

CTLA-4 (CD152) is a surface molecule on activated T-cell membrane. CTLA-4 binds B7.1 (CD80) and B7.2 (CD86) from antigen-presenting cells, leading to T-cell co-stimulation. CTLA-4 has a role on immune regulation, mainly switching from Th2 to Th1-response pattern. This effect is antagonist to CD28. Predominantly Th1 response was found in granulomatous inflammation (Csernok et al, 1999), CTLA-4 expression is increased in patients with active disease (Steiner et al, 2001) and associations with some CTLA-4 polymorphysms were found (Huang et al, 2000; Giscombe et al, 2002; Zhou et al, 2004], all in Wegener granulomatosis. In this context, CTLA-4-Ig abatacept might be a potential agent in the management of ANCA-associated vasculitis. No case reports or series have been published, but results from an ongoing trial, ABAVAS (www.clinicaltrials.gov), are awaited.

2.5 Other biological agents

We found no other reports about other biologics in ANCA-associated vasculitis. Recombinant interleukin-6 receptor tocilizumab might have a role, so as interleukin-6 levels are increased in these disorders and correlated to disease activity (Nakahama et al, 1993). Conversely, no differences in interleukin-1 levels were found between patients with active ANCA vasculitis, convalescent vasculitis and healthy controls [Nogueira E et al, 2010], making anakinra and other IL-1 antagonists unlikely to be effective.

3. Large vessel vasculitides

The primary large vessel vasculitides, Takayasu's arteritis (TA) and giant cell arteritis (GCA), are chronic inflammatory diseases of the large elastic arteries characterised by systemic inflammation and critical ischemia. GCA primarily affects temporal arteries and other extracranial branches, while in TA the aorta and its proximal branches are usually involved. TA predominates in young adults, but patients with GCA are usually older. Though these differences, some authors suggested that both entities might be two poles of the spectrum within the same disease (Maksimowicz-McKinnon et al, 2009). Glucocorticoids continue being the mainstay of initial therapy, but long-term use is associated with a great amount of adverse side effects. Both conditions can follow a chronic relapsing course, requiring long-term therapy. In addition, most patients that initially respond to glucocorticoids flare on dose reduction or discontinuation. In the Cleveland cohort (Maksimowicz-McKinnon et al., 2007), only 20% of patients persisted on remission with <10 mg prednisolone for 6 months. It is therefore common the need of an additional immunosuppressive agent to induce or maintain remission in large cohorts (Kerr et al., 1994; Vanoli et al., 2005; Park et al., 2005).

Granulomatous inflammation is one of the key histopathological features of large vessel vasculitides. Taking into account the role of tumour necrosis factor-alpha (TNFα) in the formation and maintenance of the granuloma, it could be expected that anti-TNF therapies may be beneficial in refractory forms of large vessel vasculitides. TNFα is a pro-inflammatory cytokine produced primarily by cells from monocyte-macrophage lineage. Its biologic effects include adhesion molecule expression, synthesis of chemokines and other pro-inflammatory cytokines, activation of immune system cells (T-cells, B-cells and macrophages), and inhibition of regulatory T-cells (Chung & Seo, 2009). TNFα can be found in both cell membrane-bound and soluble forms. At this time, five agents directed against TNFα are approved for use in rheumatoid arthritis and other inflammatory arthropathies: infliximab, etanercept, adalimumab, certolizumab and golimumab.

3.1 Takayasu´s arteritis

TA primarily involves the aorta and its primary branches. The inflammatory process cause wall thickening on the affected arteries. Although experience with anti-TNF agents in difficult-to-treat cases of TA is limited, multiple investigators have reported successful results.

Hoffman and associates published the first long-term study of anti-TNF therapy in TA in 2004 (Hoffmann et al., 2004). In this open-label trial, 15 patients with refractory forms of TA were enrolled. Thirteen of them had high doses requirements of glucocorticoids to maintain remission and relapsed while treated with conventional and experimental therapy; and 2 of them refused re-treatment with glucocorticoids following relapses (2 of the 15 patients). Anti-TNF agents were used, seven patients received etanercept (ETN) (25 mg twice weekly) and eight received infliximab (IFX) (from 3 to 5 mg/kg initially, and at two weeks, six weeks, and every four to eight weeks thereafter). Previous treatments included methotrexate, cyclophosphamide, mycophenolate, cyclosporin and tacrolimus. Rapid improvement was noted in 14 out 15 patients, within 2–8 weeks. Sustained remission, lasting 1 - 3.3 years, was achieved in 10 patients (75%) who were able to discontinue glucocorticoids. Four patients (27%) partially responded and were able to reduce the steroid dose by at least 50%. At 12 months, most patients required no steroids. One patient did not respond to IFX. Nine of the 14 patients with an initial response to 3 mg/kg of IFX required dose escalation to maintain disease control. Two relapses occurred with interruption of therapy, but disease control was regained when treatment was restarted.

Molloy et al (2008) reported the largest case series to date in the literature, a retrospective study examining 25 patients with active, relapsing TA. Patients were treated with IFX (n=21) or ETN (n=9) and followed for a median of 28 months. Of the nine patients initially treated with ETN, four underwent complete remission and two experienced partial remission. Two of the four patients in complete remission switched to IFX, one due to unavailability of ETN (and subsequently had a sustained remission) and the other due to a major disease flare at 67 months, but relapsed after two IFX infusions and treatment was subsequently stopped. Of the six patients in remission, three had disease relapses: two of them regained disease control with an increase in dose of ETN to 50 mg twice weekly, and the other one also required addition of prednisolone. Three patients who did not respond to ETN were switched to IFX and achieved complete remission. Of the 21 patients treated with IFX (including the five previously treated with ETN), 12 achieved complete remission and six achieved partial remission. Three patients discontinued IFX; 12 of the remaining 18 patients relapsed and required treatment with higher doses of IFX administered at shorter intervals. Median stable IFX dose was 5 mg/kg (range 4–10 mg/kg), administered at a median interval of 6 weekly (range 4–8 weekly). Of the nine patients that either permanently or temporarily discontinued IFX, eight had a disease flare at a median interval of 5 months (range 2–12); two of these patients restarted IFX treatment and again achieved remission.

Other small series have reported a similar rapid response to IFX, with dose escalation frequently needed to maintain remission (Karageorgaki et al., 2007; Tanaka et al., 2006; Jolly & Curran, 2005; Della Rossa et al., 2005). Also, a further case of refractory TA entered remission with adalimumab when infliximab was discontinued after a lupus-like reaction (Tato et al., 2005). Current data may suggest that the use of IFX compared with etanercept or adalimumab is recommendable, but one should note that doses frequently had to be escalated above the baseline 3 mg/kg dose to achieve remission.

In summary, the positive results from these case series and case reports of the use of anti-TNF agents for refractory TA are encouraging, but an adequately powered, randomized controlled trial is needed to ascertain their role.

3.2 Giant-cell arteritis

Giant-cell arteritis (GCA), also known as temporal arteritis, is an immune-mediated chronic disease characterized by granulomatous infiltrates in the wall of medium and large-sized arteries. Vessel wall inflammation leads to luminal occlusion and tissue ischemia. Patients with GCA complain of persistent unilateral headache, jaw claudication, visual disturbances, malaise and weight loss (Seo & Stone, 2004). As well as TA, GCA is characterized by granulomatous inflammation, so TNFα inhibition would appear to be an appropriate treatment approach.

Some small case series pointed that IFX might be useful as a steroid-sparing agent for GCA (Cantini et al, 2001; Andonopoulos et al, 2003; Airo et al, 2002). Based on these results, a randomized, multicenter trial of IFX versus placebo was conducted, but surprisingly failed to show efficacy (Hoffman et al, 2007). Forty-four patients newly diagnosed with GCA were randomly assigned in a 2:1 (IFX 5 mg/kg: placebo) ratio to receive infusions at weeks 0, 2, and 6, and every 8 weeks thereafter, after prednisone-induced remission. Primary outcomes were the number of relapse/recurrence free patients through week 22 and adverse events, while secondary outcomes included time to first relapse, number of relapse-free patients when prednisone was tapered to 10 mg day, and cumulative prednisone dose. Sixteen patients were assigned to prednisone plus placebo, and 28 to prednisone plus IFX. At 22 weeks, the proportion of patients without relapse was similar between the IFX and placebo groups (43 versus 50% respectively, P=0.65). In addition, IFX did not increase the proportion of patients whose prednisone dose could be tapered to 10 mg/d without relapse (61% for IFX versus 75% for placebo, P=0.31). There was a trend for more infections in the IFX (71%) than in the placebo (56%) group. Consequently, the trial was stopped early. The investigators concluded that the addition of IFX to glucocorticoids neither improve the durability of remissions nor reduce cumulative glucocorticoids requirements in GCA. This data suggests that, similarly to what has been reported in PMR (Salvarani et al., 2007), TNFα inhibition is effective to some extent in long-standing, refractory GCA, but not (or only marginally) effective in new-onset GCA. The results of these studies led the European Vasculitis Study (EUVAS) group to not recommend the use of infliximab in GCA as an adjuvant therapy to glucocorticoids (Mukhtyar et al, 2009).

The first randomized trial showed etanercept as a useful steroid-sparing agent in refractory GCA (Martinez-Taboada et al, 2008). Fifteen patients with biopsy-proven GCA, in remission with a stable dose of prednisone (median 15 mg daily) were included. Prednisone was tapered according to a predefined schedule allowing for dose adjustments in case of flares. Placebo or etanercept 25 mg were given subcutaneously twice weekly for 12 months followed by a 3-month observation period. Patients in the etanercept group discontinued more easily prednisone (although the difference did not reach significance) and the cumulative dose after 12 months of treatment was significantly lower. The number and severity of adverse events was similar in both groups. The results of this study thus appear to support the concept that TNF blockade with etanercept has a clinically relevant effect in suppressing disease activity in refractory GCA (Salvarani et al, 2008). It should be mentioned however that treatment arm only contained eight patients.

Interleukin-6 blockade with tocilizumab (a humanized anti-interleukin-6 receptor monoclonal antibody) seems to be a promising target for future randomized controlled trials; current reported uses are limited (Seitz et al, 2011). Other possible therapeutic agents include abatacept, a recombinant fusion protein that modulates CD28-mediated T-cell costimulation, and rituximab, a B-cell depleting antibody. The last has been used in one patient with GCA, with resolution of arteritis at 4.5 months (Bhatia et al, 2005). However, this patient subsequently developed pneumonia that required mechanical ventilation.

4. Behçet's disease

4.1 Introduction

Behçet's disease is a chronic multisystemic vasculitis affecting small and large arterial and venous branches (Yazici et al, 2010). The condition presents a distinctive geographical pattern, with higher incidence rates in Turkey, other Mediterranean countries and Middle and Far East countries, following the ancient "silk route" until Japan. On the other hand, it is rare in Northern Europe and United States. Genetic and environmental factors have been proposed as responsible for this unique distribution, but not fully explaining those differences (Verity et al, 1999). HLA-B51 is the strongest genetic association, but only explains 20% of disease heritability and Japanese patients with Behçet's disease do not share this association. An environmental trigger might play a role on the onset of the disease; this is suggested by the fact that the incidence rate of Behçet's disease in Turkish people living in Germany is considerably lower compared to those living in Turkey (Zouboulis et al, 1997).
Though mucocutaneous features are the most frequent clinical involvement in Behçet's disease, some patients suffers from severe eye involvement (chronic posterior uveitis), arterial aneurisms and central nervous system disease, leading to significant morbidity and mortality. Male and young patients often have a more severe disease. Management is mainly symptomatic and empiric. Drugs commonly used are topical and systemic glucocorticoids, colchicine, azathioprine or thalidomide. Severe cases may require cyclosporin, cyclophosphamide and high doses of glucocorticoids. Functional visual loss due to Behçet's disease uveitis is seen in 10-15% of patients. Mortality of pulmonary artery aneurisms is about 50%. Central nervous system is associated to 30% rate of mortality (Saadoun et al, 2010). So despite the usual schemes of management, there is ongoing morbidity and mortality in patients with Behçet's disease. Further more effective and less harmful agents are awaited, and biological agents might be this desired option; efficacy and safety data will be reviewed in this section.

4.2 TNF blockade

Tumour necrosis factor (TNF) inhibitors are the most widely used biological agents in Behçet's disease. Beside clinical, there are experimental data supporting this use: First, Behçet's disease was found to be mediated by cytokines derived from Th1 lymphocytes, including TNF (Gul, 2001). Second, patients with active disease showed an increased TNF expression (Yamashita et al, 1997; Mege et al, 1993). And third, TNF levels, both in sera and in aqueous humour, are increased in Behçet's disease (Evereklioglu et al, 2002; Chronopoulou et al, 2001).
Anti-TNF agents have been essentially tried in patients with refractory features of the disease. Case reports and retrospective case series were the initial data, but later prospective controlled studies have been reported. Generally, anti-TNF agents are recommended for patients with active disease which is refractory to conventional treatments (Sfikakis et al, 2007). But evidence level is not equal for each Behçet's feature, so we will separately review the most common or troublesome manifestations of the disease, regarding data about efficacy and safety of the anti-TNF agents.

4.2.1 Mucocutaneous and joint disease

The mainstay manifestation of Behçet's disease is the recurrent oral ulceration. It is the usual onset feature, is present in virtually all patients and is the required criteria for the diagnosis of the disease (International Study Group for Behçet's Disease, 1990). Other skin manifestations are genital ulcers (scrotum, major and minor labia), papulo-pustular acne-like lesions, subcutaneous nodules in lower limbs (remedying those of erythema nodosum), skin ulcers, pyoderma gangrenosum or palpable purpura. Oral and genital ulcers are typically mildly painful and completely heal after 1-3 weeks, but larger ones can leave a scar. The management usually includes topical glucorticoids, colchicine or thalidomide.

Patients with Behçet's disease often present with arthritis, typically simetrical or asimetrical non-erosive oligoarthitis. Commonly affects to knees, wrists, ankles or elbows. Sometimes arthritis develops in a monoarticular or polyarticular pattern. Erosive arthritis is rare and later studies have found no association with axial involvement.

Skin and joint involvement is often mild and easily controlled. But these features might be very distressing with a significant physical and psychological burden. Occasionally some patients present with a persistent and severe condition, refractory to conventional treatments. There are some reports about using anti-TNF drugs in this small group of patients. In 2001, first case reports were published. Goossens et al reported a patient with mouth, anous, praeputium and left foot ulcers, refractory to conventional treatment, who achieved a sustained remission after two infusions of infliximab 10mg/kg. A 65 year-old woman, with history of 10 years of persistent orogenital ulcers despite several treatments (glucocorticoids, colchicine, thalidomide, azathioprine, cyclosporin and dapsone), successfully responded to infliximab (5mg/kg) three infusions (0, 2 and 6 weeks) (Robertson & Hickling, 2001). Others cases of refractory Behçet's skin involvement controlled with anti-TNF have been reported (Haugeberg et al, 2004; Almoznino & Ben-Chetrit, 2007).

In 2005, a double-blind, placebo-controlled trial evaluating etanercept in Behçet's disease was published (Melikoglu et al, 2005). The aim of the authors was to evaluate the effect of etanercept in pathergy and monosodium urate (MSU) reactions, and in minor Behçet's features (patients with severe manifestations were excluded). Pathergy reaction consists in the development of a papule or pustule 48 hours after an intradermal needle prick. MSU reaction is the persistence of erythema 48 hours after an intradermal inoculation of MSU crystals. Both reactions demonstrate skin hypersensitivity and are high specific for Behçet's disease (Gilhar et al, 1989). Enrolled patients randomised to receive etanercept (25mg twice a week) or placebo. After 4 weeks of treatment and 3 months of follow-up, patients in etanercept showed lower rates of oral ulcers, subcutaneous nodules and papulo-pustular lesions, but differences disappeared after discontinuation of the drug. Inflammatory markers also decreased. Genital ulcers and arthritis showed no benefits with etanercept. Interestingly, no effect on pathergy and MSU reaction was found. Treatment was safe and well-tolerated, with no significant adverse events. Despite some bias (small size, short-term follow-up, etc.), this was the first and successful controlled study with anti-TNF drugs in Behçet's disease, focused on its skin and joint manifestations.

4.2.2 Eye disease

More than 50% of patients with Behçet's disease will present with eye involvement (Yacici et al, 2010). This may occur at every point on the course of the disease, but in male and younger patients tends to develop in first 3 years after diagnosis, leading to a worse prognosis. Behçet's eye disease is a chronic, relapsing bilateral non-granulomatous panuveitis, affecting both anterior and posterior poles of the ocular globe. Retinal occlusive vasculitis is often seen; conjunctivitis is rare. The disease runs with recurrent severe attacks, followed by spontaneous remissions. Though not associated to mortality, uveitis is one of the leading causes of morbidity in Behçet's disease. About 20-30 years ago the rate of blindness due to uveitis was higher than 75% of patients. Fortunately, better schemes of management and higher level of awareness made this outcome decrease, but still 10-15% of patients will develop functional visual loss (Kural-Seyahi et al, 2003). Loss of sight is due to permanent damage of intraocular structures by recurrent inflammatory attacks, atrophy of the optic nerve, secondary glaucoma or cataracts.

The management of patients with Behçet's eye disease should achieve rapid resolution of intraocular inflammation, prevent further attacks and preserve vision. Rapid control of inflammation is highly imperative in acute posterior uveitis (anterior pole inflammation usually is not severe and is well controlled with topical treatment). Glucocorticoids, azathioprine and cyclosporin are generally used, even in combination for refractory cases. However, despite these drugs, some patients will persist with recurrent flares leading to visual loss. In this subgroup of patients, monoclonal anti-TNF agent infliximab showed promising results in single reports and case series. In five patients with recurrent panuveitis, a single infusion of infliximab achieved a rapid remission in 24 hours and complete resolution in following 7 days (Sfikakis et al, 2001). Muñoz-Fernandez et al (2001) reported a successful outcome with infliximab 5mg/kg on a patient with sight-threatening panuveitis: inflammatory signs resolved and visual acuity significantly improved after three infusions. Another patient with severe neuroretinitis, oral and genital ulcers, arthritis, erythema nodosum and superficial thrombophlebitis, was treated with infliximab 5mg/kg at 0, 2, 4 and 8 weeks scheme. All symptoms significantly improved after first infusion, achieving remission with the second one (Triolo et al, 2002).

In 2005, a prospective evaluation of infliximab in Behçet's uveitis was published (Tugal-Tutkun et al, 2005). Thirteen male patients with recurrent posterior uveitis refractory to combination of cyclosporin, azathioprine and prednisolone were enrolled. Cyclosporin was discontinued. The authors used infliximab at 5mg/kg dose, administered at weeks 0, 2, 6 and 14 weeks. During the infusion period, lower incidence of eye flares were noted compared to pre-enrolment period, achieving 4 of them (30.8%) remission. No extraocular features of the disease occurred during this period and prednisolone dose reduced. Interestingly, the effect of infliximab got lost in the observation period (between weeks 23 and 54): there was no significant difference with the previous-treatment, and only 1 patient remained attack-free. Safety profile was acceptable, with no severe events. Since then, other prospective uncontrolled trials have been reported. Tognon et al (2007) tried infliximab in 7 patients with sight-threating uveitis refractory to several immunosuppressive agents, with excellent results: intensity and number of relapses decreased, and visual acuity improved in 30% of eyes while in the rest remained stable. Extraocular manifestation controlled as well. No safety problems were noted. Niccoli et al (2007) assessed the efficacy of infliximab 5mg/kg (9 infusions) plus prednisolone 1mg/kg over a long-term follow-up (24 months) in 12 consecutive patients with refractory posterior uveitis. A rapid response was noted after first infusion. At 12 months, 75% of the patients achieved a complete remission with no relapses detected, and at 24 months 78% of them still remained in remission. Treatment was well tolerated with no significant adverse events.

There are no prospective controlled trials evaluating infliximab in Behçet's uveitis. But two reports retrospectively evaluated infliximab against conventional immunosuppressive therapy (Tabbara & Al-Hemidan, 2008; Yamada et al, 2010). Both studies showed excellent results in the group of patients treated with infliximab, with significantly lower number of acute flares. Visual acuity improved in both groups, but only in the study by Tabbara median values were significantly higher with infliximab. It is noteworthy that more severe adverse events were noted in patients treated with conventional agents. An arguable bias for these studies is that treatment groups are not comparable - patients treated with infliximab present a more aggressive uveitis, refractory to high immunosuppression; but the fact that infliximab succeed, even better than previous agents, is an encouraging data. Infliximab is nowadays recommended for acute flares of posterior uveitis with significant reduction of visual acuity; when remission is achieved, infliximab may be switched to immunosuppressive drugs, as cyclosporin or azathioprine, with low-dose oral glucocorticoids (Sfikakis et al, 2007). As known from rheumatoid arthritis, long-term use of infliximab may lead to the development of resistances (Ito el al, 2010), as it is a chimeric, not fully humanised monoclonal antibody.

Evidence of efficacy with etanercept in Behçet's eye disease is lacking - there are scant reports and, as previously commented, in controlled trial by Melikoglu (2005) patients with active eye disease were not enrolled - so this drug cannot be recommended. Adalimumab seems to be effective in refractory Behçet's uveitis, but data only come from case reports and retrospective series (Mushtaq et al, 2007; Bawazeer & Raffa, 2010; Takase K et al, 2011), so further research is needed.

4.2.3 Gastrointestinal disease

Gastrointestinal involvement is one of the most frequent features in patients with Behçet's disease from Japan, Taiwan and Northern Europe - ranges from 30% to 50% - while the frequency in Turkey and Western Asia is low - about 5% (Ebert, 2009; Yacizi et al, 2010). Beside mouth ulcers, Behçet's disease predominantly affects small and large bowel, especially around ileocecal region. Esophageal, gastric or rectal involvement is rare. Type of intestinal involvement depends on subjacent vasculitis: small vessel vasculitis leads to mucosal inflammation and aphthous ulcers, meanwhile large vessel vasculitis associates with ischemia and infarction. Abdominal pain is the most common complaint; others are bloody stools, persistent diarrhoea or unexplained weight loss. The disease is often mild, but some patients complicates with perforation, mesenteric ischemia or major gastrointestinal bleeding. Gastrointestinal involvement typically associates with cutaneous papulo-pustular lesions and pyoderma gangrenosum.

As well as other Behçet's features, intestinal disease runs in an unpredictable course with flares and remissions. Recurrences after treatment are frequent, even after surgery, especially on the anastomotic site (Ha HK et al, 1998). In two case series from France (Saadoun et al, 2010) and Turkey (Kural-Seyahi et al, 2003) no patients died due to intestinal involvement, but in French series pancreatitis was the cause of death in one patient. Behçet's bowel disease management is similar to other features of the condition, where glucocorticoids and colchicine for mild disease and azathioprine or cyclosporin for severe disease are commonly used. Thalidomide and mesalazine could act as glucocorticoids-dose sparing agents. Anti-TNF agents have been used, but data mainly come from case reports (Hassard et al, 2001). Iwata et al (2009) tried infliximab in 10 patients with active entero-Behçet's disease refractory to conventional immunosuppressive agents or with contraindications against its use. All patients showed a rapid improvement in the intestinal manifestations, achieving remission 5 out 10 patients at 6 months, and 9 out 10 at 12 months.

Extraintestinal features of the disease improved as well and no severe adverse events were detected. Infliximab was used at dosage of 3mg/kg, but one patient required an increase to 5mg/kg due to a suspected recurrence. In another case series (Naganuma et al, 2008) 6 patients with fulminant intestinal disease were treated with infliximab with successful outcome, getting 5 of the six patients on remission. Despite limitation by lacking of controlled trials, current evidence supports the use of infliximab in refractory, severe cases of Behçet's intestinal disease. There is no data about etanercept or adalimumab, so formal recommendations cannot be done.

4.2.4 Central nervous system disease

Neurological involvement in Behçet's disease widely ranges between series, from 1.3% to 59%, with an average of about 10% of patients (Al-Araji & Kidd, 2009), usually developing a few years after the diagnosis of the disease. Men have two-three times higher risk of development compared to women. The condition specifically affects to central nervous system (CNS); peripheral involvement is uncertain. Though infrequent, it is often included in differential diagnosis in demyelinating and inflammatory CNS disorders. CNS-Behçet's disease presents with two different forms, rarely both in a same patient. First, parenchymal CNS disease is a subacute meningoencephalitis mainly located to brainstem, basal ganglia, thalamus and white matter. Hemispheres, spinal cord and other parts of CNS might be affected as well, but more common as a diffuse rather than focal involvement. And second, vessels, especially veins, are affected in non-parenchymal CNS-Behçet's disease, leading to cranial venous thrombosis and intracranial hypertension. Strokes due to arterial involvement are seldom seen. Patients complain of nonspecific symptoms (headache, malaise, fatigue, fever, etc.) and signs and symptoms derived from the area of CNS affected. A silent form has been described in asymptomatic patients but with detectable signs on the neurological examination.

Neuro-Behçet's disease is one of the most serious causes of morbidity and mortality in Behçet's. In spite of around a third of patients will present single episodes, another third will suffer further relapses and the other third a persistent, progressive involvement with aggravating neurological function (Akman-Demir et al, 1999). And how rapid the treatment is initiated probably will influence in further prognosis. Prospective controlled trials in Neuro-Behçet's disease are lacking, so treatment schemes are largely empirical. Intravenous methylprednisolone, followed by tapering prednisolone, is the first line agent after diagnosis. Initiation of an immunosuppressive agent (i.e. azathioprine, methotrexate or mycophenolate mofetil) depends on severity, previous episodes and response to glucocorticoids.

As well as in other less common Behçet's features, no adequate controlled studies have evaluated the role of anti-TNF agents in neuro-Behçet's. But results from case series are very promising. Pipitone et al (2008) retrospectively reviewed 8 patients with parenchymal neuro-Behçet's disease treated with infliximab. Dosage of 5 mg/kg was used in all patients, and adjunct drugs varied. Neurological involvement was refractory to immunosuppressive agents or developed while this treatment was being used due to other features of the disease. All 8 patients successfully responded to treatment, with rapid and marked improvement of symptoms. In one patient infliximab lost his efficacy after 5 years, with recurrence of symptoms, but improved again after initiating etanercept. No safety problems were reported. Other series (Kikuchi et al, 2008) also showed good results with infliximab 5mg/kg in 5 patients with progressive neuro-Behçet's disease refractory to glucocorticoids and methotrexate. Infliximab was added to former treatment scheme. Interestingly, the authors found marked reduction of interleukin-6 levels on cerebrospinal fluid after initiating the drug, meanwhile TNFα levels remained unchanged. One patient developed a suspected *Pneumocystis jiroveci* pneumonia during the treatment, responding to cotrimoxazole. In summary, further controlled trials are highly desirable, but we consider that anti-TNF agents should be tried in cases with refractory neurological Behçet's disease.

4.2.5 Vascular disease

Vascular involvement in Behçet's disease affects venous and arterial systems, both with an inflammatory basis (Yacizi et al, 2010). Approximately, one third of patients will present venous thrombosis on deep or superficial systems, typically on their lower limbs. Interestingly, pulmonary embolisms are very rare. Venous thrombosis can develop in other body locations, as suprahepatic veins - leading to Budd-Chiari syndrome (Seyahi et al, 2007) - or intracranial venous sinuses, as previously commented. Arterial involvement is lees frequent (<5%), but associated with poorer outcomes. Inflammatory pseudoaneurisms form in abdominal aorta, carotid, femoral or pulmonary arteries. If left untreated, mortality of pulmonary artery aneurisms is about 50% (Hamuryudan et al, 1994). Due to the inflammatory basis and the very low rate of embolism, not anticoagulation but immunosuppression is the mainstay of the management of Behçet's vascular disease, though controlled studies are lacking. Glucocorticoids and azathioprine or methotrexate may be used for venous thrombosis, but arterial involvement requires high-dose endovenous methylprednisolone and cyclophosphamide. The experience with anti-TNF agents lies on reported cases of refractory, life-threatening vascular involvement (Lee et al, 2010; Baki et al, 2006), with successful outcomes. No increased risk of atherosclerosis has been found in Behçet's disease.

4.3 Other biological agents

Rituximab, a chimeric monoclonal antibody against CD20 surface marker of B-cells, is widely used in other systemic autoimmune disorders, as rheumatoid arthritis, systemic lupus erythematosus or ANCA-associated vasculitis. Rituximab has been used in Behçet's disease as well. In 2008, Sadreddini et al communicated a patient with a severe retinal vasculitis refractory to azathioprine who developed hypersensitivity to etanercept. In this patient, rituximab (1gr, 2 infusions 2 weeks apart) improved the inflammatory signs and visual acuity in 6 weeks after the infusion. Recently, a pilot study evaluating rituximab in Behçet's eye disease has been published (Davatchi et al, 2010). Twenty patients with Behçet's uveitis and partial or absent response to cytotoxic agents were enrolled and randomised to receive rituximab (1gr, 2 infusions 2 weeks apart, plus weekly methotrexate and oral prednisolone) or an aggressive cytotoxic regime with cyclophosphamide, azathioprine and oral prednisolone. The author used the change in Total Adjusted Disease Activity Index (TADAI), a combination of different parameters of eye examination, as an outcome measure. TADAI and every single measure improved in both groups, but the difference between groups was no significant. Serious adverse events were detected in rituximab group - pneumonia in one patient and a severe infusion reaction in another. Though rituximab was as effective as cytotoxic schemes in Behçet's uveitis, further studies are needed.

As well as TNFα, interleukin–1β and other pro-inflammatory cytokines levels are elevated in sera of patients with active Behçet's disease (Duzgun et al, 2005). Furthermore, an increase in interleukin-1 receptor antagonist, one of the natural immunomodulating molecules of this cytokine, has been reported after controlling the disease (Benezra et al, 1997). In our search, we found an only report about using interleukin-1β antagonist anakinra in patients with Behçet's disease: Botsios et al [2008] communicated an excellent response to anakinra in a 75 year-old woman whose disease was previously refractory to several immunosuppressive agents and partially responded to infliximab. Further studies are clearly needed to establish formal recommendations.

The anti-interleukin 2 receptor CD25 monoclonal antibody daclizumab was tested in a prospective placebo-controlled trial in Behçet's uveitis (Buggage et al, 2007). Patients in both groups continued to receive their previous immunosuppressive agents, and endovenous infusions of daclizumab 1mg/kg or placebo was added every two weeks for six weeks (4-dose induction), then once every four weeks for a minimum of 24 months following randomization. Ocular attacks continued to happen in both groups, but rate was even higher in patients on daclizumab arm. No safety problems were reported. Daclizumab is not recommended for the management of Behçet's disease.

Auto-reactive T lymphocytes may have a role in pathogenesis of Behçet's disease, explaining the successful response to calcineurin inhibitors (as cyclosporin) seen in this disease. In 2003, a series with patients with Behçet's disease treated with the anti-CD52 humanised monoclonal antibody alemtuzumab (CAMPATH-1H) was published (Lockwood et al, 2003). Patients with different active disease features were enrolled, being thirteen of them refractory to immunosuppressive agents. After a course of 5 daily infusions of alemtuzumab (total 134mg), eight patients achieved complete remission and seven patients showed a partial remission after 3 months of follow-up. Seven patients required further immunosuppressive agents to control the disease. No serious adverse events were detected. No controlled group was used in this study, but T-cells might be a new promising target for the management of Behçet's disease.

5. Mixed cryoglobulinemic vasculitis

Mixed cryoglobulinemic vasculitis (MC) is a small-vessel vasculitis characterised by the proliferation of B-cell clones producing pathogenic IgM with rheumatoid factor activity. More than 80% of MC vasculitis cases are attributable to hepatitis C viral (HCV) infection. Patients whose manifestations are not controlled by standard therapy, could be candidates for new biological therapy.

Rituximab is a chimeric murine/human anti-CD20 monoclonal antibody that binds to the B cell surface antigen CD20, resulting in selective depletion of peripheral B cells which can last for 6 months or longer. In order to analyse the efficacy and tolerance of rituximab treatment in patients with MC vasculitis, Cacoub et al performed a systematic review (Cacoub et al., 2008), which founded 13 manuscripts that reported on a total number of 57 cases of MC secondary to hepatitis C virus (HCV) infection (43 patients, 75.4%) or essential mixed cryoglobulinemia (14 patients, 24.6%). There were two large uncontrolled series of 20 (Sansonno et al, 2003) and 15 (Zaja et al, 2003) patients, and two smaller series of 6 (Roccatello et al, 2004) and 5 (Quartuccio et al, 2006) patients. All other publications reported either single or two case reports. Most patients (48 out of 57) received four weekly consecutive intravenous infusions of 375 mg/m2 of rituximab for either unresponsiveness or intolerance to previous treatments (n=52). The duration of follow-up after rituximab therapy was 9.7 months. Partial or complete remissions were observed in 80% of patients with skin involvement, 79% of patients with arthralgias, 93% of patients with neuropathy, and 83%of patients with glomerulonephritis. A relapse of MC was noted in 14 out of 36 (39%) patients after a mean of 6.7 months; eight of these patients went into complete remission after a second course of rituximab. A relatively small number of side effects were reported. The authors concluded that rituximab therapy for patients with MC vasculitis, either HCV induced or essential, shows a great efficacy on the main vasculitis signs in the majority of reported patients. A relapse of cryoglobulinemia vasculitis was frequently noted. About 30% of MC patients undergo active disease despite treatment with rituximab or antiviral therapy alone. So the combination of rituximab with Peg-IFNα-ribavirin appears logical. The long-term follow-up of a cohort of patients with HCV–related vasculitis treated with rituximab with or without PEGylated interferon alfa-2b (PEG–IFN alfa-2b) plus ribavirin has been reported (Terrier et al., 2009). Patients received rituximab 375 mg/m2 and 40mg of intravenous methylprednisolone weekly for 4 weeks, followed by 1 year of therapy with PEG–IFN alfa-2b and ribavirin. The study group comprised 32 HCV RNA–positive patients with HCV-related vasculitis: 20 patients were treated with rituximab plus PEG–IFN alfa-2b and 12 antiviral-intolerant patients were treated with rituximab alone. Of the 20 patients with combined-treatment, 9 had not previously received antiviral treatment, while 11 were resistant to or had relapsed after combination antiviral therapy: all of them were previously enrolled in a 16-patient study (Saadoun et al, 2008), the 5 remaining patients in that study died - 1 patient - or were lost to follow-up - four patients. Complete remission was achieved in 80% of patients with combined-treatment, and partial remission in 15% of cases. A complete or partial immunologic response was observed in 67 and 33% of patients, respectively. The 12 patients who received rituximab alone because of intolerance of antiviral treatments experience complete or partial clinical response in 58 and 9% of patients respectively. Relapses were recorded in 22% of patients after a mean follow-up period of 23±12 months and these relapses were associated with loss of virologic control in all patients and with B cell recovery in 78% of cases.

6. References

Airo P, Antonioli CM, Vianelli M, Toniati P (2002). Antitumour necrosis factor treatment with infliximab in a case of giant cell arteritis resistant to steroid and immunosuppressive drugs. *Rheumatology (Oxford)* 41:347–349.

Akman-Demir G, Serdaroglu P, Tasçi B (1999). Clinical patterns of neurological involvement in Behçet's disease: evaluation of 200 patients. The Neuro-Behçet Study Group. *Brain* 122: 2171–82.

Al-Araji A, Kidd DP (2009). Neuro-Behçet's disease: epidemiology, clinical characteristics, and management. *Lancet Neurol* 8(2):192-204.

Al-Bishri J, le Riche N, Pope JE (2005). Refractory polyarteritis nodosa successfully treated with infliximab. *J Rheumatol* 32(7):1371-3.

Almoznino G, Ben-Chetrit E (2007). Infliximab for the treatment of resistant oral ulcers in Behçet's disease: a case report and review of the literature. *Clin Exp Rheumatol* 25(4 Suppl 45):S99-102.

Andonopoulos AP, Meimaris N, Daoussis D, Bounas A, Giannopoulos G (2003). Experience with infliximab (anti-TNF alpha monoclonal antibody) as monotherapy for giant cell arteritis. *Ann Rheum Dis* 62:1116.

Arbach O, Gross WL, Gause A (2002). Treatment of refractory Churg-Strauss-Syndrome (CSS) by TNF-alpha blockade. *Immunobiology*; 206(5):496-501.

Baki K, Villiger PM, Jenni D, Meyer T, Beer JH (2006). Behcet's disease with life-threatening haemoptoe and pulmonary aneurysms: complete remission after infliximab treatment. *Ann Rheum Dis* 65(11):1531-2.

Bawazeer A, Raffa LH (2010). Clinical experience with adalimumab in the treatment of ocular Behçet disease. *Ocul Immunol Inflamm* 18(3):226-32.

Benezra D, Maftzir G, Barak V (1997). Blood serum interleukin-1 receptor antagonist in pars planitis and ocular Behçet disease. *Am J Ophthalmol* 123(5):593-8.

Bhatia A, Ell PJ, Edwards JC (2005). Anti-CD20 monoclonal antibody (rituximab) as an adjunct in the treatment of giant cell arteritis. *Ann Rheum Dis* 64(7): 1099-100.

Booth A, Harper L, Hammad T, Bacon P, Griffith M, Levy J et al (2004). Prospective study of TNFalpha blockade with infliximab in anti-neutrophil cytoplasmic antibody-associated systemic vasculitis. *J Am Soc Nephrol*; 15(3):717-21.

Botsios C, Sfriso P, Furlan A, Punzi L, Dinarello CA (2008). Resistant Behçet disease responsive to anakinra. *Ann Intern Med* 149(4):284-6.

Buggage RR, Levy-Clarke G, Sen HN, Ursea R, Srivastava SK, Suhler EB et al (2007). A double-masked, randomized study to investigate the safety and efficacy of daclizumab to treat the ocular complications related to Behçet's disease. *Ocul Immunol Inflamm* 15(2):63-70.

Cacoub P, Delluc A, Saadoun D, Landau DA, Sene D (2008). Anti-CD20 monoclonal antibody (rituximab) treatment for cryoglobulinemic vasculitis: where do we stand? *Ann Rheum Dis* 67:283–287.

Cantini F, Niccoli L, Salvarani C, Padula A, Olivieri I (2001). Treatment of longstanding active giant cell arteritis with infliximab: report of four cases. *Arthritis Rheum* 44 (12): 2933-5.

Chronopoulou H, Tzavara V, Oikonomopoulos N et al (2001). High levels of TNF-a in the in the aqueous humor in patients suffering from Adamantiades-Behçet's disease: preliminary results. *Invest Ophthalmol Vis Sci* 42 (suppl 4):S708.

Chung SA, Seo P (2009). Advances in the use of biologic agents for the treatment of systemic vasculitis. *Current Opinion in Rheumatology*; 21:3–9.

Csernok E, Trabandt A, Müller A, Wang GC, Moosig F, Paulsen J et al (1999). Cytokine profiles in Wegener's granulomatosis: predominance of type 1 (Th1) in the granulomatous inflammation. *Arthritis Rheum* 42(4):742-50.

Davatchi F, Shams H, Rezaipoor M, Sadeghi-Abdollahi B, Shahram F, Nadji A et al (2010). Rituximab in intractable ocular lesions of Behcet's disease; randomized single-blind control study (pilot study). *Int J Rheum Dis* 13(3):246-52.

Deguchi Y, Shibata N, Kishimoto S (1990). Enhanced expression of the tumor necrosis factor/cachectin gene in peripheral blood mononuclear cells from patients with systemic vasculitis. *Clin Exp Immunol* 81:311-4.

Della Rossa A, Tavoni A, Merlini G, Baldini C, Sebastiani M, Lombardi M et al (2005). Two Takayasu arteritis patients successfully treated with infliximab: a potential disease-modifying agent? *Rheumatology (Oxford)* 44: 1074.

Düzgün N, Ayaşlioğlu E, Tutkak H, Aydintuğ OT (2005). Cytokine inhibitors: soluble tumor necrosis factor receptor 1 and interleukin-1 receptor antagonist in Behçet's disease. *Rheumatol Int* 25(1):1-5.

Ebert EC (2009). Gastrointestinal manifestations of Behçet's disease. *Dig Dis Sci* 54(2):201-7.

Everekliogiu C, Er H, Turkoz Y, Cekmen M (2002). Serum levels of TNF-a, sIL-2R, OL-6, and IL-8 are increased and associated with elevated lipid peroxidation in patients with Behçet's disease. *Mediators Inflamm* 11:87–93.

Ferraro AJ, Smith SW, Neil D, Savage CO (2008). Relapsed Wegener's granulomatosis after rituximab therapy--B cells are present in new pathological lesions despite persistent 'depletion' of peripheral blood. *Nephrol Dial Transplant* 23(9):3030-2.

Gilhar A, Winterstein G, Turani H, Landau J, Etzioni A (1989). Skin hyperreactivity response (pathergy) in Behçet's disease. *J Am Acad Dermatol* 21(3 Pt 1):547-52.

Giscombe R, Wang X, Huang D, Lefvert AK (2002). Coding sequence 1 and promoter single nucleotide polymorphisms in the CTLA-4 gene in Wegener's granulomatosis. *J Rheumatol* 29(5):950-3.

Goossens PH, Verburg RJ, Breedveld FC (2001). Remission of Behçet's syndrome with tumour necrosis factor alpha blocking therapy. *Ann Rheum Dis* 60(6):637.

Gul A (2001). Behçet's disease: an update on the pathogenesis. *Clin Exp Rheumatol* 19 (suppl 24):S6–12.

Ha HK, Lee HJ, Yang SK, Ki WW, Yoon KH, Shin YM et al (1998) Intestinal Behcet syndrome: CT features of patients with and patients without complications. *Radiology* 209(2):449–454.

Hagen EC, de Keizer RJ, Andrassy K, van Boven WP, Bruijn JA, van Es LA, et al (1995). Compassionate treatment of Wegener's granulomatosis with rabbit anti-thymocyte globulin. Clin Nephrol 43:351–9.

Hamuryudan V, Yurdakul S, Moral F, Numan F, Tüzün H, Tüzüner N et al (1994). Pulmonary arterial aneurysms in Behçet's syndrome: a report of 24 cases. Br J Rheumatol 33(1):48-51.

Hassard PV, Binder SW, Nelson V, Vasiliauskas EA (2001). Anti-tumor necrosis factor monoclonal antibody therapy for gastrointestinal Behçet's disease: a case report. *Gastroenterology* 120(4):995-9.

Haugeberg G, Velken M, Johnsen V (2004). Successful treatment of genital ulcers with infliximab in Behcet's disease. *Ann Rheum Dis* 63(6):744-5.

Hoffman G, Kerr G, Leavitt R, Hallahan C, Lebovics R, Travis W et al (1992). Wegener's granulomatosis: an analysis of 158 patients. *Ann Intern Med*; 116:488–98.

Hoffman, GS, Merkel, PA, Brasington, RD, Lenschow DJ, Liang P (2004). Anti-tumor necrosis factor therapy in patients with difficult to treat Takayasu arteritis. *Arthritis Rheum* 50:2296.

Hoffman GS, Cid MC, Rendt-Zagar KE, Merkel PA, Weyand CM, Stone JH et al; Infliximab-GCA Study Group (2007). Infliximab for maintenance of glucocorticosteroid-induced remission of giant cell arteritis: a randomized trial. *Ann Intern Med* 146 (9):621-30.

Huang D, Giscombe R, Zhou Y, Lefvert AK (2000). Polymorphisms in CTLA-4 but not tumor necrosis factor-alpha or interleukin 1beta genes are associated with Wegener's granulomatosis. *J Rheumatol* 27(2):397-401.

International Study Group for Behçet's Disease (1990). Criteria for diagnosis of Behçet disease. *Lancet* 335: 1078-1080.

Ito T, Sonoda KH, Hijioka K, Fujimoto T, Ishibashi T (2010). Acquired resistance to infliximab against uveitis due to Behçet's disease after one year of administration. *Jpn J Ophthalmol* 54(5):502-4.

Iwata S, Saito K, Yamaoka K, Tsujimura S, Nawata M, Suzuki K et al (2009). Effects of anti-TNF-alpha antibody infliximab in refractory entero-Behcet's disease. *Rheumatology (Oxford)* 48(8):1012-3.

Jennette JC, Falk RJ, Andrassy K, Bacon PA, Churg J, Gross WL et al (1994). Nomenclature of systemic vasculitides. Proposal of an international consensus conference. *Arthritis Rheum* 37(2):187-92.

Jolly M, Curran JJ (2005). Infliximab-responsive uveitis and vasculitis in a patient with Takayasu arteritis. *J Clin Rheumatol* 11:213–215.

Jones RB, Ferraro AJ, Chaudhry AN, Brogan P, Salama AD, Smith KG et al (2009). A multicenter survey of rituximab therapy for refractory antineutrophil cytoplasmic antibody-associated vasculitis. *Arthritis Rheum* 60(7):2156-68.

Jones RB, Tervaert JW, Hauser T, Luqmani R, Morgan MD, Peh CA et al; European Vasculitis Study Group (2010). Rituximab versus cyclophosphamide in ANCA-associated renal vasculitis. *N Engl J Med* 363(3):211-20.

Karageorgaki ZT, Mavragani CP, Papathanasiou MA, Skopouli FN (2007). Infliximab in Takayasu arteritis: a safe alternative? *Clin Rheumatol* 26:984–987

Kaushik VV, Reddy HV, Bucknall RC (2006). Successful use of rituximab in a patient with recalcitrant Churg-Strauss syndrome. *Ann Rheum Dis* 65(8):1116-7.

Keogh KA, Ytterberg SR, Fervenza FC, Carlson KA, Schroeder DR, Specks U (2006). Rituximab for refractory Wegener's granulomatosis: report of a prospective, open-label pilot trial. *Am J Respir Crit Care Med* 173(2):180-7.

Kerr GS, Hallahan CW, Giordano J, Leavitt RY, Fauci AS, Rottem M et al (1994). Takayasu arteritis. *Ann Intern Med* 120:919–29.

Kikuchi H, Aramaki K, Hirohata S (2008). Effect of infliximab in progressive neuro-Behçet's syndrome. *J Neurol Sci* 272(1-2):99-105.

Koukoulaki M, Smith KG, Jayne DR (2006). Rituximab in Churg-Strauss syndrome. *Ann Rheum Dis* 65(4):557-9.

Kural-Seyahi E, Fresko I, Seyahi N, Ozyazgan Y, Mat C, Hamuryudan V et al (2003). The long-term mortality and morbidity of Behçet syndrome: a 2-decade outcome survey of 387 patients followed at a dedicated center. *Medicine (Baltimore)* 82(1):60-76.

Lamprecht P, Voswinkel J, Lilienthal T, Nolle B, Heller M, Gross WL et al (2002). Effectiveness of TNF-alpha blockade with infliximab in refractory Wegener's granulomatosis. *Rheumatology (Oxford)* 41(11):1303-7.

Laurino S, Chaudhry A, Booth A, Conte G, Jayne D (2010). Prospective study of TNFalpha blockade with adalimumab in ANCA-associated systemic vasculitis with renal involvement. *Nephrol Dial Transplant* 25(10):3307-14.

Lee SW, Lee SY, Kim KN, Jung JK, Chung WT (2010). Adalimumab treatment for life threatening pulmonary artery aneurysm in Behçet disease: a case report. *Clin Rheumatol* 29(1):91-3.

Little MA, Nightingale P, Verburgh CA, Hauser T, De Groot K, Savage C et al; European Vasculitis Study (EUVAS) Group (2010). Early mortality in systemic vasculitis: relative contribution of adverse events and active vasculitis. *Ann Rheum Dis* 69(6):1036-43.

Lockwood CM, Hale G, Waldman H, Jayne DR (2003). Remission induction in Behçet's disease following lymphocyte depletion by the anti-CD52 antibody CAMPATH 1-H. *Rheumatology (Oxford)* 42(12):1539-44.

Ludviksson B, Sneller M, Chua K, Talar-Williams C, Langford C, Ehrhardt R et al (1998). Active Wegener's granulomatosis is associated with HLA-DR+ CD4+ T cells exhibiting an unbalanced Th1-type T cell cytokine pattern: reversal with IL-10. *J Immunol* 160:3602-9.

Lukas R, Keller F (1998). Anti-thymocyte globulin therapy in a patient with pANCA vasculitis and crescentic glomerulonephritis. *Nephron* 78:231.

Maksimowicz-McKinnon K, Clark TM, Hoffmann GS (2007). Limitations of therapy and a guarded prognosis in an American cohort of Takayasu Arteritis patients. *Arthritis Rheum* 56(3): 1000–7.

Maksimowicz-McKinnon K, Clark TM, Hoffman GS (2009). Takayasu arteritis and giant cell arteritis: a spectrum within the same disease? *Medicine (Baltimore)* 88(4):221-6.

Martinez-Taboada VM, Rodriguez-Valverde V, Carreno L, López-Longo J, Figueroa M, Belzunegui J et al (2008). A double-blind placebo controlled trial of etanercept in patients with giant cell arteritis and corticosteroid side effects. *Ann Rheum Dis* 67:625–630.

Mege JL, Dilsen N, Sanguedolce V, Gul A, Bongrand P, Roux H et al (1993). Overproduction of monocyte-derive TNF-a, IL-6, IL-8 and increased neutrophil superoxide generation in Behçet's disease. A comparative study with familial Mediterranean fever and healthy subjects. *J Rheumatol* 20:1544–9.

Melikoglu M, Fresko I, Mat C, Ozyazgan Y, Gogus F, Yurdakul S et al (2005). Short-term trial of etanercept in Behçet's disease: a double blind, placebo controlled study. *J Rheumatol* 32(1):98-105.

Molloy ES, Langford CA, Clark TM, Gota CE, Hoffman GS. (2008). Antitumour necrosis factor therapy in patients with refractory Takayasu's arteritis: long-term follow-up. *Ann Rheum Dis* 67:1567–1569.

Mukhtyar C, Guillevin L, Cid MC, Dasgupta B, de Groot K, Gross W et al; European Vasculitis Study Group (2009). EULAR recommendations for the management of large vessel vasculitis. *Ann Rheum Dis* 68(3):318-23.

Muñoz-Fernández S, Hidalgo V, Fernández-Melón J, Schlincker A, Martín-Mola E (2001). Effect of infliximab on threatening panuveitis in Behçet's disease. *Lancet* 358(9293):1644.

Mushtaq B, Saeed T, Situnayake RD, Murray PI (2007). Adalimumab for sight-threatening uveitis in Behçet's disease. *Eye (Lond)* 21(6):824-5.

Naganuma M, Sakuraba A, Hisamatsu T, Ochiai H, Hasegawa H, Ogata H et al (2008). Efficacy of infliximab for induction and maintenance of remission in intestinal Behçet's disease. *Inflamm Bowel Dis* 14(9):1259-64.

Nakahama H, Yokokawa T, Okada M, Miyazaki M, Imai N, Kubori S et al (1993). Distinct responses of interleukin-6 and other laboratory parameters to treatment in a patient with Wegener's granulomatosis. *Intern Med* 32(2):189-92.

Nassonov E, Samsonov M, Tilz G, Beketova T, Semenkova E, Baranov A et al (1997). Serum concentrations of neopterin, soluble interleukin 2 receptor, and soluble tumor necrosis factor receptor in Wegener's granulomatosis. *J Rheumatol* 24:666–70.

Niccoli L, Nannini C, Benucci M, Chindamo D, Cassarà E, Salvarani C et al (2007). Long-term efficacy of infliximab in refractory posterior uveitis of Behcet's disease: a 24-month follow-up study. *Rheumatology (Oxford)* 46(7):1161-4.

Nogueira E, Hamour S, Sawant D, Henderson S, Mansfield N, Chavele KM et al (2010). Serum IL-17 and IL-23 levels and autoantigen-specific Th17 cells are elevated in patients with ANCA-associated vasculitis. *Nephrol Dial Transplant* 25(7):2209-17.

Noronha I, Kruger C, Andrassy K, Ritz E, Waldherr R (1993). In situ production of TNF-alpha, IL-1 beta and IL-2R in ANCA-positive glomerulonephritis. *Kidney Int* 43:682–92.

Omdal R, Wildhagen K, Hansen T, Gunnarsson R, Kristoffersen G (2005). Anti-CD20 therapy of treatment-resistant Wegener's granulomatosis: favourable but temporary response. *Scand J Rheumatol* 34(3):229-32.

Park MC, Lee SW, Park YB, Chung NS, Lee SK (2005). Clinical characteristics and outcomes of Takayasu's arteritis: analysis of 108 patients using standardized criteria for diagnosis, activity assessment, and angiographic classification. *Scand J Rheumatol* 34:284–92.

Pepper RJ, Fabre MA, Pavesio C, Gaskin G, Jones RB, Jayne D et al (2008). Rituximab is effective in the treatment of refractory Churg-Strauss syndrome and is associated with diminished T-cell interleukin-5 production. *Rheumatology (Oxford)* 47(7):1104-5.

Pipitone N, Olivieri I, Padula A, D'angelo S, Nigro A, Zuccoli G et al (2008). Infliximab for the treatment of Neuro-Behçet's disease: a case series and review of the literature. *Arthritis Rheum* 59(2):285-90.

Popa ER, Stegeman CA, Bos NA, Kallenberg CG, Tervaert JW (1999). Differential B- and T-cell activation in Wegener's granulomatosis. *J Allergy Clin Immunol* 103(5 Pt 1):885-94.

Popa ER, Franssen CF, Limburg PC, Huitema MG, Kallenberg CG, Tervaert JW (2002). In vitro cytokine production and proliferation of T cells from patients with anti-proteinase 3- and antimyeloperoxidase-associated vasculitis, in response to proteinase 3 and myeloperoxidase. *Arthritis Rheum* 46(7):1894-904.

Quartuccio L, Soardo G, Romano G, Zaja F, Scott CA, De Marchi G et al (2006). Rituximab treatment for glomerulonephritis in HCV-associated mixed cryoglobulinaemia: efficacy and safety in the absence of steroids. *Rheumatology (Oxford)* 45:842.

Robertson LP, Hickling P (2001). Treatment of recalcitrant orogenital ulceration of Behçet's syndrome with infliximab. *Rheumatology (Oxford)* 40(4):473-4.

Roccatello D, Baldovino S, Rossi D, Mansouri M, Naretto C, Gennaro M et al (2004). Longterm effects of anti-CD20 monoclonal antibody treatment of cryoglobulinaemic glomerulonephritis. *Nephrol Dial Transplant* 19:3054–61.

Saadoun D, Resche-Rigon M, Sene D, Perard L, Karras A, Cacoub P (2008). Rituximab combined with peginterferon-ribavirin in refractory HCV-associated cryoglobulinemia vasculitis. *Ann Rheum Dis* 67:1431–1436.

Saadoun D, Wechsler B, Desseaux K, Le Thi Huong D, Amoura Z, Resche-Rigon M et al (2010). Mortality in Behçet's disease. *Arthritis Rheum* 62(9):2806-12.

Sadreddini S, Noshad H, Molaeefard M, Noshad R (2008). Treatment of retinal vasculitis in Behçet's disease with rituximab. *Mod Rheumatol* 18(3):306-8.

Salvarani C, Macchioni P, Manzini C, Paolazzi G, Trotta A, Manganelli P et al (2007). Infliximab plus prednisone or placebo plus prednisone for the initial treatment of polymyalgia rheumatica. *Ann Intern Med* 146:631–9.

Salvarani C, Pipitone N, Boiardi L, Hunder GG (2008). Do we need treatment with tumour necrosis factor blockers for giant cell arteritis? *Ann Rheum Dis* 67(5):577-9.

Sánchez-Cano D, Callejas-Rubio JL, Ortego-Centeno N (2008). Effect of rituximab on refractory Wegener granulomatosis with predominant granulomatous disease. *J Clin Rheumatol* 14(2):92-3.

Sansonno D, De Re V, Lauletta G, Tucci FA, Boiocchi M, Dammacco F (2003). Monoclonal antibody treatment of mixed cryoglobulinemia resistant to interferon alpha with an anti-CD20. *Blood* 101:3818–3826.

Seitz M, Reichenbach S, Bonel HM, Adler S, Wermelinger F, Villiger PM (2011). Rapid induction of remission in large vessel vasculitis by IL-6 blockade. A case series. *Swiss Med Wkly* 141:w13156.

Seo P, Stone JH (2004). Large-vessel vasculitis. *Arthritis Rheum* 51(1):128-39.

Seo P, Specks U, Keogh KA (2008). Efficacy of rituximab in limited Wegener's granulomatosis with refractory granulomatous manifestations. *J Rheumatol* 35(10):2017-23.

Seyahi E, Hamuryudan V, Hatemi G, Melikoglu M, Celik S, Fresko I et al (2007). Infliximab in the treatment of hepatic vein thrombosis (Budd-Chiari syndrome) in three patients with Behcet's syndrome. *Rheumatology (Oxford)* 46(7):1213-4.

Sfikakis PP, Theodossiadis PG, Katsiari CG, Kaklamanis P, Markomichelakis NN (2001). Effect of infliximab on sight-threatening panuveitis in Behçet's disease. *Lancet* 358(9278):295-6.

Sfikakis PP, Markomichelakis N, Alpsoy E, Assaad-Khalil S, Bodaghi B, Gul A et al (2007). Anti-TNF therapy in the management of Behcet's disease--review and basis for recommendations. *Rheumatology (Oxford)* 46(5):736-41.

Specks U, Fervenza FC, McDonald TJ, Hogan MC (2001). Response of Wegener's granulomatosis to anti-CD20 chimeric monoclonal antibody therapy. *Arthritis Rheum* 44(12):2836-40.

Stasi R, Stipa E, Del Poeta G, Amadori S, Newland AC, Provan D (2006). Long-term observation of patients with anti-neutrophil cytoplasmic antibody-associated vasculitis treated with rituximab. *Rheumatology (Oxford)* 45(11):1432-6.

Steiner K, Moosig F, Csernok E, Selleng K, Gross WL, Fleischer B et al (2001). Increased expression of CTLA-4 (CD152) by T and B lymphocytes in Wegener's granulomatosis. *Clin Exp Immunol* 126(1):143-50.

Stone JH, Uhlfelder ML, Hellmann DB, Crook S, Bedocs NM, Hoffman GS (2001). Etanercept combined with conventional treatment in Wegener's granulomatosis: a six-month open-label trial to evaluate safety. *Arthritis Rheum* 44(5):1149-54.

Stone JH, Merkel PA, Spiera R, Seo P, Langford CA, Hoffman GS et al; RAVE-ITN Research Group (2010). Rituximab versus cyclophosphamide for ANCA-associated vasculitis. *N Engl J Med* 363(3):221-32.

Tabbara KF, Al-Hemidan AI (2008). Infliximab effects compared to conventional therapy in the management of retinal vasculitis in Behçet disease. *Am J Ophthalmol* 146(6):845-50.e1.

Takase K, Ohno S, Ideguchi H, Uchio E, Takeno M, Ishigatsubo Y (2011). Successful switching to adalimumab in an infliximab-allergic patient with severe Behçet disease-related uveitis. *Rheumatol Int* 31(2):243-5.

Tamura N, Matsudaira R, Hirashima M, Ikeda M, Tajima M, Nawata M et al (2007). Two cases of refractory Wegener's granulomatosis successfully treated with rituximab. *Intern Med* 46(7):409-14.

Tanaka F, Kawakami A, Iwanaga N, Tamai M, Izumi Y, Aratake K et al (2006). Infliximab is effective for Takayasu arteritis refractory to glucocorticoid and methotrexate. *Intern Med* 45:313–316.

Tato F, Rieger J, Hoffmann U (2005). Refractory Takayasu's arteritis successfully treated with the human, monoclonal antitumor necrosis factor antibody adalimumab. *Int Angiol* 24:304–307.

Tektonidou MG, Skopouli FN (2006). Sustained 3-year remission after Rituximab treatment in a patient with refractory Wegener's granulomatosis. *Clin Exp Rheumatol* 24(2 Suppl 41):S103.

Terrier B, Saadoun D, Sene D, Sellam J, Pérard L, Coppéré B et al (2009). Efficacy and tolerability of rituximab with or without PEGylated interferon alfa-2b plus ribavirin in severe hepatitis C virus-related vasculitis: a long-term followup study of thirty-two patients. *Arthritis Rheum* 60: 2531-40.

Tognon S, Graziani G, Marcolongo R (2007). Anti-TNF-alpha therapy in seven patients with Behcet's uveitis: advantages and controversial aspects. *Ann N Y Acad Sci* 1110:474-84.

Triolo G, Vadalà M, Accardo-Palumbo A, Ferrante A, Ciccia F, Giardina E et al (2002). Anti-tumour necrosis factor monoclonal antibody treatment for ocular Behçet's disease. *Ann Rheum Dis* 61(6):560-1.

Tugal-Tutkun I, Mudun A, Urgancioglu M, Kamali S, Kasapoglu E, Inanc M et al (2005). Efficacy of infliximab in the treatment of uveitis that is resistant to treatment with the combination of azathioprine, cyclosporine, and corticosteroids in Behçet's disease: an open-label trial. *Arthritis Rheum* 52(8):2478-84.

Vanoli M, Daina E, Salvarani C, Sabbadini MG, Rossi C, Bacchiani G et al (2005). Takayasu's arteritis: a study of 104 Italian patients. *Arthritis Rheum* 53(1): 100–7.

Verity DH, Marr JE, Ohno S, Wallace GR, Stanford MR (1999). Behçet's disease, the Silk Road and HLA-B51: historical and geographical perspectives. *Tissue Antigens* 54(3):213-20.

Walsh M, Chaudhry A, Jayne D (2008). Long-term follow up of relapsing/refractory anti-neutrophil cytoplasm antibody associated vasculitis treated with the lymphocyte depleting antibody alemtuzumab (CAMPATH-1H). *Ann Rheum Dis* 67: 1322-1327.

Wegener's Granulomatosis Etanercept Trial (WGET) Research Group (2005). Etanercept plus standard therapy for Wegener's granulomatosis. *N Engl J Med* 352(4):351-61.

Yamada Y, Sugita S, Tanaka H, Kamoi K, Kawaguchi T, Mochizuki M (2010). Comparison of infliximab versus ciclosporin during the initial 6-month treatment period in Behçet disease. *Br J Ophthalmol* 94(3):284-8.

Yamashita N, Kaneoka H, Kaneko S, Takeno M, Oneda K, Koizumi H et al (1997). Role of gamma-delta T lymphocytes in the development of Behçet's disease. *Clin Exp Immunol* 107:241–7.

Yazici Y, Yurdakul S, Yazici H (2010). Behçet's syndrome. *Curr Rheumatol Rep* 12(6):429-35.

Zaja F, De Vita S, Mazzaro C, Sacco S, Damiani D, De Marchi G et al (2003). Efficacy and safety of rituximab in type II mixed cryoglobulinemia. *Blood* 101:3827-3834.

Zhou Y, Huang D, Paris PL, Sauter CS, Prock KA, Hoffman GS (2004). An analysis of CTLA-4 and proinflammatory cytokine genes in Wegener's granulomatosis. *Arthritis Rheum* 50(8):2645-50.

Zouboulis CC, Kötter I, Djawari D, Kirch W, Kohl PK, Ochsendorf FR et al (1997). Epidemiological features of Adamantiades-Behçet's disease in Germany and in Europe. *Yonsei Med J* 38(6):411-22.

8

Intravenous Immunoglobulin Therapy in Primary Vasculitides

Norbert Lukán
4th Internal Department Medical Faculty, Safarik University, Košice
Slovak Republic

1. Introduction

Vasculitis is defined as chronic blood vessel inflammation confirmed by histologic evidence. The typical course of the disease may lead to blood vessel stenosis/occlusion causing organ ischemia, or to thinning of the blood vessel which results in aneurysm formation or hemorrhage. Although in 1994 the American College of Rheumatology introduced morphological and histopathological classification criteria for the most common forms of vasculitides at the Chapel Hill Consensus Conference (CHCC) (Jennette et al., 1994), vasculitides are generally divided into two main categories. Primary vasculitides represent the first group, are the entities of unknown cause in which blood vessel inflammation is the pathologic basis of tissue injury. Secondary vasculitides constitute the second, heterogeneous and much bigger group, in which inflammatory process occurs in association with an underlying disease or exposure.

The pathophysiology of the vasculitides is based on immunologic mechanisms. These mechanisms appear to play an active role in mediating the inflammatory response, but precise mechanisms still remain poorly understood. Although the primary events that initiate this process remain largely unknown, recent investigations have brought us closer to understanding some of the critical pathways involved in disease and provided a rationale for the study of novel therapeutic agents (Langford, 2010).

Intravenous immunoglobulin (IVIG) represents one of the novel alternative choices for the treatment as the standard regimen and IVIG has now become an important option in a number of clinical indications beyond primary immunodeficiency, including vasculitides.

2. Mechanisms of action

When Burton in 1951 for the first time published experience with the use of immunoglobulins in the replacement therapy for patients with primary immunodeficiencies and later other authors for secondary immunodeficiencies, no one would have expected that it could lead to the contemporary wide use of IVIG. Immunoglobulins can be applied in several immunomodulatory and anti-inflammatory indications as well. However, the exact mechanisms of action are only tentative. Some pathogenetic aspects have been already described, but during last fifteen years of intensive research new perspectives in understanding immunologic mechanisms of IVIG effects were introduced.

Basic immunomodulatory mechanisms of IVIG in autoimmune and inflammatory diseases could be devided into two groups. The first group involves mechanisms of humoral immunity and the second one involves mechanisms of cell-mediated immunity. Both groups interdependently involve modulation of expression and function of Fc receptors, interference with complement activation and the cytokine network, provision of antiidiotypic antibodies, modulation of dendritic cells, T and B-cell activation and differentiation and their effector functions (Negi et al., 2007).

Intravenous immunoglobulins are prepared from pooled normal polyspecific human IgG obtained from large numbers of healthy donors. IVIG thus contains the wide spectrum of natural antibodies that far exceeds spectrum present in individual subjects. Essential roles of natural antibodies in healthy subject are: first line defense against infection, clearance of aging cells, antigen presentation to T-cells, anti-tumoral surveillance, anti-inflammatory activity and selection of immune repertoires and homeostasis of autoreactivity (Lacroix-Desmazes et al., 1998).

2.1 Natural antibodies in IVIG

Immunomodulatory effect of IVIG is probably dependent on the content of natural antibodies in treatment preparations because it is hypothesized that the presence of natural antibodies in healthy subjects control autoreactivity and maintain immune homeostasis. IVIG preparations contain sampling from the entire array of variable regions of antibodies, so they play an important role in selection of autoreactive B-cells and prevent uncontrolled expansion of specific autoreactive clones in disease. In addition, natural antibodies may play a role in prevention of the occurrence of pathological autoimmune reactions by binding to microbial epitopes that are similar or identical to self antigens (Cohen & Cooke, 1986). Superantigens trigger the activation of autoreactive cells. IVIG contain anti-antibodies which could eliminate superantigens such as toxic shock syndrome toxin 1 and Staphylococcal enterotoxins. These superantigens are generally considered to be the triggers of exacerbation in Wegener´s granulomatosis (WG) (Stegeman et al., 1994, Boros et al., 2005).

2.2 Effect on Fc receptor modulation and anti-inflammatory activity

In order to prevent intracellular degradation of immunoglobulins in normal conditions Fc-receptor (FcRn) binds the molecule IgG inside the lysosome. During IVIG treatment oversaturation of normal molecules result in the accelerated catabolism of IgG and therefore reduce the level of pathogenic autoantibodies. In addition such IgG saturation leads to downregulation of FcRn in lysosomes and amplifies the effect of such treatment (Yu & Lennon, 1999). This hypothesis was supported in an experimental model, where in FcRn knockout mice, IVIG did not increase the clearance of antibodies, while in the wild type animals it did (Hansen & Balthasar, 2002). Analogous to normal circulating immunoglobulins intravenous immunoglobulins have also anti-inflammatory properties which modulate systemic inflammation during various inflammatory pathologies. Kaneko et al., (2006) showed that distinct properties of the Fc segment of IgG result from differential sialylation of the Fc core polysaccharide. IgG acquires anti-inflammatory properties upon Fc sialylation, which is reduced upon the induction of an antigen-specific immune response.

2.3 Immunomodulatory role of antiidiotypic antibodies

IVIG contains anti-idiotypes which are capable to neutralize pathogenic autoantibodies as described in antiphospholipid syndrome (Sherer et al., 2000) and idiopathic trombocytopenic purpura (Hoffmann et al., 2000). Interaction between antiidiotypes (Fab binding site) from IVIG and idiotype receptors on B-cells is probably responsible for the regulatory effect on autoreactive B-cell clones in patients with autoimmune and inflammatory disorders. Leucht et al., (2001) showed selective (VH gene origin) B-cell activation after IVIG treatment on patient with Kawasaki disease (KD). Sequence analysis has revealed that the most frequently used germ-line gene segments of all IVIG-bound Fabs were identical to those observed for many other autoantibodies and also represent the most frequently rearranged VH genes among human B-cells. It suggests that anti-idiotypic interactions may have an important role for the development and the control of the B-cell repertoire (Sibéril et al., 2007).

2.4 Dendritic cells as a target of immunomodulatory effect

Defective functions of dendritic cells have also been attributed for predisposition in vasculitis pathology. Bayary et al. (2006) have shown that dendritic cells are influenced by IVIG at therapeutic concentrations (25 - 35 mg/ml) in terms of modulation of differentiation, maturation and function of dendritic cells. They observed that IVIG abrogates secretion of IL-12, downregulates the capacity of mature and immature dendritic cells to express costimulatory molecules (CD80, CD86, CD40) which results in inhibition of auto- and alloreactive T-cell activation and proliferation. Providing that the suppression of these signals is necessary for optimal antigen presentation and T-cell activation, it could be plausible explanation of the efficacy of IVIG in many immuno-inflammatory diseases including vasculitides.

2.5 Regulation of cytokine production

IVIG shows anti-inflammatory effect in vasculitis by modulation of cytokine antagonists and Th1 and Th2 cytokine production. Andersson et al. (1996) published that the addition of IVIG (6 mg/ml) to stimulated cell cultures of peripheral blood mononuclear cells caused a marked inhibition of proliferation and blast transformation despite unaffected cell survival. These cells exhibited a significant inhibition of production of T-cell derived cytokines IL-2, IL-10, TNF-beta, IFN-gamma. Gupta et al. (2001) found reduction of proinflammatory cytokines Il-6, Il-8 and TNF-alfa in patients with KD. Lau et al. (2009) confirmed in murine model of KD that IVIG in therapeutic concentrations, but not salicylate, effectively reduced the immune response leading to TNF-alpha expression. Possible mechanism published Siedlar et al. (2011) when in vitro exposure of the healthy individuals' monocytes to the IVIG preparation resulted in reduced TNF production, which was overcome by blockade of the FcγRIIB in the CD14(+) CD16(++) CD32B(high) monocytes. Reduction in the number of CD14(+) CD16(++) monocytes and the blockade of their cytokine production via triggering CD32B can contribute to the anti-inflammatory action of IVIG. Regulation of cytokine and cytokine antagonists production is supposed to be one of the major anti-inflammatory mechanisms of intravenous immunoglobulins.

2.6 Attenuation of complement activation

Pathomechanisms of some vasculitides are closely associated with complement activation. Cryoglobulinemic vasculitis (glomerulonephritis) in patients with hepatitis C is associated with hypocomplementemia caused by its consumption (D´Amico & Fornasieri, 1995). In these patients various complement components such C3 and C1q has been detected in the different tissues (Haydey et al., 1980). IgA deposition, as well as complement factors (C3, properdin, and complement membrane attack), were detected in mesangion in patients with Henoch-Schönlein purpura (HSP) complicated by nephritis (Bene & Faure, 1987). Deposition of C3, C4, MBL but no C1q were detected in an other study (Hisano et al., 2005). Association of complement activation in vasculitides is not clearly understood. The mentioned studies showed that the complement system could be activated both through the alternative and classical/lectin pathway in patients with HSP. In ANCA-associated vasculitides interaction among ANCA, neutrophils and complement suggests a role of these components in the development of the disease. The ANCA-activated neutrophils release factors that can directly damage the endothelium but also activate the alternative complement pathway with the generation of the powerful neutrophil chemoattractant C5a. C5a and neutrophil C5aR may thus compose an amplification loop for ANCA-mediated neutrophil activation. Complement activation amplifies neutrophil influx and activation eventually culminates in severe necrotizing inflammation of the vessel wall in ANCA-associated vasculitides (Chen et al., 2010).

2.7 Regulation of T and B-cells

In normal condition T-cells and B-cells are important for the control of autoreactivity and induction of tolerance. In vasculitides, as well as in other autoimmune diseases, T-cells most likely play a role in delivering proper signals to autoreactive B-cells for the production of autoantibodies (Negi et al., 2007). T-cells probably also participate in granuloma formation in Wegener´s granulomatosis (Heeringa et al., 2005). In granulomatous lesions of WG T-cells with fenotype CD4+, CD28- represents a major source of proinflammatory cytokines (TNF-alfa, IFN-gamma) and may function as an essential driving force for perpetuating inflammation (Holle & Gross, 2009). These interactions indicate that an aberrant signaling cascade could be activated. Membrane molecules of T and B-cells could react with IVIG. In the last two decades many authors described that IVIG contain antibodies against variable membrane molecules variable such as CD4, CD5, CD40, CD95 and cytokine receptors and a variable amount of solubilised CD4, CD8, HLA-I and HLA-II molecules (Ephrem et al., 2005). Pool of antibodies stored in intravenous immunoglobulins directed to such functional molecules of lymphocytes is important for the immunomodulatory effects of IVIG and may interfere with antigen recognition by the T-cells (Blasczyk et al., 1993).

2.8 Modulation of Th17 cell function

Recently discovered regulatory Th17-cells and cell-derived cytokines play an important role in the pathogenesis of several autoimmune/inflammatory diseases including vasculitides. In Wegener´s granulomatosis, regulatory T-cells display impaired suppressor activity potentially favouring inflammation and break of tolerance (Abdulahad et al., 2007). Th17 - cells produce several cytokines such as Il-17, Il-21, IL-22, CCL-20 which induce massive inflammatory tissue reactions and these cytokines also stimulate nonimmune cells (fibroblasts, endothelial and epithelial cells) to the production of other proinflammatory mediators (Il-6, TNF-alfa, prostaglandins, NO, MMP and chemokines (Miossec et al., 2009). Maddur et al. (2011) published their results concerning the inhibition of differentiation, amplification and function of Th17-cells by IVIG treatment. The inhibitory effect depends on Fab2 receptor on Th17-cells. Maddur concluded that inhibition of effector cytokine release (Il-17A, IL-17F, IL-21) by these cells could demonstrate efficacy of IVIG in patient with autoimmune diseases by newly discovered mechanism.

3. Clinical indications

Intravenous immunoglobulins contain many different types of immune globulins (differentiated on the basis of structure and biological activity) that target different specific immune functions of the body. In this way, immunoglubulins imparts several types of immune fighting antibodies simultaneously. Seeing that the precise mechanism of IVIG are still largely unknown, the therapeutic mechanism of low-dose and high-dose regimen, as well as the short-and long-term effects are not the same for each condition. In low-dose and long term regimen IVIG were initially used to treat immunodeficiencies. Controversial knowledge about effectivity of high-dose treatment regimens leads to organizing several scientific meetings where attempt for treatment guidelines has been emphasized. In 2007 EULAR recommendations for the management of primary vasculitides were published in two parts according to CHCC classification - recommendations for small & medium vessel vasculitides and recommendations for large vessel vasculitides. These recommendations have been developed according to standardized operating procedures by EULAR standing committees. The guidance needs to be tailored to meet individual requirements. It is intended for use by healthcare professionals, medical students and specialist trainees, and pharmaceutical industries and drug regulatory organizations (Mukhtyar et al., 2009a, b). The British Society for Rheumatology published by Lapraik et al. (2007) guidelines for the management of adult ANCA-associated vasculitides. The main need for guidelines was to review the current treatment protocols and to highlight where there is an evidence base for treatment protocols and where treatment is based on individual preference. Recommendations are classified according to the level of evidence and the strength of recommendation. For large vessel vasculitides there is no place for IVIG according to EBM recommended treatment choice. For small and medium vessel vasculitides in statement 11 - "Alternative immunomodulatory therapy" - for patients who fail to achieve remission and have persistent low activity intravenous immunoglobulin can be used to achieve remission. These patients should be referred to an expert centre for further management and enrolment in clinical trials (level of evidence 3, grade of recommendation C). Contraindications of such treatment protocol are patients with selective IgA deficiency who may develop an anaphylactic reaction and patients with hypergamaglobulinaemia with risk of hyperviscosity state. Accorging to BSR guidelines (Lapraik et al., 2007) IVIG may be considered as an alternative therapy in patients with refractory disease or in patients for whom conventional therapy is contraindicated, for example, in the presence of infection, in the severely ill patient or in pregnancy (grade of recommendation B). In the management of refractory vasculitis it is important to identify drives for vasculitis, such as, intercurrent infection or malignancy, or non-compliance.

3.1 Kawasaki disease

Clinical criteria and the exclusion of other conditions, including sepsis define the diagnosis of Kawasaki disease (Brogan et al. 2002). After the estimation of correct diagnosis the treatment regimes are focused on reducing inflammation and preventing vascular complications. Coronary artery abnormalities develop within 8 weeks of Kawasaki disease onset. Males and young children are most at risk. No IVIG treatment is considered to be one of the positive risk factor for Kawasaki disease cardiac complications (Phillip & Luqmani, 2008). So that, besides the standard regimes IVIG represent approved choice of treatment in KD with one basic aim - directly reduce the risk of developing coronary artery abnormalities. The highest doses of IVIG were associated with the lowest risk late coronary complications. Meta-analysis study (Durongpisitkul et al., 1995) of treatment studies showed that a single high-dose of IVIG (>1g/kg) in combination with aspirin reduced coronary artery abnormality formation from 23% to 2.3%. Japan research committee reported one trial using low-dose of IVIG (100 mg/kg as a single dose) which showed no significant difference between the treatment groups in term of the occurrence of coronary artery abnormalities. It should emphasized that high-dose IVIG treatment in acute phase of KD have to start as soon as possible after diagnosis (Newburger et al., 1986).

3.2 Polyarteritis nodosa

Polyarteritis nodosa (PAN) is a systemic necrotizing vasculitis affecting medium or small arteries characterized by a wide variety of clinical features including fever, constitutional symptoms, and systemic involvement (muscles, joints, intestines, nerves, kidneys, and skin). Asano et al. (2006) postulated that the effect of IVIG therapy on PAN is temporary, but in situation that PAN is induced by infections, IVIG therapy leads to a complete remission of the disease due to the neutralization of immune activation triggers, such as Parvovirus B19 and Streptococcus. Also Girisgen et al. (2011) based on the case report of 7 years old girl with polyarteritis nodosa and Henoch–Schönlein purpura nephritis suggested that IVIG might an important adjunct therapy in selected patients with polyarteritis nodosa, especially in the lack of response to steroids and immunosuppressive drugs. On the contrary González-Fernández & García-Consuegra (2007) published the case-report of a child with polyarteritis nodosa that was unresponsive to conventional treatment, as well as IVIG treatment during her first and second hospitalizations. Treated child was successfully improved after the addition of iloprost and bosentan.

3.3 Wegener´s granulomatosis and microscopic polyangiitis

Wegener's granulomatosis is a rare disorder which is characterized by necrotizing granulomatous vasculitis of small vessels. WG mainly affects the upper and lower respiratory tract, the kidneys, joints, skin and eyes in contrary to microscopic polyangiitis (MPA) which is characterized by pauci-immune, necrotizing, small-vessel vasculitis without clinical or pathological evidence of necrotizing granulomatous inflammation. MPA usually affects the kidneys, nervous system (particularly the peripheral nerves), skin, and lungs. Some authors mention that WG, MPA even the Churg-Strauss syndrome (CSS) form a part of a spectrum of one disease rather than entirely different entity (Kallenberg, 2005) and PAN. In a view of such classification more accurately criteria are expected. Watts et al. in 2007 published reclassification of ANCA-associated vasculitides and PAN which would be applied into clinical research in the future. This classification allows less unclassified patients and overlapping diagnosis in epidemiological studies as well as in pharmacological trials of various treatment regimes. Until present no study was realized by using this criteria and the evaluation of IVIG treatment in ANCA-associated vasculitides allows us to join WG and MPA under one condition. Moreover the role of IVIG for the treatment of ANCA associated vasculitides has not been clearly defined. IVIG treatment of these entities is frequently discussed subject of many scientific contributions. Jayne et al. (2000) published the only randomized placebo controlled trial of 34 patients with WG/MPA and found that a single course of IVIG reduced disease activity in persistent ANCA associated vasculitides, but this effect was not maintained beyond three month. Side effects were frequent, but mild and reversible. Authors advise IVIG as an alternative treatment in persistent disease after standard therapy. Martinez et al. (2008) published results of multicenter, prospective, open-label study of 22 patients (19 with WG and 3 with MPA) and concluded that IVIG induced complete remissions of relapsed ANCA-associated vasculitides in 13 of 22 patients at nine months. Because of the good safety and tolerance profiles of IVIG, these agents can be included in a therapeutic strategy with other drugs used to treat relapses of WG or MPA. In 2009 Fortin et al. reanalyzed data from 187 publications and found the only randomized controlled trial published by Jayne et al. in 2000. The main aim of Frontin´s review was to determine if intravenous immunoglobulin adjuvant therapy provides a therapeutic advantage over treatment with systemic corticosteroids in combination with immunosuppressants for the treatment of WG. After data extraction and statistical analysis Frontin concluded that there were no significant differences between adjuvant IVIG and adjuvant placebo in mortality, serious adverse events, time to relapse, open-label rescue therapy and infection rates. The fall in disease activity score, derived from patient-reported symptoms, was slightly greater in the IVIG group than in the placebo group after one month. Total adverse events in the IVIG group were increased 3,5 times (relative risk (RR) 3.50; 95% CI 1.44 to 8.48, $P < 0.01$). General conclusion from published Cochrane review is that there is insufficient evidence for comparing the advantages of IVIG adjuvant therapy to the treatment using the combination of steroids and immunosuppressants for patients with WG. Hiemstra & Jayne (2009) recommended in situations where glucocorticoids and immunosuppressives are contraindicated or represent an unacceptably high infection risk that IVIG may be considered; these include the presence of sepsis, a patient in intensive care unit or in pregnancy. IVIG cannot be recommended for routine use in ANCA-associated vasculitides, but can be considered where conventional agents are ineffective or contraindicated. Chung & Seo (2009) in general evaluation of advances in use of biological agents for the treatment of systemic vasculitides summarized that IVIG is not a panacea but play a role as adjunctive therapy for disease refractory to routine immunosuppression. IVIG may also be useful for patients in whom immunosuppression is undesirable or contraindicated (pregnancy).

3.4 Churg-Strauss syndrome

Churg-Strauss syndrome (CSS) is characterized by the presence of asthma, eosinophilia, and small vessel vasculitis with granuloma. Hamilos & Christensen first reported in 1991 that a 33-year-old man with CSS, who was resistant to conventional steroid treatment, showed a marked improvement of vasculitis symptoms and normalization of eosinophil count after IVIG therapy. However, there have been only a few reports on the use of IVIG therapy for CSS (Taniguchi et al., 2007). In 2004 Tsurikisawa et al. reported that neurological and cardiac manifestations in 15 patients with CSS, who were not responsive to corticosteroids with or without cyclophosphamide, were significantly improved after IVIG therapy. Intravenous immunoglobulin therapy may also be considered as a second-line treatment for CSS patients, particularly in the case of neuropathy or cardiomyopathy, which are resistant to conventional therapy. There is not much evidence supporting the effectiveness of IVIG in CSS, however, the mechanisms underlying the action of IVIG remain unclear. (Baldini et al., 2010). In 2004 Danieli et al. published the long term effectiveness of intravenous immunoglobulin and plasmapheresis associated with prednisone and cyclophosphamide in Churg-Strauss syndrome. Complete clinical and functional recovery with a long term stable remission and a low incidence of side effects can be achieved by intravenous immunoglobulin associated with plasmapheresis in patients with Churg-Strauss syndrome. Churg-Strauss syndrome (CSS) is an extremely rare disease, and even less common in women of childbearing age. Hot et al. (2007) in their case report not only supports the beneficial effect of IVIG in CSS, but also illustrates its successful and safe use in a patient who was pregnant. They concluded alternative indication of IVIG in ANCA associated vasculitides during the pregnancy.

3.5 Behçet´s syndrome

Behçet's syndrome is a systemic vasculitis with an unknown etiology affecting the small and large vessels of the venous and arterial systems. Recent European League Against Rheumatism guidelines are useful for the management of the disease in organ systems distinct from the vascular, neurological, and gastrointestinal systems. This is because of a lack of controlled studies evaluating such vascular, neurological, and gastrointestinal complications (Yazici et al., 2010). Seider et al. (2001) reported their results in the group of four patients in which the use of an immunoglobulin had brought the acute inflammation, uncontrolled by corticosteroids and/or cyclosporine A, under control and preserved the remission for a period of at least 1 year. Beales (1998) reported a case report of Behçet's colitis. Such gastrointestinal involvement in Behçet's syndrome is relatively rare, but could bring significant complications (Yurdakuk et al. 1996). Treatment may be difficult and published report suggests intravenous immunoglobulin to be beneficial. Behçet's colitis rapidly responded to IVIG, initially when the patient had failed steroid and immunosuppressive therapy and subsequently when IVIG was used as primary therapy. Leong et al. (2008) according to various reviewing american organisations calculated score for treatment of Behçet´s syndrome to zero (not recommended), but above mentioned reports advise IVIG treatment in specific situations.

3.6 Henoch-Schönlein purpura

Most studies concerning IVIG treatment in Henoch-Schönlein purpura are case reports and bring repugnant conclusions. Orbach et al. (2004) reported that IgA nephropathy and HSP with poor prognosis may improve with IVIG, but 5/15 patients suffered from progressive renal failure after treatment. Hamidou et al. (1996) reported the efficacy of intravenous immunoglobulin in severe gastrointestinal manifestations. Fagbemi et al. (2007) described one patient with massive gastrointestinal haemorrhage in isolated intestinal Henoch-Schönlein purpura with prompt response to intravenous immunoglobulin infusion. They concluded that in severe cases where there is significant gastritis, IVIG provides an effective alternative to corticosteroids that may be employed as first-line therapy. In an open prospective cohort study Rostoker et al. (1994) treated 2 patients with HSP (from the group of 11 patients with IgA nephropathy) and concluded for all eleven patients that IVIG should protect renal function. On the contrary, other authors reported 3 more cases of HSP who did not show improvement in renal function, but rather deterioration (Orbach et al., 2004).

3.7 Mixed cryoglobulinaemia

Mixed cryoglobulinemia type II causes small vessel vasculitis. Vasculitis in skin, peripheral nerve, kidneys, gastrointestinal tract and joints is evoked by presence of circulating cryoglobulins of both polyclonal IgG and a monoclonal IgM rheumatoid factor that are directed against the IgG. The use of IVIG in mixed cryoglobulinaemia type II has been reported without favorable effect and could lead to the induction of cryoglobulinaemia (cryoglobulinemic vasculitis) (Odum et al., 2001). In the presence of peripheral neuropathy vasculitis IVIG treatment showed beneficial effect (Almog et al., 2010). Until present, there is lack of supporting information, but according to Levy et al. (2005) IVIG may be beneficial in cases of resistant vasculitic peripheral neuropathy usually connected with cryoglobulinaemia. IVIG should probably be considered as a sole or adjuvant treatment in patients for whom conventional treatment is contraindicated, or for patients in whom conventional treatment is failed.

4. Economic, supervising and supply implications

IVIG is an expensive blood product that has been used in clinical praxis. IVIG preparations are derived from donor blood with potential risk of such infections as hepatitis and HIV. The process used to prepare final products for use in humans is monitored by the manufacturer and the supervising institutions of particular countries for the presence of dangerous infectious agents. The monitoring starts with the screening of potential donors. Under processing, a multi-step approach that extracts the desired immunoglobulins and attempts to remove all other substances is used. At the end, samples of each batch are tested for the presence of infectious particles. While all attempts are taken to reduce the risk of infection, some small risk still exists.

In last recent years, there was a marked limitation in their supply from manufacturers. This can be caused by several reasons, but main reason is supposed to be the increased use of immunoglobulin for the treatment of assorted new clinical indications, often used without evidence of benefit in the literature. Other liable factory which have affected supply and production costs have been are lack of donors and possible contamination of these human plasma products by infectious agents. It may carry a risk of transmitting infectious agents, e.g. viruses (hepatitis C) (Bjoro et al., 1994) and theoretically, the Creutzfeldt-Jakob disease caused by prions (Will et al., 1996).

For example, UK Department of Health published from November 2007 to May 2008 the programme related to manufacturing, distribution and use of intravenous immunoglobulins in the country. The Demand Management Programme is a three-part initiative that consists of: 1) National Clinical Guidelines for the appropriate use of IVIG, 2) Demand Management Plan and 3) National Immunoglobulin Database. Published material also includes requirement for the major UK supplier of immunoglobulin to buy plasma from the USA. This fact significantly increased production costs. Plasma was previously sourced within the UK as a by-product of voluntary blood donations. Second requirement was to close a UK manufacturer, Scottish National Blood Transfusion Service, also resulting in reduced local supply. Some additional problems increasing the price of IVIG is shortage availability of therapeutic immunoglobulin due to reduced imports by commercial companies who market intravenous immunoglobulins and acute shortages caused by unexpected withdrawals of batches of immunoglobulin for safety reasons e.g. the introduction of further measures to reduce the risk of disease transmission by immunoglobulin infusions (Department of Health UK, 2008). The UK demand management plan restricts IVIG use where benefit is unproved (Vaitla & McDermott, 2010).

In many European countries use of IVIG is mostly limited for treatment primary immune deficiencies where such treatment has been known to be life saving. Even though use of intravenous immunoglobulins in inflammatory diseases has been increased and a recent

literature search revealed more than 150 off-label usages of IVIG, which included 6781 patients in clinical trials and 362 patients in case reports (Leong et al., 2008).
Due to shortage at the same time also in the USA, prices for IVIG have been on an upward trend, most notably in the secondary market. Many medical professionals have reported that the majority of their IVIG use was applied for off-label indications. Off-label use seems to be increased, contributing to rising demand.

Name	Producer	Indications	Last update EMA
Flebogamma	Grifols	RT, BMT, KD, ITP,GBS	09/2010
Kiovig	Baxter	RT, BMT, KD, ITP,GBS	05/2008
Privigen	CSL Behring	RT, BMT, KD, ITP,GBS	03/2008
*Orfagen	Orfagen	PM	10/2003

Table 1. a. IVIG indications exceeded RT in EU (EMA)

Name	Producer	Indication	Last update FDA
Gammagard S/D	Baxter	RT, KD, ITP	10/2008
Gammagard Liquid	Baxter	RT	04/2005
Iveegam E/N	Baxter	RT, KD	N/A
Polygam S/D	Baxter	RT, ITP	N/A
Carimune	CSL Behring	RT, ITP	10/2008
Privigen	CSL Behring	RT, ITP	07/2007
Panglobulin NF	CSL Behring	RT, ITP	N/A
Gamamr-P I.V.	CSL Behring	RT	N/A
Flebogamma DIF	Grifols	RT	07/2010
Venoglobulin-S	Gfrfols	RT, ITP, KD	N/A
Gammaplex	Bio Products	RT	10/2009
Octagam	Octapharma	RT	02/2006
Gamunex - C	Talecris	RT, ITP, CIDP	09/2008

Table 1. b. IVIG indications exceeded RT by FDA in USA. (N/A - without actual FDA approval)

Unexpected development in last years led all responsible representatives (EMA, FDA, medical professional societies, manufacturers) to coop with arose situation and postulate exact indications in Europe and USA respectively (Table 1a and 1b). There are less IVIG products with limited indications in summary of product characteristics at present market in comparison with the eighties. Uncertain role of IVIG in unlabeled indications is well established in UK Department of Health Clinical Guidelines for Immunoglobulin Use. The goal of submitted material is to ensure best practice across all indications, based on available evidence and expert opinion. Table 2 shows approved, potentially approved (grey) indications of IVIG in vasculitis treatment in UK (Department of Health UK, 2008).

5. Dosage implications

Generally accepted dosing regimes can be divided into two main groups. The first labeled group represents substitution (replacement) therapy used in primary and secondary

immunodeficiencies and the second group represents immunomodulatory therapy in idiopathic thrombocytopenic purpura, Kawasaki disease, Gullain-Barré syndrome, chronic inflammatory demyelinating polyneuropathy and polymyositis. All these indications are approved by EMA and FDA in Europe and USA respectively (Table 2 and 3). In replacement therapy (low-dose) group recommended dosis ranges from 0,2 to 0,8 g per kg of body weight and in immunomodulatory (high-dose) group ranges from 1,0 to 2,0 g/kg.
The labeled use of IVIG is at present widely overlapped by unlabeled indications. These indications include the treatment of many immunological and idiopathic diseases involving nearly all organ systems. Man could say "gunshot into the unknown". Leong et al. (2008) analyzed over 150 unlabeled uses of IVIG, including the most studied indications (e.g. multiple sclerosis, antiphospholipid syndrome in miscarriage, ...) and concluded that evidence for unlabeled use of IVIG has been interpreted in different ways by various reviewing subjects.

Condition	Recommended - short term	Recommended - long term	Evidence (grade)	Alternatives
KD	Yes	No	A, Ia	None
DM, JDM	Selected	Seleted	B, IIa	CS, IS, PE
CNS vasculitis	N/A	N/A	IIb	CS, IS
PM	N/A	N/A	III	CS, IS, PE
SV, AAV	N/A	N/A	III	IS
SLE, JSLE	N/A	N/A	III	CS, IS

Table 2. UK Department of Health guidelines for using IVIG in vasculitis (adapted).

Indication	Ratko	Orange	Ahme d	Aetna	BC	MLD T	Score
KD (labeled)	NI	2	NI	2	2	2	2,0
Unlabeled							
Behçet´s syndrome	0	NI	NI	0	NI	NI	0,0
CCS	NI	NI	NI	2	NI	NI	2,0
PAN	NI	NI	NI	0	NI	NI	0,0
Systemic vasculitides	1	1	NI	0	NI	NI	0,7
Secondary vasculitides	NI	NI	NI	0	NI	NI	0,0
WG	NI	NI	NI	0	NI	NI	0,0

Table 3. Indication score of various US guidelines for using IVIG in vasculitis (adapted according to Leong et al., 2008).

Until present immunological mechanisms of immunomodulatory effect of IVIG are not clearly known. In such context a question of adequate dosage appears in the relation of cost/benefits of unlabeled treatment. We published (Lukán et al., 2008) an adequate response in a case of Wegener´s granulomatosis after lower "high-dose" regimen (1 g/kg) which lasts until present without any therapy, only with mild increase of cANCA and no clinical recurrency. Many authors published effectiveness of such lower dose regime also in other rheumatological and hematological indications. Genevay et al. (2001) published effective use of IVIG in lower doses (0,8 g/kg) but only for maintenance treatment in polymyositis and concluded considerable reduction in treatment costs without a negative influence on patient´s health conditions. Sherer et at. (2008) reported a retrospective analysis the medical records of 62 patients who received low-dose of IVIG and concluded that low-dose IVIG is a possible therapeutic option which is associated with lower cost, however treatment did not improved vasculitis in analyzed patients. Authors recommend IVIG only as an add-on therapy. Mori et al. (1988) concluded that in the treatment of acute idiopathic thrombocytopenic purpura there was no difference in therapeutic efficacy between the high and the low-dose IVIG regimen. Boman et al. (1995) achieved dramatic responses to IVIG in two cases of cerebral vasculitis even after the administration of the first dose (1 g/kg). One of the patients improved within 24 h of the administration, treatment continued at 4-week intervals and the patient was stable for 13 month, in spite of halving the dose of IVIG. Gedalia et al. (1995) reported in cutaneous polyarteritis nodosa combined with streptococcal infection in a dose 1 g/kg and Asano et al. (2006) in female patient with polyarteritis nodosa without any infection in a dose of 0,5 g/kg rapid and dramatic improvement after the first administration of IVIG. Monova et al. (2002) collected data on 116 patients with lupus nephritis who were treated with intravenous immunoglobulins. IVIG was applied in a dose of 0,255 g/kg. Depending on the clinical improvement afterwards the courses were repeated after 1 month (and every 3 months for maintenance of remission) to 7 years. Full remission was achieved in 36 patients. Partial remission was present in 48 patients. 32 patients went into end-stage renal failure and/or died. In 13/34 patients with impaired renal function serum creatinine levels returned to normal after treatment. Recher et al. (2010) reported a case report on unexpectedly successful a low-dose regimen (0,6 g/kg) in female patient with inclusion body myositis which costs approximately fourfold less than high-dose IVIG. In Henoch-Schönlein purpura some authors (Heldrich et al., 1993, Rostoker et al., 1995, Ruellan et al., 1997) administered low-dose or lower limit of high-dose regimens, others (Rostoker et al., 1994, Lamireau et al., 2001, Fagbemi et al., 2007) strictly apply 2 g/kg. Apart from the dose applied all authors emphasize dramatic improvement of IVIG treatment already after 24 hours after beginning (Girisgen et al., 2011).

It could be supposed that patients who respond to high-dose IVIG therapy would probably also respond to much lower doses, in many rheumatological indications vasculitides not excluded. In addition to economic reasons, low-dose regimen would likely help to reduce treatment related side effects. The lack of validated and generally accepted outcome measures as well as prospective clinical studies, makes it difficult to compare the effect of different interventions in different cases (Yu & Lennon, 1999).

6. Conclusion

Biological complexity of vasculitides and their contemporary nomenclature complicates not only the estimation of appropriate diagnosis but also hampers effective treatment.. Intravenous immunoglobulins represent one of the very often discussed alternative treatment modality of vasculitides. For patients who fail to achieve remission, have persistent low activity of inflammation and relapse, intravenous immunoglobulins could be used as an alternative/adjuvant immunomodulatory therapy. Mechanism of action of intravenous immunoglobulins is complex and its effects are not clearly understood.

Even though many questions remain unanswered, intravenous immunoglobulins could be considered as an effective treatment regimen in many "off label" indications particularly in the cases when standard immunosuppressive regimes fail or could be harmful. In spite of evidence of efficacy, dosage and timing IVIG therapy, questions of costs/benefits still remain insufficiently documented and controlled trials with consecutive formation of common guidelines are required.

7. Acknowledgment

Prof. Ivan Tkac M.D., PhD., Head of the IV. Internal 4th Internal Department Medical Faculty, Safarik University, Košice, Slovakia is acknowledged for his help with manuscript.

8. Abbreviations used in text and tables (in alphabetic order)

BMT - bone marrow transplantation, BSR - British Society for Rheumatology , CHCC - Chapel Hill Consensus Conference, CIDP - chronic inflammatory demyelinating polyneuropathy, CS- corticosteroids, CSS - Churg-Strauss syndrome, EBM - evidence based medicine, EULAR - European League Against Rheumatism, GBS - Gullain-Barré syndrome, HSP - Henoch-Schönlein purpura, IS - immunosuppressives, ITP - idiopathic trombocytopenic purpura, IVIG - intravenous immunoglobulin(s), KD - Kawasaki disease, MPA - microscopic polyangiitis, PAN - polyarteritis nodosa, PE - plasma exchange, PM - polymyositis, RT - replacement therapy, WG - Wegener´s granulomatosis.

9. References

Abdulahad, W., H., Stegeman, C., A., van der Geld, Y., M., Doornbos-van der Meer, B., Limburg, P., C., Kallenberg, C., G. (2007). Functional defect of circulating regulatory CD4+ T cells in patients with Wegener's granulomatosis in remission. *Arthritis Rheum.* Vol.56, No.6, pp. 2080-2091.

Almog, O., Berlin, T., Rotman-Pikielny, P., Levy, Y. (2010). A dramatic response to intravenous immunoglobulin in a patient with mixed cryoglobulinemia. *Isr Med Assoc J.* Vol.12, No.1, pp. 53-54.

Andersson, J., Skansén-Saphir, U., Sparrelid, E., Andersson, U. (1996). Intravenous immune globulin affects cytokine production in T lymphocytes and monocytes/ macrophages. *Clin Exp Immunol.* Vol.104, Suppl 1, pp. 10-20.

Asano, Y., Ihn, H., Maekawa, T., Kadono, T., Tamaki, K. (2006). High-dose intravenous immunoglobulin infusion in polyarteritis nodosa: report on one case and review of the literature. *Clin Rheumatol.* Vol.25, No.3, pp. 396-398.

Baldini, C., Talarico, R., Della Rossa, A., Bombardieri, S. (2010). Clinical manifestations and treatment of Churg-Strauss syndrome. *Rheum Dis Clin North Am.* Vol.36, No.3, pp. 27-43.

Bayary, J., Dasgupta, S., Misra, N., Ephrem, A., Duong Van Huyen, J., P., Delignat, S., Hassan, G., Caligiuri, G., Nicoletti, A., Lacroix-Desmazes, S., Kazatchkine, M., D., Kaveri, S. (2006). Intravenous immunoglobulin in autoimmune disorders: an insight into the immunoregulatory mechanisms. *Int Immunopharmacol.* Vol.6, No.4, pp. 528-534.

Beales, I., L. (1998). Gastrointestinal involvement in Behçet's syndrome. *Am J Gastroenterol.* Vol.93, No.12, p.2633.

Bene, M., C., Faure, G., C. (1987). Composition of mesangial deposits in IgA nephropathy: complement actors. *Nephron.* Vol.46, No.2, p. 219.

Bjoro, K.; Froland, S.. S.; Yun, Z,; Samdal, H., H.; Haaland, T. (1994) Hepatitis C infection in patients with primary hypogammagobulinemia after treatment with contaminated immunoglobulin. *N Engl J Med.* Vol.331, No.24, pp. 1607–1611.

Blasczyk, R., Westhoff, U., Grossewilde, H. (1993). Soluble CD4, CD8, and HLA molecules in commercial immunoglobulin preparations. *Lancet* Vol.341, No.8848 , pp. 789–790.

Boman, S., Ballen, J., L., Seggev, J., S. (1995). Dramatic responses to intravenous immunoglobulin in vasculitis. *J Intern Med.* Vol.238, No.4, pp. 375-377.

Boros, P., Gondolesi, G., Bromberg, J., S. High dose intravenous immunoglobulin treatment: mechanisms of action. (2005) *Liver Transpl.* Vol.11, No.12, pp. 1469-1480.

Brogan, P., A., Bose, A., Burgner, D., Shingadia, D., Tulloh, R., Michie, C., Klein, N., Booy,R., Levin, M., Dillon, M., J. (2002). Kawasaki disease: an evidence based approach to diagnosis, treatment, and proposals for future research. *Arch Dis Child.* Vol.86, No.4, pp. 286-290.

Chen, M., Daha, M., R., Kallenberg, C., G. (2010). The complement system in systemic autoimmune disease. *J Autoimmun.* Vol.34, No.3, pp. :J276-286.

Chung, S., A., Seo, P. (2009). Advances in the use of biologic agents for the treatment of systemic vasculitis. *Curr Opin Rheumatol.* Vol.21, No.1, pp. 3-9.

Cohen, I., R., Cooke, A. (1986). Natural autoantibodies might prevent autoimmune disease *Immunol. Today* Vol.7, No.12, pp. 363-364.

D'Amico, G., Fornasieri, A. (1995). Cryoglobulinemic glomerulonephritis: membrano-proliferative glomerulonephritis induced by hepatitis C virus. *Am J Kidney Dis.* Vol.25, No.3, pp. 361-369.

Danieli, M., G., Cappelli, M., Malcangi, G., Logullo, F., Salvi, A., Danieli, G. (2004). Long term effectiveness of intravenous immunoglobulin in Churg-Strauss syndrome. *Ann Rheum Dis.* Vol.63, No.12, pp. 1649-1654.

Department of Health. (2008). http://www.dh.gov.uk/en/Publicationsandstatistics/Publications/ PublicationsPolicyAndGuidance/DH_085237.

Durongpisitkul, K., Gururaj, V., J., Park, J., M., Martin, C., F. (1995). The prevention of coronary artery aneurysm in Kawasaki disease: a meta-analysis on the efficacy of aspirin and immunoglobulin treatment. *Pediatrics.* Vol.96, No.6, pp. 1057-1061.

Ephrem, A., Misra, N., Hassan, G., Dasgupta, S., Delignat, S., Duong Van Huyen, J., P., Chamat, S., Prost, F., Lacroix-Desmazes, S., Kavery, S., V., Kazatchkine, M., D. (2005). Immunomodulation of autoimmune and inflammatory diseases with intravenous immunoglobulin. *Clin Exp Med.* Vol.5, No.4, pp. 135-140.

Fagbemi, A., A., Torrente, F., Hilson, A., J., Thomson, M., A., Heuschkel, R., B., Murch, S., H. (2007). Massive gastrointestinal haemorrhage in isolated intestinal Henoch-Schönlein purpura with response to intravenous immunoglobulin infusion. *Eur J Pediatr.* Vol.166, No.9, pp. 915-919.

Fortin, P., M,, Tejani, A,. M., Bassett, K., Musini, V., M. (2009). Intravenous immunoglobulin as adjuvant therapy for Wegener's granulomatosis. *Cochrane Database Syst Rev.* Issue.3, CD007057.

Gedalia, A., Correa, H., Kaiser, M., Sorensen, R. (1995). Case report: steroid sparing effect of intravenous gamma globulin in a child with necrotizing vasculitis. *Am J Med Sci.* Vol.309, No.4, pp. 226-228.

Genevay, S., Saudan-Kister, A., Guerne, P., A. (2001). Intravenous gammaglobulins in refractory polymyositis: lower dose for maintenance treatment is effective. *Ann Rheum Dis.* Vol.60, No.6, pp. 635–636.

Girisgen, I., Sonmez, F., Koseoglu, K., Erisen, S., Yılmaz, D. (2011). Polyarteritis nodosa and Henoch-Schönlein purpura nephritis in a child with familial Mediterranean fever: a case report. *Rheumatol Int.* Jan 23. [Epub ahead of print]

González-Fernández, M., A., García-Consuegra, J. (2007). Polyarteritis nodosa resistant to conventional treatment in a pediatric patient. *Ann Pharmacother.* Vol.41, No.5, pp. 885-890.

Gupta, M., Noel, G., J., Schaefer, M., Friedman, D., Bussel, J., Johann-Liang, R. (2001). Cytokine modulation with immune gamma-globulin in peripheral blood of normal children and its implications in Kawasaki disease treatment. *J Clin Immunol.* Vol.21, No.3, pp. 193-199.

Hamidou, M., A., Pottier, M., A., Dupas, B. (1996). Intravenous immunoglobulin in Henoch-Schönlein purpura. *Ann Intern Med.* Vol.125, No.12, pp. 1013-1014.

Hamilos, D., L., Christensen, J. (1991). Treatment of Churg-Strauss syndrome with high-dose intravenous immunoglobulin. *J Allergy Clin Immunol.* Vol.88, No.5, pp. 823-824.

Hansen, R., J., Balthasar, J., P. (2002). Intravenous immunoglobulin mediates an increase in anti-platelet antibody clearance via the FcRn receptor. *Thromb Haemost.* Vol.88, No.6, pp. 898-899.

Haydey, R., P., Patarroyo de Rojas, M., Gigli, I. (1980). A newly described control mechanism of complement activation in patients with mixed cryoglobulinemia (cryoglobulins and complement). *J Invest Dermatol.* Vol.74, No.5, pp. 328-332.

Heeringa, P., Huugen, D., Tervaert, J., W. (2005). Anti-neutrophil cytoplasmic autoantibodies and leukocyte-endothelial interactions: a sticky connection? *Trends Immunol.* Vol.26, No.11, pp. 561-564.

Heldrich, F., J., Minkin, S., Gatdula, C., L. (1993). Intravenous immunoglobulin in Henoch-Schönlein purpura: a case study. *Md Med J.* Vol.42, No.6, pp. 577- 579.

Hiemstra, T., F., Jayne, D. (2009). Newer therapies for vasculitis. *Best Pract Res Clin Rheumatol.* Vol.23, No.3, pp. 379-389.

Hisano, S., Matsushita, M., Fujita, T., Iwasaki, H. (2005). Activation of the lectin complement pathway in Henoch-Schönlein purpura nephritis. *Am J Kidney Dis.* Vol.45, No.2, pp. 295-302.

Hoffmann, M., Uttenreuther-Fischer, M., M., Lerch, H., Gaedicke, G., Fischer, P. (2000). IVIG-bound IgG and IgM cloned by phage display from a healthy individual reveal the same restricted germ-line gene origin as in autoimmune thrombocytopenia. *Clin Exp Immunol.* Vol.121, No1, pp. 37-46.

Holle, J., U., Gross, W., L. (2009). ANCA-associated vasculitides: pathogenetic aspects and current evidence-based therapy. *J Autoimmun.* Vol.32, No.3-4, pp. 163-171.

Hot, A., Perard, L., Coppere, B., Simon, M., Bouhour, F., Ninet, J. (2007). Marked improvement of Churg-Strauss vasculitis with intravenous gamma globulins during pregnancy. *Clin Rheumatol.* Vol.26, No.12, pp. 2149-2151.

Jayne, D., R., Chapel, H., Adu, D., Misbah, S., O'Donoghue, D., Scott, D., Lockwood, C., M. (2000). Intravenous immunoglobulin for ANCA-associated systemic vasculitis with persistent disease activity. *QJM.* Vol.93, No.7, pp. 433-439.

Jennette, J., C.; Falk, R., J.; Andrassy, K.; Bacon, P., A.; Churg, J.; Gross, W., L.; Hagen, E., C.;

Hoffman, G., S.; Hunder, G., G.; Kallenberg, C., G. et al. (1994). Nomenclature of systemic vasculitides. Proposal of an international consensus conference. *Arthritis Rheum.,* Vol.37, No.2, pp. 187-192.

Kallenberg, C., G. (2005). Churg-Strauss syndrome: just one disease entity? *Arthritis Rheum.* Vol.52, No.9, pp. 2589-2593.

Kaneko, Y., Nimmerjahn, F., Ravetch, J., V. (2006). Anti-inflammatory activity of immunoglobulin G resulting from Fc sialylation. *Science.* Vol.313, No.5787, pp. 670-673.

Lacroix-Desmazes, S., Kaveri, S., V., Mouthon, L., Ayouba, A., Malanchere, E., Coutinho, A., Kazatchkine, M., D. (1998). Self-reactive antibodies (natural autoantibodies) in healthy individuals. *Journal of Immunological Methods.* Vol.216, No.1-2, pp. 117-137.

Lamireau, T., Rebouissoux, L., Hehunstre, J., P. (2001). Intravenous immunoglobulin therapy for severe digestive manifestations of Henoch–Schönlein purpura. *Acta Paediatr.* Vol.90, No.9, pp. 1081-1082.

Langford, C., A. (2010) Vasculitis. *J Allergy Clin Immunol.* Vol.125, No.2, Suppl.2, pp. S216-S225.

Lapraik, C., Watts, R., Bacon, P., Carruthers, D., Chakravarty, K., D'Cruz, D., Guillevin, L., Harper, L., Jayne, D., Luqmani, R., Mooney, J., Scott, D. (2007). BSR and BHPR Standards, Guidelines and Audit Working Group. BSR and BHPR guidelines for the management of adults with ANCA associated vasculitis. *Rheumatology (Oxford).* Vol.46, No.10, pp. 1615-1626.

Lau, A., C., Duong, T., T., Ito, S., Yeung, R., S. (2009). Intravenous immunoglobulin and salicylate differentially modulate pathogenic processes leading to vascular damage in a model of Kawasaki disease. *Arthritis Rheum.* Vol.60, No.7, pp. 2131-2141.

Leong, H., Stachnik, J., Bonk, M., E., Matuszewski, K., A. (2008). Unlabeled uses of intravenous immune globulin. *Am J Health Syst Pharm.* Vol.65, No.19, pp. 1815-1824.

Leucht, S., Uttenreuther-Fischer, M., M., Gaedicke, G., Fischer, P. (2001). The B cell superantigen-like interaction of intravenous immunoglobin (IVIG) with Fab fragments of V(H) 3-23 and 3-30/3-30.5 germline gene origin cloned from a patient with Kawasaki disease is enhanced after IVIG therapy. *Clin Immunol.* Vol.99, No.1, pp. 18-29.

Levy, Y., Uziel, Y., Zandman, G., Rotman, P., Amital, H., Sherer, Y., Langevitz, P., Goldman, B., Shoenfeld, Y. (2005). Response of vasculitic peripheral neuropathy to intravenous immunoglobulin. *Ann N Y Acad Sci.* Vol.1051, pp. 779-786.

Lukan, N., Lazurova, I., Racz, O., Kristofova, B., Tkac, I. (2008). An intravenous immunoglobulin therapy of serious autoimmune rheumatic diseases. *Bratisl Lek Listy.* Vol.109, No.11, pp. 489-492.

Maddur, M., S., Vani, J., Hegde, P., Lacroix-Desmazes, S., Kaveri, S., V., Bayry, J. (2011). Inhibition of differentiation, amplification, and function of human T(H)17 cells by intravenous immunoglobulin. *J Allergy Clin Immunol.* Vol.127, No.3, pp. 823-830.

Martinez, V., Cohen, P., Pagnoux, C., Vinzio, S., Mahr, A., Mouthon, L., Sailler, L., Delaunay, C., Sadoun, A., Guillevin, L. (2008). French Vasculitis Study Group. Intravenous immunoglobulins for relapses of systemic vasculitides associated with antineutrophil cytoplasmic autoantibodies: results of a multicenter, prospective, open-label study of twenty-two patients. *Arthritis Rheum.* Vol.58, No.1, pp. 308-317.

Miossec, P., Korn, T., Kuchroo, V., K. (2009). Interleukin-17 and type 17 helper T cells. *N Engl J Med.* Vol.361, No.9, pp. 888-898.

Monova, D., Belovezhdov, N., Altunkova, I., Monov, S. (2002). Intravenous immunoglobulin G in the treatment of patients with chronic glomerulonephritis: clinical experience lasting 15 years. *Nephron.* Vol.90, No.3, pp. 262-266.

Mori, P., G., Lanza, T., Mancuso, G., De Mattia, D., Catera, P., Miano, C., Del Principe, D., Cottafava, F. (1988). Treatment of acute idiopathic thrombocytopenic purpura (AITP): cooperative Italian study group results. *Pediatr Hematol Oncol.* Vol.5, No.3, pp. 169-178.

Mukhtyar, C., Guillevin, L., Cid, M., C., Dasgupta, B., de Groot, K., Gross, W., Hauser, T., Hellmich, B., Jayne, D., Kallenberg, C., G., Merkel, P., A., Raspe, H., Salvarani, C., Scott, D., G., Stegeman, C., Watts, R., Westman, K., Witter, J., Yazici, H., Luqmani, R. (2009). European Vasculitis Study Group. EULAR recommendations for the management of primary small and medium vessel vasculitis. *Ann Rheum Dis.* Vol.68, No.3, pp. 310-317.

Mukhtyar, C., Guillevin, L., Cid,, M., C., Dasgupta, B., de Groot, K., Gross, W., Hauser, T., Hellmich, B., Jayne, D., Kallenberg, C., G., Merkel, P., A., Raspe, H., Salvarani, C., Scott, D., G., Stegeman, C., Watts, R., Westman, K., Witter, J., Yazici, H., Luqmani, R. (2009). European Vasculitis Study Group. EULAR recommendations for the management of large vessel vasculitis. *Ann Rheum Dis.* Vol.68, No.3, pp. :318-323.

Negi, V., S., Elluru, S., Sibéril, S., Graff-Dubois, S., Mouthon, L., Kazatchkine, M., D., Lacroix-Desmazes, S., Bayry, J., Kaveri, S., V. (2007). Intravenous immunoglobulin: an update on the clinical use and mechanisms of action. *J Clin Immunol.* Vol.27, No.3, pp. 233-245.

Newburger, J., W., Takahashi, M., Burns, J., C., Beiser, A., S., Chung, K., J., Duffy, C., E., Glode, M., P., Mason, W., H., Reddy, V., Sanders, S., P., et al. (1986). The treatment of Kawasaki syndrome with intravenous gamma globulin. *N Engl J Med.* Vol.315, No.6, pp. 341-347.

Odum, J., D'Costa, D., Freeth, M., Taylor, D., Smith, N., MacWhannell, A. (2001). Cryoglobulinaemic vasculitis caused by intravenous immunoglobulin treatment. *Nephrol Dial Transplant.* Vol.16, No.2, pp. 403-406.

Orbach, H., Tishler, M., Shoenfeld, Y. (2004). Intravenous immunoglobulin and the kidney – a two-edged sword. *Semin Arthritis Rheum.* Vol.34, No.3, pp. 593-601.

Phillip, R., Luqmani, R. (2008). Mortality in systemic vasculitis: a systematic review. *Clin Exp Rheumatol.* Vol.26, No.5, Suppl 51, pp. S94-104.

Recher, M,, Sahrbacher, U., Bremer, J., Arndt, B., Steiner, U., Fontana, A. (2010). Treatment of inclusion body myositis: is low-dose intravenous immunoglobulin the solution? *Rheumatol Int.* Jan 1. [Epub ahead of print]

Rostoker, G., Desvaux-Belghiti, D., Pilatte, Y., Petit-Phar, M., Philippon, C., Deforges, L., Terzidis, H., Intrator, L., André, C., Adnot, S., Bonin, P., Bierling, P., Remy, P., Lagrue, G., Lang, P., Weil, B. (1994). High-dose immunoglobulin therapy for severe IgA nephropathy and Henoch-Schönlein purpura. *Ann Intern Med.* Vol.120, No.6, pp. 476-484.

Rostoker, G., Desvaux-Belghiti, D., Pilatte, Y., Petit-Phar, M., Philippon, C., Deforges, L., Terzidis, H., Intrator, L., André, C., Adnot, S., et al. (1995). Immunomodulation with low-dose immunoglobulins for moderate IgA nephropathy and Henoch-Schönlein purpura. Preliminary results of a prospective uncontrolled trial. *Nephron.* Vol.69, No.3, pp. 327-334.

Ruellan, A., Khatibi, M., Staub, T., Martin, T., Storck, D., Christmann, D. (1997) . Purpura rhumatoide et immunoglobulines intraveineuses. *Rev Med Interne.* Vol.18, No.9, pp. 727-729.

Seider, N., Beiran, I., Scharf, J., Miller, B. (2001). Intravenous immunoglobulin therapy for resistant ocular Behçet's disease. *Br J Ophthalmol.* Vol.85, No.11, pp. 1287-1288.

Sherer, Y., Y., Levy, Y., Shoenfeld, Y. (2000). Intravenous immunoglobulin therapy of antiphospholipid syndrome. *Rheumatology (Oxford)* Vol.39, No.4, pp. 421–426.

Sherer, Y., Kuechler, S., Jose Scali, J., Rovensky, J., Levy, Y., Zandman-Goddard, G., Shoenfeld, Y. (2008). Low dose intravenous immunoglobulin in systemic lupus erythematosus: analysis of 62 cases. *Isr Med Assoc J.* Vol.10, No.1, pp. 55-57.

Sibéril, S., Elluru, S., Graff-Dubois, S., Negi, V., S., Delignat, S., Mouthon, L., Lacroix-Desmazes, S., Kazatchkine, M., D., Bayary, J., Kaveri, S., V. (2007). Intravenous immunoglobulins in autoimmune and inflammatory diseases: a mechanistic perspective. *Ann N Y Acad Sci.* Vol.1110, pp. 497-506.

Siedlar, M., Strach, M., Bukowska-Strakova, K., Lenart, M., Szaflarska, A., Węglarczyk, K., Rutkowska, M., Baj-Krzyworzeka, M., Pituch-Noworolska, A., Kowalczyk, D., Grodzicki, T., Ziegler-Heitbrock, L., Zembala, M. (2011). Preparations of intravenous immunoglobulins diminish the number and proinflammatory response of CD14(+)CD16(++) monocytes in common variable immunodeficiency (CVID) patients. *Clin Immunol.* Jan 15. [Epub ahead of print]

Stegeman, C., A., Cohen-Tervaert, J., W., Sluiter, W., J., Manson, W., L., de Jong, P., E., Kallenberg, C., G., M. (1994). Association of chronic nasal carriage of staphylococcus aureus and higher relapse rates in Wegener granulomatosis. *Ann Intern Med.* Vol.120, No.1, pp. 12-17.

Taniguchi, M., Tsurikisawa, N., Higashi, N., Saito, H., Mita, H., Mori, A., Sakakibara, H., Akiyama, K. (2007). Treatment for Churg-Strauss syndrome: induction of remission and efficacy of intravenous immunoglobulin therapy. *Allergol Int.* Vol.56, No.2, pp. 97-103.

Tsurikisawa, N., Taniguchi, M., Saito, H., Himeno, H., Ishibashi, A., Suzuki, S., Akiyama, K. (2004). Treatment of Churg-Strauss syndrome with high-dose intravenous immunoglobulin. *Ann Allergy Asthma Immunol.* Vol.92, No.1, pp. 80-87.

Vaitla, P., M.; McDermott, E., M. (2010). The role of high-dose intravenous immunoglobulin in rheumatology. *Rheumatology (Oxford).* Vol.49, No.6, pp. 1040-1048.

Watts, R., Lane, S., Hanslik, T., Hauser, T., Hellmich, B., Koldingsnes, W., Mahr, A., Segelmark, M., Cohen-Tervaert, J., W., Scott, D. (2007). Development and validation of a consensus methodology for the classification of the ANCA-associated vasculitides and polyarteritis nodosa for epidemiological studies. *Ann Rheum Dis.* Vol.66, No.2, pp. 222-227.

Will, R., G.; Ironside, J., W.; Zeidler, M.; Cousens, S., N.; Estibeiro, K.; Alperovitch, A.; Poser, S.; Pocchiari, M.; Hofman, A.; Smith, P., G. (1996). A new variant of Creutzfeldt-Jakob disease in the UK. *Lancet.* Vol.347, No.9006, (Apr 6), pp. 921-925.

Yazici, Y., Yurdakul, S., Yazici, H. (2010). Behçet's syndrome. *Curr Rheumatol Rep.* Vol.12, No.6, pp. 429-435.

Yu, Z., Lennon, V., A. (1999). Mechanism of intravenous immune globulin therapy in antibody-mediated autoimmune diseases. *N Engl J Med.* Vol.340, No.3, pp. 227-228.

Yurdakul, S., Tüzüner, N., Yurdakul, I., Hamuryudan, V., Yazici, H. (1996). Gastrointestinal involvement in Behçet's syndrome: a controlled study. *Ann Rheum Dis.* 1996 Vol.55, No.3, pp. 208-210.

Immunopathogenesis Based Adamantiades-Behcet Disease Vasculitis Treatment

Panagiota Boura, Konstantinos Tselios,
Ioannis Gkougkourelas and Alexandros Sarantopoulos
*Clinical Immunology Unit, 2nd Department of Internal Medicine,
Hippokration General Hospital, Aristotle University of Thessaloniki
Greece*

1. Introduction

All immune cell lineages arise from the multipotent stem cells in the bone marrow. The development and regulation of immune system cells (immune homeostasis) depends on the programmed appearance of specific cell surface molecules (e.g. receptors) and responsiveness to certain cytokines and chemokines. After maturation, the immune system cells include antigen presenting cells (APCs), other phagocytic cells like neutrophils, eosinophils, basophils and lymphocytes which include T lymphocytes, B lymphocytes and natural killer (NK) cells. Depending on an initial stimulus and the microenvironmental conditions at a given time, each lymphocyte lineage can be subdivided to different populations with discrete specialized functions. Subpopulations of crucial importance are CD4+ T cells (mainly Th1, Th2, Th17 and T regulatory cells) and CD8+ T cells, CD16- and CD16+ NK cells and CD5+ and CD5- B cells.

As a structure, the immune system consists of central locations of immune cell production and differentiation (bone marrow and thymus) and peripheral organs, where encounter with antigen and response to it occurs, that is the spleen, lymph nodes, tonsils and mucosa-associated lymphoid tissue (MALT). Mucosal surfaces and the skin provide the main primary access for foreign antigens to meet cells of the immune system, where they first react primarily with APCs.

Innate immunity includes skin and mucosal barriers, as well as the innate immune cells that are triggered and react in minutes after they encounter 'foreign' material. The innate immune system, as it represents the first line of host defense against foreign entities, is regarded as a nonspecific system and its main role is to engulf and eliminate pathogens, trigger pro-inflammatory responses and present antigens to adaptive immune cells, which are subsequently activated. More recently it has been shown that the innate immune system has a necessary degree of specificity that enables it to discriminate between self and foreign particles (e.g. microorganisms). Germline encoded and constitutively expressed *pattern recognition receptors (PRRs)*- like Toll receptors on innate immune cells, help them to discriminate highly conserved *pathogen associated molecular patterns (PAMPs)*, which activate specific signaling pathways that lead to robust but well-defined innate immune responses.

Research on innate immunity is progressively uncovering molecular and cellular mechanisms by which it recognizes environment and reacts to it, leading to protective or pathological and harmful immune responses. Understanding innate and adaptive immunity pathways in detail will have a great impact on revealing the immunopathology of immune-mediated diseases like Adamantiades-Behcet Disease (ABD) and developing more targeted immunotherapeutic agents to manipulate, even life-threatening, ABD vasculitis.

2. General considerations in ABD immunopathogenesis

ABD owes its name to Benediktos Adamantiades (Greek ophthalmologist), who had described it first in 1930 and Hulusi Behcet (Turkish dermatologist), who described hypopyon, iritis and orogenital aphthosis in 1937 (Adamantiades, 1931; Behcet, 1937). However, the first description of the disease dates back, 2500 years, to Hippokrates, to the 5th century BC, in the Epidemion book, case 7, where it is described as aphthous ulceration, genital ulceration and iridocyclitis.

There were other forms of fever…
Many developed aphthae, ulcerations…
Many ulcerations about the genital parts…
Watery ophthalmies of a chronic character, with pains…

Since the early descriptions, additional clinical features have been described and added to disease spectrum. ABD can be manifested with different organ involvement, articular, neurological, pulmonary and gastrointestinal, besides the classical clinical triad proposed by the International Study Group for Behcet's Disease.

Nowadays, ABD diagnosis rests upon a set of established criteria, where no single clinical or laboratory feature is pathognomonic (International Study Group for Behcet's Disease, 1990, Table 1).

Recurrent oral ulcerations plus two	Recurrent genital ulcers Skin lesions (erythema nodosum, acne, folliculitis) Ocular lesions (uveitis) Positive pathergy test

Table 1. Diagnostic Criteria for ABD

From early descriptions, it was shown that patients with ABD cluster according to a geographic pattern that coincides with the ancient "Silk Route". It has a higher incidence (100 times more common) in the countries of the Mediterranean Basin, Middle East and Far East, which includes Greece, Turkey, Saudi Arabia, Iran, Korea ,China and Japan while it is rare in North America. Although sporadic cases are described, there is an increased frequency among relatives (familial aggregation), mainly in HLA-B51 class I gene positive relatives. Genetic susceptibility factors seem to be connected with more severe disease expression. Particularly, in Asia, up to 80% of patients are HLA-B51 positive. Recent studies focus on new genetic markers that could amplify immune responses responsible for disease expression (HLA and non-HLA genes), probably under an environmental challenge e.g. an infectious agent (the infectious model), (Fietta, 2005; Kaklamani et al, 1998; Verity et al, 2003; Yazici H et al, 1999).

ABD etiopathogenesis still remains a mystery to be elucidated. There is substantial evidence for an infectious background participating in disease initiation, especially, in genetically predisposed individuals. A number of viruses like HSV, Parvovirus B19 or bacteria like uncommon serotypes of Streptococcus have been implicated. At the moment there is no concrete proof of the existence of certain microorganisms in the etiology of ABD and the initiation of the immunological process. Molecular mimicry between bacterial (HSV, streptococci) and human heat shock proteins (HSP), due to significant peptide homology between bacterial and human HSPs has been widely accepted, might be the basic link between infection and (auto)immunity in predisposed subjects, and could initiate and augment T and B cell immune responses. Besides, the option of exposure to chemicals was not supported for long. However, although immunological abnormalities concerning innate and adaptive immunity in ABD have been extensively studied, there is no adequate proof that ABD is either a typical autoimmune disease- it does not fulfill substantial criteria- or an auto-inflammatory disease- it is a very weak hypothesis at the moment (Direskeneli & Saruhan-Direskeneli, 2003; Kapsimali et al, 2010; Mumcu et al, 2007; Zouboulis & May, 2003).

ABD is a systemic vasculitis which may affect arteries and veins of all sizes in any organ and underlies disease manifestations. To a great extent, disease pathology points to a vascular inflammation. Biopsies of affected organs usually reveal vasculitis, where intense infiltrations of neutrophils predominate and CD4+ T lymphocytes are present in the early stages.

Venous vascular involvement and thrombosis is the characteristic feature of the disease, probably responsible for most of the tissue damage seen. Inflammatory changes in large arteries are typical of vasculitis, lack wall thickening and granuloma formation and have a tendency towards aneurysm formation. It is more severe in males. ABD lacks an increased risk of atherosclerosis. The term 'vasculo-Behcet' has been adopted to describe cases where vascular features dominate in disease expression. After initial vascular lesion (usually venous thrombosis), other vascular lesions may follow and lead to progressive, multifocal vascular disease with an unfavorable prognosis (Melikoglu et al, 2008).

Vascular inflammation is mainly due to complex innate-immune, pro-inflammatory mechanisms which activate and perpetuate adaptive/specific immune responses against antigens not identified clearly. Endothelial dysfunction, partly due to anti-endothelial autoimmune reactions and non-specific coagulation/fibrinolytic abnormalities, has also been demonstrated and participates in disease pathophysiology to some extent. In such cases aggressive treatment consisting of immunosuppressive drugs is recommended (Calamia et al, 2011; Calamia & Kaklamanis, 2008).

Management decisions are often difficult to take and there is a lack of controlled trials. A sequential therapeutic approach, based on ABD immunopathology and the immunomodulatory action achieved by immunosuppressive drugs is discussed.

2.1 Innate immunity cells abnormalities in ABD

Neutrophil involvement in ABD pathogenesis represents a challenging issue, as neutrophil hyperactivation seems to play a pivotal role in the inflammatory vasculitic characteristics of disease lesions. Neutrophils are the dominant subpopulation of the inflammatory infiltrates in the vessel wall (Hayasaki et al, 2004).

Neutrophil hypereactivity is a major contributor to the well-known pathergy skin reaction, which might be positive during periods of active disease. Pathergy reaction is a non-specific skin hyper-reactivity to minor trauma, such as a needle prick (Boura et al, 2007; Ozdemir et al, 2007).

At the tissue level, neutrophils were described to be present in the anterior chamber of the eye and the corneal epithelium, as well as in the ciliary body and chorioid tissue (Mendoza-Pinto et al, 2010).

These cells are reported to be functionally impaired in the disease. Eksioglu-Demiralp et al described specific defects concerning neutrophil activation, oxidative burst and phagocytic activity (Eksioglu-Demiralp et al, 2001). On the other hand, increased synthesis of reactive oxygen species (ROS) has been reported in ABD. ROS-mediated oxidative stress seems to play an important role in pathogenesis, as advanced oxidation protein products were described to correlate with disease activity (Yazici C et al, 2004). This contradiction might mean that functional activity of neutrophils might correlate to disease activity or other, poorly defined, parameters.

Additionally, it has been postulated that endothelial cells cooperate with neutrophils and monocytes in the vasculitic process. Endothelial cell activation and subsequently increased expression of cell adhesion molecules is a characteristic feature of the disease, which can trigger neutrophils and monocytes to initiate natural immune responses on the vessel wall. Recently, a novel mechanism by which neutrophils may interact with cytokine-activated endothelial cells in the presence of anti-endothelial cell antibodies has been described. Main receptors were Fc-gamma-RIIa and CXCR1/2. Moreover, endothelium activation leads to excessive thrombin formation and impaired fibrinolytic function, thus contributing to the generation of a prothrombotic state in ABD (Florey et al, 2007; Lee MT et al, 2007; Probst et al, 2004).

Furthermore, neutrophils are primed by overproduced pro-inflammatory cytokines, secreted by antigen presenting cells (APCs) and the endothelium (e.g. TNF-α, IL-1, IL-6, IL-8 etc). Under such conditions, they secrete other cytokines that prime themselves, cause Th1 polarization and maintain a non-specific, pro-inflammatory microenvironment to retain enhanced activity (Carletto et al, 1997; Katsantonis et al, 2000; Zouboulis et al, 2000).

Recently, the role of matrix metalloproteinases, particularly MMP-2 and MMP-9 was underlined in ABD. Pay et al found increased levels of these molecules in the serum of ABD patients and this was strongly correlated to vasculo-Behcet disease, especially aneurysm formation. Other investigators confirmed the elevated MMP-9 levels in the cerebrospinal fluid of ABD patients, suggesting that they might be involved in the pathogenesis of neuro-ABD (Hamzaoui K et al, 2009; Pay et al, 2007).

It is reported that neutrophils are more resistant to spontaneous apoptosis (via Fas/Fas ligand interactions) during the remission of ABD uveitis, while resistance was restored in the active phase of the disease (Fujimori et al, 2008).

Monocytes are also involved in ABD pathogenesis. Recent studies support the possible role of bacterially-induced innate immune responses through monocyte Toll-like receptor (TLR) activation. It was reported that TLR-2 was decreased after stimulation with LPS and HSP-60, or increased after bacterial lipoteichoic acid stimulation. TLR-6 expression was found to be enhanced after stimulation with HSP-60 and Streptococcus sanguis (Neves et al, 2009; Yavuz et al, 2008). As mentioned above, HSP-60 and Streptococcus sanguis represent candidate antigens in ABD pathogenesis.

Antigen-presenting cells are reported to be activated in ABD patients, since ex vivo cultured monocytes were able to produce increased amounts of TNF-α, IL-6 and IL-8 (Mege et al, 1993). Moreover, there is strong evidence suggesting that APCs may be primarily involved in ABD immunopathogenesis. Early data comes from pathergy reaction histology, where

Saito et al showed that Langerhans cells were increased in the dermis layer shortly after needle prick (Saito et al, 1980).
However, it has not been clarified whether APC hypereactivity is a primary defect of these cells or the result of disease related conditions. Nevertheless, IL-12 and IL-18, cytokines mostly produced by APCs, are known to strongly promote Th1 polarization of immune responses. Both these cytokines have been found in increased levels during active disease, implying a central role for APCs in ABD pathogenesis (Hamzaoui K et al, 2002).
Finally, Pay et al described decreased numbers of peripheral plasmacytoid dendritic cells, along with decreased levels of IFN-β and suggested that this cell subset may also participate in disease pathogenesis (Pay et al, 2007).

2.1.1 Gamma-delta (γδ) T cells

These specialized T cells (TCR comprising of γ and δ heterodimer) have been increasingly investigated during recent years. They are thought to play a critical role in mucosal immunity, being the first line of defense against invading micro-organisms, as well as the link between innate and adaptive immune response (Casetti et al, 2008).
A subset of γδ T cells (Vgamma9+Vdelta2+) was found in increased numbers in the blood of active ABD patients. These cells were reported to express IL-2 receptor and HLA-DR surface molecules, indicating a high activation status. The Vgamma9+Vdelta2+ T cells were described to infiltrate target organs, such as the eye, while other studies found that they strongly proliferate after stimulation with bacterial extracts of the oral flora (Bank et al, 2003; Verjans et al, 2002; Yamashita et al, 1997).
The critical role of gammadelta T cells in ABD is underlined in the study of Treusch et al, who found a decrease in their numbers after treatment with interferon-alpha-2a (Treusch et al, 2004).
Later, it was shown that expanded CD56+ and CD8+ gammadelta T cells in ABD were capable of secreting IFN-γ and TNF-α. Data is further supported by the fact that these cells seem to be polyclonally rather than oligoclonally activated in ABD patients with oral ulcers. Probably because of repeated inflammation of the oral mucosa, due to a wide variety of antigenic stimuli, activation and proliferation of these cells might play a role in disease clinical heterogeneity (Freysdottir, 1999, 2006).

2.1.2 NK and NKT cells

Early studies reported an increase in NK cell numbers in ABD patients. However, others described a decrease in their cytotoxic activity in the active phase of the disease, which was restored in remission periods. However, recent studies reported that, although increased in active disease, NK cells do not seem to exert impaired cytotoxic activity, as they were shown to adequately suppress IFN-γ production by CD4+ T cells, thus regulating a Th1 response in ABD (Onder et al, 1994; Suzuki et al, 1992; Yamaguchi et al, 2010).
Natural killer T cells (NKT) comprise a sublineage of T cells that share characteristics of conventional T cells and NK cells and bridge innate and adaptive immunity. Their activation is restricted by the MHC molecule CD1d. Early studies reported an increase of CD4+CD16+ and CD4+CD56+ T cells in ABD. Other investigators confirmed the presence of increased CD56+ T cells in the periphery of patients with active ABD uveitis, in contrast with other forms of immune-mediated uveitis (Eksioglu-Demiralp et al, 1999; Yato & Matsumoto, 1999).

In the tissue level, NKT cells were found to be increased in the aqueous humor of uveitis patients. Additionally, in neuro-ABD patients, NKT cells were reported to be decreased in the periphery and increased in the cerebrospinal fluid, thus suggesting a recruitment of these cells in the site of inflammation. It should be mentioned that these cells were strongly Th1 polarized. Further studies demonstrated that CD8+CD56+ T cells represent potent cytotoxic effectors in ABD uveitis, as they were found to express both surface FasL and preformed intracellular perforin (Ahn et al, 2005; Hamzaoui K et al, 2006; Yu et al, 2004).

2.2 Adaptive immunity cells abnormalities in ABD

Although the exact pathogenetic mechanisms behind ABD remain to be fully elucidated, much evidence has been accumulated regarding the involvement of adaptive immune response in the disease. Recent studies have revealed the central role of T-cell mediated immunity; in parallel, histopathological studies have demonstrated, mainly, T-cell-dominated perivascular infiltrates in skin, oral lesions and retina, as well as in choroids and periretinal scar tissue (Charteris et al, 1992a, 1992b; Gul et al, 1995, Poulter & Lehner, 1989).

2.2.1 T cell abnormalities

CD4+ T helper cells differentiate into, at least, four distinctive functional subsets, namely Th1, Th2, Th17 and T regulatory cells (Mucida & Cheroutre, 2010). For all of these lymphocyte subpopulations quantitive and/or qualitive abnormalities have been shown in ABD (Chi et al, 2008; Hamzaoui K et al, 2006, Ilhan et al, 2008; Mantas et al, 1999).

Genetic and environmental factors may have an influence independently or in association with other parameters, such as the ligation of T-cell receptor (TCR), the activation of co-stimulatory molecules, the predominance of a given cytokine in the microenvironment and others (Direskeneli et al, 1999).

Many investigators suggest that a Th1 polarization of the immune response is present, at least, in active ABD. Th1 type proinflammatory cytokines, such as IL-2 and IFN-γ, are reported not only to be increased in peripheral blood of patients with ABD, but also to correlate with disease activity. Additionally, IL-12, which drives Th1 immune response from naïve T cells, is also reported to be elevated in ABD. Interleukin-12 is suggested to play a substantial role in ABD; when recombinant IL-12 was added to peripheral blood lymphocytes from patients with active disease, it prevented spontaneous and Fas-induced apoptosis, resulting to proliferation of autoreactive Th1 lymphocytes that could contribute to a prolonged autoimmune inflammation (Esin et al, 1997; Frassanito et al, 1999; Nara et al, 2008; Sugi-Ikai et al, 1998).

Recently, IL-15 was reported to be increased in ABD, either in serum or in the aqueous humor of uveitis patients; IL-15 is able to induce pro-inflammatory cytokines, such as TNF-α and IL-1β, and facilitate maintenance of auto-reactive CD8+ T cells (Curnow et al, 2008; Waldman, 2004).

The Th1 cells were proven to expand with high individual variability of the Vβ TCR, suggesting that there is no single antigen responsible for T cell activation (Direskeneli et al, 1999).

Histopathological studies also point to a Th1 type tissue infiltration in ABD, possibly driven by the highly expressed IL-12 and IL-23 in intestinal and cutaneous lesions. Interestingly, both streptococcal antigens and auto-antigens, such as aB-crystallin also drive an IL-12 mediated response in ABD (Imamura et al, 2005; Kulaber et al, 2007; Lew et al, 2008; Yanagihori et al, 2006).

Concerning Th2 type of immune response, both, cells and signature cytokines, such as IL-4, IL-10 and IL-13 are reported to be unaffected or decreased in ABD by most researchers in the serum or in the aqueous humor. However, other studies reported a significant expression of IL-4 in oral ulcers from ABD patients, suggesting the presence of a more complex antigenic stimulus during the disease (Ahn et al, 2006; Dalghous et al, 2006, Mantas et al, 1999).

Th17 cells represent a relatively new functional subset of T helper cells, which mainly produce IL-17A-F, IL-22, IL-23 and TNFa. Interleukin-6 and TGF-β are considered to be the major cytokines responsible for the differentiation of these cells from naïve T cells. Recent studies have shown a possible role for these cells in the majority of systemic and organ-specific autoimmune diseases (Mesquita et al, 2009).

Concerning ABD, active disease is characterized by high serum levels of IL-6 and IL-17, compared to patients in remission, while serum levels of IL-23 and IL-17 are reported to be elevated in active uveitis. However, an increased Th17 response is not confirmed by all studies (Chi et al, 2008; Ferrante et al, 2010; Saruhan-Direskeneli et al, 2003).

Recent papers underline Th17 involvement in disease pathogenesis in the context of their ratio to Th1 cells. Kim et al reported an increased peripheral Th17/Th1 ratio, especially in uveitis and folliculitis patients, while there were no significant differences concerning Th1/Th2 and Th17/Th2 ratios (Kim et al, 2010). Histopathological studies, however, did not confirm these results in the tissue level (Canete et al, 2009).

Cytotoxic T cells are also reported to be activated in ABD, probably as a response to a profound inflammation. CD8+ T cells were also found in increased numbers in the aqueous humor in uveitis patients. Furthermore, recent studies support that these cells play a fundamental role in ABD flares, as they were found in increased numbers in active disease, along with γδT cells. Additionally, CD8+ T cells were shown to express the CD69 molecule (early activation marker), while their numbers and function returned to normal after successful management of the disease flare (Houman et al, 2004; Yasuoka et al, 2008).

2.2.2 Immune regulation in ABD

Firstly described by Sakaguchi et al in the '70s, T regulatory cells represent potent regulators of the immune response. These cells are divided into two broad categories, namely the "naturally occurring" and the "inducible" T regulatory cells (Sakaguchi et al, 1995).

Interest for immune regulation in ABD intensified as early as 1982, when Victorino et al and Sakane et al independently reported abnormal T cell suppressor activity (Sakane et al, 1982; Victorino et al, 1982). Recent studies were not able to definitely shed light in this issue. Paradoxically, CD4+CD25+FoxP3+ T regulatory cells were reported to be increased in active ABD compared to inactive disease and healthy controls, while they could suppress their T effector cell counterparts. The authors suggested that this may be due to the need for inflammation suppression in ABD (Hamzaoui K et al, 2006).

On the other hand, other investigators showed that T regulatory cells were significantly decreased before ocular attack in ABD patients, suggesting that they may serve as a predictive marker in ocular disease, thus, allowing treatment intensification before relapse (Nanke et al, 2008).

The exact interactions between T regulatory cells and other immune cells in ABD are not well understood. Hamzaoui suggested a possible cross talk between these cells and NKT cells, as these subpopulations can modulate each other through cell-to-cell contact and IL-2 dependent mechanisms, respectively (Hamzaoui K, 2007). Furthermore, other cells with possible regulatory activity, such as gammadelta-T-cells were reported to be incapable of maintaining a regulatory profile in ABD (Clemente et al, 2010).
T regulatory cells represent a promising therapeutic target for suppressing inflammation in ABD. Recently, Sugita et al reported T-reg expansion after in vitro stimulation with infliximab and significant suppression of bystander T effector cells in active ABD uveitis (Sugita et al, 2011). Additionally, other investigators reported that vitamin D is an important promoter of T cell regulation in vivo in ABD patients, as its levels were strongly correlated to T regulatory cells (Hamzaoui K et al, 2010).

2.2.3 B cell abnormalities and autoantibodies in ABD

Although not a typical autoimmune disease, ABD is characterized by B cell activation, despite the absence of disease-specific autoantibodies. Early studies demonstrated that the total numbers of B cells were normal during the disease; however, an increased expression of activation markers, such as CD13, CD133, CD80 and memory marker CD45RO was reported. Despite the presumed B cell activation, plasma cells were found in low levels, in contrast to other well-defined autoantibody-mediated disorders. These results suggest a modified B cell function in ABD, although it is not known if it is related to a weak stimulus by an unknown external antigen or it represents an epiphenomenon in the context of the general dysfunction of the immune system (Eksioglu-Demiralp et al, 1999).
After the identification of the multiple roles of B cells in the immune response, such as antigen presentation and cytokine release, newer studies reported some interesting results. B cells (along with plasma cells) were found in histopathological studies in the synovium, the central nervous system and the vessel wall of patients with ABD (Hirohata, 2008; Hirohata & Kikuchi, 2009; Suh et al, 2001).
Furthermore, it was recently reported that B-cell activating factor (BAFF) receptor was upregulated on B cells in patients with ABD vasculitis, as well as serum BAFF levels and mRNA in skin biopsies. Later, Hamzaoui A et al showed that BAFF, along with IL-6 and IL-13, were, also, increased in the broncho-alveolar lavage (BAL) fluid from ABD patients with active pulmonary involvement; All these factors are known to actively participate in the maturation and activation of B cells (Hamzaoui A, 2010; Hamzaoui K, 2008).
Consequently to B cell activation, various autoantibodies have been detected in the sera of ABD patients; however, their role in disease pathogenesis remains to be defined. Antinuclear antibodies (ANA) and rheumatoid factors are typically absent. On the other hand, autoantibodies against cell surface antigens, such as anti-endothelial cells antibodies (AECA), or against mucosal antigens have repeatedly been reported. Recent studies, based on proteomics, have revealed the presence of antibodies against more specific antigens, such as α-enolase, α-tropomyosin, kinectin, selenium-binding protein, esterase-D and carboxy-terminal subunit of Sip-1 (Delunardo et al, 2006; Direskeneli et al, 1995; Lee KH et al, 2003; Lu et al, 2005; Mahesh et al, 2005; Michelson et al, 1985; Mor et al, 2002; Okunuki et al, 2007, 2008).

Concerning AECA, their prevalence in ABD is reported to vary from 18-50%; however, difficulties in method standardization led to significant discrepancy between the different studies and raised concerns about their clinical utility. Furthermore, other studies confirmed that AECA were not quite specific for the disease; instead, they are frequently detected in other systemic vasculitides and/or autoimmune diseases. Despite their inspecificity, AECA were shown to mediate enhanced polymorphonuclear adhesion to activated endothelial cells, thus promoting tissue injury during systemic inflammation. An association between IgG-AECA and central nervous system involvement in ABD was reported (Dinc et al, 2003; Souza et al, 2007; Zeng et al, 2004).

Alpha-enolase represents a target antigen of IgM AECA, reported to be detectable in approximately half of ABD patients, especially in those with overt vascular involvement; however, its specificity is not satisfying (Lee JH et al, 2009).

3. Coagulation and fibrinolytic abnormalities in ABD

Although no specific defect in the coagulation cascade has so far been detected, ABD is characterized by thrombotic manifestations in 7-38% of the patients. In most studies, both coagulation and fibrinolytic pathways seem to be activated (Leiba et al, 2004).

Various pro-coagulant conditions, such as deficiencies of protein C, protein S, antithrombin III and factor V Leiden and prothrombin G20210A mutations have been described in ABD patients (Ates et al, 2003; Caramaschi et al, 2010). Additionally, higher levels of homocysteine, factor VIII, thrombin-antithrombin III complexes (TAT) and prothrombin fragment 1+2 maintain the intravascular generation of thrombin in these patients (Espinosa et al, 2002; La Regina et al, 2010). Despite all these data, it seems that thrombophilic factors do not play a major role in the thrombotic tendency of ABD. Leiba et al, in a tightly designed study, showed that the only factor that was strongly correlated to thrombosis in these patients was hypertriglyceridemia (Leiba et al, 2004). Other studies reported that active ABD patients were characterized by hypertriglyceridemia, low HDL and high Lp(a) levels (Musabak et al, 2005).

Regarding the fibrinolytic cascade, most studies have revealed defective fibrinolysis with lower levels of tissue plasminogen activator (t-PA) and increased thrombin activatable fibrinolysis inhibitor (TAFI) and thrombomodulin. Other studies involve the plasminogen activator inhibitor (PAI), as this molecule appears to be increased in ABD, resulting in defective tPA/PAI complex formation (Donmez et al, 2010; Ozturk et al, 2004). Furthermore, the endothelial dysfunction due to immune-mediated vasculitis may also play an important role in the thrombotic tendency of the disease.

Another important thrombogenic factor in ABD is the presence of antiphospholipid antibodies. Indeed, anticardiolipin (ACA) and anti-β2-glycoprotein 1 (anti-β2-GPI) antibodies, as well as lupus anticoagulant (LA) have been described in selected ABD patients (Bonnet et al, 2004; Kandolf-Sekulovic et al, 2005). Additionally, newer epitopes, such as antibodies against the phosphatidylserine-prothrombin complex (anti-PS/PT) or annexin V, have also been reported to be associated with thrombosis in these patients (Aslan et al, 2004; Kawakami et al, 2009). The significance of these antibodies in thrombotic manifestations of ABD remains to be fully elucidated.

In Table 2, a synopsis of the main abnormalities of the immune cells in ABD is presented.

Neutrophils	Hyperactivation Cytokine and MMPs secretion Resistance to apoptosis Tissue infiltration
Monocytes/Macrophages	Altered TLR expression Secretion of IFN-γ, IL-1, IL-8, IL-12, TNF-α
Gammadelta T cells	Vgamma9+Vdelta2+ expansion Secretion of IFN-γ, TNF-α Polyclonal proliferation
NK cells	Increased numbers Impaired cytotoxic activity? Abnormal KIR repertoire
NKT cells	Recruitment to the site of inflammation High expression of FasL and perforin Interaction with T regulatory cells?
CD8+ T cells	Increased numbers Highly activated (CD69)
CD4+ T cells (Th1 polarized)	Secretion of IL-2, IL-12, IFN-γ Resistance to apoptosis Tissue infiltration
CD4+ T cells (Th17 polarized)	Disease initiation? Secretion of IL-17, IL-23 Increased Th17/Th1 ratio
T regulatory cells	Probably low numbers during active disease Impaired suppressive activity?
B cells	Normal numbers, but activated Increased expression of BAFF receptor Autoantibody production (AECA and others)

Table 2. Main abnormalities in immune cells in ABD

A proposed model for ABD vasculitis pathogenesis

(schematic representation -1, -2, -3)
In genetically predisposed individuals, due to an exogenous stress, e.g. an infectious insult, a systemic or local non-specific immune response is mediated via innate immune cells and the endothelium.
Respiratory burst products and proinflammatrory cytokines and chemokines secreted at the site of the initial insult further attract monocytes, neutrophils and dendritic cells around the area and the blood-endothelial barrier breaks down (schematic representation -1).
Initial insult is neutralized, but HSPs derived from bacterial load, as well as HSPs from affected tissue/s give rise to a second, more specific T-cell-mediated immune response, according to molecular mimicry and/or epitope spreading model. These events might be augmented and spread out in case of repeated antigenic stimuli (second hit). Endothelial-innate cell contact and activation perpetuates the proinflammatory milieu and along with

local tissue injury produces a 'danger model' situation, where APCs, through PAMP-PRR cross-talk, are activated and induce downstream Th1 and Th17 polarization of the specific immune response. Main cytokines mediating this process are IL-1, TNF-α, IL-6, IL-8, IL-12, IL-18 and others, (schematic representation -2).

T cells, through this antigen-driven activation, are committed and clonally expanded against certain candidate peptides via well known mechanisms of molecular cross-reactivity. The orchestrated immune reaction involves B cells activated by CD4+ T cells to produce autoantibodies (AECA?) that are able to induce endothelial damage and contribute to neutrophil migration as well.

Gammadelta-T-cells probably contribute to the pathogenetic process, by cytokine secretion which augments Th1 polarization. The role of cell-mediated cytotoxicity is not clear at the moment. Probably, CD8+, NK and NKT cells are recruited in the site of inflammation and mediate a cytotoxic immune response.

Hyperactivated neutrophils, primed by cytokines and the activated endothelium (overexpressing cell adhesion molecules), migrate into the vessel wall and produce reactive oxygen species and MMPs, thus contributing to vasculitic lesions and aneurysm formation.

Additionally, low numbers or defective function of T regulatory cells probably cannot adequately regulate the hyperactivation status of effector cells, (schematic representation -3).

Finally, during disease perpetuation, tissue damage may produce new epitopes (damage-associated molecular patterns, DAMPs) that can further augment immune cells activation and contribute to the clinical heterogeneity of the disease.

This pathogenetic model is briefly presented in Figure 1.

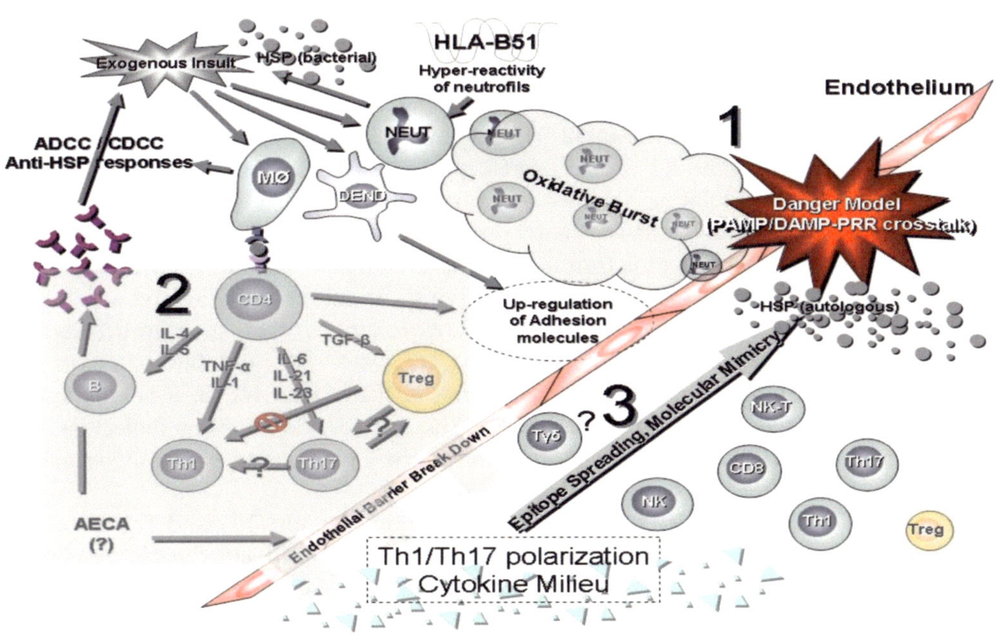

Fig. 1. Proposed pathogenetic model of ABD vasculitis

4. Therapeutic approach to ABD vasculitis

4.1 General principles

Although treatment of ABD was reviewed recently, management of complicated cases, especially those with vascular involvement, still poses a great challenge to experienced physicians. Nowadays, the recently published EULAR (European League Against Rheumatism) recommendations are considered to be the accepted guidelines for the management of the disease. Nonetheless, treatment concerning vascular involvement, either major vessel or visceral disease (medium-small vessel vasculitis) is largely based on expert opinion and uncontrolled evidence from open trials and observational studies. So the need for further properly designed controlled clinical trials is obvious (Hatemi et al, 2008).
In general, topical therapy should be applied in mucocutaneous lesions and should be the only treatment for mild symptoms. Although antiseptics seem to prevent secondary infections and reduce pain intensity, antibiotics face antigen burden and they are important in identifying disease relapses as well. Drugs with anti-inflammatory action are used as adjuvants but, beyond this, it is imperative to emphasize that the physician must be vigilant for alarming clues of systemic vasculitis and ready to implement immunomodulating regimen (Alpsoy, 2005; Alpsoy et al, 2007).
Treatment decisions depend on the age, sex, comorbidities, patient's willingness to cooperate and other parameters, such as the site and severity of involvement, as well as the frequency of recurrences. Fortunately, a part of disease burden can be managed with mild systemic immunosuppression. Early and aggressive immunosuppression is mandatory in severe or life- threatening cases. Below, the most commonly used immunomodulating drugs for the management of major vessel disease or visceral involvement will be discussed. (Table 3)

4.2 Glucocorticosteroids (C/S)

It is well known that glucocorticosteroids modify immune response to diverse stimuli by suppressing inflammatory reactions in general. They have profound metabolic effects and they affect the replication, movement and activity of virtually all cells involved in inflammatory process. Although C/S exert cytotoxic effects to activated T cells at high doses, their immunomodulating effects are probably mostly attributed to their ability to modify cellular immune functions when low doses are used orally. At the cellular level C/S bind to their intracellular receptor forming an active complex. The complex moves to the nucleus, where it binds to DNA sequences modifying chromatin structure and altering the transcription machinery. Another mechanism of action is that glucocorticosteroids-glucocorticosteroids receptor complex directly increases IκB (inhibitory factor κB) expression. IκB inhibits the actions of transcription nuclear factor NFκB. It is well known that NFκB promotes gene induction of cytokines, chemokines and adhesion molecules, thus amplifying lymphocyte proliferation and leading to the perpetuation of the inflammatory process (Bruton et al, 2005; Rhen & Chidlowski, 2005).
Through these mechanisms C/S suppress cellular immunity, both Th17 and Th1 responses. This action explains their therapeutic use in ABD. Although more detailed trials are needed, worldwide clinical experience has shown that C/S are the cornerstone of treatment for many ABD complications. High oral doses, up to 100mg/day for a long period of time, or pulse treatment with 1gr/day for 3 consecutive days or more are given, in serious or life-threatening cases, like aneurysm formation or cavernous sinus thrombosis (Hatemi et al,

2008). It was demonstrated that in large-vessel arterial disease (arterial occlusion or aneurysm) high dose glucocorticosteroids alone did not improve occlusive disease and mortality (Li Thi Huong et al, 1995). On the contrary, other studies have shown that C/S in combination with other immunosuppressants had a significant beneficial effect in vascular complications of ABD (Alpsoy & Alkman, 2009, Sharaf & Yazici, 2009). In another recently conducted randomized trial, low dose intramuscular depot C/S was used and proved to be beneficial in milder manifestations, like erythema nodosum, but no for genital ulcers. The trial used the drug in depot form for intramuscular injection, so no conclusions can be drawn for the efficacy of the usual oral or intravenous regimen (Mat et al, 2006).
Adverse effects such as osteoporosis, metabolic disturbances, psychosis must been taken into account. EULAR committee recommends the use of C/S as a first line therapy for managing all ABD manifestations. Different level of evidence for every case is probably attributed to data availability. Based on immunopathology and clinical data, we suggest the administration of high dose intravenous corticosteroids for the achievement of remission in large vessel or CNS vasculitis, followed by a slow tapering schedule to the lowest effective dose which sustains remission, under close clinical and laboratory follow up (Bruton et al, 2005; Hatemi et al, 2008; Li Thi Huong, 1995; Sharaf & Yazici, 2009).

4.3 Azathioprine

Azathioprine is a prodrug of 6-mercaptopurine, containing an imidazole ring and acts like an antimetabolite. Azathioprine and mercaptopurine appear to induce immunosuppression by interfering with purine nucleic acid metabolism. The drug intervenes with the process of cell division at steps that are required for lymphoid cell proliferation following antigenic stimulation. Stimulated lymphoid cells incapable of entering cell mitotic phase undergo apoptosis, establishing a relevant state of immunosuppression. Although RNA synthesis is blocked at the same time, these agents appear to have less effect on cell function if implemented after antigen exposure than on nucleic acid synthesis in proliferating, antigen encountering, T cells (Bruton et al, 2005).
The efficacy of azathioprine in ABD is well established. The usual dose is 1-2.5 mg/kg/day (not exceeding 200 mg/day) and an average of 3 months is required for its effect to be established. This slow immunomodulating action limits the use of azathioprine as a sole agent of therapy in acute vasculitis presentation. However, it can be used additionally in the acute phase as a corticosteroid sparing agent, as well as prophylactically. Yazici H et al propose azathioprine as a first line therapy for non-life-threatening cases of neurological complications (Yazici H et al, 1990). According to the EULAR recommendations, azathioprine should be used in any ABD patient having inflammatory eye disease with posterior segment involvement (Hatemi et al, 2008). Its efficacy and safety was evaluated in a randomized, double-blind, placebo-controlled trial. In this trial, there were fewer new cases of ocular involvement in azathioprine plus corticosteroids group comparative to corticosteroids alone (one versus eight). Additionally, the patients taking azathioprine had less frequent oral ulcers, genital ulcers and arthritis (Yazici H et al, 1990). Contemplating the pathophysiology of ABD (see above), immunosuppressants like azathioprine may play a role in the management of vessel thrombosis through anti-inflammatory action on vessel wall. Results from Sharaf et al confirm the clinical experience that by dampening immune system activation, pro-thrombotic diathesis can be, at least partially, reversed (Sharaf & Yazici, 2009).

In general, azathioprine could be used as a first line treatment in combination with corticosteroids in almost all serious manifestations of the disease and is preferable for maintenance therapy after remission induction. Common side effects are gastrointestinal disturbances, liver toxicity and bone marrow suppression but rarely do they lead to drug discontinuation. In parallel, due to B cell impairment and mild hypoglobulinemia, humoral immunity can be weakened by these cytotoxic agents as well.

4.4 Cyclophosphamide (CyP)

Cyclophosphamide is a highly active alkylating agent, which impairs DNA duplication and cell division. Although it is not a cell specific drug, the greater effect is observed upon rapidly proliferating cells, such as T cell clones after their encounter with the antigen. Initially, cyclophosphamide has proven a reliable agent in management of lupus nephritis and ANCA associated vasculitis and, eventually, has found a distinguished place in ABD vasculitis (Bruton et al, 2005).

It has been known that pulse CyP, combined with intravenous C/S regimen, help to achieve remission in ABD vascular and/or visceral involvement (Du et al, 1990; Hamza et al, 1992). According to EULAR recommendations, large vessel vasculitis, such as pulmonary and/or peripheral aneurysms, need to be treated with CyP for at least 2 years (Hatemi et al, 2008). The drug may be administrated either intravenously, as pulse treatment in doses 400-700mg/m^2, or orally in doses of 1-3 mg/day. The exact dose depends upon the severity of the disease and considerations of renal and hepatic impairment. Deep immunosuppression following CyP administration has a life-saving effect. Also in a double-blind cross over trial, CyP has proven beneficial in patients with intractable uveitis (Davatchi et al, 1999).

Due to its severe toxicity (bone marrow suppression, mucositis, neurotoxicity, syndrome of inappropriate ADH secretion, cancer), this drug must be used in life-threatening or non-responding cases. We prefer to administer CyP intravenously, as monthly or 3-weekly pulses of 500-1000mgr bolus, in order to partially avoid bladder toxicity. For safety reasons, mesna (chelic agent) and adequate fluids must be administered concurrently.

4.5 Cyclosporine

Cyclosporine is a cyclic polypeptide, which forms a complex with cyclophylin, an intracellular factor mediating signaling pathways. This complex binds to calcineurin and inhibits Ca2+-stimulated dephosphorylation of the cytosolic component of the transcription factor NFAT. Activated cytoplasmic NFAT translocates to the nucleus and binds to nuclear components required for complete T-cell activation, blocking of IL-2 and other Th1 cytokine producing genes (Th1 to Th2 switch). Besides this, calcineurin also possess peptidyl-prolyl cis-trans-isomerase enzymatic activity. The peptidyl-prolyl cis-trans-isomerase domain of calcineurin facilitates binding to CD147, also known as an inducer of extracellular-matrix metalloproteinases (MMPs). This binding causes CD147 to translocate to the cell surface, where it plays a critical role in stimulating matrix-metalloproteinase activity, leading to matrix degradation. Thus, this agent inhibits the enzymatic activation of MMPs, which leads to vessel wall thinning (Weintraub, 2009). Cyclosporine is effective against T-cell–dependent immune reactions and a suitable drug for immune intervention in the pathophysiological process of ABD vasculitis (see above). Additionally, cyclosporine, in synergy with C/S, downregulates the activity of NKT cells controlling inflammatory process (Bruton et al, 2005; Chi et al, 2010).

The efficacy of cyclosporine in ABD has been evaluated primarily in patients with ocular, mucocutaneous and articular manifestations. Approximately 50% of patients showed clinical remission when treated with cyclosporine. Two well designed trials proved that cyclosporine protects ocular degeneration and visual acuity better than conventional regimen containing prednisolone (Atmaca, 1994; Ernakova, 2003). A direct comparison of the therapeutic potential of cyclosporine to oral cyclophosphamide was conducted by Ozyazgan Y et al in patients with ocular inflammation. Therapeutic superiority concerning visual acuity was seen in the cyclosporine group at six months, but similar results were noted for both agents at two years (Ozyazgan et al, 1992). Similarly, comparison of cyclosporine with glucocorticoids or chloramboucil indicates its superiority to control ocular symptoms. EULAR recommendations suggest cyclosporine or infliximab in combination with azathioprine and corticosteroids for refractory eye involvement and major vessel disease as well (strength of recommendation C) (Hatemi et al, 2008).
Side effects are hypertension, nephrotoxicity and predisposition to infections. Furthermore, the role of cyclosporine in vascular neurological involvement in ABD has not been clarified yet and its use is discouraged (Bruton et al, 2005).

4.6 Colchicine

Colchicine exerts a variety of pharmacological effects, especially in cellular immunity. The drug arrests cell division in G1 phase by interfering with microtubule and spindle formation. This anti-mitotic effect is greatest on cells with rapid turnover (e.g. neutrophils and expanding lymphocyte clones). Colchicine also renders cell membranes more rigid and decreases the secretion of chemotactic factors from activated neutrophils, thus inhibiting inflammation in many ways (Actulga et al, 1980; Bruton et al, 2005).
Clinical experience and randomized trials support that the use of colchicine, alone or in combination with penicillin, is beneficial in reducing the number of episodes of aphthous mucositis and arthritis (Al Waiz et al, 2005). According to the authors' opinion and EULAR recommendations, colchicine has no role in severe large vessel vasculitis management and in acute relapses. Slow onset of action and lack of T cell specificity render this drug improper for use in severe cases. Beyond that, there is strong recommendation (category Ib) for the management of cases where the dominant lesion is erythema nodosum (medium size vasculitis) (Hatemi et al, 2008).
Side effects of colchicine such as nausea, vomiting, diarrhea and hematologic disturbances are well controlled with stepwise use of the drug.

4.7 Methotrexate (MTX)

Methotrexate competitively inhibits dihydrofolate reductase (DHFR), an enzyme that participates in the tetrahydrofolate synthesis. Methotrexate acts specifically during DNA and RNA synthesis and, thus, it is cytotoxic during the S-phase of the cell cycle. MTX, by inhibiting the enzymes involved in purine metabolism, and leads to intracellular accumulation of adenosine and suppression of intercellular adhesion molecule expression by T cells. These two mechanisms provoke T cell inhibition (Bruton et al, 2005; Johnston et al, 2005).
Concerning ABD vasculitis, literature for MTX is relatively poor. However, Borhani Haghighi A proposes MTX as a first line therapy in neurological complications (Borhani Haghighi, 2009). The relatively low cost and the acceptable safety profile make MTX a preferable choice (Davatchi et al, 2003; Kikuchi et al, 2003). EULAR committee recommends

MTX for CNS involvement (strength of recommendation C), but no distinction is made between vascular and parenchymal involvement (Hatemi et al, 2008). Common side effects are liver toxicity and macrocytosis.

4.8 Biologic agents

4.8.1 Interferon

Although interferons (alpha, beta, and gamma) were identified by their antiviral activity, these agents also have important immunomodulatory functions. Interferons bind to membrane receptors type I and II and produce their immunomodulating effects through a cascade of gene induction and transcriptional changes. The final result is enhancement of macrophage phagocytic activity and augmentation of specific cytotoxicity by CD8+T lymphocytes. How these changes modify immune system reaction in ABD has not been clarified. Possible mechanisms include reduction of viral antigen load and antiproliferative properties on lymphocytes and damaged tissue cells. Another probable mechanism of action is the up-regulation of sTNF-α-RII (soluble TNF-α receptor) and IL-1ra (interleukin 1 receptor antagonist). It should be emphasized that other studies entangle IFN-α action in the induction and propagation of autoimmune process (Kotter et al, 2004; Theofilopoulos et al, 2005).

In a systematic review by Kotter I et al, the authors concluded that nearly all patients with mucocutaneous symptoms and/or arthritis and/ or uveitis responded to IFN-α administration in a dose related manner (Kotter et al, 2004). Additionally, in other studies including cases of refractory uveitis, IFN-α had similar positive results. These reports were confirmed by Tugal-Tutkun et al, although they reported lower rates of complete response (Tugal-Tutkun et al, 2006). EULAR committee justifies the use of IFN-α with or without corticosteroids for eye disease, instead of cyclosporine or azathioprine. On the contrary, EULAR recommendations do not consider the use of IFN-α for major artery vasculitis due to insufficient data from large studies (Hatemi et al, 2008). We consider that potent, traditional immunosuppressants are preferable in these cases and that administration of an agent with parallel immunostimulant properties in full-blown inflammation is ambiguous (Boura et al, 2006). Side effects of IFN-α include psychosis, nausea, vomiting, diarrhea, hematologic changes, liver toxicity and leucoencephalopathy (Bruton et al, 2005).

4.8.2 Anti – TNF- α (tumor necrosis factor) agents

TNF-α, as a pro-inflammatory cytokine, promotes immune reactions and inflammation. Infliximab is a chimeric anti–TNF-α monoclonal antibody, which binds with high affinity to TNF-α and prevents the cytokine from binding to its receptors. A number of studies (uncontrolled, open labeled, case series and reports) indicate that infliximab control mucocutaneous, joint, neural, gastrointestinal and eye manifestations of disease, inducing remission (Boura et al, 2006; Sfikakis et al, 2001, 2004). Additionally, in these studies, infliximab proved adequate to sustain remission in cases refractory to azathioprine and/or cyclosporine. Sfikakis et al propose infliximab as a second line therapy for ABD relapses when usual therapy fails or as a first line regimen in severe sight-threatening uveitis (Sfikakis et al, 2004). Our experience is in agreement.

Etanercept contains the ligand binding portion of a human TNF-α receptor fused to the Fc portion of human IgG1, and binds to TNF-α, thus preventing it from interacting with its receptors. Melikoglu M et al conducted a controlled study using etanarcept in ABD.

Etanercept was superior to placebo in controlling oral ABD manifestations, whereas the rate of genital ulcers healing, joint symptoms and papulopustular skin lesions were not statistically different between the two groups (Melikoglu et al, 2005). Different results were reported from the Study Group on Autoimmune Diseases (GEAS), who published an impressive rate of response in ABD using etanercept (96%), (Ramos-Casals et al, 2008). These contradictory results indicate that more studies need to be undertaken in order to assess etanercept in ABD.

Like infliximab and etanercept, adalimumab binds to TNF-α, preventing it from activating TNF-α receptors. There is an increasing number of reports that adalimumab is promising on patients with symptoms refractory to other agents (Bawazeer et al, 2010). EULAR recommendations include anti TNF-α agents in possible therapeutic regimens for gastrointestinal and CNS involvement, but no mention is made for major vessel inflammation (Hatemi et al, 2008).

Side effects (infections, cancer) and cost must be taken into account. TNF-α antagonists could be reserved as a second line therapy in intractable posterior uveitis and CNS vascular disease as well.

4.8.3 Anakinra (anti-interleukin-1)

IL-1 mediates its pro-inflammatory actions through IL-1 receptor binding on the surface of immunocompetent cells. For homeostatic reasons there is a naturally occurring IL-1 receptor antagonist (IL-1ra) in serum, which competes with IL-1 for receptor binding, blocks IL-1 activity and ameliorates its pro-inflammatory actions. The balance between IL-1 and IL-1ra may contribute to the extent of an inflammatory response. Anakinra, a recombinant non-glycosylated version of human IL-1 receptor antagonist, may have a therapeutic role in ABD. Although literature is limited, a case report of a patient with severe vascular and gastrointestinal ABD, refractory to conventional treatment, who responded only to anakinra has been published (Botsios et al, 2008). However, later reports question the long term efficacy of anakinra in preventing secondary complications, such as amyloidosis (Bilginer et al, 2010). These ambiguous results confirm the view that further studies are needed.

4.9 Other treatments

There are limited data available regarding the use of alternative therapeutic options in ABD. Intravenous immunoglobulins have been tested either in a small number of patients or in a heterogeneous group of patients with eye inflammation (Seider et al, 2001).

IL-6 plays a central role in disease pathophysiology. IL-6 levels have been reported to be elevated in the cerebrospinal fluid of patients with active CNS disease. Probably anti–IL-6 treatment could be useful in vascular manifestations of ABD. In fact, Borhani Haghighi A proposed tocilizumab (anti-interleukin-6 agent), as an additional weapon to the therapeutic armentarium (Borhani Haghighi & Safari, 2008).

Lim SH and de Cata A reported resolution of ABD manifestations after non myeloablative hematopoietic stem cell transplantation (autologous or derived from allogeneic bone marrow or umbilical cord blood). There is an increasing number of studies proposing this practice as an upcoming treatment for refractory ABD. The rational is the depletion of activated immune cells from the body (De Cata et al, 2007; Lim et al, 2009)

All these therapeutic modalities have not been tested adequately and are not mentioned in current guidelines.

5. Specific considerations for vascular inflammation in ABD

5.1 Major vessel involvement

Although large artery disease is uncommon in ABD, it can lead to significant morbidity and mortality. The percentage of ABD patients with arterial damage varies from 5 to 18%. The two main presentations of arterial involvement is lumen stenosis, or more likely, aneurysm formation.

Although pathogenesis is yet unclear, the hypothetical model already proposed for other large vessel vasculitides might be of value. According to this model, IL-1 and TNF-α secretion from dendritic cells, macrophages and neutrophils results in the production of radical oxygen species and mettalloproteinases with subsequent elastic fiber destruction, thinning of media layer and expansive remodeling of the artery (Weyand & Goronzy, 2003). Chronic uncontrolled inflammation also leads also to arterial occlusions due to intimal thickening. These two forms of vessel remodeling may be detected in the same patient (Buggage et al, 2005).

Aneurysm formation and/or occlusive lesions may require combined medical and surgical intervention under the supervision of an experienced clinical immunologist. Urgent surgery is mandatory in case of enlarging or ruptured aneurysms or due to organ-threatening ischemia. Equally significant is the implementation of postoperative immunosuppressive therapy, to prevent relapse and common complications after arterial bypass surgery, such as graft occlusion and new aneurysm formation at the site of anastomosis (Calamia et al, 2011; Tuzun et al, 1997).

The first goal is to achieve remission with immunosuppressive drugs. We suggest aggressive therapy with methylprednisolone 1000mg x 3 or more consecutive days, followed by oral C/S and CyP in intravenous pulse treatment (4-8mg/kg) until clinical and laboratory remission.

A number of patients with major-vessel arterial disease were studied in a retrospective manner. This study illustrated that C/S, even in high doses, did not improve occlusive disease when fibrosis of intima was irreversible, emphasizing the importance of early immune intervention (Le Thi Huong, 1999).

Anticoagulation is employed successfully in several cases, but EULAR committee do not recommend anticoagulants or antiplatelet drugs due to lack of evidence from randomized controlled trials and possible danger of bleeding in sites of aneurysmal rupture (Hatemi et al, 2008). (see algorithm 1)

5.2 Medium - small vessel involvement

Although large vessel involvement is responsible for deaths in ABD, small and medium vessel vasculitis maintains the main characteristic in disease pathophysiology. Pathological findings compatible with vasculitis from different anatomical sites have been reported. More specifically, the histopathological findings range from minor neutrophilic vascular infiltration to true leukocytoclastic (oral lesions) or lymphocytic (genital lesions) vasculitis. Although such interesting clues indicate a variance in the pathophysiologic process, there are no data to suggest different therapeutic approaches in patients with different type of lesions (Chun et al, 1990; Nazarro et al, 1966).

Retinal vasculitis is a serious finding in posterior uveitis of ABD patients. EULAR committee recommends a treatment regimen that includes azathioprine and systemic corticosteroids for the management of the first attack. Doses of prednisone up to 1 mg/kg/day for one month with tapering thereafter as tolerated proved to be adequate in most of the cases. Furthermore, long term follow-up of patients proves that local and/or systemic corticosteroids and azathioprine are beneficial for maintenance treatment as well (Hatemi et al, 2008; Iscan et al, 2005; Yazici et al, 2010).

In severe relapsing or refractory eye inflammation, initial pulse therapy with intravenous methylprednisolone (1 g/day for three days or more) is needed. A number of observational studies have suggested efficacy of infliximab for the treatment of inflammatory eye disease. Combination of the above agents with cyclosporine or IFN-α can be used for intractable eye inflammation (EULAR recommendations 1 and 2), although the level of evidence is low (grade of evidence III) (Hatemi et al, 2008; Yazici et al, 2010).

Alternatively, the addition of cyclophosphamide pulse treatment prior to infliximab in refractory ocular ABD could be used. There is a possible synergistic effect of cyclophosphamide and infliximab in controlling ocular inflammation when used consecutively (submitted for publication).

In general, neurological complications could be treated in the same manner as posterior uveitis. The combination of high-dose C/S (3–7 pulses of intravenous methylprednisolone 1 g/day) with another immunosuppressive agent (preferably azathioprine) is required. Cyclophosphamide, methotrexate and TNF-α antagonists represent quite useful alternatives in severe parenchymal disease. For dural sinus thrombosis, short pulses of intravenous C/S are usually adequate. In neurological involvement, cyclosporine should not be introduced due to its potential neurotoxicity (strength of recommendation C) (Borhani Haghighi, 2009; Borhani-Haghighi & Safari, 2010; Hatemi et al, 2008; Kotter et al, 2006).

Serious renal lesions are rare and range from minor IgA deposits in glomerulus to catastrophic crescentic glomerulonephritis. In case of clinically important glomerulonephritis, treatment varies according to other organ involvement. A reasonable approach is cyclophosphamide 750-1000 mg /month plus glucocorticosteroids 500-1000 mg /day for three days and 60-100 mg oral prednisolone in tapering doses until clinical remission (Altiparmak et al, 2001). (see algorithm 2)

5.3 Venous thrombosis

Deep vein thrombosis (DVT) is the most frequent vascular manifestation of ABD. DVT is believed to result from endothelial inflammation leading to thrombosis through pro-thrombotic alterations in the vessel wall, upregulation of adhesion molecules and endothelial dysfunction. DVT can occur in any site of the vascular tree, most commonly in lower extremities, but also in hepatic veins, cerebral venous sinuses, superior and inferior vena cava (Ames et al, 2001).

Thrombotic events are prevented by ameliorating systemic inflammation, rather than by the institution of primary anticoagulation (Kuzu et al, 1994; Mader et al, 1999; Sarica-Kucukoglu et al, 2006). EULAR does not recommend the use of antiplatelet drugs, anticoagulants or fibrinolytic agents for thrombotic events in ABD, due to insufficient data from large studies (Hatemi et al, 2008).

The authors suggest that venous thrombosis must be faced on case-by-case basis, through cooperation with appropriate subspecialists. When anti-thrombotic intervention is considered, aspirin is a rational choice. Acetylosalicylic acid interferes with the transcriptional activation of the interferon-γ gene, a mechanism of action that may be particularly useful in inhibiting T-cell function in ABD. Furthermore, from the pathophysiological models of giant cell arteritis, we know that IFN-γ favor intimal hyperplasia and endothelial dysfunction. (see algorithm 1)

Target	Therapeutic Goals	Current or emerging approach
Interleukin-1	Suppression of acute phase response Inhibition of macrophages	Anakinra, C/S
Interleukin-6	Suppression of acute phase response Inhibition of macrophages	Tocilizumab, C/S
Interferon-γ or interferon- γ inducing genes	Disruption of adaptive T-cell response	acetosalicylic acid, C/S
Metalloproteinases	Inhibition of matrix degradation- -inhibition of expanding remodeling	Cyclosporine
Innate immune responses	Inhibition of nuclear factor k-B	C/S, Interferons
Adaptive immune responses	Inhibition of T cell clones activation	Cyclophosphamide, Cyclosporine
Vascular thrombosis	Inhibition of prothrombotic changes of endothelium	acetosalicylic acid, anticoagulants, immunosuppressants
TNF-α	Inhibition of TNF-α mediated immune response	etanercept, infliximab, adalimumab

Table 3. Therapeutic targets for pathogenic pathways in Adamantiades- Behcet disease and indicative approaches

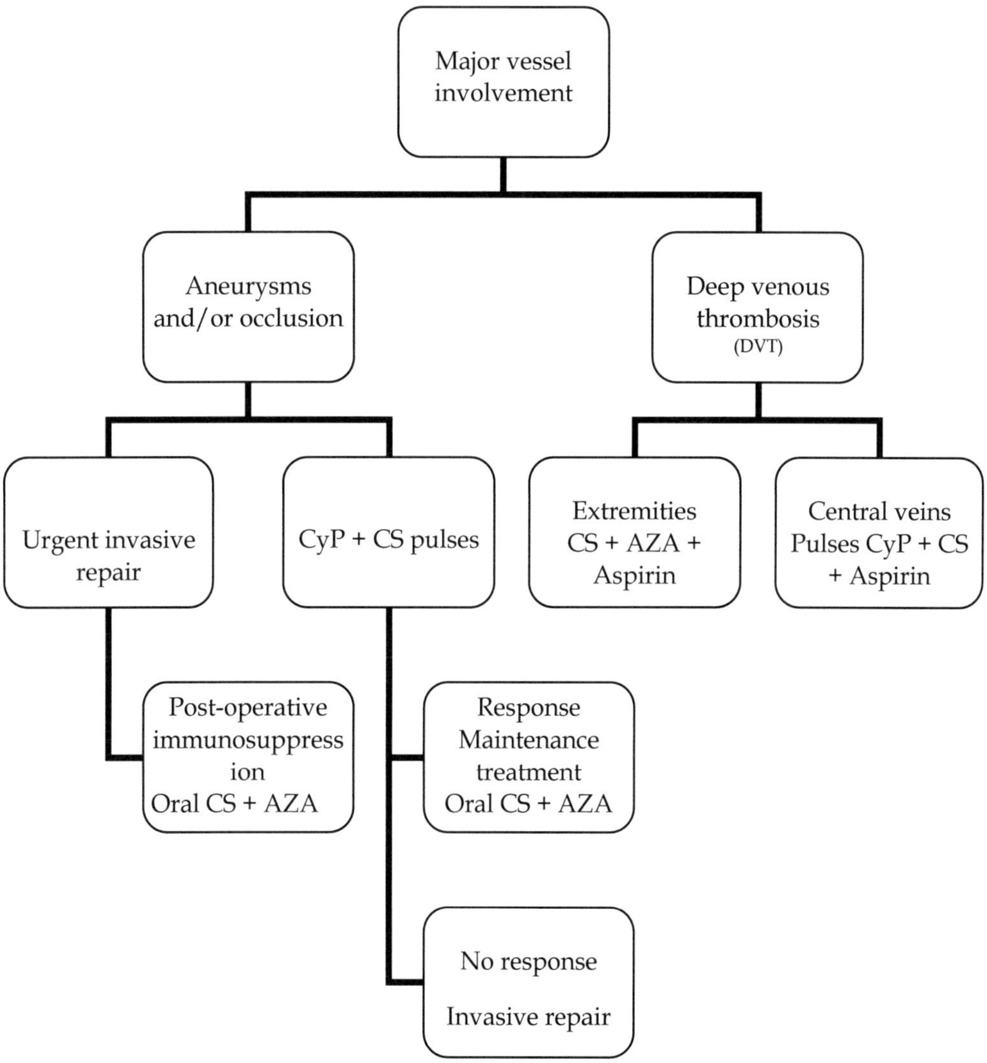

Algorithm 1. Therapeutic intervention for major vessel involvement in ABD.

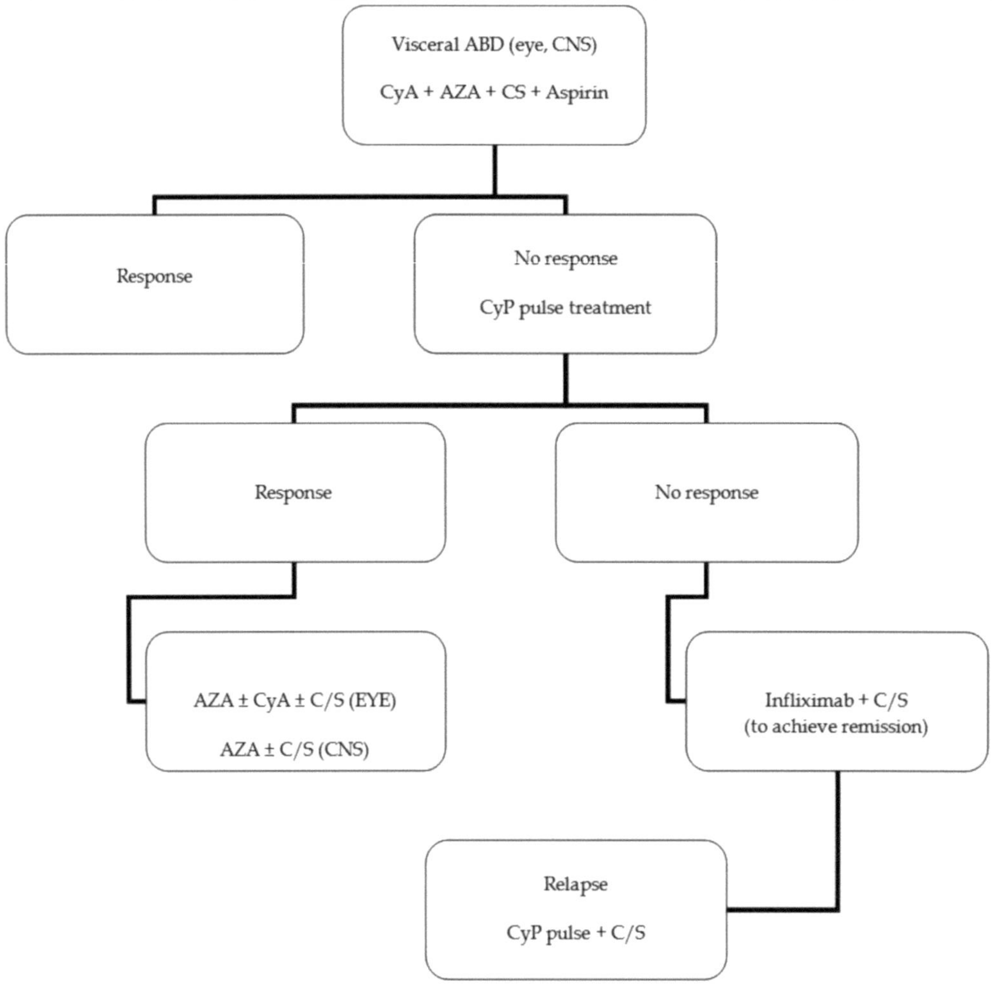

Algorithm 2. Therapeutic intervention for visceral involvement (eye, CNS) in ABD.

6. Conclusions

The multi-level pathogenetic process of visceral ABD implies that inflammation control by one single agent is seemingly impossible; indeed, various combinations of immunomodulating agents are proposed.

Early administration of immunosuppressive therapy is critical before permanent damage is established. Invasive approaches must be implemented when needed.

Urgent intervention is mandatory in life threatening circumstances.

Although there is an increasing amount of data from controlled trials regarding specific issues in ABD therapy (targeting management of early ABD and particular disease mechanisms), current guidelines are largely based on the opinion of experts.

7. References

Adamantiades B. ((1931) Sur un cas d'iritis a hypopion recidivant. *Ann Ocul (Paris)* 168: 271-8

Ahn JK, Chung H, Lee DS, Yu YS & Yu HG. (2005) CD8brightCD56+ T cells are cytotoxic effectors in patients with active Behcet's uveitis. *J Immunol* 175: 6133-42

Ahn JK, Yu HG, Chung H & Park YG. (2006) Intraocular cytokine environment in active Behcet uveitis. *Am J Ophthalmol* 142: 429-34

Aktulga E, Altac M, Muftuoglu A et al. (1980) A double blind study of colchicine in Behcet's disease. *Haematologica* 65: 399–402

Alpsoy E. (2005) Behçet's disease: treatment of mucocutaneous lesions. *Clin Exp Rheumatol* 23: 532–9

Alpsoy E, Zouboulis CC & Ehrlich CE. (2007) Mucocutaneous lesions of Behçet's disease. *Yonsei Med J* 48: 573–85

Alpsoy E & Alkman A. (2009) Behçet's disease: an algorithmic approach to its treatment. *Arch Dermatol Res* 301: 693-702

Altiparmak MR, Tanverdi M, Pamuk ON, Tunu R & Hamuryudan V. (2002) Glomerulonephritis in Behcet's disease: report of seven cases and review of the literature. *Clin Rheumatol* 21: 14-8

Al-Waiz MM, Sharquie KE, A-Qaissi MH & Hayani RK. (2005) Colchicine and benzathine penicillin in the treatment of Behcet disease: a case comparative study. *Dermatol Online J* 11: 3

Ames PR, Steuer A, Pap A & Denman AM. (2001) Thrombosis in Behçet's disease: a retrospective survey from a single UK centre. *Rheumatology (Oxford)* 40: 652–5

Aslan H, Pay S, Gok F et al. (2004) Antiannexin V autoantibody in thrombophilic Behcet's disease. *Rheumatol Int* 24: 77-9

Ates A, Duzgun AN, Ulu A, Tiryaki AO & Akar N. (2003) Factor V gene (1691A and 4070G) and prothrombin gene 20210A mutations in patients with Behcet's disease. *Pathophysiol Haemost Thromb* 33: 157-63

Atmaca LS & Batioglu F. (1994) The efficacy of cyclosporin-a in the treatment of Behcet's disease. *Ophthalmic Surg* 25: 321-7

Bank I, Duvdevani M & Livneh A. (2003) Expansion of gammadelta T-cells in Behcet's disease: role of disease activity and microbial flora in oral ulcers. *J Lab Clin Med* 141: 33-40

Bawazeer A, Raffa LH & Nizamuddin. (2010) Clinical experience with adalimumab in the treatment of ocular Behçet disease. *Ocul Immunol Inflamm* 18: 226-32

Behcet H. (1937) Uber rezidivierende, aphthose, durch ein Virus verursachte Geschwure im Mund, am Auge und an den Genitalien. *Dermatol Wochenschr* 105: 1152-7

Bilginer Y, Ayaz NA & Ozen S. (2010) Anti-IL-1 treatment for secondary amyloidosis in an adolescent with FMF and Behçet's disease. *Clin Rheumatol* 29: 209-10

Bonnet F, Debruxelles S, Dubourguet L et al. (2004) Lupus anticoagulant and Behcet's disease: increase of vascular risk? *Rev Med Interne* 25: 835-6

Borhani Haghighi A & Safari A. (2008) Tocilizumab may be a potential addition to our weapons against neuro-Behçet's disease. *Med Hypotheses* 71: 156-7

Borhani Haghighi A. (2009) Treatment of neuro-Behçet's disease: an update. *Expert Rev Neurother* 9: 565-74

Borhani Haghighi A & Safari A. (2010) Proposing an algorithm for treatment of different manifestations of neuro-Behcet's disease. *Clin Rheumatol* 29: 683-6

Botsios C, Sfriso P, Furlan A, Punzi L & Dinarello CA. (2008) Resistant Behçet disease responsive to anakinra. *Ann Intern Med* 149: 284-6

Boura P, Tselios K, Kamali S, Skendros P, Sarantopoulos A & Topouzis F. (2006) Concurrent relapsing central nervous system and ocular involvement in a case of life-threatening Adamantiades-Behçet Disease (ABD). *Neurol Sci* 27: 432-5

Boura P, Tselios K, Skendros P, Kamali S, Sarantopoulos A & Raptopoulou-Gigi M. (2007) Adamantiades-Behcet disease (ABD) in northern Greece: experience from a single center. *Hippokratia* 11: 210-5

Bruton L. Lazo J & Parker K. (2005) In: *Goodman & Gilman's "The pharmacological basis of therapeutics"*. 11th edition McGrawHill, pp 1408-17

Buggage RR, Levy-Clarke G, Sen HN et al. (2005) Major vessel involvement in Behcet disease. *Curr Opin Rheumatol* 17:1-8

Calamia KT & Kaklamanis PG. (2008) Behcet's disease: recent advances in early diagnosis and effective treatment. *Curr Rheumatol Rep* 10: 349-55

Calamia KT, Schirmer M & Melikoglu M. (2011) Major vessel involvement in Behçet's disease: an update. *Curr Opin Rheumatol* 23: 24-31

Canete JD, Celis R, Noordenbos T et al. (2009) Distinct synovial immunopathology in Behcet's disease and psoriatic arthritis. *Arthritis Res Ther* 11: R17

Caramaschi P, Poli G, Bonora A et al. (2010) A study on thrombophilic factors in Italian Behcet's patients. *Joint Bone Spine* 77: 330-4

Carletto A, Pacor ML, Biasi D et al. (1997) Changes of neutrophil migration without modification of in vitro metabolism and adhesion in Behcet's disease. *J Rheumatol* 24: 1332-6

Casetti R & Martino A. (2008) The plasticity of γδ T cells: innate immunity, antigen presentation and new immunotherapy. *Cell Mol Immunol* 5: 161-70

Charteris DG, Champ C, Rosenthal AR & Lightman SL. (1992) Behcet's disease: activated T lymphocytes in retinal perivasculitis. *Br J Ophathlmol* 76: 499-501

Charteris DG, Barton K, McCartney AC & Lightman SL. (1992) CD4+ lymphocyte involvement in ocular Behcet's disease. *Autoimmunity* 12: 201-6

Chi W, Zhu X, Yang P et al. (2008) Upregulated IL-23 and IL-17 in Behcet's patients with active uveitis. *Invest Ophthalmol Vis Sci* 49: 3058-64

Chi W, Yang P, Zhu X et al. (2010) Production of interleukin-17 in Behcet's disease is inhibited by cyclosporin A. *Mol Vis* 16: 880-6

Chun SI, Su WP & Lee S. (1990) Histopathologic study of cutaneous lesions in Behçet's syndrome. *J Dermatol* 17: 333–41

Clemente A, Cambra A, Munoz-Saa I et al. (2010) Phenotype markers and cytokine intracellular production by CD8+

gammadelta T lymphocytes do not support a regulatory T profile in Behcet's disease patients and healthy controls. *Immunol Lett* 129: 57-63

Curnow SJ, Pryce K, Modj N et al. (2008) Serum cytokine profiles in Behcet's dsease : is there a role for IL-15 in pathogenesis? *Immunol Lett* 121: 7-12

Dalghous AM, Freysdottir J & Fortune F. (2006) Expression of cytokines, chemokines and chemokine receptors in oral ulcers of patients with Behcet's disease (BD) and recurrent aphthous stomatitis is Th1 associated, although Th2 association is also observed in patients with BD. *Scand J Rheumatol* 35: 472-5

Davatchi F, Shahram F, Chams H & Akbarian M. (1999) Pulse cyclophosphamide for ocular lesions of Behçet's disease: double blind crossover study. *Arthritis Rheum* 42: 320

Davatchi F, Shahram F, Chams H et al. (2003) High dose methotrexate for ocular lesions of Behcet's disease. Preliminary short-term results. *Adv Exp Med Biol* 528: 579-84

De Cata A, Intiso D, Bernal M et al. (2007) Prolonged remission of neuro-Behçet's disease following autologous transplantation. *Int J Immunopathol Pharmacol* 20: 91–6

Delunardo F, Conti F, Margutti P et al. (2006) Identification and characterization of the carboxy-terminal region of Sip-1, a novel autoantigen in Behcet's disease. *Arthritis Res Ther* 8: R71

Dinc A, Takafuta T, Jiang D, Melikoglu M, Saruhan-Direskeneli G & Shapiro SS. (2003)Anti-endothelial cell antibodies in Behcet's disease. *Clin Exp Rheumatol* 21(suppl 30): S27-30

Direskeneli H, Keser G, D'Cruz D et al. (1995) Antiendothelial cell antibodies, endothelial proliferation and von Willebrand factor antigen in Behcet's disease. *Clin Rheumatol* 14: 55-61

Direskeneli H, Eksioglu-Demiralp E, Kibaroglu A, Yavuz S, Ergun T & Akoglu T. (1999) Oligoclonal T cell expansions in patients with Behcet's disease. *Clin Exp Immunol* 117: 166-70

Direskeneli H & Saruhan-Direskeneli G. (2003) The role of heat shock proteins in Behcet's disease. *Clin Exp Rheumatol* 21(suppl 30): S44-8

Donmez A, Aksu K, Advin H et al. (2010) The plasma levels of activated thrombin activatable fibrinolysis inhibitor and thrombomodulin in Behcet's disease and their association with thrombosis. *Thromb Res* 126: 207-10

Du LT, Fain O, Wechsler B et al. (1990) Value of "bolus" cyclophosphamide injections in Behcet's disease. Experience of 17 cases. *Presse Med* 19: 1355-8

Eksioglu-Demiralp E, Direskeneli H, Ergun T, Fresko I & Akoglu T. (1999) Increased CD4+CD16+ and CD4+CD56+ T cell subsets in Behcet's disease. *Rheumatol Int* 19: 23-6

Eksioglu-Demiralp E, Kibaroglu A, Direskeneli H et al. (1999) Phenotypic characteristics of B cells in Behcet's disease: increased activity in B cell subsets. *J Rheumatol* 26: 826-32

Eksioglu-Demiralp E, Direskeneli H, Kibaroglu A, Yavuz S, Ergun T & Akoglu T. (2001) Neutrophil activation in Behcet's disease. *Clin Exp Rheumatol* 19(suppl 24): S19-24

Ermakova NA. (2003) Efficacy of corticosteroids and cyclosporin in the treatment of retinal vasculitis in patients with Behcet's disease. *Adv Exp Med Biol* 528: 563–5

Esin S, Gul A, Hodara V et al. (1997) Peripheral blood T cell expansions in patients with Behcet's disease. *Clin Exp Immunol* 107: 520-7

Espinosa G, Font J, Tassies D et al. (2002) Vascular involvement in Behcet's disease: relation with thrombophilic factors, coagulation activation and thrombomodulin. *Am J Med* 112: 37-43

Ferrante A, Ciccia F, Principato A et al. (2010) A Th1 but not a Th17 response is present in the gastrointestinal involvement of Behcet's disease. *Clin Exp Rheumatol* 28 (suppl 60): S27-S30

Fietta P. (2005) Behcet's disease: familial clustering and immunogenetics. *Clin Exp Rheumatol* 23(suppl 38): S96-105

Florey OJ, Johns M, Esho OO, Mason JC & Haskard DO. (2007) Antiendothelial cell antibodies mediate enhanced leukocyte adhesion to cytokine-activated endothelial cells through a novel mechanism requiring cooperation between Fc-gamma-RIIa and CXCR1/2. *Blood* 109: 3881-9

Frassanito M, Dammacco R, Cafforio P & Dammacco F. (1999) Th1 polarization of the immune response in Behcet's disease: a putative pathogenetic role of interleukin-12. *Arthritis Rheum* 42: 1967-74

Freysdottir J, Lau S & Fortune F. (1999) Gammadelta T cells in Behcet's disease (BD) and recurrent aphthous stomatitis (RAS). *Clin Exp Immunol* 118: 451-7

Freysdottir J, Hussain L, Farmer I, Lau SH & Fortune F. (2006) Diversity of gammadelta T cells in patients with Behcet's disease is indicative of polyclonal activation. *Oral Dis* 12: 271-7

Fujimori K, Ohi K, Takeuchi M et al. (2008) Circulating neutrophils in Behcet's disease are resistant for apoptotic cell death in the remission phase of uveitis. *Graefes Arch Clin Exp Ophthalmol* 246: 285-90

Gul A, Esin S, Dilsen S, Konice M, Wigzell S & Biberfeld P. (1995) Immunohistology of skin pathergy reaction in Behcet's disease. *Br J Dermatol* 132: 901-7

Hamza M, Meddeb S, Mili I & Ouertani A. (1992) Bolus of cyclophosphamide and methylprednisolone in uveitis in Behcet's disease. Preliminary results with the use of new criteria of evaluation. *Ann Med Interne (Paris)* 143: 438-41

Hamzaoui K, Hamzaoui M, Guemira F, Bessioud M, Hamza M & Ayed K. (2002) Cytokine profile in Behcet's disease patients. Relationship with disease activity. *Scand J Rheumatol* 31: 205-10

Hamzaoui K, Kamoun M, Houman H et al. (2006) Discrepancies of NKT cells expression in peripheral blood and in cerebrospinal fluid from Behcet's disease. *J Neuroimmunol* 175: 160-8

Hamzaoui K, Hamzaoui A & Houman H. (2006) CD4+CD25+ regulatory T cells in patients with Behcet's disease. *Clin Exp Rheumatol* 24(suppl 42): S71-8

Hamzaoui K. (2007) Paradoxical high regulatory T cell activity in Behcet's disease. *Clin Exp Rheumatol* 25(suppl 45): s107-13

Hamzaoui K, Houman H, Ben Dhifallah I, Kamoun M & Hamzaoui A. (2008) Serum BAFF levels and skin mRNA expression in patients with Behcet's disease. *Clin Exp Rheumatol* 26(suppl 50): S64-71

Hamzaoui K, Maitre B & Hamzaoui A. (2009) Elevated levels of MMP-9 and TIMP-1 in the cerebrospinal fluid of neuro-Behcet's disease. *Clin Exp Rheumatol* 27(Suppl 53): S52-7

Hamzaoui A, Chelbi H, Sassi FH & Hamzaoui K. (2010) Release of B-cell activating factor of the TNF family in bronchoalveolar lavage from Behcet's disease with pulmonary involvement. *Oxid Med Cell Longev* 3: 122-8

Hamzaoui K, Ben Dhifallah I, Karray E, Sassi FH & Hamzaoui A. (2010) Vitamin D modulates peripheral immunity in patients with Behcet's disease. *Clin Exp Rheumatol* 28(suppl 60): S50-7

Hatemi G, Silman A, Bang D et al. (2008) EULAR Expert Committee. EULAR recommendations for the management of Behçet disease. *Ann Rheum Dis* 67: 1656-62

Hayasaki N, Ito M, Suzuki T et al. (2004) Neutrophilic phlebitis is characteristic of intestinal Behcet's disease and simple ulcer syndrome. *Histopathology* 45: 377-83

Hippocrates. (1993) *Endemic Diseases. Third Book. Case 7.* Kaktos (ed). 13: 209

Hirohata S. (2008) Histopathology of central nervous system lesions in Behcet's disease. *J Neurol Sci* 267: 41-7

Hirohata S & Kikuchi H. (2009) Histopathology of the ruptured pulmonary artery aneurysm in a patient with Behcet's disease. *Clin Exp Rheumatol* 27(Suppl 53): S91-5

Houman H, Hamzaoui A, Ben Ghorbal I, Khanfir MS, Feki M & Hamzaoui K. (2004) Tc1/Tc2 ratio in the inflammatory process in patients with Behcet's disease. *Mediators Inflamm* 13: 247-53

Ilhan F, Demir T, Turkcuoglu P, Turgut B, Demir N & Godekmerdan A. (2008) Th1 polarization of the immune response in uveitis in Behcet's disease. *Can J Ophthalmol* 43: 105-8

Imamura Y, Kurokawa MS, Yoshikawa H et al. (2005) Involvement of Th1 cells and heat shock protein 60 in the pathogenesis of intestinal Behcet's disease. *Clin Exp Immunol* 139: 371-8

International Study Group for Behcet's disease. (1990) Criteria for diagnosis of Behcet's disease. *Lancet* 335: 1078-80

Iscan ZH, Vural KM & Bayazit M. (2005) Compelling nature of arterial manifestations in Behcet disease. *J Vasc Surg* 41: 53-8

Johnston A, Gudjonsson JE, Sigmundsdottir H, Runar LB & Valdimarsson H. (2005) The anti-inflammatory action of methotrexate is not mediated by lymphocyte apoptosis, but by the suppression of activation and adhesion molecules. *Clin Immunol* 114: 154–63

Kaklamani VG, Vaiopoulos G & Kaklamanis PG. (1998) Behcet's disease. *Semin Arthritis Rheum* 27: 197-217

Kandolf-Sekulovic L, Pavlovic MD, Glisic B et al. (2005) Adamantiades-Behcet's disease, deep venous thrombosis and anticardiolipin antibodies: report of two cases. *J Eur Acad Dermatol Venereol* 19: 484-6

Kapsimali VD, Kanakis MA, Vaiopoulos GA & Kaklamanis PG. (2010) Etiopathogenesis of Behcet's disease with emphasis on the role of immunological aberrations. *Clin Rheumatol* 29: 1211-6

Katsantonis J, Adler Y, Orfanos CE & Zouboulis CC. (2000) Adamantiades-Behcet's disease: serum IL-8 is a more reliable marker for disease activity than C-reactive protein and erythrocyte sedimentation rate. *Dermatology* 201: 37-9

Kawakami T, Yamazaki M, Mizoguchi M & Soma Y. (2009) Antiphosphatidylserine-prothrombin complex antibodies in 3 patients with Behcet's disease involving superficial vein thrombophlebitis. *Arch Dermatol* 145: 171-5

Kikuchi H, Aramaki K & Hirohata S. (2003) Low dose MTX for progressive neuro-Behcet's disease. A follow-up study for 4 years. *Adv Exp Med Biol* 528: 575-8

Kim J, Park JA, Lee EY, Lee YJ, Song YW & Lee EB. (2010) Imbalance of Th17 to Th1 cells in Behcet's disease. *Clin Exp Rheumatol* 28(suppl 60): S16-9

Kotter I, Gunaydin I, Zierhut M & Stobiger N. (2004) The use of interferon alpha in Behcet's disease: review of the literature. *Semin Arthritis Rheum* 33: 320-35

Kotter I, Gunaydin I, Batra M et al. (2006) CNS involvement occurs more frequently in patients with Behcet's disease under cyclosporin A (CSA) than under other medications - results of a retrospective analysis of 117 cases. *Clin Rheumatol* 25: 482–6

Kulaber A, Tugal-Tutkun I, Yentur SP et al. (2007) Proinflammatory cellular immune response in Behcet's disease. *Rheumatol Int* 27: 1113-8

Kuzu MA, Ozaslan C, Koksoy C, Gürler A & Tüzüner A. (1994) Vascular involvement in Behçet's disease: 8 year audit. *World J Surg* 18: 948–53

La Regina M, Orlandini F, Prisco D & Dentali F. (2010) Homocysteine in vascular Behcet's disease: a meta-analysis. *Arterioscler Thromb Vasc Biol* 30: 2067-74

Lee JH, Cho SB, Bang D et al. (2009) Human anti-alpha-enolase antibody in sera from patients with Behcet's disease and rheumatologic disorders. *Clin Exp Rheumatol* 27(suppl 53): S63-6

Lee KH, Chung HS, Kim HS et al. (2003) Human alpha-enolase from endothelial cells as a target antigen of anti-endothelial cell antibody in Behcet's disease. *Arthritis Rheum* 48: 2025-35

Lee MT, Hooper LC, Kump L et al. (2007) Interferon-beta and adhesion molecules (E-selectin and s-ICAM-1) are detected in sera from patients with retinal vasculitis and are induced in retinal vascular endothelial cells by Toll-like receptor-3 signalling. *Clin Exp Immunol* 147: 71-80

Leiba M, Seligsohn U, Sidi Y et al. (2004) Thrombophilic factors are not the leading cause of thrombosis in Behcet's disease. *Ann Rheum Dis* 63: 1445-9

Lew W, Chang JY, Jung JY & Bang D. (2008) Increased expression of interleukin-23 p19 mRNA in erythema nodosum-like lesions of Behçet's disease. *Br J Dermatol* 158: 505–11

Li Thi Huong D, Wechsler B, Du LT et al. (1989) Arterial manifestations of Behçet's disease. 12 cases. *Rev Med Interne* 10: 303–11

Li Thi Huong D, Wechsler B, Papo T et al. (1995) Arterial lesions in Behcet's disease. A study in 25 patients. *J Rheumatol* 22: 2103-13

Lim SH, Hulsey M & Esler WV. (2009) Resolution of Behcet's disease after non-myeloablative allogeneic stem cell transplant for acute myeloid leukaemia. *Rheumatology (Oxford)* 48: 88-9

Lu Y, Ye P, Chen SL, Tan EM & Chan EK. (2005) Identification of kinectin as a novel Behcet's disease autoantigen. *Arthritis Res Ther* 7: R1133-9

Mader R, Ziv M, Adawi M, Mader R & Lavi I. (1999) Thrombophilic factors and their relation to thromboembolic and other clinical manifestations in Behcet's disease. *J Rheumatol* 26: 2404-8

Mahesh SP, Li Z, Buggage R et al. (2005) Alpha-tropomyosin as a self-antigen in patients with Behcet's disease. *Clin Exp Rheumatol* 140: 368-75

Mantas C, Direskeneli H, Eksioglu-Demiralp E & Akoglu T. (1999) Serum levels of Th2 cytokines IL-4 and IL-10 in Behcet's disease. *J Rheumatol* 26: 510-2

Mat C, Yurdakul S, Ozyazgan Y, Uysal S, Uysal O & YazBcB H. (2006) A double-blind trial of depot corticosteroids in Behçet's syndrome. *Rheumatology (Oxford)* 45: 348–52

Mege JL, Dilsen N, Sanguedolce V et al. (1993) Overproduction of monocyte derived tumor necrosis factor alpha, interleukin (IL)-6, IL-8 and increased neutrophil superoxide generation in Behcet's disease. A comparative study with familial Mediterranean fever and healthy subjects. *J Rheumatol* 20: 1544-9

Melikoglu M, Fresko I, Mat C et al. (2005) Short-term trial of etanercept in Behcet's disease: a double blind, placebo controlled study. *J Rheumatol* 32: 98-105

Melikoglu M, Kural-Seyahi E, Tascilar K & Yazici H. (2008) The unique features of vasculitis in Behcet's syndrome. *Clin Rev All Immunol* 35: 40-6

Mendoza-Pinto C, Garcia-Carrasco M, Jimenez-Hernandez M et al. (2010) Etiopathogenesis of Behcet's disease. *Autoimmun Rev* 9: 241-5

Mesquita D, Cruvinel WM, Camara NOS, Kallas EG & Andrade LEC. (2009) Autoimmune diseases in the Th17 era. *Braz J Med Biol Res* 42: 47-86

Michelson JB, Chisari FV & Kansu T. (1985) Antibodies to oral mucosa in patients with ocular Behcet's disease. *Ophthalmology* 92: 1277-81

Mor F, Weinberger A & Cohen IR. (2002) Identification of alpha-tropomyosin as a target self-antigen in Behcet's syndrome. *Eur J Immunol* 32: 356-65

Mucida D & Cheroutre H. (2010) The many face-lifts of CD4 T helper cells. *Adv Immunol* 107: 139-52

Mumcu G, Inanc N, Yavuz S & Direskeneli H. (2007) The role of infectious agents in the pathogenesis, clinical manifestations and treatment strategies in Behcet's disease. *Clin Exp Rheumatol* 25(suppl 45): S27-33

Musabak U, Baylan O, Cetin T et al. (2005) Lipid profile and anticardiolipin antibodies in Behcet's disease. *Arch Med Res* 36: 387-92

Nanke Y, Kotake S, Goto M, Ujihara H, Matsubara M & Kamatani N. (2008) Decreased percentages of regulatory T cells in peripheral blood of patients with Behcet's disease before ocular attack: a possible predictive marker of ocular attack. *Mod Rheumatol* 18: 354-8

Nara K, Kurokawa MS, Chiba S et al. (2008) Involvement of innate immunity in the pathogenesis of intestinal Behcet's disease. *Clin Exp Immunol* 152: 245-51

Nazarro P. (1966) Cutaneous manifestations of Behçet's disease. Clinical and histopathological findings. In: Monacelli M, Nazzaro P. International symposium on Behçet's disease. Rome. Karger, Basel. pp 15–41

Neves FS, Carrasco S, Goldenstein-Schainberg C, Concalves CR & De Mello SB. (2009) Neutrophil hyperchemotaxis in Behcet's disease: a possible role for monocytes orchestrating bacterial-induced innate immune responses. *Clin Rheumatol* 28: 1403-10

Okunuki Y, Usui Y, Takeuchi M et al. (2007) Proteomic surveillance of autoimmunity in Behcet's disease with uveitis: selenium-binding protein is a novel autoantigen in Behcet's disease. *Exp Eye Res* 84: 823-31

Okunuki Y, Usui Y, Kezuka T et al. (2008) Proteomic surveillance of retinal auto-antigens in endogenous uveitis: implication of esterase-D and brain type creatine kinase as novel autoantigens. *Mol Vis* 14: 1094-1104

Onder M, Bozkurt M, Gurer MA, Gulekon A, Sezgin P && Imir T. (1994) Natural cellular cytotoxicity in Behcet's disease. *J Dermatol* 21: 239-43

Ozdemir M, Balevi S, Deniz F & Mevlitoglu I. (2007) Pathergy reaction in different body areas in Behcet's disease. *Clin Exp Dermatol* 32: 85-7

Ozturk MA, Ertenli I, Kiraz S et al. (2004) Plasminogen activator inhibitor-1 as a link between pathological fibrinolysis and arthritis of Behcet's disease. *Rheumatol Int* 24: 98-102

Ozyazgan Y, Yurdakul S & Yazici H. (1992) Low dose cyclosporin A versus pulsed cyclophosphamide in Behcet's syndrome: a single masked trial. *Br J Ophthalmol* 76: 241-3

Pay S, Simsek I, Erdern H et al. (2007) Dendritic cell subsets and type I interferon system in Behcet's disease: does functional abnormality in plasmacytoid dendritic cells contribute to Th1 polarization? *Clin Exp Rheumatol* 25(suppl 45): S34-40

Pay S, Abbasov T, Erdem H et al. (2007) Serum MMP-2 and MMP-9 in patients with Behcet's disease: do their higher levels correlate to vasculo-Behcet's disease associated with aneurysm formation? *Clin Exp Rheumatol* 25(Suppl 45): S70-5

Poulter LW & Lehner T. (1989) Immunohistology of oral lesions from patients with recurrent oral ulcers and Behcet's syndrome. *Clin Exp Immunol* 78: 189-95

Probst K, Fijnheer R & Rothova A. (2004) Endothelial cell activation and hypercoagulability in ocular Behcet's disease. *Am J Ophthalmol* 137: 850-7

Ramos-Casals M, Brito-Zeron P, Munoz S & Soto MJ. (2008) A systematic review of the off-label use of biological therapies in systemic autoimmune diseases. *Medicine (Baltimore)* 87: 345-64

Rhen T & Cidlowski JA. (2005) Antiinflammatory action of glucocorticoids--new mechanisms for old drugs. *N Engl J Med* 353: 1711-23

Saito T, Honma T & Saigo K. (1980) Epidermal Langerhans cells after the prick test for Behcet's disease. *Dermatologica* 161: 152-6

Sakaguchi S, Sakaguchi N, Asano M, Itoh M & Toda M. (1995) Immunologic self-tolerance maintained by activated T cells expressing IL-2 receptor alpha-chains (CD25). Breakdown of a single mechanism of self-tolerance causes various autoimmune diseases. *J Immunol* 155: 1151-64

Sakane T, Kotani H, Takada S & Tsunematsu T. (1982) Functional aberration of T cell subsets in patients with Behcet's disease. *Arthritis Rheum* 25: 1343-51

Sarica-Kucukoglu R, Akdag-Kose A, Kayabali M et al. (2006) Vascular involvement in Behçet's disease: a retrospective analysis of 2319 cases. *Int J Dermatol* 45: 919–21

Saruhan-Direskeneli G, Yentur SP, Akman-Demir G, Isik N & Serdaroglu P. (2003) Cytokines and chemokines in neuro-Behcet's disease compared to multiple sclerosis and other neurological diseases. *J Neuroimmunol* 145: 127–34

Seider N, Beiran I, Scharf J & Miller B. (2001) Intravenous immunoglobulin therapy for resistant ocular Behcet's disease. *Br J Ophthalmol* 85: 1287-8

Sfikakis PP, Theodossiadis PG, Katsiari CG, Kaklamanis P & Markomichelakis NN. (2001) Effect of infliximab on sight-threatening panuveitis in Behçet's disease. *Lancet* 358: 295–6

Sfikakis PP, Kaklamanis PH, Elezoglou A et al. (2004) Infliximab for recurrent, sight-threatening ocular inflammation in Adamantiades–Behçet disease. *Ann Intern Med* 140: 404–6

Sharaf PH & Yazici Y. (2009) Necrotizing vasculitis--a 2009 update. *Bull NYU Hosp Jt Dis* 67: 303-5

Souza RC, Lage L, Goldenstein-Schainberg C, Macedo AR, Carrasco S & Concalves CR. (2007) Anti-endothelial cell antibodies and central nervous system involvement in Behcet's disease. *Clinics (Sao Paulo)* 62: 685-90

Sugi-Ikai N, Nakazawa M, Nakamura S, Ohno S & Minami M. (1998) Increased frequencies of interleukin-2 and interferon-gamma-producing T cells in patients with active Behcet's disease. *Invest Ophthalmol Vis Sci* 39: 996-1004

Sugita S, Yamada Y, Kaneko S, Horie S & Mochizuki M. (2011) Induction of regulatory T cells by infliximab in Behcet's disease. *Invest Ophthalmol Vis Sci* 52: 476-84

Suh CH, Park YB, Song J, Lee CH & Lee SK. (2001) Oligoclonal B lymphocyte expansion in the synovium of a patient with Behcet's disease. *Arthritis Rheum* 44: 1707-12

Suzuki Y, Hoshi K, Matsuda T & Mizushima Y. (1992) Increased peripheral blood gammadelta+ T cells and natural killer cells in Behcet's disease. *J Rheumatol* 19: 588-92

Theofilopoulos AN, Baccala R, Beutler B & Kono DH. (2005) Type I interferons (alpha/beta) in immunity and autoimmunity. *Annu Rev Immunol* 23: 307-36

Treusch M, Vonthein R, Baur M et al. (2004) Influence of human recombinant interferon-alpha-2a on altered lymphocyte subpopulations and monocytes in Behcet's disease. *Rheumatology (Oxford)* 43: 1275-82

Tugal-Tutkun I, Güney-Tefekli E & Urgancioglu M. (2006) Results of interferon-alpha therapy in patients with Behçet uveitis. *Graefes Arch Clin Exp Ophthalmol* 244: 1692-5

Tuzun H, Besirli K, Sayin A et al. (1997) Management of aneurysms in Behçet's syndrome: an analysis of 24 patients. *Surgery* 121: 150–6

Verjans GM, van Hagen PM, van der Kooi A, Osterhaus AD & Baarsma GS. (2002) Vgamma9Vdelta2 T cells recovered from eyes of patients with Behcet's disease recognize non-peptide prenyl pyrophosphate antigens. *J Neuroimmunol* 130: 46-54

Victorino RM, Ryan P, Hughes GR & Hodgson HJ. (1982) Cell-mediated immune functions and immunoregulatory cells in Behcet's syndrome. *Clin Exp Immunol* 48: 121-8

Waldman TA. (2004) Targeting the interleukin-15/interleukin-15 receptor system in inflammatory autoimmune diseases. *Arthritis Res Ther* 6: 174-7

Weintraub NL. (2009) Understanding abdominal aortic aneurysm. *N Engl J Med* 361: 1114-6

Weyand CM & Goronzy JJ. (2003) Medium- and large-vessel vasculitis. *N Engl J Med* 349: 160-9

Yamaguchi Y, Takahashi H, Satoh T et al. (2010) Natural killer cells control a T-helper 1 response in patients with Behcet's disease. *Arthritis Res Ther* 12: R80

Yamashita N, Kaneoka H, Kaneko S et al. (1997) Role of gammadelta T lymphocytes in the development of Behcet's disease. *Clin Exp Immunol* 107: 241-7

Yanagihori H ,Oyama N, Nakamura K, Mizuki N, Oguma K & Kaneko F. (2006) Role of IL-12B promoter polymorphism in Adamantiades-Behcet's disease susceptibility: an involvement of Th1 immunoreactivity against Streptococcus sanguinis antigen. *J Invest Dermatol* 126: 1534-40

Yasuoka H, Yamaguchi Y, Mizuki N, Nishida T, Kawakami Y & Kuwana M. (2008) Preferential activation of circulating CD8+ and gammadelta T cells in patients with active Behcet's disease and HLA-B51. *Clin Exp Rheumatol* 26(suppl 50): S59-63

Yato H & Matsumoto Y. (1999) CD56+ T cells in the peripheral blood of uveitis patients. *Br J Ophthalmol* 83: 1386-8

Yavuz S, Elbir Y, Tulunay A, Eksioglu-Demiralp E & Direskeneli H. (2008) Differential expression of Toll-like receptor-6 on granulocytes and monocytes implicates the role of micro-organisms in Behcet's disease etiopathogenesis. *Rheumatol Int* 28: 401-6

Yazici C, Kose K, Calis M, Demir M, Kirnap M & Ates F. (2004) Increased advanced oxidation protein products in Behcet's disease: a new activity marker? *Br J Dermatol* 151: 105-11

Yazici H, Pazarli H, Barnes CG et al. (1990) A controlled trial of azathioprine in Behcet's syndrome. *N Engl J Med* 322: 281-5

Yazici H, Yurdakul S & Hamuryudan V. (1999) Behcet's syndrome. *Curr Opin Rheumatol* 11: 53-7

Yazici Y, Yurdakul S & Yazici H. (2010) Behçet's syndrome. *Curr Rheumatol Rep* 12: 429-35

Yu HG, Lee DS, Seo JM et al. (2004) The number of CD8+ T cells and NKT cells increases in the aqueous humor of patients with Behcet's uveitis. *Clin Exp Immunol* 137: 437-43

Zeng XJ, Zhu WG, Deng XX, Tang FL & Dong Y. (2004) Anti-endothelial cell antibodies in systemic vasculitis: detection and correlation with disease activity. *Zhongua Yi Xue Za Zhi* 84: 1629-32

Zouboulis CC, Katsantonis J, Ketteler R et al. (2000) Adamantiades-Behcet's disease: interleukin-8 is increased in serum of patients with active oral and neurological manifestations and is secreted by small vessel endothelial cells. *Arch Dermatol Res* 292: 279-84

Zouboulis CC & May T. (2003) Pathogenesis of Adamantiades-Behcet's disease. *Med Microbiol Immunol* 192: 149-55

10

Bypass for the Treatment of Vasculitis Affecting the Central Nervous System

Ana Rodríguez-Hernández[1],
S. Andrew Josephson[2] and Michael T. Lawton[1]
[1]*Department of Neurological Surgery. University of California, San Francisco*
[2]*Department of Neurology. University of California, San Francisco*
USA

1. Introduction

Vasculitis affecting the central nervous system (CNS) comprises a large group of diseases characterized by inflammation of arteries that narrows the arterial lumen, compromises cerebral blood flow, and causes a variety of ischemic symptoms. These diseases share similar pathology, but differ in their ages of onset and involved arteries (Begelman & Olin, 2000; Sheikhzadeh et al., 2002; Weyand & Goronzy, 2003). Large-vessel vasculitides are characterized by inflammation of the aorta and the carotid arteries. Giant-cell arteritis, for example, affects patients older than 50 years, while Takayasu's arteritis affects women in their second and third decades of life. With giant-cell arteritis, incidences range from 15 to 25 cases per 100,000 with a predilection for people of northern European descent; Takayasu's arteritis is most commonly seen in Japan, Southeast Asia, India, and Mexico and has an annual incidence in North America of 2.6 per million people. Large-vessel vasculitides in the pediatric population are rare (Gardner-Medwin et al., 2002). Nevertheless, most childhood vasculitides, such as Henoch-Schonlein purpura, Kawasaki disease, polyarteritis nodosa, Wegener granulomatosis, and Behcet disease, are medium- and small-vessel syndromes that often present pathognomonically and rarely, if ever, lead to aortitis or large-vessel obliterative arteriopathy.

Management of vasculitis is almost always medical and individualized to the presenting symptoms, involving a combination of corticosteroids, cytotoxic immunosuppressive agents (intended to decrease inflammation and prevent arterial occlusion) and antibiotics in infectious causes. In the later stages of these diseases, cerebral ischemia may result from chronic scarring or occlusion of arteries rather than acute inflammation. Therefore, revascularization is sometimes necessary to prevent cerebral ischemia and infarction, and bypass surgery has an important role in the treatment of selected cases of vasculitis outside of the acute inflammatory phase.

The aforementioned variable pattern of involvement of different vasculitides can affect conventional donor and recipient sites for common extracranial-intracranial bypasses. Consequently, bypasses for vasculitis often require unusual and complex reconstructions that are not part of the standard bypass repertoire. In this chapter, we review the special techniques and nuances of bypass for vasculitis patients and we demonstrate our experience with case examples.

2. Ilustrative cases

Case 1

A previously healthy 10-month old boy presented with sudden right-sided hemiparesis. Magnetic resonance imaging (MRI) and magnetic resonance angiography (MRA) demonstrated acute ischemia in the left middle cerebral artery territory. Cerebral angiography demonstrated severe obliterative arteriopathy of the great vessels with complete occlusion of all vessels originating from the aortic arch and reconstitution of the cerebral perfusion through unique collateralization patterns. The cerebral vasculature appeared to be structurally unaffected by the underlying vascular pathology.

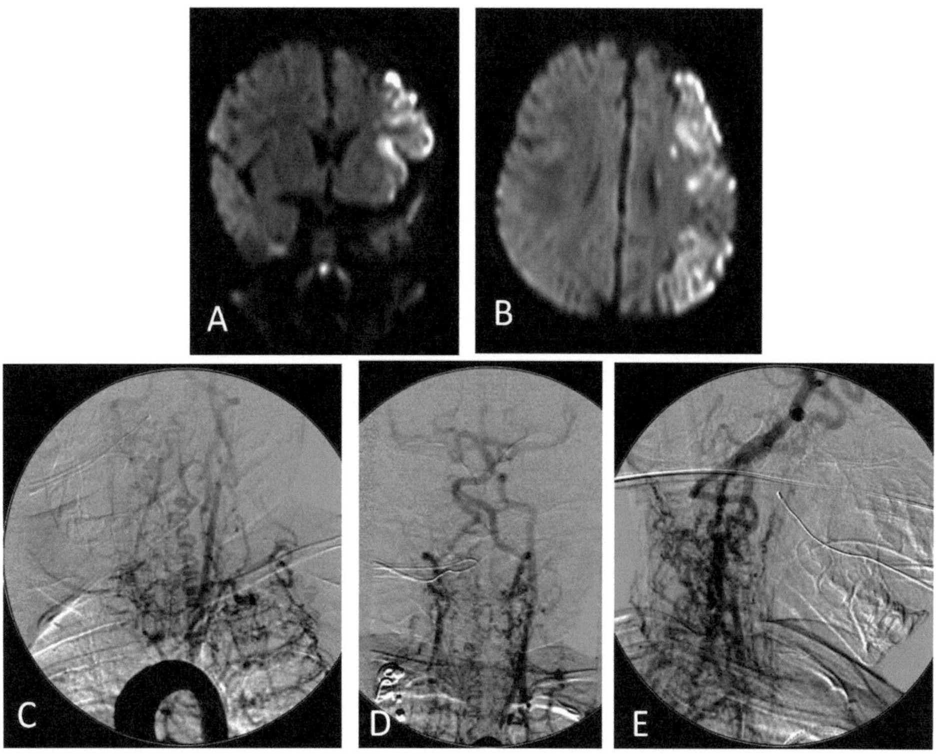

Fig. 1. Magnetic resonance imaging demonstrated acute ischemia in the left MCA territory (diffusion-weighted images, (A) coronal and (B) axial views). (C) Catheter angiography (aortic injection, anteroposterior view) revealed severe obliterative arteriopathy of the great vessels originating from the aortic arch. Cerebral blood flow was reconstituted by collaterals from the anterior spinal artery to the vertebral arteries, and from intercostal and cervical arteries to the left CCA. Delayed phase of the angiogram showed late filling of the left ICA and vertobasilar circulation (aortic injection, (D) anteroposterior and (E) lateral views)

The patient's hemiparesis improved with hypervolemic therapy and pressor agents, but his deficits returned when these pressor agents were weaned. Despite reconstitution of blood flow in his left carotid system by his native cervical collateral vessels, his left hemisphere remained the symptomatic side. After several unsuccessful attempts to wean him from hypertensive therapy, a revascularization procedure was planned to address his hemispheric hypoperfusion and inadequate collateral blood flow.

Microsurgical Technique

An aortocarotid bypass from the aortic arch to the common carotid artery was determined to be the shortest and best method of augmenting blood flow to the ischemic left hemisphere. An oblique incision along the medial border of the left sternomastoid muscle was made just above the clavicle and the proximal left common carotid artery was exposed, revealing an indurated and completely obstructed artery. The aortic arch was then exposed through a median sternotomy. The aortic arch appeared normal, but the common carotid artery was also indurated and completely obstructed. The origin of the common carotid artery was occluded with a Weck clip and transected from the arch. There was no retrograde flow from the CCA, and a longitudinal incision was made along the carotid until a lumen with back bleeding was encountered. The lumen was probed with a 4-mm dilator and back-bleeding became more brisk. The end of the CCA was cleaned and prepared for the distal anastomosis.

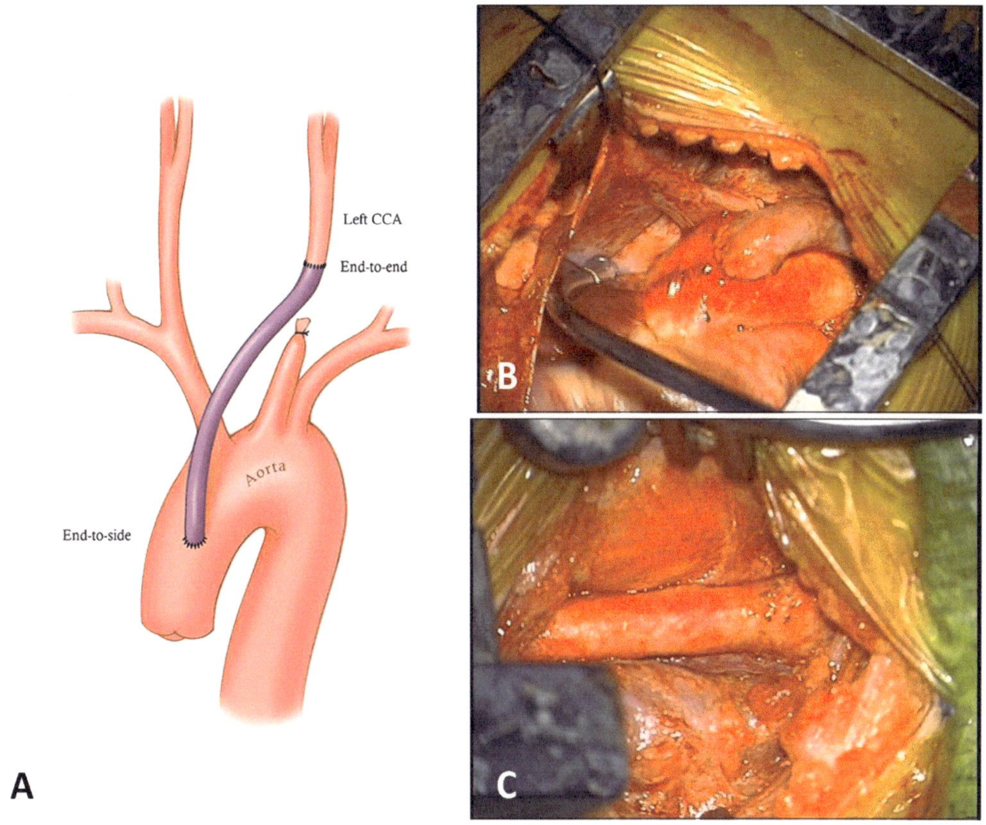

Fig. 2. (A) Illustration showing the aortocarotid bypass from the aortic arch to the proximal left CCA, using a cryopreserved saphenous vein allograft. (B) The aortic arch was exposed through a median sternotomy and a proximal end-to-side anastomosis was performed using a side-biting clamp on the aorta. (C) The graft was tunneled to a cervical incision and an end-to-end anastomosis to the CCA completed the bypass, with strong pulsations in the carotid bifurcation.

The boy's saphenous vein was considered for the bypass, but the caliber was too small and instead, a 5-mm diameter, cryopreserved, allograft saphenous vein was selected (CryoLife, Kennesaw, GA). The ends of the vein graft and the common carotid artery were beveled and anastomosed end-to-end. The vein graft was then tunneled to the mediastinum and trimmed to reach the aorta. A side-biting clamp was placed on the aortic arch, obviating the need for cardiopulmonary bypass. A small incision was made in the aorta and the proximal end of vein graft was sewn to the aorta in an end-to-side fashion. After completing the anastomosis, the side-clamp was removed and flow was established in the bypass with good pulsation in the vein graft and in the downstream carotid artery. Heparin (1mg/kg) was used during the procedure and was not reversed.

Clinical Course

Postoperatively, the patient continued to improve and his hemiparesis resolved completely. His pressor agents were weaned and he remained neurologically intact, independent of his blood pressure. An angiogram demonstrated the widely-patent interpositional vein graft between the aortic arch and left common carotid artery. Furthermore, the arterial vessels of the cerebral vasculature appeared well-perfused via the left internal carotid artery.
At last clinical follow-up 12 months after presentation, the bypass remained patent based on carotid ultrasound examination, and the patient demonstrated no new neurological symptoms. He was advancing steadily with his developmental milestones and his language function was normal.

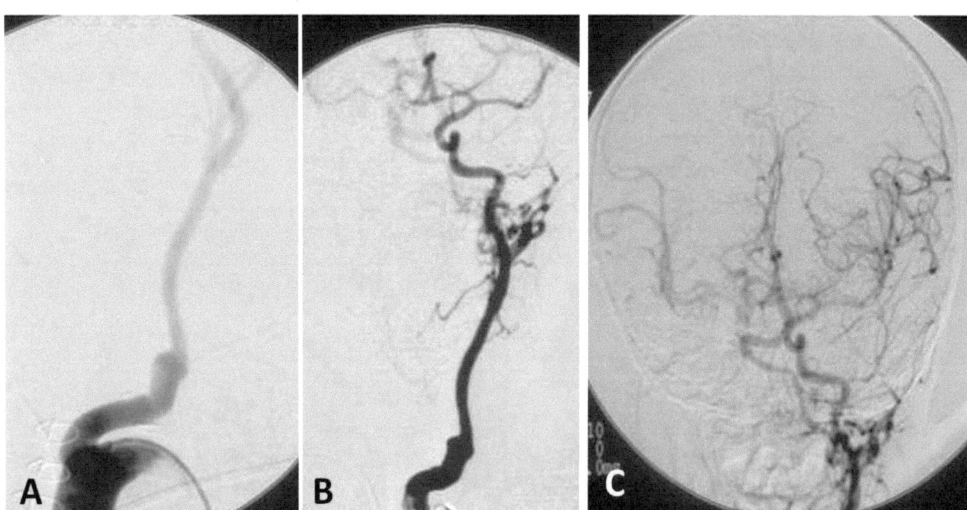

Fig. 3. Postoperative catheter angiography demonstrated a patent aortocarotid bypass ((A) aortic injection, anteroposterior view) and improved cerebral perfusion through the left ICA ((B) graft injection, anteroposterior view). (C) Delayed phase of the angiogram showed filling of the right carotid circulation via anterior communicating artery and the basilar circulation via the posterior communicating artery.

Case 2

A 48 year-old female with a history of Takayasu's arteritis presented to the ER with a sudden, severe headache. CT scan demonstrated subarachnoid hemorrhage. Cerebral angiography revealed a fusiform aneurysm at the basilar apex. Both common carotid arteries and her right vertebral artery were occluded. Her entire cerebral circulation was supplied by the left vertebral artery. Since microsurgical clipping of the aneurysm would likely require some temporary occlusion of the basilar artery, a revascularization procedure was planned.

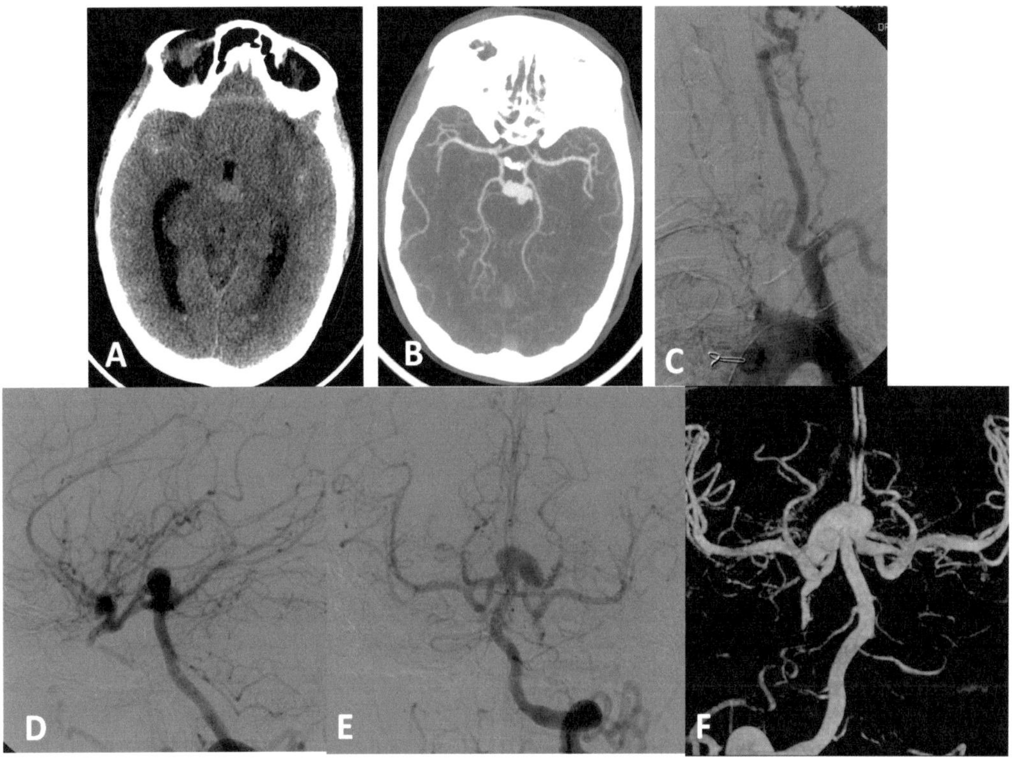

Fig. 4. (A) A brain CT scan revealed subarachnoid hemorrhage and (B) CT angiography revealed a fusiform basilar tip aneurysm. (C) Angiography showed that her innominate artery and left common carotid artery were occluded from her prior disease and surgery (aortic arch injection, anteroposterior view), and only her right vertebral artery was supplying her cerebral circulation. Two large posterior communicating arteries were collateralizing the anterior circulation (D, vertebral artery injection, lateral and (E) anteroposterior views). (F) Angiography with 3D reconstruction depicted the fusiform aneurysm at the basilar apex.

Microsurgical technique

A subclavian-middle cerebral artery bypass was thought to be the most suitable revascularization option. A saphenous vein graft was harvested from the thigh and down into the midcalf using endoscopic technique. The subclavian donor site was prepared by reopening a prior surgical incision from previous aorto-subclavian bypass that had occluded. After trimmed appropriately, the vein graft was first anastomosed to the recipient M2 branch. It was tunneled underneath the inferior edge of the craniotomy incision down to the previously prepared subclavian site, cut to the appropriate size, and sewn in and end-to-side fashion to the subclavian artery.

Having placed the bypass, a temporary clip on the basilar trunk softened the aneurysm which allowed complete dissection of the neck and its definitive clipping occluding the rupture site. A fusiform segment of the basilar artery apex was also reinforced with cotton wrapping.

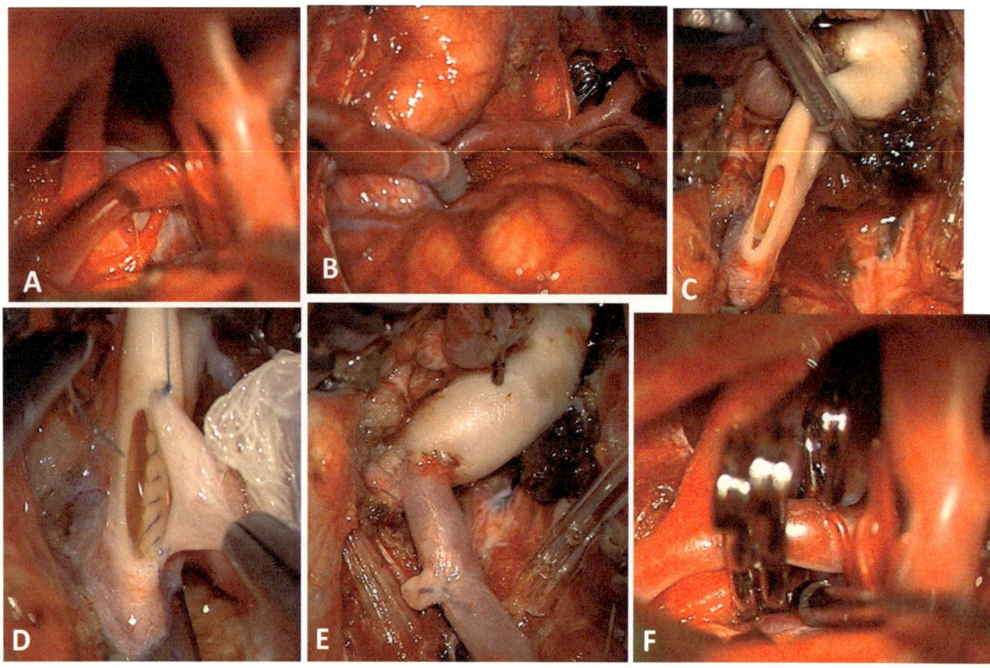

Fig. 5. (A) A left orbitozygomatic approach exposed the basilar apex aneurysm and the need for temporary occlusion was confirmed. (B). A shapenous vein graft was harvested and anastomosed first to the recipient M2 branch. (C) The subclavian artery was exposed through a supraclavicular incision and an arteriotomy was made with an aortic punch. (D,E) The tunneled graft was anastomosed with running 9-0 sutures end-to-side. (F) With the bypass in place, a temporary clip on the basilar trunk softened the aneurysm and allowed complete dissection of the neck. The aneurysm was clipped with fenestrated clips transmitting the PCA and its perforators.

Clinical course

Postoperatively, the patient developed a pulmonary embolism which required the placement of a vena cava filter. However, she recovered well and was discharged home after a 2 week hospitalization without any neurological symptom. At last follow-up 4 years after the procedure, the patient remained neurologically asymptomatic and an angiogram demonstrated the patent vein graft between the left subclavian and left middle cerebral artery.

Case 3

A 43-year-old woman presented with right sided neglect and expressive aphasia due to left parietal stroke. An angiogram showed an occluded left internal carotid artery with compromised blood flow to the left hemisphere. The right internal carotid artery had a high-grade stenosis in the proximal half of the cervical segment, but restored caliber in the distal cervical segment and normal blood flow to the right hemisphere. These findings suggested large vessel vasculitis and a revascularization procedure was planned with a STA-MCA bypass.

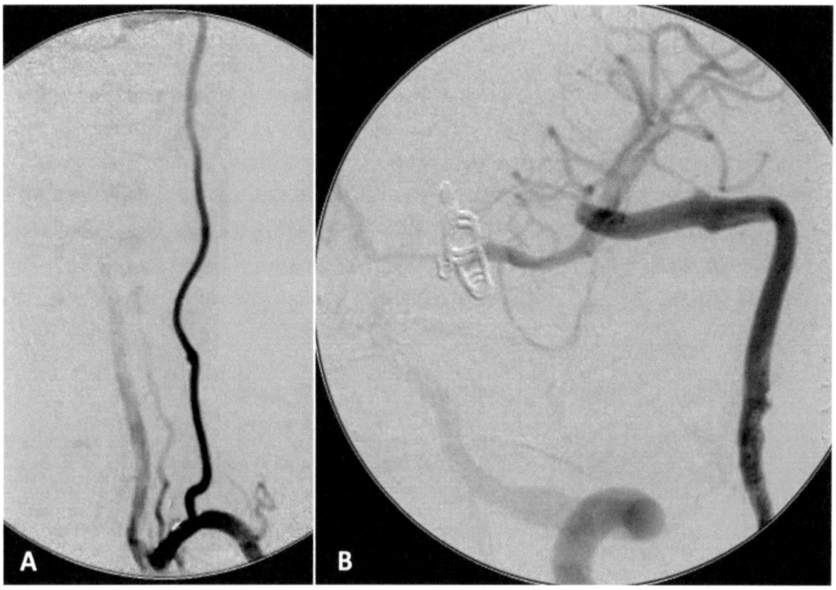

Fig. 6. Postoperative angiogram showed a patent subclavian-MCA bypass ((A) left subclavian injection, anteroposterior cervical view) with good filling of the left MCA territory distally ((B) left subclavian injection, anteroposterior cranial view).

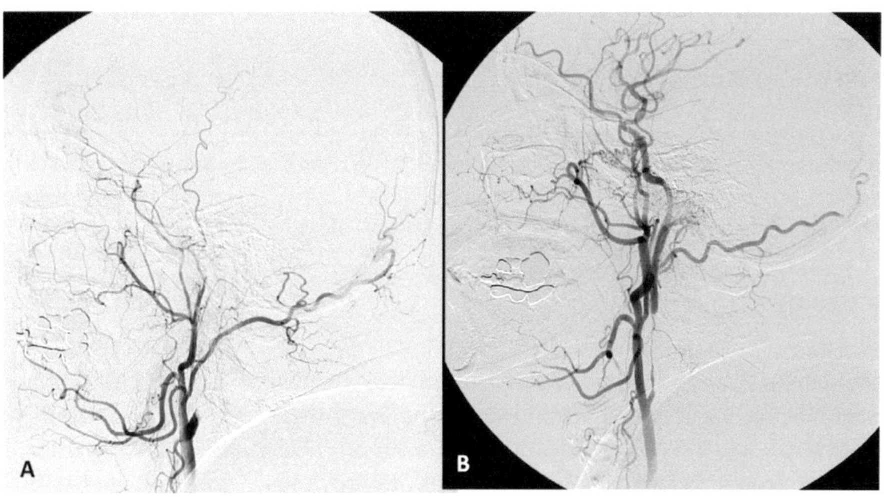

Fig. 7. (A) Angiography showed a completely occluded left internal carotid artery (left common carotid artery injection, anteroposterior view) and (B) a high grade stenosis in the cervical segment of the right internal carotid artery (right common carotid artery injection, anteroposterior view.

Microsurgical technique

The left temporal artery was harvested from the zygoma all the way up to the superior temporal line. A small fronto-temporal craniotomy was then performed and the possible recipient arteries on the cortical surface were exposed. As previously noticed on the angiogram and most likely related to the patient vasculitis, all the cortical vessels had a smaller caliber than usually observed. An adequate recipient branch was dissected and the temporal artery was swung to it in and end-to- side fashion. An ICG videoangiography confirmed the patency of this technically demanding anastomosis.

Clinical course

Postoperatively, a control angiogram demonstrated patency of the left STA-MCA bypass. The patient´s vasculitis was diagnosed as Takayasu´s arteritis. She was discharged home with no neurological deficits.

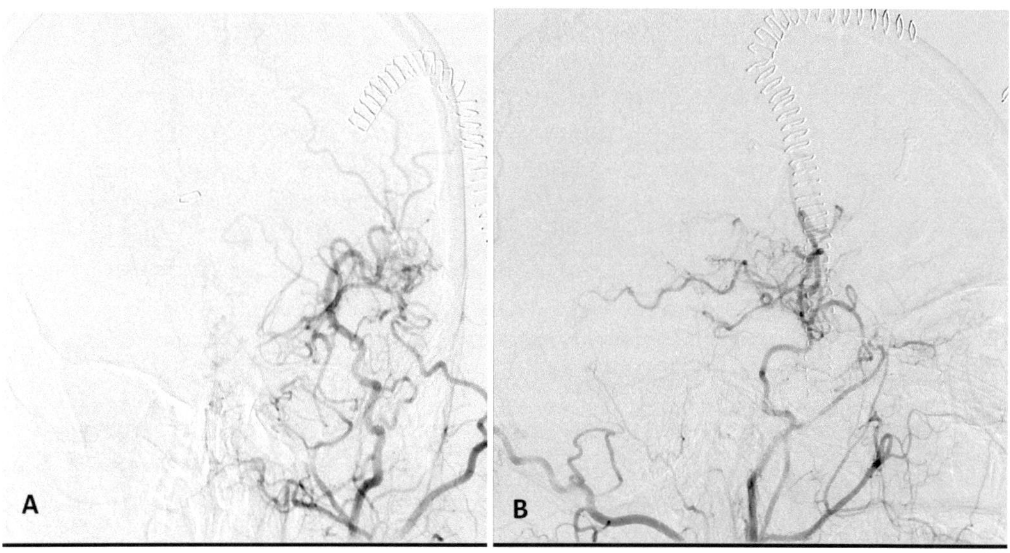

Fig. 8. Postoperative angiogram showed a patent left STA-MCA bypass with good filling of the left MCA territory distally (A) Left common carotid artery injection, anteroposterior view. (B) Left common carotid artery injection, lateral view.

3. Discussion

3.1 Indications for bypass

The treatment of vasculitis in the acute phases begins with medical therapy with corticosteroids and/or cytotoxic immunosuppressants, the specific medication depending on the type of vasculitis. The indications for brain revascularization in vasculitis are symptomatic cerebral ischemia despite medical therapy, caused by significant reduction in blood flow that is not compensated by collateral circulation.

Catheter angiography helps defining a patient's underlying vasculopathy, but also his or her compensatory collateral circulation. An intact circle of Willis can compensate for a carotid occlusion with cross-filling from the contralateral ICA through the anterior communicating artery (ACoA) and from the vertebrobasilar circulation through the posterior communicating artery (PCoA). Retrograde flow in the ophthalmic artery can provide collateral circulation from the external carotid artery (ECA). Leptomeningeal collaterals can be recruited over the cerebral convexity connecting PCA and MCA territories as well as ACA and MCA territories. Other less common sources of collateral circulation include: anterior, middle, and posterior meningeal arteries in the dura mater connecting to cortical arteries; ACA-PCA connections through a "limbic loop;" extracranial connections between ECA or vertebral artery branches and the distal ICA; and anterior spinal artery collateralizing the vertebrobasilar circulation. Well developed collateral circulation can compensate for severe occlusive vasculitis, whereas the absence of collateral circulation may indicate surgical bypass (Hofmeijer et al, 2002; Yamauchi et al, 2004).

In addition to the diagnosis of an underlying vasculopathy and the evaluation of the collateral circulation, confirming the presence of ischemic tissue that is at risk for stroke, but still salvageable, is another important criterion for bypass surgery. A large evolving or completed stroke on CT scans or MR imaging contraindicates bypass surgery because this brain tissue is not salvageable and revascularization could precipitate hemorrhagic conversion of an acute infarction. Bypass candidates have small or no strokes and significant areas of ischemia that can be rescued by revascularization. The ability to identify mismatches between blood supply and brain demand helps facilitate patient selection and increases the likelihood of a benefit to those who undergo bypass surgery. Perfusion CT (PCT) imaging is a simple, quick, and accessible technique that provides physiological, qualitative information about those mismatches called the ischemic penumbra (Hemphill et al., 2005; Kamath et al, 2008). PCT imaging uses a bolus injection of iodinated contrast and spiral CT imaging during the passage of the contrast bolus through the brain. Perfusion maps show parameters including: time to peak (TTP, the time between the first arrival of contrast intracranially and its peak concentration), mean transit time (MTT, the average time for blood to travel through a volume of brain), cerebral blood flow (CBF), and cerebral blood volume (CBV). In acute stroke, ischemic penumbra has increased TTP and MTT, relatively normal CBV due to vasodilation and recruitment of collateral flow, and decreased CBF. In contrast, infarcted brain has increased TTP and MTT, but CBV and CBF are both decreased. The identification of ischemic but salvageable penumbra encourages stroke intervention. Measuring salvageable tissue via PET is a more quantitative method that is more difficult to obtain due to limited availability.

Our current algorithm for surgical selection identifies patients with symptomatic lesions refractory to medical management, no significant infarction in the involved vascular territories, and poor collateral circulation on angiography. PCT imaging then identifies hemodynamic insufficiency as increased MTT, typically with near normal CBV and decreased CBF.

3.2 Surgical technique

Selecting the appropriate donor and recipient vessels can be challenging due to the distribution of disease, the lack of normal anatomy, and the lack in some cases of an autologous graft that is available or unaffected by the disease. For example, traditional donor arteries like the STA may be involved with the pathology and therefore, alternative bypasses are needed.

STA-MCA bypass

STA-MCA bypass is by far the most common bypass for any stroke patient, whatever the etiology. The patient is positioned supine and with the head turned 90 degrees to align the lateral convexity parallel to the floor. The course of the STA is mapped with a Doppler flow probe and the posterior limb is usually selected. The anterior limb is used only when the posterior limb is too small. The microscope is used to dissect the STA from zygoma to the superior temporal line. The artery is left in continuity and vasodilated with papaverine extraluminally. Temporalis muscle is divided under the STA and mobilized to each side. Alternatively, temporalis can be flapped anteriorly to expose directly over or in the Sylvian fissure for a larger recipient artery. A small craniotomy is made by working under the STA and staying below the superior temporal line. Dura is opened in flap that preserves middle meningeal arteries if they have developed collateral circulation.

MCA vessels exiting the Sylvian fissure are inspected under the microscope and a recipient artery is selected with suitable size and accessibility. The STA is transected, stripped of its adventitia, cut at a 60 degree angle, and spatulated with an axial incision in the arterial wall. After the patient is placed into propofol-induced EEG burst suppression, the recipient artery is trapped between temporary clips, arteriotomized, and flushed with heparinized saline. Two 10-0 sutures are placed on either end of the arteriotomy to approximate the STA and MCA. Running continuous sutures are placed from one end of the arteriotomy to the other, then tightened and tied. The opposite wall is sutured similarly. The temporary clips are removed and hemostasis is achieved with fibrillar Nu-Knit packing. Indocyanine green videoangiography confirms the patency of the bypass.

The closure must avoid compromising flow in the bypass. The dural closure should not constrict the STA is it passes through. A small passageway for the STA is rongeured from the bone flap. Temporalis muscle is closed loosely around the graft, and galea sutures and skin staples are placed carefully to avoid pinching the graft.

High-flow bypasses

Vasculitis patients have variable and multifocal disease. Traditional donor arteries like the STA may be involved with the pathology and, therefore, alternative bypasses are needed. Bypasses with interposition grafts like saphenous vein or radial artery have higher flow than traditional EC-IC bypasses.

The cervical carotid artery is an accessible donor artery, with anastomotic sites on the ICA, ECA, and common carotid artery (CCA). The ICA is used when a patent stump is available and collateral circulation from the ECA must be preserved. ECA is used when the cerebral circulation is critically dependent on ICA flow and temporary ICA or CCA occlusion during the anastomosis would be poorly tolerated. CCA is used when the carotid bifurcation is high-riding and exposure is compromised by the mandible (Auguste et al., 2001; Sanai et al., 2008). High-flow bypasses connect the ICA, ECA, or CCA with the MCA, typically along the M2 segment distal to the lenticulostriate arteries originating from the M1 segment.

A similar bypass can be constructed for high-flow bypasses to the posterior circulation. The PCA is preferred over SCA because its caliber matches that of the bypass graft. A shorter bypass alternative is the MCA-PCA bypass, which uses the MCA as the donor site rather than the cervical carotid artery. This bypass is entirely intracranial (IC-IC), spares the patient a cervical incision, and requires only a short radial artery graft. Shorter grafts generally have higher long-term patency rates than longer grafts to the neck.

Vasculitis can also compromise patency of cervical carotid arteries. In these rare cases, a more proximal donor artery is needed (**see case 1**). The subclavian artery can be accessed through a supraclavicular incision and serve as a proximal donor. The distance to the recipient site is much longer than with other high-flow bypasses involving the cervical carotid artery, and therefore saphenous vein interposition grafts are typically required. The subclavian artery-to-MCA bypass can be used in these vasculitis patients and those with previous surgical carotid sacrifice for aneurysm, tumor, or other intervention.

4. Conclusion

Bypass surgery has an infrequent, but important role in the treatment of symptomatic vasculitis refractory to medical therapy causing cerebral ischemia. Vasculitis patients with symptomatic cerebral ischemia caused by significant reduction in blood flow that is not compensated by collateral circulation should be considered for revascularization procedures. However, bypass techniques can be especially challenging in these heterogeneous diseases and neurosurgeons should be aware of the technical difficulties associated with these procedures.

5. References

Auguste KI, Quiñones-Hinojosa A, Lawton MT. The tandem bypass: subclavian artery-to-middle cerebral artery bypass with dacron and saphenous vein grafts. Technical case report. *Surg Neurol*. 2001;56(3):164-169

Begelman SM, Olin JW: Nonatherosclerotic arterial disease of the extracranial cerebrovasculature. *Semin Vasc Surg* 13:153–164, 2000

Gardner-Medwin JM, Dolezalova P, Cummins C, Southwood TR: Incidence of Henoch-Schönlein purpura, Kawasaki disease, and rare vasculitides in children of different ethnic origins. *Lancet* 360:1197–1202, 2002

Hemphill JC 3rd, Smith WS, Sonne DC, Morabito D, Manley GT. Relationship between brain tissue oxygen tension and CT perfusion: feasibility and initial results. *Am J Neuroradiol*. 2005 May;26(5):1095-1100.

Hofmeijer J, Klijn CJ, Kappelle LJ, Van Huffelen AC, Van Gijn J. Collateral circulation via the ophthalmic artery or leptomeningeal vessels is associated with impaired cerebral vasoreactivity in patients with symptomatic carotid artery occlusion. *Cerebrovasc Dis*. 2002;14(1):22-26

Kamath A, Smith WS, Powers WJ, Cianfoni A, Chien JD, Videen T, Lawton MT, Finley B, Dillon WP, Wintermark M. Perfusion CT compared to H(2) (15)O/O (15)O PET in patients with chronic cervical carotid artery occlusion. *Neuroradiology*. 2008 Sep;50(9):745-751.

Sanai N, Fullerton H, Karl TR, Lawton MT. Aortocarotid bypass for hemispheric hypoperfusion in a child. *J Neurosurg Pediatr*. 2008 Apr;1(4):343-347

Sheikhzadeh A, Tettenborn I, Noohi F, Eftekharzadeh M, Schnabel A: Occlusive thromboaortopathy (Takayasu disease): clinical and angiographic features and a brief review of literature. *Angiology* 53:29–40, 2002

Weyand CM, Goronzy JJ: Medium- and large-vessel vasculitis. *N Engl J Med* 349:160–169, 2003

Yamauchi H, Kudoh T, Sugimoto K, Takahashi M, Kishibe Y, Okazawa H. Pattern of collaterals, type of infarcts, and haemodynamic impairment in carotid artery occlusion. *J Neurol Neurosurg Psychiatry*. 2004(12):1697-1701

11

Therapeutic Vascular Angiogenesis for Vasculitis Related Peripheral Artery Disease

Gen Takagi[1], Masaaki Miyamoto[1], Yasuhiko Tabata[2] and Kyoichi Mizuno[1]

[1]Nippon Medical School,
[2]Kyoto University
Japan

1. Introduction

The increasing morbidity due to peripheral artery disease (PAD) has given rise to a recent focus in cardiovascular medicine, and strategies for peripheral intervention have proliferated. For example, distal bypass, and catheter intervention for below-knee arteries have been performed aggressively. Also, there has been detailed research on the mortality of peripheral artery disease. In fact, it is reported that the mortality of PAD is higher than that of colon cancer. In a the patient with complicated PAD, even leg amputation does not prevent adverse events (Cruz, 2003; Aulivola, 2004). In this context, the discovery of other options for peripheral intervention is an impending. Also, patients may have various other diseases or a condition underlying the ischemic insult. Among these, vasculitis and collagen disease are often associated with difficult ischemic conditions. In these cases, there are limited options for treatment. Here we describe new techniques to achieve peripheral circulation including vascular angiogenesis, and explain the potential mechanism and effectiveness including that in vasculitis patients.

2. Guidelines for peripheral artery disease

Guidelines for peripheral artery disease have been published by the Trans Atlantic Inter-Society Consensus (Hirsch, 2006). In these guidelines, a treatment strategy was precisely determined. However, there is still no established evidence regarding treatment for below-knee arterial ischemia, especially for patients with critical limb ischemia (CLI), which is intractable limb ischemia due to PAD, who immediately face limb amputation. Catheter intervention and distal bypass grafting are well known to improve distal ischemia; however, however in specific conditions such as vasculitis or collagen disease, which is the focus of this chapter, the location of the occluded artery is mainly distal to the ankle or wrist which makes it difficult to treat with these strategies, and also, due to the pathogenesis of the original disease, the target vessels often become reoccluded soon after treatment.

3. Diagnosis and definition of severity

Definitive diagnosis should be made by documentation of the affected tissue. In order to make the correct diagnosis, biopsy of abnormal or symptomatic tissue is reliable. In patients with proven vasculitis, the diagnostic yield from biopsies of clinically normal sites is considerably less than 20%. In addition, when a wound is complicated by vasculitis or collagen disease, the invasive nature of by biopsy itself worsens the wound, and it is usually difficult to obtain a tissue sample unless amputation tissue is available.

In order to perform correct diagnosis and appropriate treatment, it is necessary to define the severity of ischemia using a reliable and safe method. Ankle-brachial index (ABI) is one of the useful screening methods for PAD. However, the data are inconsistent when the artery is severely calcified, which is known as Mönckeberg sclerosis (figure 1), which shows a pseudo-normalized value. Also, ABI is not a suitable method to define the amputation level. Skin perfusion pressure(SPP), obtained by digitized quantification of blood flow, is a reliable method that is also useful to define the amputation level. However, in vasculitis or collagen disease, it is difficult to apply because most patients experience excruciating pain, and cuff inflation may worsen the patient's condition. Thus, there is no clear consensus regarding an evaluation method for CLI. One of the potential less invasive approaches to analyze blood flow level is, analyze radio-isotope imaging by ^{99m}technetium-tetrofosmin (^{99m}Tc-TF) perfusion scintigraphy (Miyamoto, 2004). Furthermore, in consideration of repeatability, cost effectiveness, and minimum stimulation to the ischemic area, we propose transcutaneous oxygen tension ($TcPO_2$) as the most useful method. It requires only electrode placement on the skin surface, and is suitable to examine distal ischemia even if the ischemic region is located below the ankle. The disadvantage of $TcPO_2$ is the influence of the environment such as surrounding temperature or patient condition. In order to avoid possible error in detection, we propose that "maximum $TcPO_2$" could clarify the result, and we believe the environmental influence could be minimized by data acquisition during 100% oxygen inhalation (Tara, 2011a).

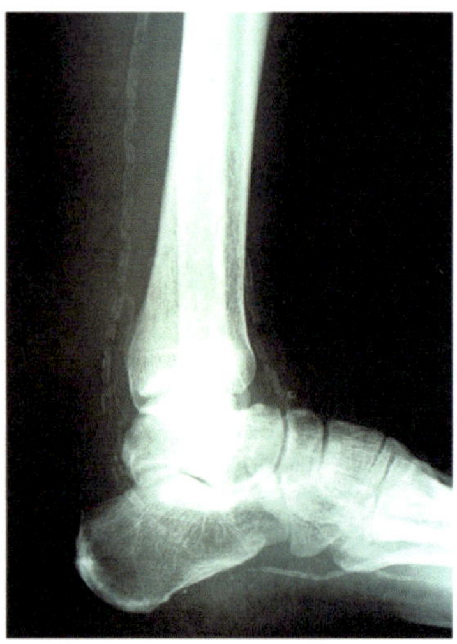

Fig. 1. X-ray of leg. Representative case of Mönckeberg sclerosis. Vascular calcification and its location are well defined without contrast medium.

4. Novel approach

Due to pathogenesis of vasculitis, such as rheumatoid arthritis or collagen disease, vascular involvement mainly occurs in distal microvessels. Furthermore, the vasculitides are defined by the presence of an inflammatory process in the vessel wall, with reactive damage to mural structures. Often direct vascular stimulation by surgical or catheter intervention of small vessels causes acute thrombosis or closure of the vessels. Also, according to the TASC guidelines, an intervention strategy has not been established for vasculitis. One of the recent topics is vascular regenerative therapy for PAD through the implantation of autologous bone marrow mononuclear cells into the ischemic area. In this context, the topic has been extended to secondary PAD due to vasculitis. In Japan, there has been a pilot study regarding bone marrow-derived stem cell implantation for collagen disease-related peripheral ischemia (Kamata, 2007; Takahashi, 2009). On the other hand, it was reported that endothelial progenitor cell function is inhibited, in collagen disease such as SLE patients treated with corticosteroids (Grisar, 2008), and also production of angiogenic factors from bone marrow cells is suppressed (Greenberger; Nauck, 1998). In addition, collected bone marrow would include a substantial amount of activated dendrocytes and immune stimulating cytokines such as interferon gamma which may worsen an ischemic ulcer. Thus, we focused on a more specific approach to vasculitis or collagen disease in order to establish a more safe and effective approach.

5. Growth factor approach

One strategy is to deliver recombinant proteins directly to the ischemic tissue by intramuscular or intraarterial injection. An alternate strategy is to use gene therapy, by direct transfer of expression vectors with either virus or naked plasmid. An optimal delivery strategy has not been established, and the approach of using a large amount of protein or gene as a therapeutic agent has several disadvantages. Also, the outcomes of early-phase clinical trials with a particular molecule have been less than encouraging, possibly because of factors such as the selection and formulation of the growth factor, duration of exposure, route of administration, and selection of patients. On the basis of our experiences, bone marrow mononuclear cell implantation in patients with complicated CLI is effective (Miyamoto, 2004). Regarding the mechanism, our colleague demonstrated potential cytokines produced from bone marrow mononuclear cells in response to ischemia (Uemura, 2006). Among these growth factors such as basic fibroblast growth factor (b-FGF), vascular endothelial growth factor (VEGF), and insulin-like growth factor (IGF), only b-FGF has a strong angiogenic property (Doi, 2007) and human recombinant b-FGF is available to purchase for clinical use in Japan. Furthermore, as b-FGF is a water soluble compound, Tabata et al (Tabata, 1998) developed a drug delivery system (DDS), utilizing b-FGF conjugated with gelatin hydrogel by chemical cross-linking that enables slow release of b-FGF over two weeks. The precise method of gelatin hydrogel preparation (Figure 2) has been previously described (Tara, 2011b), in brief, gelatine microspheres were impregnated with an aqueous solution containing recombinant human b-FGF followed by leaving at 4 °C for over 12 hours to obtain b-FGF-incorporated gelatine hydrogel. Under general anesthesia, we injected prepared b-FGF (600 μg)-incorporated gelatin hydrogel directly into the calf muscle at twenty sites around the ulcer under Doppler echo-guidance.

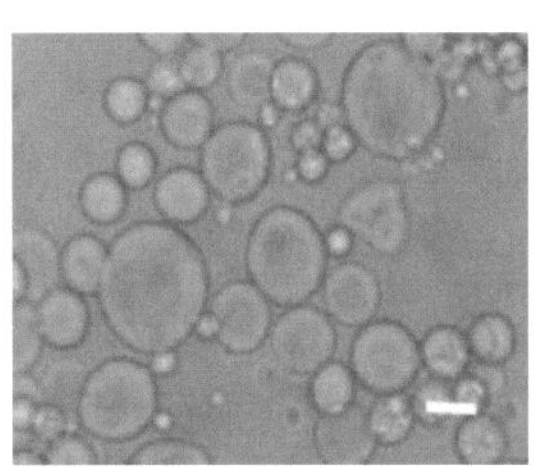

Fig. 2. Gelatin microspheres. White bar indicates 20μm.

6. Our experience of novel treatment for vasculitis

6.1 Churg-Strauss syndrome

Churg-Strauss syndrome (CSS; allergic angitis and granulomatosis) is a rare syndrome that is occasionally complicated by cutaneous, and vascular involvement which shows characteristic histopathologic findings (Figure 3-A). Vasculitis involves the microcirculation, often with intractable cutaneous ulcers (Figure 3-B), and when vascular involvement occurs at the visible artery level (Figure 3-C), standard corticosteroid treatment is less effective. Often the ulcer is complicated by antibiotics-resistant bacterial infection, which makes it difficult to continue or increase the corticosteroid dose. We injected 600μg b-FGF protein into the calf muscle, and the ulcer had healed 15 weeks later (Figure 3-D) (Kawanaka, 2009).

6.2 Systemic lupus erythematosus (SLE)

SLE is a systemic autoimmune disease characterized by the presence of immune complexes, autoantibodies and anti-nuclear antibody ANA), sometimes with cardiovascular involvement such as coronary arteritis or small arterial disease. Our case had an intractable ulcer above the lateral malleolus (Figure 4-A). Digital subtraction angiography revealed total occlusion of the right anterior tibial artery, right posterior tibial artery and right peroneal artery. The dorsalis pedis artery showed hardly any flow, and was supplied by collateral circulation (Figure 4-B). We injected 600μg b-FGF protein into the calf muscle and the ulcer had healed 4 weeks later (Figure 4-C) (Tara, 2011b).

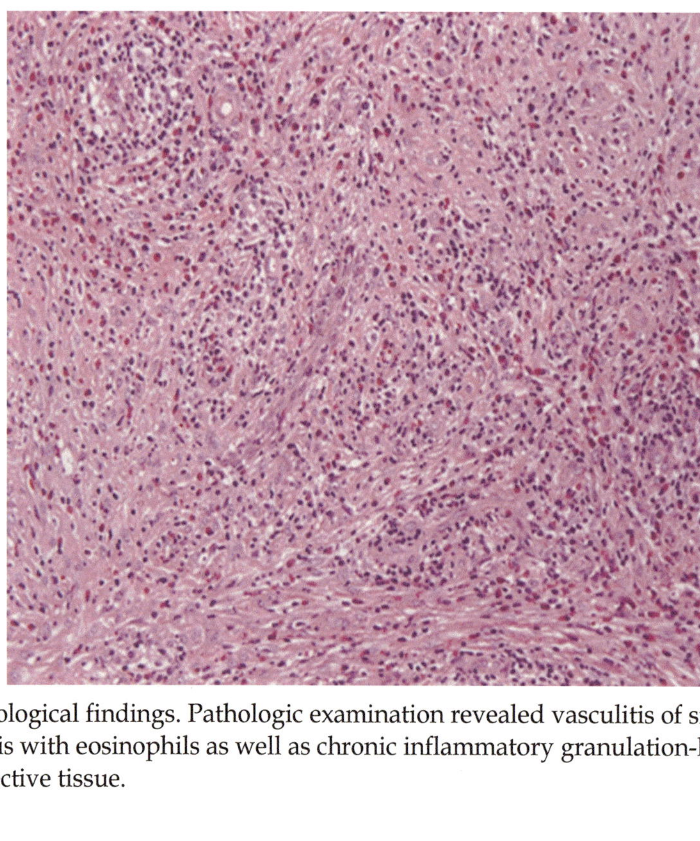

Fig. 3.A. Histological findings. Pathologic examination revealed vasculitis of small arteries and capillaritis with eosinophils as well as chronic inflammatory granulation-like changes in fibrous connective tissue.

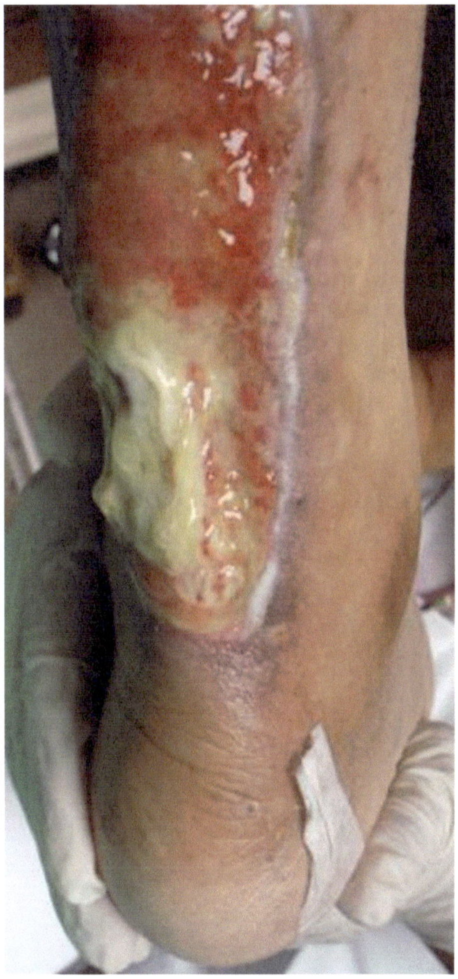

Fig. 3. B. Patient with Churg-Strauss syndrome. Photographs show right lower calf ulcer that did not respond to topical and medical treatment.

7. Discussion

Among the vasculitides, we experienced cases of Churg-Strauss syndrome and SLE complicated by intractable ulcers. A DDS designed to provide controlled- release b-FGF protein mono-therapy successfully improved those ulcers and avoided major amputation. Leg ulcers complicate many conditions including ischemia and infection, and the location of ischemia varies among different diseases. Considering the pathogenesis of vasculitis, this protein - based angiogenesis therapy is less invasive, repeatable, safe and effective. Utilization of this DDS approach would be a powerful approach for vasculitis - related intractable ulcer. We recommend this controlled-release b-FGF protein therapy when the ulcer does not respond to usual corticosteroid therapy and when ischemia is documented angiographically. In the future, we plan to establish a multi-growth factor approach to enhance local circulation and wound healing in intractable ulcers.

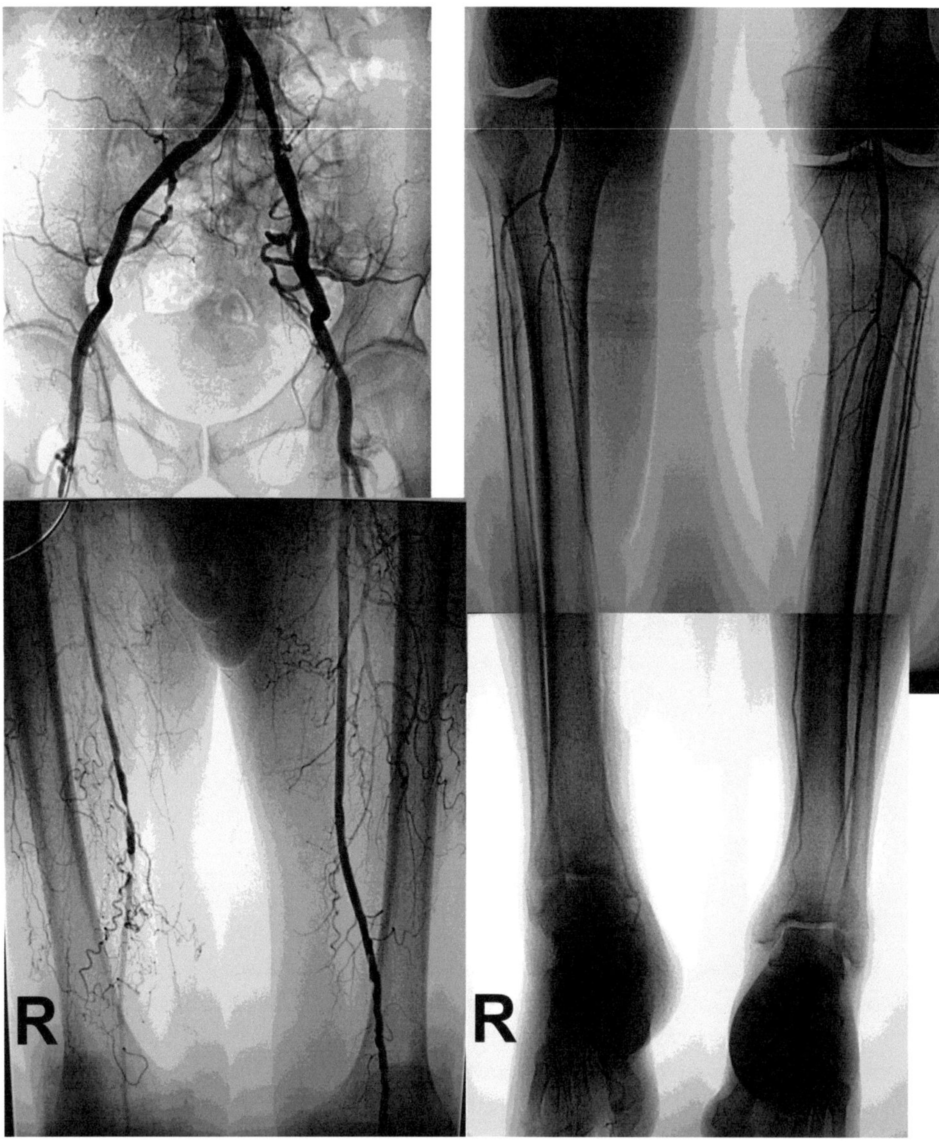

Fig. 3. C. Digital subtraction angiographic findings. Total occlusion of the right superficial femoral artery is shown.

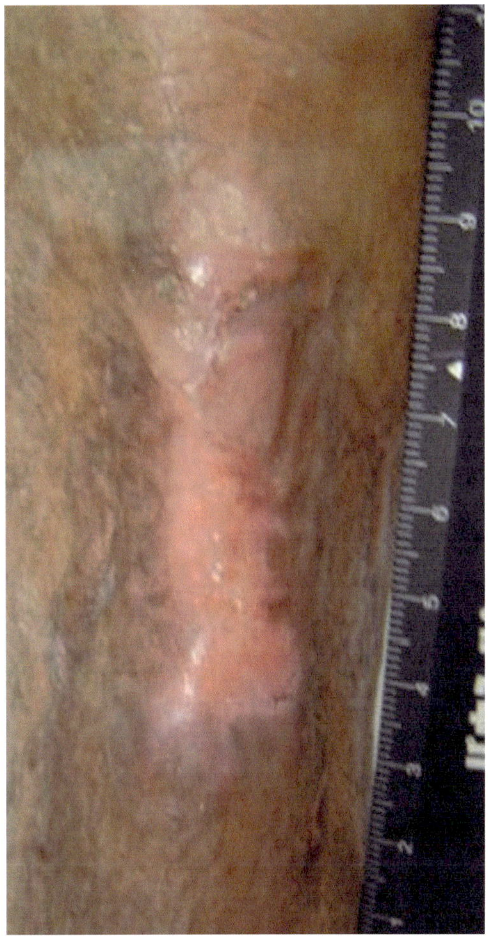

Fig. 3. D. Skin ulcer after treatment. The skin ulcer had healed completely 15 weeks after treatment.

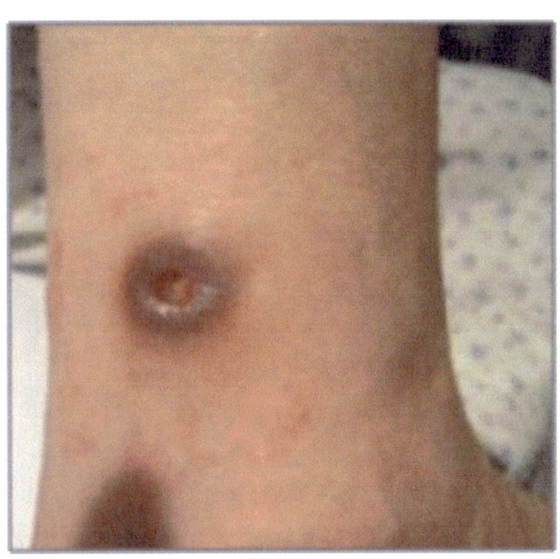

Fig. 4. A. Patient with SLE. The photograph shows a skin ulcer above the right lateral malleolus.

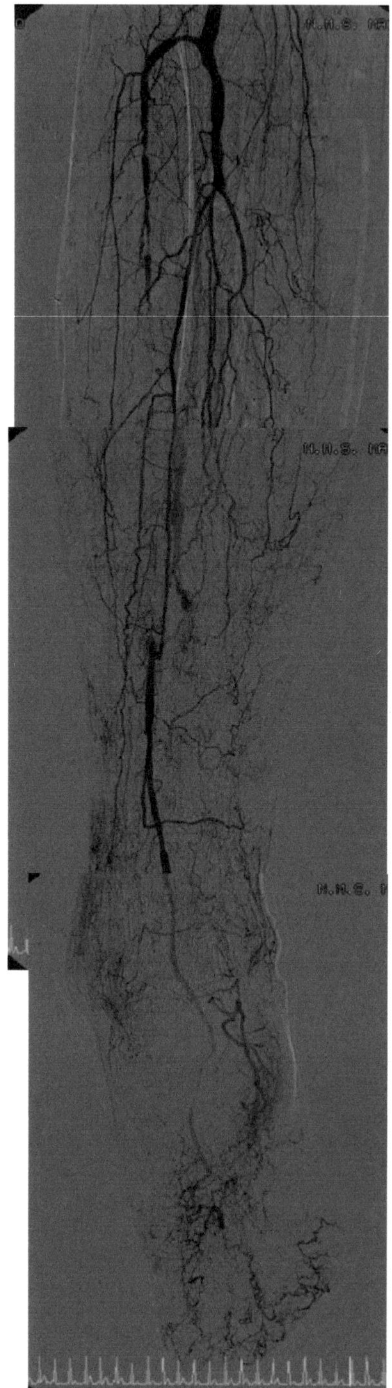

Fig. 4. B. Digital subtraction angiographic findings. Total occlusion of the right anterior tibial artery, right posterior tibial artery and right peroneal artery is shown. The dorsalis pedis artery was enhanced by collateral circulation

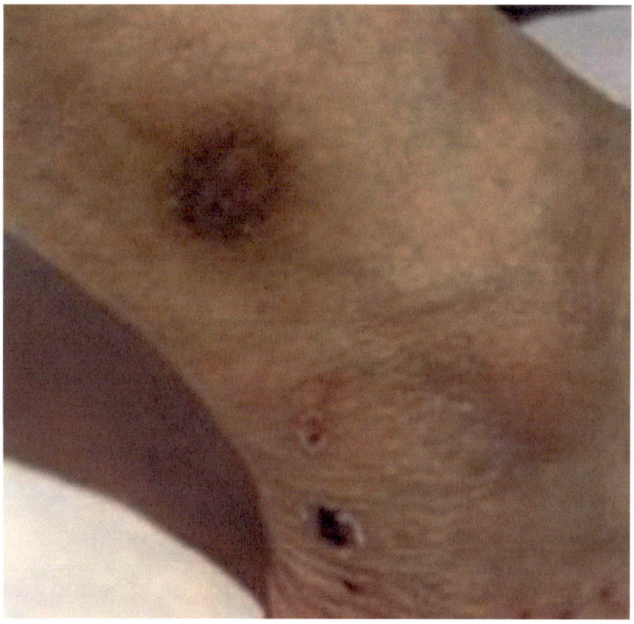

Fig. 4. C. SLE ulcer after treatment. The skin ulcer had healed completely 4 weeks after treatment.

8. Conclusion

Controlled-release b-FGF administration successfully healed ischemic skin ulcers and improved local skin blood perfusion in patients with vasculitis or collagen disease. Our findings suggest a novel clinical approach for ischemic skin ulcer associated with vasculitis or collagen disease.

9. References

Aulivola B, Hile CN, Hamdan AD, Sheahan MG, Veraldi JR, Skillman JJ, Campbell DR, Scovell SD, LoGerfo FW & Pomposelli FB, Jr. (2004). Major lower extremity amputation: outcome of a modern series. *Arch Surg* 139, 395-399; discussion 399.

Cruz CP, Eidt JF, Capps C, Kirtley L & Moursi MM. (2003). Major lower extremity amputations at a Veterans Affairs hospital. *Am J Surg* 186, 449-454.

Doi K, Ikeda T, Marui A, Kushibiki T, Arai Y, Hirose K, Soga Y, Iwakura A, Ueyama K, Yamahara K, Itoh H, Nishimura K, Tabata Y & Komeda M. (2007). Enhanced angiogenesis by gelatin hydrogels incorporating basic fibroblast growth factor in rabbit model of hind limb ischemia. *Heart Vessels* 22, 104-108.

Greenberger S, Boscolo E, Adini I, Mulliken JB & Bischoff J. Corticosteroid suppression of VEGF-A in infantile hemangioma-derived stem cells. *N Engl J Med* 362, 1005-1013.

Grisar J, Steiner CW, Bonelli M, Karonitsch T, Schwarzinger I, Weigel G, Steiner G & Smolen JS. (2008). Systemic lupus erythematosus patients exhibit functional deficiencies of endothelial progenitor cells. *Rheumatology (Oxford)* 47, 1476-1483.

Hirsch AT, Haskal ZJ, Hertzer NR, Bakal CW, Creager MA, Halperin JL, Hiratzka LF, Murphy WR, Olin JW, Puschett JB, Rosenfield KA, Sacks D, Stanley JC, Taylor LM, Jr., White CJ,

White J, White RA, Antman EM, Smith SC, Jr., Adams CD, Anderson JL, Faxon DP, Fuster V, Gibbons RJ, Hunt SA, Jacobs AK, Nishimura R, Ornato JP, Page RL & Riegel B. (2006). ACC/AHA 2005 guidelines for the management of patients with peripheral arterial disease (lower extremity, renal, mesenteric, and abdominal aortic): executive summary a collaborative report from the American Association for Vascular Surgery/Society for Vascular Surgery, Society for Cardiovascular Angiography and Interventions, Society for Vascular Medicine and Biology, Society of Interventional Radiology, and the ACC/AHA Task Force on Practice Guidelines (Writing Committee to Develop Guidelines for the Management of Patients With Peripheral Arterial Disease) endorsed by the American Association of Cardiovascular and Pulmonary Rehabilitation; National Heart, Lung, and Blood Institute; Society for Vascular Nursing; TransAtlantic Inter-Society Consensus; and Vascular Disease Foundation. *J Am Coll Cardiol* 47, 1239-1312.

Kamata Y, Takahashi Y, Iwamoto M, Matsui K, Murakami Y, Muroi K, Ikeda U, Shimada K, Yoshio T, Okazaki H & Minota S. (2007). Local implantation of autologous mononuclear cells from bone marrow and peripheral blood for treatment of ischaemic digits in patients with connective tissue diseases. *Rheumatology (Oxford)* 46, 882-884.

Kawanaka H, Takagi G, Miyamoto M, Tara S, Takagi I, Takano H, Yasutake M, Tabata Y & Mizuno K. (2009). Therapeutic angiogenesis by controlled-release fibroblast growth factor in a patient with Churg-Strauss syndrome complicated by an intractable ischemic leg ulcer. *Am J Med Sci* 338, 341-342.

Miyamoto M, Yasutake M, Takano H, Takagi H, Takagi G, Mizuno H, Kumita S & Takano T. (2004). Therapeutic angiogenesis by autologous bone marrow cell implantation for refractory chronic peripheral arterial disease using assessment of neovascularization by 99mTc-tetrofosmin (TF) perfusion scintigraphy. *Cell Transplant* 13, 429-437.

Nauck M, Karakiulakis G, Perruchoud AP, Papakonstantinou E & Roth M. (1998). Corticosteroids inhibit the expression of the vascular endothelial growth factor gene in human vascular smooth muscle cells. *Eur J Pharmacol* 341, 309-315.

Tabata Y, Yamada K, Miyamoto S, Nagata I, Kikuchi H, Aoyama I, Tamura M & Ikada Y. (1998). Bone regeneration by basic fibroblast growth factor complexed with biodegradable hydrogels. *Biomaterials* 19, 807-815.

Takahashi M, Izawa A, Ishigatsubo Y, Fujimoto K, Miyamoto M, Horie T, Aizawa Y, Amano J, Minota S, Murohara T, Matsubara H & Ikeda U. (2009). Therapeutic neovascularization by the implantation of autologous mononuclear cells in patients with connective tissue diseases. *Curr Pharm Des* 15, 2778-2783.

Tara S, Miyamoto M, Takagi G, Fukushima Y, Kirinoki-Ichikawa S, Takano H, Takagi I, Mizuno H, Yasutake M, Kumita S & Mizuno K. (2011a). Prediction of limb salvage after therapeutic angiogenesis by autologous bone marrow cell implantation in patients with critical limb ischemia. *Ann Vasc Dis* 4, 24-31.

Tara S, Takagi G, Kirinoki-Ichikawa S, Yamamoto T, Takano H, Takagi I, Yasutake M, Miyamoto M, Tabata Y & Mizuno K. (2011b). Novel approach to ischemic skin ulcer in systemic lupus erythematosus: Therapeutic angiogenesis by controlled-release basic-fibroblast growth factor. *Geriatr Gerontol Int* in press.

Uemura R, Xu M, Ahmad N & Ashraf M. (2006). Bone marrow stem cells prevent left ventricular remodeling of ischemic heart through paracrine signaling. *Circ Res* 98, 1414-1421.

12

Oral Delivery of DNA Vector Conjugated with Chitosan and Its Effect on Th1 Polarized Inflammation

Bunsoon Choi[1], Ju Young Choi[1], Do-Hyun Jo[2] and Seonghyang Sohn[1]
[1]*Laboratory of Cell Biology, Institute for Medical Sciences,*
[2]*Department of Molecular Science and Technology, Ajou University, Suwon, Korea*

1. Introduction

Gene therapy can be defined as the transfer of genetic materials to specific cells in order to exert a therapeutic effect. Gene therapy is a promising approach to the treatment of a wide range of diseases by compensating for defective genes or producing beneficial proteins (Zhao et al., 2009; Mansouri et al., 2004). Gene vectors play many important roles in gene therapy. Recently, nonviral vectors have been increasingly proposed as safer alternatives to viral vectors because of their potential advantages such as ease of synthesis, cell/tissue targeting, low immune response, and unrestricted plasmid size (Leong et al., 1998). Among nonviral systems, cationic polymers have attracted a great deal of attention because they can easily form self-assembling polyelectrolyte complexes between plasmid DNA and cationic polymers and mediate transfection via condensing DNA into nanoparticles, protecting DNA from enzymatic degradation, and facilitating cell uptake and endolysosomal escape (Wang et al., 2002). Among cationic polymers, polyethylenimine (PEI) and chitosan are widely used as nonviral vectors for gene delivery. These compounds have the same ability to enter cells by binding to proteoglycans on cell surfaces and undergoing endocytosis (Lungwitz et al., 2005; Köping-Höggard et al., 2001; Mansouri et al., 2006). However, after uptake, they have very different transfection efficiencies. PEI is considered to be the most effective cationic polymer for gene delivery (Densmore et al., 2009). However, PEI is also associated with dose-dependent toxicity, especially at high molecular weights, which probably explains why it has not yet been used in human studies (Kunath et al., 2003). Conversely, chitosan is degraded in the endosome and the material is then released into the cytoplasm. The material is then transported to the nucleus. Therefore, chitosan is generally considered less effective in gene delivery systems than PEI *in vitro* and *in vivo*. However, it is well known as a biocompatible, biodegradable, and relatively non toxic material with high cationic potential (Lee et al.,1998). Therefore, chitosan nanoparticles could be applied to vectors for gene delivery. In addition, chitosan is a widely available orally administered protein that can also be readily formed into nanoparticles able to entrap plasmid DNA and promote gene expression (Bowman & Leong , 2006).

The purpose of this study was to evaluate chitosans of different molecular weights as DNA complexing agents based on their efficiency at transfecting RAW 264.7 cells and their *in vivo* effects following oral administration to mice. Additionally, chitosan-pcDNA-EGFP-mIL4 nanoparticle complexes administered to mice were evaluated to determine if they can up-regulate the serum level of IL-4, and therefore ameliorate T helper type 1 polarized inflammation in herpes simplex virus induced inflammation.

2. Methods

2.1 Preparation of vector particle

The pCIN-mIL4 vector was constructed by inserting IL-4 cytokine genes into pCI-neo (pCIN; Gibco-Invitrogen, Rockville, MD). The IL-4 gene was amplified by PCR from MFG-muIL-4 plasmids with specific IL-4 primers and then inserted into pCIN to generate pCIN-mIL4 (Lee et al., 1999). Plasmid DNA was purified on Qiagen columns (Qiagen, Chatsworth, CA), after which it was mixed with chitosan or precipitated onto nanoparticles (Gan & Wang, 2007). Next, 2 µL of different molecular weight (3kDa, 10 kDa, 50 kDa) 2% chitosans dissolved in 0.1% acetic acid were mixed with 1 µg of pCIN-mIL4 DNA vector. To produce chitosan-DNA nanoparticles, chitosan was dissolved in 1% acetic acid (chitosan acetate) (0.35%w/v), after which chitosan-DNA nanoparticle complexes were precipitated by centrifugation and confirmed by agarose gel electrophoresis. Briefly, 50 µg of pCIN-mIL4 DNA was dissolved in 5 ml of 20% sodium sulfate, after which an equal volume of chitosan acetic acid and DNA solution was mixed and centrifuged. The supernatant was then discarded and stored at 4 °C.

2.2 Chitosan treatment

Chitosan with different molecular weights (3, 10, and 50 kDa) was dissolved in 0.1 M acetic acid solution and then filtered to remove the insoluble particles. The pH was subsequently adjusted to 8.0 with 1 M NaOH, which resulted in the formation of white precipitates. The precipitated chitosan was subsequently washed thoroughly using deionized water until a neutral pH was attained, at which point the product was vacuum dried at room temperature for 24 h (Gan & Wang, 2007).

2.3 *In vitro* transfection of RAW 264.7 cells with IL-4 DNA

RAW 264.7 cells, which are a murine macrophage cell line, were cultured in Dulbecco's modified Eagle's medium (DMEM) supplemented with 10% fetal bovine serum (FBS) and 1% penicillin/streptomycin. Before transfection, cells were harvested, washed twice, and resuspended in 12-well plates at a density of $1x10^5$ cells per well. Cells were then transfected with a total of 1 µg of pCIN-mIL4 vector using 2 µL of oligofectamine (Gibco-Invitrogen, Rockville, MD) and/or chitosan. Finally, cells were cultured for 48 h in medium containing 10% FBS, harvested, and analyzed for IL-4 expression.

2.4 *In vivo* administration of IL-4 DNA

The pCIN-mIL4 or pCIN DNA vector was administered orally once a day for two to three days. Each dose carried 20 µg of DNA into the mice. In normal mice, intestinal tissues and serum were collected day 2 and 5 after the last administration. In herpes simplex virus induced inflammatory Behcet's disease mice, 20 µg of pCIN-EGFP-mIL4 was mixed with chitosan and then orally administered for three consecutive days. At 20 days after last administration, the mice were sacrificed and the intestinal tissues were collected for confocal microscopy. Mice were bred in temperature and light controlled conventional rooms (20-22

°C, 12 h light cycle starting at 8:00 a.m.) during which time they had free access to food and water. During the experimental period, the animals were closely observed. Mice were handled in accordance with protocols approved by our institutional animal care committee.

2.5 RNA isolation & RT-PCR

Total RNA was isolated by acid guanidium thiocyanate - phenol - chloroform extraction (Chomczynski & Sacchi, 1987). Spleen tissues were homogenized in 1 mL of extraction buffer, which was composed of 4 M guanidine solution (Aldrich, Milwaukee, WI, USA), 25 mM sodium citrate pH 7.0, 0.5% sodium N-lauroyl sarcosinate (Fisher, Pittsburgh, PA), and 0.1 M 2-mercaptoethanol (Sigma, St. Louis, MO). A 1/10 volume of chloroform: isoamyl alcohol (49: 1) was added to the samples, which were incubated on ice for five minutes, then centrifuged at 10,000 x g for 15 minutes at 4 °C. RNA contained in the upper aqueous phase was collected, precipitated with an equal volume of isopropanol, and washed twice in 70% EtOH. RNA pellets were dissolved in distilled water, quantified by OD 260/280, and then visualized in an ethidium bromide stained agarose gel. Two micrograms of total RNA were reverse transcribed using a cDNA kit (Gibco BRL, Grand Island, NY, USA), oligo dT primers and AMV reverse transcriptase to generate cDNA for use as a template in PCR amplifications. Two microliters from the reverse transcriptase reaction were then added to PCR reaction mixtures composed of 50 mM KCl pH 8.4, 20 mM Tris-HCl, 2.5 mM $MgCl_2$, 200 μM dNTPs, 2.5 U of Taq polymerase (Gibco BRL), and 1.2 μM primers. The specific primers were as follows:

β-actin (Murray et al., 1990)	(S) 5' - TGGAATCCTGTGGCATCCATGAAAC - 3'
	(A) 5' - TAAAACGCAGCTCAGTAACAGTCCG - 3'
IL-4 (Lee et al., 1986)	(S) 5' - ACGCCATGCACGGAGATGGAT - 3'
	(A) 5' - CAAGCATGGAGTTTTCC - 3'

2.6 Determination of IL-4 levels in mice

The serum levels of IL-4 in mice administered pCIN-mIL4 or chitosan-pCIN-mIL4 nanoparticles were measured by ELISA using commercially available IL-4 ELISA kits (R&D systems Inc., Minneapolis, MN).

2.7 Confocal microscopy

Intestinal tissues isolated from mice administered chitosan-pcDNA-EGFP-mIL4 mixture were sectioned in cryostat for confocal microscopy. Sectioned tissues were observed under a confocal microscope (Zeiss, Germany).

2.8 Animals, introduction of Behcet's disease symptoms and treatment of Behcet's disease mice with chitosan-pcDNA-EGFP-mIL4

Four to five-week-old male ICR mice were used for this experiment. The earlobes of the mice were scratched with a needle and then inoculated with 1.0 x 10^6 plaque forming units/ml of HSV type 1 (F strain). Virus inoculation was conducted twice with a 10-day interval between treatments, after which the mice were observed for 16 weeks. Mice were bred in temperature- and light-controlled conventional rooms (20-22 °C, 12 h light cycle starting at 8:00 a.m.) with free access to food and water. During the experimental period, the animals were closely observed and photographed. Animals were handled in accordance to a protocol approved by our institutional animal care committee.

A revised Japanese classification with minor modifications was used to classify symptomatic mice with Behcet's disease. Briefly, oral, genital and other skin ulcers (including bulla and crust) and eye symptoms were classified as major symptoms, while arthritis, gastrointestinal ulcers and neurological disorders were identified as minor symptoms. Mice with at least one major and one minor symptom were classified as having Behcet's disease. Of the total number of HSV-injected mice, 15% developed Behcet's disease -like symptoms. Treatments that led to the disappearance of symptoms or a decrease in the lesion size of greater than 20% were classified as effective. Scoring of the severity of Behcet's disease was followed by determination of the Behcet's disease activity index, as outlined in the Behcet's disease Activity Forum (www.behcet.ws/pdf/BehcetsDiseaseActivityForm pdf). Among the symptoms in patients, mouth ulceration, genital ulceration, erythema, skin pustules, skin ulceration, joints-arthritis, diarrhea, red eye (right, left), reduced vision (right, left), loss of balance, discoloration, and swelling of the face were selected and analyzed in the Behcet's disease mouse model. The score of each symptom was one, and after the score was computed the total was used to determine the severity of Behcet's disease. Symptomatic mice were photographed on the starting day of drug administration and on day 20 after chitosan-DNA vector administration. Chitosan-pcDNA-EGFP-mIL4 was orally administered to Behcet's disease-like mice for three consecutive days. Placebo was administered to Behcet's -like disease mice in an identical manner.

2.9 Statistical analysis

All data are represented as the mean ± SE. Statistical differences between control and IL-4 vector injected groups were determined using the Student *t* test and Bonferroni correction. Statistical analysis was conducted using MedCalc® version 9.3.0.0.

3. Results

3.1 pCIN-mIL4 vector was mixed with chitosan *in vitro*

1 µg of pCIN-mIL4 DNA vector and 2 µL of 2% of chitosan (3 kDa, 10 kDa, and 50 kDa) were mixed and loaded into 1% agarose gel. The DNA vector was well complexed with chitosan as shown in Figure 1.

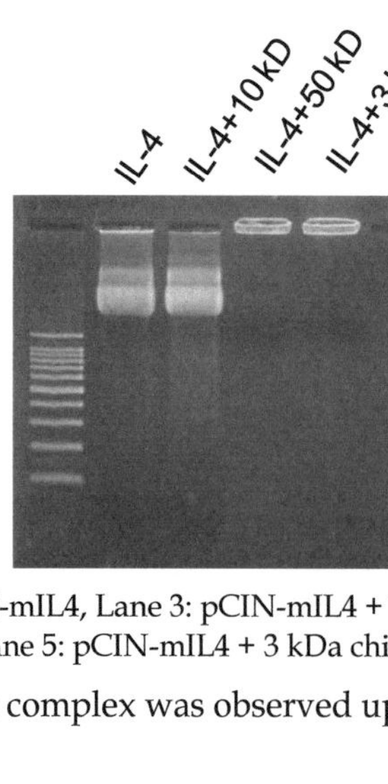

Lane 1: DNA marker, Lane 2: pCIN-mIL4, Lane 3: pCIN-mIL4 + 10 kDa chitosan mixture, Lane 4: pCIN-mIL4 + 50 kDa chitosan mixture, Lane 5: pCIN-mIL4 + 3 kDa chitosan mixture

Fig. 1. pCIN-mIL4 and chitosan complex was observed upon agarose gel electrophoresis.

3.2 pCIN-mIL4 DNA vector was transfected into RAW 264.7 cells with or without chitosan

To determine if the Chitosan-pCIN-mIL4 DNA vector mixture could deliver pCIN-mIL4 DNA vector into the cells and if the delivered DNA could be expressed to mRNA, pCIN-mIL4 DNA vector was transfected into RAW 264.7 cells with or without chitosan. The mixture containing 50 kDa chitosan-pCIN-mIL4 strongly increased IL-4 mRNA expression in RAW 264.7 cells when compared to 10 kDa chitosan or 3 kDa chitosan or untreated groups based on analysis by reverse transcriptase PCR (RT-PCR) (Figure 2).

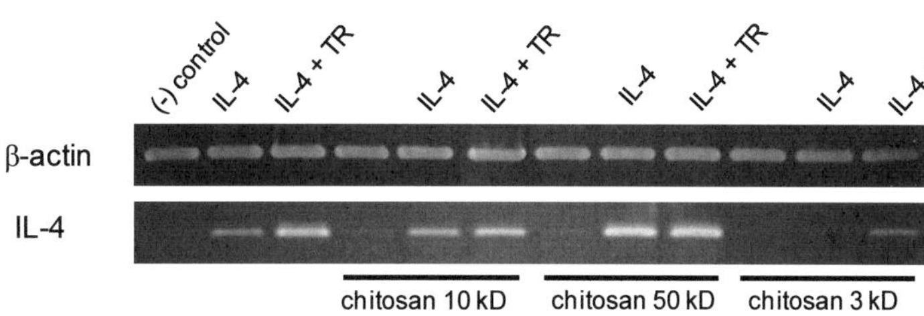

Fig. 2. pCIN-mIL4 DNA vectors mixed with three kinds of chitosan were transfected into RAW 264.7 cells. IL-4 mRNA expression was detected by RT-PCR. Oligofectamin was used as a transfection reagent, and compared to chitosan.

3.3 Chitosan-pCIN-mIL4 DNA vector nanoparticles were transfected to RAW 264.7 cells without oligofectamin

To compare the efficiency of delivery of DNA vector between the chitosan-DNA vector mixture and chitosan-DNA vector nanoparticles, pCIN-mIL4 DNA vector dissolved in sodium sulfate was mixed with 50 kDa chitosan-acetic acid solution, and then transfected to RAW 264.7 cells without oligofectamin. After 48 h, the cells were harvested and analyzed for IL-4 expression by RT-PCR. Chitosan-pCIN-mIL4 DNA nanoparticle transfected cells strongly expressed IL-4 mRNA when compared to the pCIN control vector, chitosan-pCIN nanoparticle, pCIN-mIL4 vector and chitosan transfected groups (Figure 3). The mRNA expression of IL-4 did not differ between chitosan-pCIN-mIL4 mixture and chitosan-pCIN-mIL4 nanoparticle group. There was also no difference between groups treated with 1 μg and 2 μg of pCIN-mIL4 DNA-chitosan nanoparticles. The efficiency of delivery of the DNA vector was similar between the chitosan-DNA vector mixture and chitosan-DNA vector nanoparticles.

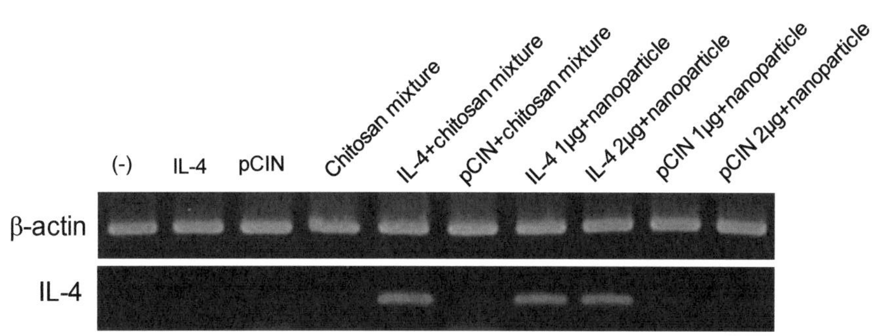

Fig. 3. Comparison of the chitosan-pCIN-mIL4 DNA vector mixture and chitosan-pCIN-mIL4 DNA vector nanoparticles in *in vitro* transfection of IL-4 vector by RT-PCR.

3.4 Chitosan-pCIN-mIL4 DNA vector mixture was orally administered to normal mice

After oral administration of the 50 kDa chitosan-pCIN-mIL4 DNA vector mixture to normal mice, the serum level of IL-4 was detected by ELISA (n=5 per each bar). Two doses of chitosan-pCIN-mIL4 DNA mixtures (5 μg DNA vector + 15 μg chitosan/mouse, 10 μg DNA vector + 30 μg chitosan/mouse) were applied to normal mice for two consecutive days. In addition, DNA vector (5 μg, 10 μg DNA vector/mouse) or chitosan (15 μg, 30 μg chitosan/mouse) was separately administered to mice as controls. The mice were sacrificed on day 5 after the last administration, and the sera were collected and subjected to ELISA. In addition, the intestinal tissues were isolated on day 2 and 5 after treatment and analyzed for the presence of IL-4 mRNA in the 10 μg DNA vector + 30 μg chitosan/mouse treated group. Administration of the 10 μg pCIN-mIL4 DNA vector + 30 μg chitosan mixture led to a significant increase in the serum level of IL-4 (10.25±2.9 pg/ml) when compared to mice that received 10 μg pCIN-mIL4 DNA vector alone (7.0±0.99 pg/ml; p=0.035) (Figure 4A). The

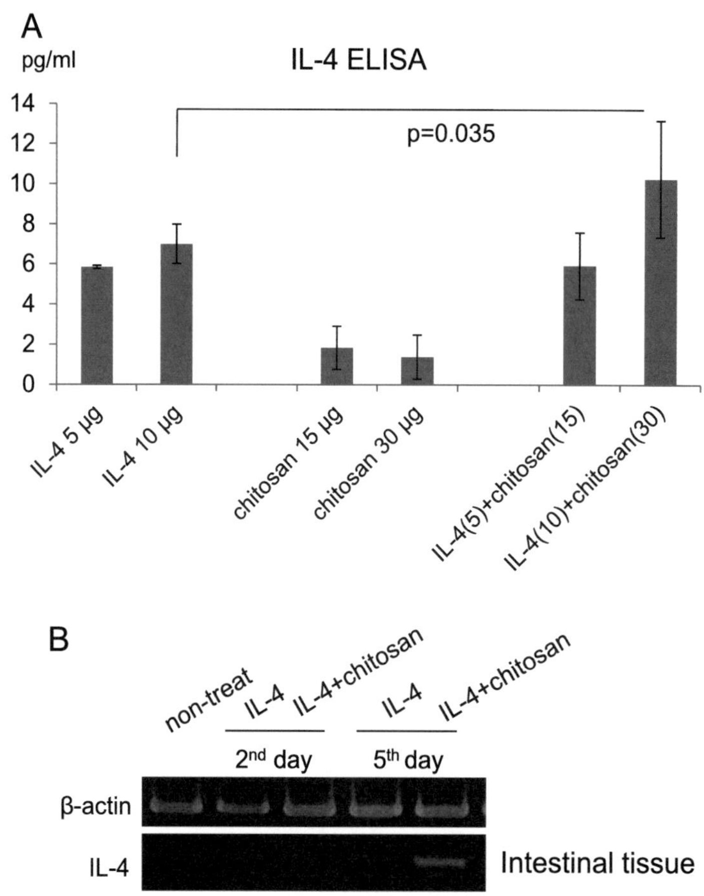

Fig. 4. Oral administration of the chitosan-pCIN-mIL4 DNA vector mixture to normal mice up-regulated the serum level of IL-4 and IL-4 mRNA expression in intestinal tissues.

intestinal tissues isolated on day 2 and 5 after administration showed increased IL-4 mRNA expression when compared to non-treated mice (Figure 4B). Specially, IL-4 mRNA was strongly expressed on day 5 after administration of the chitosan-pCINmIL4 DNA vector mixture when compared to the pCINmIL4 DNA vector administered group.

3.5 Confocal microscopy in intestinal tissues of normal mice treated with chitosan-pcDNA-EGFP-mIL4 DNA vector mixture

To confirm the aforementioned results microscopically, the pcDNA-EGFP-mIL4 DNA vector was mixed with chitosan, after which 20 μg of the mixture was administered once a day for two consecutive days. At 10 and 20 days after last administration, the intestinal tissues were isolated and cryosectioned for subsequent observation under the confocal microscope. GFP was strongly observed in the intestinal tissue at day 10 after administration and remained day 20 (Figure 5). GFP was not detected in the mice treated with chitosan or pcDNA vector alone, nor was it detected in the mice treated with pcDNA-EGFP-mIL4 DNA vector.

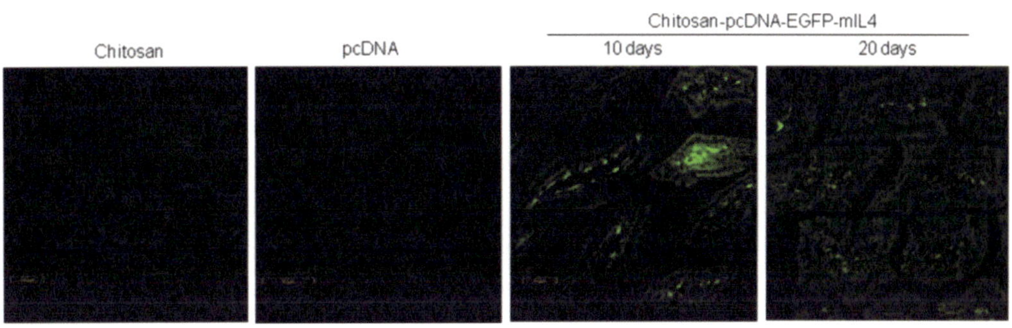

Fig. 5. Oral administration of the chitosan-pcDNA-EGFP-mIL4 DNA vector mixture to normal mice resulted in GFP in the intestinal tissues as determined by confocal microscopy.

3.6 Confocal microscopy in intestinal tissues of chitosan-pcDNA-EGFP-mIL4 DNA vector mixture treated Behcet's Disease (BD)-like mice

To confirm the aforementioned results microscopically and determine if the treatment could improve herpes simplex virus induced inflammatory BD symptoms, 20 μg of pcDNA-EGFP-mIL4 DNA vector was mixed with chitosan, and then administered to BD mice orally once a day for three consecutive days. At day 20 after the last administration, the intestinal tissues were isolated and cryosectioned for subsequent observation under the confocal microscope. GFP was strongly observed in the intestinal tissue (Figure 6A). However, GFP was not detected in the chitosan or pcDNA vector treated mice. Moreover, 20 days after last administration, the change in cutaneous ulceration of BD symptoms was photographed and compared to the symptoms before treatment. The symptoms improved after the treatment (Figure 6B), and the increased IL-4 level likely influenced this improvement.

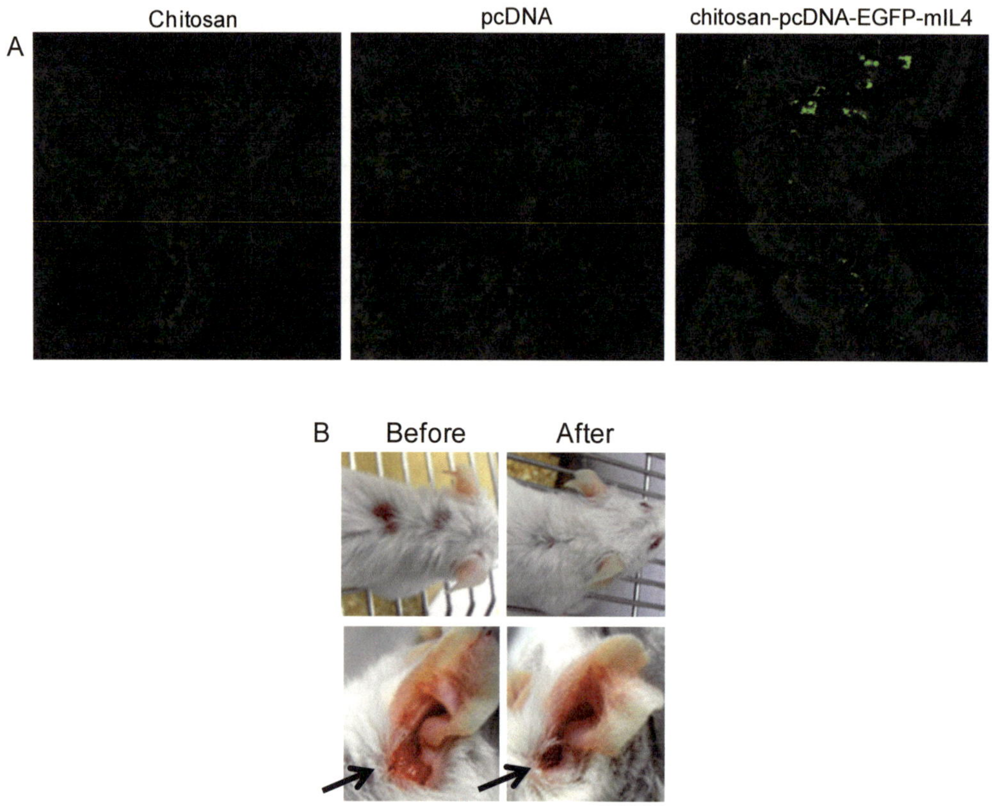

Fig. 6. Oral administration of the chitosan-pcDNA-EGFP-mIL4 DNA vector mixture to Behcet's disease mice resulted in GFP in the intestinal tissues (A) and improved the cutaneous symptoms of BD (B).

4. Discussion

In recent years, gene transfer technology has been shown to increase and evolve (Evans, 2004); however, the development of an effective non-viral gene delivery system has not yet been accomplished (Fernandes et al., 2000). Chitosan can encapsulate DNA vector to form complexes that are absorbed to the cell surface. The complexes are then endocytosed and transported to the nucleus by escaping the endosomal and lysosomal systems (Ishii et al., 2001). There are several indications that the transfection activity of chitosan-DNA vector complexes is dependent on the cell line being transfected (Erbacher et al., 1998). Several factors, including the molecular mass of chitosan, plasmid concentration, stoichiometry of the complex, serum concentration and pH of the transfection medium, can affect the transfection activity and cell uptake (Ishii et al., 2001). In the present study, we used chitosan with three different molecular weights as nanoparticles for *in vitro* transfection experiments. Among the treatments, the 50 kDa chitosan was the most effective agent for delivery of pCIN-mIL4 vector into the RAW 264.7 cells.

Oral delivery is attractive due to factors such as ease of administration, convenience to the patient, and improved compliance (Tighe et al., 1998). The oral delivery of biomaterials such as peptides, proteins, DNA vectors, and siRNA is the greatest challenge facing the drug delivery system. Chitosan is a natural cationic polysaccharide obtained from deacetylation of chitin that is found in crustacean shells. Chitosan is a biocompatible, non-toxic, biodegradable and mucoadhesive polymer, with the ability to form gels at low pH. In addition, the degradation of chitosan occurs via the microflora available in the colon. These properties could provide a basis for the preparation of controlled release formulations, particularly for colon-specific drug delivery (Tavakol et al., 2009; Hejazi & Amiji, *2003*). Chitosan has been shown to increase the transcellular and paracellular transport of macromolecules across intestinal epithelial monolayers (Angelova & Hunkeler, 2001). Chitosan has more recently been used successfully to deliver a reporter gene encoding chloramphenicol acetyl transferase orally to enterocytes, Peyer's patches and mesenteric lymph nodes (MacLaughlin et al., 1998). Roy et al. confirmed the effectiveness of orally delivered chitosan-DNA nanoparticles for inducing protective immunity in the peanut allergy mouse model (Roy et al., 1999).

In the present study, we constructed a chitosan-pCIN-mIL4 DNA vector mixture. Our results demonstrated that the chitosan-pCIN-mIL4 mixture was able to deliver DNA vector to the cell and that oral administration of chitosan-pCIN-mIL4 mixture increased the IL-4 mRNA level and serum protein level of IL-4 significantly when compared to treatment with pCIN-mIL4 alone. The administration of chitosan pCIN-mIL4 DNA vector to mice *in vivo* more strongly increased the mRNA expression in intestinal tissues and protected against degradation until DNA vector reach tothe intestinal tissue. GFP intensity was still very strong in the intestinal tissues when compared to DNA vector alone.

In summary, our results demonstrate that chitosan is a good candidate for the development of novel gene delivery systems. Treatment with an oral chitosan- pCIN-mIL-4 mixture can lead to expression of IL-4 mRNA and protein in intestinal tissues and increased serum levels of IL-4. Chitosan can encapsulate and protect pDNA, enabling effective transfer of the GFP gene into cells *in vivo*. Thus, chitosan-DNA vector mixture could be a promising method for gene therapy by oral administration.

5. Acknowledgements

This work was supported from the National Research Foundation of Korea (NRF) by the Ministry of Education, Science and Technology (2010-0011130) and the Korean Health Technology R&D Project, Ministry for Health, Welfare & Family Affairs, Republic of Korea. (A100535).

6. References

Angelova N & Hunkeler D. Effect of preparation conditions on properties and permeability of chitosan-sodium hexametaphosphate capsules. *Journal of*

Biomaterials Science, Polymer Edition, Vol.12, No.12, (2001), pp. 1317-1337, ISSN 0920-5063

Bowman K & Leong KW. Chitosan nanoparticles for oral drug and gene delivery. *International Journal of Nanomedicine*, Vol.1, No.2, (June 2006), pp. 117-128, ISSN 1178-2013

Chomczynski P & Sacchi N. Single step methods of RNA isolation by acid guanidium thiocyanate-phenol-chloroform extraction. *Analytical Biochemistry*, Vol.162, No.1, (April 1987), pp. 156-159, ISSN 0003-2697

Densmore CL, Orson FM, Xu B, Kinsey BM, Waldrep JC, Hua P, Bhogal B & Knight V. Aerosol delivery of robust polyethyleneimine-DNA complexes for gene therapy and genetic immunization. *Molecular Therapy*, Vol.1, No.2, (February 2000), pp. 180-188, ISSN 1525-0016

Erbacher P, Zou S, Bettinger T, Steffan AM & Remy JS. Chitosan based vector/DNA complexes for gene delivery: biophysical characteristics and transfection ability. *Pharmaceutical Research*, Vol.15, No.9, (September 1998), pp. 1332-1339, ISSN 0724-8741

Evans CH. Gene therapies for osteoarthritis. *Current Rheumatology Reports*, Vol.6, No.1, (February 2004), pp. 31-40, ISSN 1523-3774

Fernandes JC, Pelletier JP & Martel-Pelletier J. 2003. Gene therapy for osteoarthritis: new perspectives for the twenty-first century. *Clinical Orthopaedics and Related Research*, Vol.379, (October 2000), pp S262-S272, ISSN 0009-921X

Gan Q & Wang T. Chitosan nanoparticle as protein delivery carrier--systematic examination of fabrication conditions for efficient loading and release. *Colloids Surface B Biointerfaces*, Vol.59, No.1, (September 2007), pp. 24-34, ISSN 0927-7765

Hejazi R & Amiji M. *Chitosan-based gastrointestinal delivery systems, Journal of Controlled Release, Vol.89, No.2, (April* 2003), pp. 151-165, ISSN 0168-3659

Ishii T, Okahata Y & Sato T. Mechanism of cell transfection with plasmid/chitosan complexes. *Biochimica et Biophysica Acta - Biomembranes*, Vol.1514, No.1, (September 2001), pp. 51-64, ISSN 0005-2736

Köping-Höggard M, Tubulekas I, Guan H, Edwards K, Nilsson M, Varum KM & Artursson P. Chitosan as a nonviral gene delivery system. Structure-property relationships and characteristics compared with polyethylenimine in vitro and after lung administration in vivo. *Gene Therapy*, Vol.8, No.14, (July 2001), pp. 1108-1121, ISSN 0969-7128

Kunath K, Harpe A, Fischer D, Petersen H, Bickel U, Voigt K & Kissel T. Low-molecular-weight polyethylenimine as a non-viral vector for DNA delivery: comparison of physicochemical properties, transfection efficiency and in vivo distribution with high-molecular-weight polyethylenimine. *Journal of Controlled Release*, Vol.89, No.1, (April 2003), pp. 113-125, ISSN 0168-3659

Lee F, Yokota T, Otsuka T, Meyerson P, Villaret D, Cottman R, Mosmann T, Rennick D, Roehm N, Smith C, Zlotnik A & Arai K. Isolation and characterization of a mouse interleukin cDNA clone that expresses B-cell stimulatory factor 1 antivities and T-cell- and mast-cell-stimulating activities. *Proceedings of the National Academy of*

Sciences of the United States of America, Vol.83, No.7, (April 1986), pp. 2061-2065, ISSN 1091-6490

Lee KY, Kwon IC, Kim YH, Jo WH & Jeong SY. Preparation of chitosan self-aggregates as a gene delivery system. *Journal of Controlled Release*, Vol.51, No.2-3, (February 1998), pp. 213-220, ISSN 0168-3659

Lee SW, Youn JW, Seong BL & Sung YC. IL-6 induces long-term protective immunity against a lethal challenge of influenza virus. *Vaccine*, Vol.17, No.5, (February 1999), pp. 490-496, ISSN 0264-410X

Leong KW, Mao HQ, Truong-Le VL, Roy K, Walsh SM & August JT. DNA-polycation nanospheres as non-viral gene delivery vehicles. *Journal of Controlled Release*, Vol.53, No.1-3, (April 1998), pp. 183-193, ISSN 0168-3659

Lungwitz U, Breunig M, Blunk T & Gopferich A. Polyethylenimine-based non-viral gene delivery systems. *European Journal of Pharmaceutics and Biopharmaceutics*, Vol.60, No.2, (July 2005), pp. 247-266, ISSN 0939-6411

MacLaughlin FC, Mumper RJ, Wang J, Tagliaferri JM, Gill I, Hinchcliffe M & Rolland AP. Chitosan and depolymerized chitosan oligomers as condensing carriers for *in vivo* plasmid delivery. *Journal of Controlled Release*, Vol.56, No.1-3, (December 1998), pp. 259-272, ISSN 0168-3659

Mansouri S, Cuie Y, Winnik F, Shi Q, Lavigne P, Benderdour M, Beaumont E & Fernandes JC. Characterization of folate-chitosan-DNA nanoparticles for gene therapy. *Biomaterials*, Vol.27, No.9, (March 2006), pp. 2060-2065, ISSN: 0142-9612

Mansouri S, Lavigne P, Corsi K, Benderdour M, Beaumont E & Fernandes JC. Chitosan-DNA nanoparticles as non-viral vectors in gene therapy: strategies to improve transfection efficacy. *European Journal of Pharmaceutics and Biopharmaceutics*, Vol.57, No.1, (January 2004), pp. 1-8, ISSN 0939-6411

Murray LJ, Lee R & Martens C. In vivo cytokine gene expression in T cell subsets of the autoimmune MRL/MP-lpr/lpr mouse. *European Journal of Immunology*, Vol.20, No.1, (January 1990), pp. 163–170, ISSN 1521-4141

Roy K, Mao HQ, Huang SK & Leong KW. Oral gene delivery with chitosan--DNA nanoparticles generates immunologic protection in a murine model of peanut allergy. *Nature Medicine*, Vol.5, No.4, (April 1999), pp. 387-391, ISSN 1078-8956

Tavakol M, Vasheghani-Farahani E, Dolatabadi-Farahani T & Hashemi-Najafabadi, S. Sulfasalazine release from alginate-N,O-carboxymethyl chitosan gel beads coated by chitosan. Carbohydrate Polymers, Vol.77, No.2, (June 2009), pp. 326-330 ISSN 0144-8617

Tighe H, Corr M, Roman M & Raz E. Gene vaccination: plasmid DNA is more than just a blueprint. Immunology Today, Vol.19, No.2, (February 1998), pp. 89-97, ISSN 0167-5699

Wang J, Zhang PC, Lu HF, Ma N, Wang S, Mao HQ & Leong KW. New polyphosphoramidate with a spermidine side chain as a gene carrier. *Journal of Controlled Release*, Vol.83, No.1, (September 2002), pp. 157-168, ISSN 0168-3659

Zhao QQ, Chen JL, Lv TF, He CX, Tang GP, Liang WQ, Tabata Y & Gao JQ. N/P ratio significantly influences the transfection efficiency and cytotoxicity of a polyethylenimine/chitosan/DNA complex. *Biological & Pharmaceutical Bulletin*, Vol.32, No.4, (April 2009), pp. 706-710, ISSN 0918-6158

Part 3

Miscellaneous Overviews in Vasculitis

13

Churg Strauss Syndrome: Clinical and Pathogenetic Approach to Therapy

Giovanni Rolla, Monica Boita, Enrico Heffler and Giuseppe Guida
Allergy and Clinical Immunology University of Torino and AO Ordine Mauriziano
Italy

1. Introduction

The Churg-Strauss syndrome (CSS), also called allergic granulomatosis and angiitis, is a multisystem disorder characterized by allergic rhinitis, asthma, and prominent peripheral blood eosinophilia. CSS is classified as a vasculitis of the small and medium sized arteries, which commonly involve the lung, the skin and the peripheral nerves and it is associated to ANCA in 40-60 percent (Sinico & Bottero 2009). Among the three anti-neutrophil cytoplasmic antibodies (ANCA)-associated vasculitides (CSS, Wegener's granulomatosis, and microscopic polyangiitis), CSS is least common. In the general population, the frequency of the disorder has been estimated at 2.4–6.8 per 1 000 000 patient-years, while the incidence of CSS in asthma drug users has been estimated to be 14-52 per million person-years (Watts RA et al. 2000). The mean age at diagnosis of CSS is 40 years, with no gender predominance.

Diagnosis of Churg-Strauss syndrome can be difficult, because the syndrome may arise at first as a common association between asthma and allergic rhinitis. Because asthma itself might be associated with sinusitis, occasional pulmonary infiltrates (eg, mucus plugging, atelectasis, or intermittent infection), and corticosteroid dependency, a clear diagnosis of Churg-Strauss syndrome might not be made until extra respiratory system become involved, such as the abdominal viscera, heart, or nervous system.

2. Diagnostic criteria

The ACR has established six criteria for the classification of CSS in a patient with documented vasculitis (Masi AT et al.1990). The presence of four or more of these criteria had a sensitivity of 85 percent and a specificity of 99.7 percent for CSS:

- Asthma (a history of wheezing or the finding of diffuse high pitched wheezes on expiration)
- Greater than 10 percent eosinophils on the differential leukocyte count
- Mononeuropathy (particularly multiplex) or polyneuropathy
- Migratory or transient pulmonary opacities detected radiographically
- Paranasal sinus abnormality
- Biopsy containing a blood vessel showing the accumulation of eosinophils in extra-vascular areas.

Chapel Hill Consensus Conference (Jennette JC et al 1994) analyzed pathological and clinical findings to define CSS as an eosinophil-rich and granulomatous inflammation involving the

respiratory tract and necrotising vasculitis affecting small-to-medium-size vessels and associated with asthma and eosinophilia.
A clinical approach to define Churg-Strauss syndrome was that of Lanham and colleagues (Lanham JG 1984) at the Hammersmith Hospital, London, who have defined the disorder as a syndrome including:
(1) a history of asthma; (2) blood eosinophilia (>1500 cells/mcl); and (3) systemic vasculitis involving two or more organs.
Unfortunately, the involvement of two or more than two organs is difficult to assess without doing a biopsy—an invasive procedure in patients who may be very ill and need initiation of aggressive systemic corticosteroid treatment. An important clinical clue to the diagnosis of CSS in patients with chronic rhinosinusitis associated with the eosinophilic phenotype of asthma is to pay particular attention to every extra-respiratory manifestations , such as paresthesias, skin eruption or systemic symptoms.
The detection of ANCA, particularly P-ANCA (perinuclear pattern at indirect immnofluorescence) with anti-myeloperoxidase (anti MPO) specificity (ELISA assay) supports the diagnosis, but ANCA are present in only 35-40 % of patients.

3. The phases of CSS

In many patients, the disease follows a characteristic 3-stage course (Lanham JG 1984). Asthma and/or allergic rhinitis with or without nasal polyposis precedes full development of the syndrome, usually by many years. Significant blood eosinophilia, an unusual finding in uncomplicated asthma may also be present at this early stage of disease.
In the next stage, tissue infiltration by eosinophils, with or without granuloma formation, occurs in various organs, particularly in the upper and lower respiratory tract, the gastrointestinal tract, and the myocardium. Clinically, this stage is characterized by symptoms and findings related to tissue eosinophilia. Vasculitis is still absent at this stage.
The third phase of disease is defined by the onset of systemic vasculitis, which usually develops several years after the onset of asthma. Necrotizing small-vessel vasculitis may be clinically apparent in peripheral nerves (mono- or polyneuropathy, mononeuritis multiplex), skin (purpura), and kidneys (necrotizing and crescentic glomerulonephritis) (Gross WL. 2002).
Although these phases are conceptually helpful, they might not be clinically identifiable in all patients, and they often do not occur in sequence. The eosinophilic phase of the disease is the most challenging phase from the clinical diagnostic point of view. Tissue infiltration by eosinophils is observed in a variety of other conditions, including drug hypersensitivity, parasitic infections, malignancies, and allergic conditions. Chronic eosinophilic pneumonia (PEC) which frequently occurs in association with asthma and peripheral blood eosinophilia, may mimic CSS, with the only differences that necrotizing lesions are less apparent. Gastrointestinal eosinophilic disease may cause important symptoms even in the absence of vasculitis, while the development of vasculitis can be revealed by catastrophic abdominal complications, such as bowel perforation. Thus, there is no general consensus for classifying patients with this non-vasculitic second stage of CSS.
Another intriguing aspect is the differential diagnosis with the hypereosinophilic syndrome (HES). HES is defined by severe blood eosinophilia ($>1.5 \times 10^9$ cells/litre for > 6 months) and tissue infiltration by eosinophils resulting in organ dysfunction after exclusion of other causes of hypereosinophilia. Diffuse necrosis and vasculitis are generally absent, and a

history of asthma is rare in HES. Nevertheless, the clinical differentiation of HES from CSS is not always easy, particularly in the absence of apparent small-vessel vasculitis. Besides eosinophilia, HES and CSS share many common clinical features, such as neuropathy, dyspnea, fatigue, fever, and skin rashes. The role of eosinophilic granulocytes as the primary effector cells and the clinical similarities, may suggest a common etiology and pathogenesis for CSS and HES (Roufosse FE et al 2007), and raises the question whether CSS is simply the third disease stage of HES in patients with asthma.

Immunophenotype, T-cell clonal and cytogenetic studies, and molecular analysis to detect Fip1-like 1 (FIP1L1)–platelet-derived growth factor receptor-a (PDGFRA) gene fusion , the molecular markers in the most common form of HES, should therefore probably be performed for every patient suspected of having CSS, at least those who are ANCA-negative and/or without histologically proven vasculitis.

4. Etiology

4.1 The controversial association of drug treatment with CSS

Several exogenous triggering factors for the onset of disease have been suspected, including vaccinations, desensitizations, and drugs, such as macrolides, carbamazepine, quinine, and anti-asthma medications, like leukotriene-receptor antagonists (LTRAs) (Bibby et al 2010) and omalizumab, a monoclonal anti IgE antibody recently approved for severe allergic asthma (Wechsler ME et al 2009). It is more likely that anti-asthma medications unmask the underlying disease rather than cause the disease.

Systemic glucocorticoid withdrawal is facilitated by LTRAs, as well by increased dose of inhaled corticosteroids or omalizumab, leading CSS disease manifestations in those patients with undiagnosed but escalating CSS.

However, it is difficult to completely exclude the possibility that LTRAs play a causal role in the development of CSS in some patients.

An unusual CSS-like vasculitis has been associated with the use of free base cocaine (Orriols R et al. 1996) . The diagnosis of CSS in patients who use cocaine is a complicated issue because both acute and chronic eosinophilic pneumonia are manifestations of cocaine toxicity and antineutrophil cytoplasmic antibodies are detected in the majority of patients with cocaine-induced midline destructive lesions of the nose, even if the ANCAs associated with cocaine use are generally cANCA (cytoplamic pattern at indirect immnofluorescence), with anti-proteinase 3 (anti Pr3) specificity (ELISA assay).

4.2 Genetics

Whereas asthma often clusters in families, familial cases of CSS are exceptional, diminishing the role the genes may play in favor of environmental factors . Some studies, pooling CSS patients with WG and MPA, found a not significant association with a lower frequency of *HLA-DRB1*03*(Boki KA, 1997). More recent genetic studies suggested some predisposing hereditary factors, like the *HLA-DRB1*04* and *HLA-DRB1*07* alleles and the *HLA-DRB4* gene, which would be more frequent in Churg-Strauss syndrome patients than in healthy controls (Vaglio A. et al 2007). *HLA-DRB4* positive patients were associated with a higher number of vasculitis symptoms, in particular in the ANCA positive group. The interleukin IL10.2 haplotype, which is associated with enhanced IL-10 expression, and possibly the CD226 Gly307Ser polymorphism have been suggested as important genes in CSS (Wieczorek S et al, 2010) An attempt to undiscover the complex genome transcription profile of CSS has been performed by using focused microarray analysis of PBMCs in which a limited number of mRNA has been tested. Up regulation of a different number of PREP (Prolyl endopeptidase) genes suggest an enhanced immune response that might cause vascular damage (Tougan T et al, 2008).

5. Immunopatogenesis

The actual pathogenetic model of CSS is mainly incomplete.

The prodromic phase, characterized by asthma and allergic manifestations is thought to be related to a prominent Th2-lymphocyte activity. The second phase is characterized by eosinophilic infiltration into tissues. Eosinophils, when activated by Th2 related cytokines (interleukin (IL)-4, IL-5, IL-10 and IL-13), release major basic protein, eosinophilic cationic protein, eosinophil derived neurotoxin and eosinophil peroxidase, which may cause direct tissue and endothelial damage, and trigger the oxidative stress cascade.

The systemic phase, with the development of necrotizing vasculitis is associated with ANCA production, with the contribution of eosinophils. It is thought that IgE containing immune complexes (Manger BJ et al, 1985), surrounded by eosinophils and / or ANCA production would amplify and/or facilitate the development of vasculitic lesions in some patients.

5.1 The role of T cells

5.1.1 T helper cells

The pathogenic role of T cells in Churg Strauss Syndrome is suggested by different observations. First, T cells are commonly present in biopsies of active lesions, both vasculitic and granulomatous. A study of the clinicopathological features of neuropathy associated with the syndrome showed that CD8+ and CD4+ T cell outnumber eosinophils in neuronal biopsy specimen, suggesting a T-cell mediated damage of epineural vessels. (Hattori N et al, 1999).

Second, CSS shows a strong Th2-type immune response; T cell lines from CSS patients, generated *in vitro* by polyclonal stimulation, are polarized towards a Th2 phenotype (IL-4 and IL-13), which may explain the eosinophilia, the hallmark of the disease. The same cells have also been shown to release significant amounts of IFN-γ, which may be related to the granuloma formation (Kiene M et al, 2001). Current understanding of CSS implies that Th2-cells drive the activation of eosinophils, which secrete a variety of harmful mediators such as major basic protein, ECP, and eosinophil-derived neurotoxin. Interleukin-5 produced by Th2-cells is one of the key inducers of eosinophilia in CSS. Another molecule, which is supposed to play an important role , is CCL17/thymus and activation–related chemokine (TARC), a CC chemokine secreted from peripheral blood mononuclear cells (PBMCs) and various subsets of monocyte-derived dendritic cells (DCs). It is the ligand for CCR4 and CCR8 chemokine receptors on human PBMCs and T cells, respectively. Given the expression profile of its receptors and the ability of CCL17/TARC to selectively induce migration of CD4+CD45RO+ T cells producing Th2 cytokines , it may be crucial for the specific recruitment and trafficking of Th2 cells, which are known to be activated in CSS. CCL17/TARC in the affected tissue of CSS patients is readily identified by immuno-histochemical analysis, thus it may contribute to CSS pathogenesis by recruitment of Th2 cells into affected tissue (Dallos T et al, 2010).

T cells contribute to the pathogenesis of CSS by secretion of cytokines and chemokines, but they need to be functionally activated to accomplish this. Increases in serum concentration of eosinophilic cationic protein (suggesting eosinophil activation) and soluble thrombomodulin (indicating endothelial-cell damage) have been shown to correlate with soluble IL-2 receptor, suggesting T-cell activation (Schmitt WH et al, 1998).

5.1.2 T regulatory cells and Th17 populations

During the past decade, CD4+CD25+ regulatory T-cells (Tregs) have emerged as key players in the development of immunological tolerance. It has been proposed that onset of autoimmune diseases is determined by a dysfunction/deficiency of naturally occurring Treg cells and by an imbalance between self-reactive T-cells and natural Tregs. CSS patients at disease onset or relapse have fewer T regulatory cell subsets (CD4+CD25+ T cells) producing IL-10 (Tr1) than the patients in remission or patients with asthma. Moreover, the number of organs involved has been shown to correlate negatively with the number of T reg cells. This lower percentage of T reg cells during active CSS would, at least in part, explain the breakdown of immunological tolerance that leads to CSS onset. According to this hypothesis, maintenance of the numbers of regulatory T cells in patiens with chronic eosinophilic pneumonia (CEP) with asthma might inihibit CSS development (Tsurikisawa N et al, 2008).

T helper 17 cells (Th17) are a newly discovered subset of T helper cells producing interleukin 17 (IL-17) which are thought to play a role in inflammation and tissue injury (Steinman L, 2007). The percentage of Th17 in peripheral blood has been reported to be significantly higher in patients with active CSS than in healthy subjects or in patients with inactive disease (Saito H et al, 2009). An imbalance in the Th17/Treg ratio is associated to the immune suppressive degree of treated CSS patients (Jakiela B et al, 2011). These findings suggest Th17 and regulatory T cells may play important roles in the pathogenesis of CSS.

5.1.3 CD4+ and CD8+ T cell subsets

T cells normally recognize antigens as short peptides using their T cell receptor (TCR) specifically binding to MHC molecules on the surface of antigen-presenting cells. TCR recognition of the antigen results in stimulation and clonal proliferation of the activated T cell. Oligoclonal expanded T cells reflect conventional antigen (Ag) stimulation involving one every million T cells. In immune-mediated diseases where the antigen is unknown, studies of the TCR repertoire of expanded T cells can give clues to the nature of the antigen. Superantigen (SAg) are peptides that differ in several ways from conventional peptide antigens, in that they characteristically activate a much higher proportion of T cells than conventional antigens. Typically SAgs will stimulate up to 20% of circulating T cells. SAg stimulation of T cells bearing specific Vβ (Wei S et al, 1997) T-cell receptors (TCR) results in the polyclonal expansion of selected Vβ families in CD4+ and CD8+ cells, followed by T cell restricted deletion (Fraser J et al, 2000). Whether lymphocytes activation in CSS is induced by antigen (Ag) or superantigen (SAg) is not presently known. Oligoclonal expanded T cell have been actually found in CSS patients by immunoscope technique, but it is not known whether these expanded T cells are CD4+ or CD8+ (Muschen M et al, 1999). Immunoscope-based analysis of TCR repertoires in 7 CSS patients revealed clonal expansion (one or more dominant picks) of Vβ 21(7/7) , Vβ 11 (3/7) and Vβ 12 (2/7) families.

One or more Vβ families were found numerically expanded by flow cytometry among CD8 T cells population of all CSS patients who were investigated, both in clinical remission and during treatment for active disease. These expanded T cells were mostly represented by CD8+ lymphocytes with effector memory phenotype. Each CD8+/Vβ+ expanded population has been shown to be the result of the proliferation of a clonal T cell bearing a defined TCR, as detected by analysis of TCR-V-Jγ rearrangement (Guida G et al, 2008).

These CD8+/Vβ+ expanded populations have an effector memory (TEM) phenotype, as evidenced by flow cytometric analysis of CD45RA expression combined to CD62L, CCR7 or CD28 (Morice WG et al, 2004; Sallusto F et al, 1999). It has been suggested that circulating CD8+/Vβ+ TEM are antigen driven cells which may infiltrate target organs and participate to the inflammatory cascade of both vasculitic and granulomatous lesions (Guida G et al, 2008).

A few preliminary reports (Boita M et al, 2010), showed an increased expression of CCR5 and CXCR3 in CD8+ lymphocytes compared to healthy controls, both in Vβ expanded families and in total CD8+ cells, suggesting Th1 polarization. On the other hand, increased expression of CCR4 and CRTH2 was present in CD4+ cells, suggesting Th2 polarization. An oligoclonal pattern was present in most Vβ families of CD8+ lymphocytes, whereas the number of oligoclonal families of the CD4 subset was lower. TCR studies on cloned CD8 lymphocytes showed the presence of a unique TCR in each of the expanded CD8+/Vbeta+ populations.

Based on these preliminary data, it is hypotizable that monoclonal/oligoclonal expanded populations of effector CD8+ lymphocytes with a Th1/proinflammatory profile are involved in vasculitic damage, whereas CD4+ cells with a Th2 profile mediate eosinophil-rich inflammation and asthma.

5.2 The role of ANCA and B cells

Antineutrophil cytoplasmic antibodies (ANCA) are predominantly IgG autoantibodies directed against constituents of primary granules of neutrophils and monocytes' lysosomes. They exist in two forms: c-ANCA that has a Immuno Fluorescent (IF) citoplasmatic pattern against proteinase-3 (Pr-3) and p- ANCA that consists of a IF perinuclear pattern directed against myeloperoxidase (MPO). In studies with large cohort of patients with small vessel vasculitis, ANCA were detected in about 38-59% of patients with Churg-Strauss syndrome (Guillevine L et al, 1999; Cohen P et al, 1995). ANCA appearance might precede CSS clinical onset in some patients, but the primum movens for their synthesis remains unknown. In this context, B cells could play a role as autoreactive cells producing ANCA auto antibodies.

There is no uniform theory explaining how ANCA may cause pauci-immune vasculitides but the common pathogenetic model suggests that binding of ANCA causes activation of neutrophils, with subsequent increased adhesion and migration to endothelium, release of proteolytic granule enzymes and proinflammatory cytokines, generation of respiratory burst, and, eventually, endothelial cell damage. ANCA-mediated neutrophil activation disrupts apoptosis of neutrophils which undergo secondary necrosis with subsequent release of inflammatory mediators, hence amplifying the process (Csernok E, 2003) . ANCA promote the interaction between neutrophils and endothelial cells through β2 integrins (CD11a/CD18 and CD11b/CD18) and GTP binding protein chemokine receptors. Afterwards, noxious neutrophils' constituents—reactive oxygen species and proteolytic enzymes—are secreted, damaging vessel walls. Proinflammatory cytokines secreted by neutrophils as a result of ANCA binding include IL-1β, TNF-α, IL-6, IL-8, monocyte chemoattractant protein 1, and leukotriene B4. ANCA-mediated cytokine secretion will activate and recruit inflammatory cells, amplifying and perpetuating the inflamatory response, with monocytes and T cells participating later in the process (Jennette JC et al, 2006).

5.3 The role of eosinophils

CSS is defined by blood eosinophilia usually >10% and eosinophilic infiltration into affected tissues. According to this, IL-5 and other Th2 cytokines may in fact play an important role in the pathogenesis of CSS.

The production of IL-5 and other cytokines before and after stimulation with T cell-specific stimuli (anti- CD3 and anti-CD28) have been analyzed in peripheral blood mononuclear cells (PBMCs) obtained from patients with CSS, showing significant increased IL-5 level in CSS compared with healthy controls. However, IL-5 production in PBMCs cultured without T cell-specific stimuli (anti-CD3) and costimulatory signals (anti-CD28) was low both in CSS patients and controls suggesting that PBMCs in CSS require T cell activation to secrete large amounts of IL-5 (Kiene M et al, 2001; Hellmick B, 2005).

IL5 is the most potent cytokine which induces terminal differentiation of committed eosinophil precursors. Moreover, IL-5 prolongs the survival of mature eosinophils. In addition, IL-5 activates mature eosinophils and selectively induces degranulation and antibody-dependent cytotoxicity of eosinophils. Of particular interest with regard to the pathogenesis of CSS and vasculitis is the capability of IL-5 to promote the adhesion of eosinophils to vascular endothelium and CC chemokine receptor 3 (CCR3)-dependent migration of eosinophils from the vasculature into the tissues.

Because organ damage in CSS is at least partially mediated by direct invasion and degranulation of eosinophils into the tissues, other mediators than IL-5 might also be important. Recently, a chemokine family specifically mediating trafficking of eosinophils to inflammatory sites has been characterized. Currently, CCL11, CCL24, and CCL26 are grouped together as eotaxins. They all bind to a common receptor CCR3. As to be expected for eosinophil chemotactic proteins, eotaxins are induced by Th-2 associated cytokines such as IL-4 and IL-13. Heavy tissue eosinophilia is found in most biopsies from active CSS patients. Serum eotaxin-3, but not eotaxin-1 and eotaxin-2, levels have been found greatly elevated in active CSS patients compared to healthy controls. The elevated eotaxin-3 serum levels rapidly decreased upon efficient immunosuppression (Polzer K et al, 2008). Thus, eotaxin-3 constitutes a possible target for the pharmacotherapy of CSS.

6. Markers of disease

The CHCC classification introduced the concept of surrogate markers of vasculitis but a list of markers was not provided and ANCA were not included. Conflicting results of studies relating titers of ANCA to disease activity of ANCA associated vasculitides (ASV) have been reported. A recent retrospective study suggested that acute rise in ANCA titer is highly predictive of a relapse of ASV (Lurati-Ruiz F et al, 2005; Baldini C et al, 2009). When the ANCA titer remains positive during immunosuppressive treatment for induction of remission, relapses within 5 years are more likely to occur (Sanders JS et al, 2006).

The presence of ANCA was associated with renal disease, peripheral neuropathy, and biopsy-proven vasculitis. Absence of ANCA was associated with heart involvement and fever. This demonstrates that ANCA-positive Churg-Strauss syndrome differs phenotypically from ANCA negative Churg-Strauss syndrome (Sable-Fourtassou R et al,

2005; Sinico RA et al, 2005). Furthermore, ANCA might possibly indicate more severe disease at diagnosis, as assessed by the proportion of patients with poor scores in FFS and the Birmingham vasculitis activity score (BVAS).
Several research teams are attempting to identify reliable marker(s) of CSS activity. Promising markers of the disease are those referring to activity and survival of eosinophils, like serum eosinophil cationic protein (Guilpain P et al, 2007), IL-5 (Tsukadaira A et al, 1999) or eotaxin-3 (CCL26), an eosinotactic chemokine mainly expressed on vascular endothelial cells and dermal fibroblasts (Polzer K et al, 2008).
Recently, serum levels of TARC have been reported to be significantly elevated in CSS patients with active disease, and to correlate with the clinical course of the disease and with the absolute eosinophil counts, as well as with IgE levels (Dallos T et al, 2010). No confirmatory data are otherwise reported about the role of other eosinophil survival related molecules and interaction with the endothelium.
It has been suggested that the detection of clonal expanded peripheral $V\beta^{+}/CD8+$ T cell populations (assessed by flow cytometry combined to analysis of TCR-γ gene rearrangement) is stable over time and might be useful in the differential diagnosis of CSS, as suggested by the negative findings in asthmatic controls (Guida G et al, 2008).
Many of these observations require further validation and all the above-mentioned laboratory tests are not yet widely available outside highly specialized centers. Attempts to individualize CSS subgroups remain highly valuable and may further help to elucidate and understand its different underlying physio-pathogenetic mechanisms.

7. Clinical presentation and classification of severity

The most typical clinical presentation of Churg-Strauss syndrome is the appearance of vasculitic manifestations in a patient with known allergic rhinitis, sinus polyposis, and late-onset asthma, usually preexisting for 5-10 years. General symptoms (i.e., fever or weight loss), mononeuritis multiplex, and/or necrotic cutaneous purpura are the most frequent manifestations at disease onset, in combination with elevated blood eosinophilia and inflammatory syndrome.

7.1 Systemic symptoms and laboratory findings

Fever is quite frequent , as well weight loss, which is often great and might herald onset of the vasculitic phase, as do fatigue and malaise. Arthralgias are common, but frank arthritis is rare. Abnormal laboratory findings in patients with Churg-Strauss syndrome include anaemia, leukocytosis, increased peripheral blood eosinophil count, and a raised erythrocyte sedimentation rate. Rarely, eosinophilia is not present, and wide-ranging and rapid changes in eosinophil counts happen. Use of corticosteroids to treat asthma may result in failure to detect eosinophilia in a patient with undiagnosed Churg-Strauss syndrome. Blood chemistry and urinalysis findings might show occult renal disease. Antineutrophil cytoplasmic antibodies are present in more than half of patients with a perinuclear staining pattern. Antineutrophil cytoplasmic antibody-positivity needs to be confirmed by demonstration of anti-myeloperoxidase (MPO) antibodies in serum.

7.2 Skin

Skin lesions are common and variable, occurring 40-81% of CSS patients and being the presenting sign in 14% of the patients (Bosco L et al 2011). In the majority of these patients, skin lesions allowed for the histopathological diagnosis of CSS. The most common clinical features are papulo-nodules with the histological picture of extravascular Churg-Strauss granuloma followed by purpuric and/or necrotic lesions in the lower limbs corresponding to small-vessel vasculitis with eosinophils. Less common lesions include urticarial lesions and livedo reticularis. Therefore, a high index of suspicion on skin lesions and the proper lesion selection for histological examination may be very important for early diagnosis of CSS. Clinical-pathological correlation is essential, as both clinical and histological features are not pathognomonic.

7.3 Respiratory system

Upper airway

Overall, 80% of CSS patients have active sinonasal symptoms at the time of presentation and worsening of their nasal symptoms may be the main event leading to their diagnosis (Srouji I et al. 2008) . Nearly half CSS patients had undergone nasal surgery. Nasal symptoms that are of particolar interest are nasal obstruction , rhinorrhea , anosmia , and excessive sneezing . Other symptoms include nasal crusting, purulent nasal discharge, and epistaxis. Sinonasal symptoms are common at initial presentation of CSS, emphasizing the role of otolaryngologists in its diagnosis. Overall, CSS-related sinonasal morbidity is significant and comparable with that of the general rhinosinusitis population. It predominantly results from symptoms of allergic rhinitis, but a significant proportion of CSS patients also report milder forms of crusting, epistaxis, and of purulent sinusitis, symptoms which are more commonly attributed to patients with Wegener Granulomatosis.

Asthma

Asthma is one of the key features of Churg-Strauss syndrome, usually it is adult-onset asthma, preceded by sinusitis in all the patients and nasal polyposis in most of them. Asthma at its onset is generally severe and very poorly controlled. Atopy is present in more than half of patients. Onset of vasculitic symptoms is often accompanied by asthma exacerbation and lung involvement. After introducing the treatment and achieving stable remission, asthma severity/control and lung function tests improved, but systemic low-dose corticosteroid therapy is often required to maintain asthma control in most of CSS patients (Szczeklik W et al. 2011) .

Lung involvement

The lung is the most commonly involved organ. Pulmonary hemorrhage is much less common than in the other small-vessel vasculitides. At histopathologic analysis, both necrotizing small-vessel vasculitis and an eosinophil-rich inflammatory infiltrate with necrotizing granulomas are seen (Katzenstein AL 2000). The most common lung radiographic manifestations of CSS consist of transient, bilateral, nonsegmental areas of consolidation without predilection for any lung zone (Silva CI et al 2005) . The areas of consolidation can be transient, resembling Löffler syndrome, or predominantly peripheral , resembling chronic eosinophilic pneumonia or organizing pneumonia . The most common abnormality at high-resolution CT, seen in up to 90% of patients, is bilateral areas of ground-glass opacity or consolidation (Worthy SA et al 1998). These usually have a symmetric distribution and often a peripheral predominance; less commonly, they have a peri-bronchial or patchy random distribution . Another relatively common finding is the presence of septal lines, seen in approximately 50% of patients. Interlobular septal thickening may reflect the presence of edema secondary to cardiac involvement or eosinophilic infiltration of the septa.

7.4 Heart

Cardiovascular involvement is the leading cause of morbidity and death in Churg-Strauss syndrome. Heart manifestations of Churg-Strauss syndrome (CSS) are varied. In the early stages of the disease, it is difficult to distinguish between lesions that are specific to CSS and those of other etiologies. A specific physiopathology that is not mediated by ANCA seems to be involved in the genesis of CSS-related heart lesions. A negative antineutrophil cytoplasmic antibodies (ANCA) test and much higher eosinophil counts distinguish patients with cardiac involvement from those without (Neumann T et al 2009). Detailed cardiac evaluation revealed a unexpectedly high prevalence (more than 50%) of cardiac involvement in CSS patients. Impaired left ventricular function, mild to severe valvular insufficiencies , and pericardial effusions are common findings in these patients. Endomyocarditis may be found by cardiac MRI, cardiac thrombus formation, and endomyocardial biopsy, and is associated with impaired cardiac function. After therapy, most patients may regain or maintain good cardiac function. However, patients with endomyocarditis have a more severe outcome. Cardiac MRI is a sensitive, non-invasive method to detect cardiac lesions in patients whose conventional investigations indicated no cardiac disease and to assess the extent of cardiac involvement in symptomatic patients. Cardiac MRI can help to evaluate the therapeutic effect of immunosuppressants in CSS (Marmursztejn J et al 2010)

7.5 Central nervous system

Central nervous system (CNS) involvement account for 20% of neuropathy in CSS, including arachnoid hemorrhage, cerebrovascular neuropathy, meningitis, and diffuse brain damage, which may respond to treatment with high dose of prednisone plus immunosuppressants (Zhang W et al 2009).

7.6 Peripheral nervous system

A peripheral neuropathy is seen in up to 75 percent of patients with CSS. Mononeuritis multiplex and distal symmetrical and asymmetrical sensorimotor neuropathy are equally frequent. Severe neuropathic pain may accompany the peripheral neuropathy. The diagnosis of polyneuropathy is based on clinical and electrophysiologic studies, but precise histology, immuno-histochemistry and morphometric study of the peripheral nerve biopsy may be decisive in establishing the diagnosis (Kararizou E et al 2011) . There may be 2 pathogenetic mechanisms of neuropathy with CSS: ANCA-related vascular fibrinoid necrosis, and a toxic eosinophilic effect on nerve fibers which is independent of ANCA. Therapy targeting activated eosinophils may be a possible treatment for intractable neuropathy of CSS (Oka N et al. 2010).

7.7 Gastrointestinal tract

An eosinophilic gastroenteritis, characterized by abdominal pain, diarrhea, gastrointestinal bleeding, and colitis, may precede or coincide with the vasculitic phase of CSS. Gastrointestinal involvement may result in acute abdomen, acute acalculous cholecystitis, pancreatitis, mesenteric vasculitis, and bowel perforation due to necrotizing vasculitis (Rolla

G et al. 2007). Severe gastrointestinal tract involvement is a well-recognized important negative prognostic factor. With severe gastrointestinal disease, including intestinal bleeding, perforation, and pancreatitis, survival was approximately 65% at 78 months compared with nearly 90% without such involvement (Guillevin L et al 1999).

7.8 Renal

The frequency of renal involvement varies among studies , from 15 to 30% (Sinico RA et al. 2006). A few patients have rapidly progressive or acute renal insufficiency (plasma creatinine concentration >1.4 mg/dL), while most patients have isolated proteinuria or microscopic hematuria. Nephrotic syndrome is rarely reported. In the severe cases, renal biopsy shows necrotizing glomerulonephritis. A positive test for antineutrophil cytoplasmic antibodies (ANCA) is found in all patients with glomerulonephritis. Systemic hypertension affects approximately 10 to 30 percent of patients with CSS and may reflect renal involvement with CSS or be a complication of glucocorticoid therapy.

8. Assessment of prognosis

The 1996 Five-Factor Score (FFS) for systemic necrotizing vasculitides (polyarteritis nodosa, microscopic polyangiitis , and Churg-Strauss syndrome) is used to evaluate prognosis at diagnosis. Recently (Merkel PA et al 2009) the FFS have been revisited, including Wegener granulomatosis (Guillevin L et al 2011).Clinical, laboratory, and immunologic manifestations present at diagnosis of systemic necrotizing vasculitides for 1108 consecutive patients registered in the French Vasculitis Study Group database were evaluated.Overall mortality was 19.8% (219/1108); mortality for each of the systemic necrotizing vasculitides was: 27.5 % for microscopic polyangiitis, 24.6 % for polyarteritis nodosa,13.9 % for CSS and 13.2 % for WG. The following factors were significantly associated with higher 5-year mortality: age >65 years, cardiac symptoms, gastrointestinal involvement, and renal insufficiency (stabilized peak creatinine ≥150 μmol/L). All were disease-specific ($p < 0.001$); the presence of each was accorded +1 point. Ear, nose, and throat (ENT) symptoms, affecting patients with WG and CSS, were associated with a lower relative risk of death, and their absence was scored +1 point ($p < 0.001$). Only renal insufficiency was retained (not proteinuria or microscopic hematuria) as impinging on outcome. According to the 2009 FFS, 5-year mortality rates for scores of 0, 1, and ≥2 were 9%, 21% ($p < 0.005$), and 40% ($p < 0.0001$), respectively.The revised FFS for the 4 systemic necrotizing vasculitides now comprises 4 factors associated with poorer prognosis and 1 with better outcome. The retained items demonstrate that visceral involvement weighs heavily on outcome.

9. Therapy

9.1 Corticosteroids

The primary therapy for CSS is systemic glucocorticoids. An additional immunosuppressive agent is typically added in patients with more advanced or refractory disease and in those whose disease flares with tapering of systemic glucocorticoids .

Systemic glucocorticoid therapy is the most important treatment for CSS.Treatment is generally initiated with prednisone at a dose of 0.5 to 1.5 mg/kg per day, the higher dose used for patients with more severe vasculitis .Intravenous glucocorticoid (eg,

methylprednisolone 1 g daily for three days) is used for initial therapy, followed by oral glucocorticoid therapy in the most severe cases.
The majority of patients with CSS achieve a remission with glucocorticoid therapy alone, but relapses were common, and up to one-third of patients require additional immunosuppressive therapy (Ribi C et al.). In CSS patients with an FFS of 0, survival is excellent, confirming the predictive value of the FFS in this disease. Once disease manifestations have come under control, the glucocorticoid dose is gradually tapered over approximately 12 to 18 months, as tolerated. Unfortunately, over the long term, most patients continued to take oral CS, which might explain the high rate of CS-related adverse events.

9.2 Cyclophosphamide

The addition of cyclophosphamide is recommended for patients with a "five factors score" of 1, particularly in the presence of cardiac or central nervous system involvement .
Cyclophosphamide may be administered orally every day or intravenously once a month . Extrapolating from Wegener's granulomatosis, outcomes with daily and monthly regimens were similar; a slightly greater risk of bladder toxicity with the daily regimen and a slightly greater risk of relapse with the monthly regimen have been noted. The duration of cyclophosphamide therapy remains controversial. When used to treat Wegener's granulomatosis, typically a six month regimen is used.

9.3 Alternative immunosuppressive therapy

An alternative regimen for patients with milder non life-threatening disease, would be initial treatment with glucocorticoids plus either azathioprine (Bosch X et al 2007) or methotrexate (De Groot K et al 2005). In the latter study of 100 patients with early systemic ANCA-positive vasculitides (including CSS) that compared glucocorticoids plus methotrexate with glucocorticoids plus cyclophosphamide, the remission success rate was similar at six months (90 and 94 percent, respectively). However, the methotrexate regimen was less successful for patients with more extensive disease or pulmonary involvement.
Interferon-alpha appeared to be an effective and well-tolerated treatment for induction of remission in patients with refractory Churg-Strauss syndrome in a phase II study (Metzler C. et al 2008). . Recombinant interferon-alpha has been reported to be partially effective in the prevention of major relapses in patients with Churg-Strauss syndrome (Metzler C. et al 2010). Due to numerous side effects and infections during long-term administration its use should be restricted to patients with contraindications against conventional immunosuppressive therapies.

9.4 Immunosoppressive maintenance tharapy

Once remission is induced with cyclophosphamide and glucocorticoid therapy (which usually occurs within six to twelve months), patients are switched to maintenance therapy with less toxic immunosuppressive drugs, usually azathioprine or methotrexate, in combination with a tapering dose of glucocorticoids. For patients whose disease is not severe enough to require cyclophosphamide, but requires long-term therapy with moderate to high dose prednisone (more than 10 mg daily), an immunosuppressive agent is often added for a glucocorticoid sparing effect.

9.5 New promising therapeutic approach: the monoclonal antibodies

Rituximab

B cell depletion with rituximab has allowed remissions in relapsing or refractory antineutrophil cytoplasmic antibody (ANCA)-associated vasculitis in small studies. A multicenter survey of rituximab therapy for refractory ANCA-associated vasculitis has been recently published (Jones RB et al. 2009). This permitted comparison of rituximab dosing regimens, the value of continuing immunosuppression, and investigation of ANCA and B cell levels as re-treatment biomarkers. Retrospective, standardized data collection from 65 sequential patients receiving rituximab for refractory ANCA-associated vasculitis at 4 centers in the UK was used. All patients achieved B cell depletion. Complete remission occurred in 49 of the 65 patients (75%), partial remission in 15 (23%), and no response in 1 (2%). The prednisolone dosage was reduced from 12.5 mg/day (median) to 9.0 mg/day at 6 months (P = 0.0006). Immunosuppressive therapy was withdrawn in 37 of 60 patients (62%). Twenty-eight of 49 patients who achieved full remission (57%) experienced relapse (median 11.5 months). B cell return preceded relapse in 14 of 27 patients (52%). Although ANCA levels fell after rituximab therapy, relapse was not associated with ANCA positivity or a rise in ANCA levels. Neither the initial rituximab regimen (4 infusions of 375 mg/m(2) each given 1 week apart or 2 infusions of 1 gm each given 2 weeks apart) nor withdrawal of immunosuppressive therapy (37 of 60 patients [62%]) influenced the timing of relapse. Thirty-eight patients received>or=2 courses of rituximab, and complete remission was induced or maintained in 32 of them (84%). IgM levels fell, although IgG levels remained stable. Forty-six serious adverse events occurred, including 2 episodes of late-onset neutropenia, which were attributed to rituximab. Rituximab seems to be effective for inducing remission in refractory ANCA-associated vasculitis. Nevertheless, relapses may occurr, but re-treatment has been found effective and safe. ANCA and B cell levels lacked sufficient sensitivity to guide the timing of re-treatment.
Severe bronchospasm associated with rituximab for refractory Churg-Strauss syndrome has been reported (Bouldouyre MA et al 2009).

Mepolizumab

Levels of IL-5, a cytokine regulating eosinophils, can be increased in patients with CSS. Mepolizumab, a humanized monoclonal anti-IL-5 antibody, decreases steroid requirements in patients with non-CSS hypereosinophilic syndromes. Recently, whether mepolizumab would safely allow corticosteroid tapering in patients with steroid-dependent CSS while decreasing serum markers of disease activity has been investigated in an open-label pilot study (Kim S et al 2010). Seven patients received 4 monthly doses of mepolizumab to assess whether it safely decreased CSS disease activity and permitted tapering of systemic corticosteroids. Mepolizumab was safe and well tolerated in patients with CSS. Mepolizumab reduced eosinophil counts and allowed for safe corticosteroid reduction in all 7 subjects. On cessation of mepolizumab, CSS manifestations recurred, necessitating corticosteroid bursts. Mepolizumab is a safe and well-tolerated therapy in patients with CSS, offering clinical benefit by enabling corticosteroid tapering while maintaining clinical stability.

Omalizumab

The anti-IgE monoclonal antibody omalizumab is approved as add-on therapy of severe allergic asthma . Besides the IgE blockage effect, studies have shown antiallergic and anti-inflammatory properties of anti-IgE, among which is the reduction in circulating and tissue eosinophils.

Efficacy of omalizumab therapy in some cases of CSS have been reported. In two patients whose disease was not controlled by systemic glucocorticoid , omalizumab obtained disease control (Pabst S et al 2008). Another report described similar results with anti-IgE in a patient with Churg–Strauss syndrome (CSS) who still presented with asthma which was difficult to control. The asthma did not improve despite the use of high-dose inhaled corticosteroids, long-acting β2 agonists and several courses of steroid pulse therapy. Omalizumab was given and his asthma was controlled and a marked improvement in eosinophilia was observed (Giavina-Bianchi P et al 2007).

On the other hand, there are at least three cases of temporal association between anti-IgE use and the development of CSS. CSS was probably caused by systemic steroid tapering in these cases, rather than anti-IgE use.

Omalizumab can be used in patients with CSS to treat and control asthma, but it is probable that anti-IgE alone is not enough to control CSS activity. Although we are getting more evidence about the safety of omalizumab in patients with asthma and CSS, larger long-term studies are needed before the widespread use of anti-IgE can be recommended and also to verify if it is effective in the treatment of CSS.

10. References

Baldini C, Della Rossa A, Grossi S, et al. Churg–Strauss syndrome: outcome and long-term follow-up of 38 patients from a single Italian centre [in Italian]. Reumatismo; 61:118–124. 2009

Bibby S, Healy B, Steele R, Kumareswaran K, Nelson H, Beasley R. Association between leukotriene receptor antagonist therapy and Churg-Strauss syndrome: an analysis of the FDA AERS database. *Thorax* 65(2):132-8, 2010

Boita M, Guida G, Circosta P, Heffler E, Stella S, Elia AR, Rolla G, Cignetti A. Functional and molecular characterization of monoclonal T cell expansions in Churg Strauss Syndrome. Abstract, WIRM IV (World Immune Regulation Meeting), Davos, Switzerland, 2010

Boki KA, Dafni U, Karpouzas GA, Papasteriades C, Drosos AA, Moutsopoulos HM. Necrotizing vasculitis in Greece: clinical, immunological and immunogenetic aspects. A study of 66 patients. Br J Rheumatol. 1997 Oct;36(10):1059-66.

Bosch X, Guilabert A, Espinosa G, Mirapeix E. Treatment of antineutrophil cytoplasmic antibody associated vasculitis: a systematic review. JAMA. 2007;298(6):655

Bosco L, Peroni A, Schena D, Colato C, Girolomoni G. Cutaneous manifestations of Churg-Strauss syndrome: report of two cases and review of the literature. Clin Rheumatol. 2011 Apr;30(4):573-80. Epub 2010 Oct 15.

Bouldouyre MA, Cohen P, Guillevin L. Severe bronchospasm associated with rituximab for refractory Churg-Strauss syndrome. Ann Rheum Dis. 2009;68(4):606.

Clinical Research Consortium. Comparison of disease activity measures for anti-neutrophil cytoplasmic autoantibody (ANCA)-associated vasculitis. Ann Rheum Dis. 2009 Jan;68(1):103-6. Epub 2008 Jul 29.

Cohen P, Guillevin L, Baril L, Lhote F, Noel LH, Lesavre P. Persistence of antineutrophil cytoplasmic antibodies (ANCA) in asymptomatic patients with systemic polyarteritis nodosa or Churg-Strauss syndrome: follow-up of 53 patients. Clin Exp Rheumatol. 1995 Mar-Apr;13(2):193-8.

Csernok E. Anti-neutrophil cytoplasmic antibodies and pathogenesis of small vessel vasculitides. Autoimmun Rev; 2: 158 - 64.2003.Kararizou E, Davaki P, Spengos K, Karandreas N, Dimitracopoulos A, Vassilopoulos D.

Churg-Strauss syndrome complicated by neuropathy: a clinicopathological study of clinicopathological study of nine cases.Clin Neuropathol. 2011 Jan-Feb;30(1):11-7.

Dallos T, Heiland GR, Strehl J, Karonitsch T, Gross WL, Moosig F, Holl-Ulrich C, Distler JH, Manger B, Schett G, Zwerina J.CCL17/thymus and activation-related chemokine in Churg-Strauss syndrome. Arthritis Rheum. 2010 Nov;62(11):3496-503.

De Groot K, Rasmussen N, Bacon PA, Tervaert JW, Feighery C, Gregorini G, Gross WL, Luqmani R, Jayne DR. Randomized trial of cyclophosphamide versus methotrexate for induction of remission in early systemic antineutrophil cytoplasmic antibody-associated vasculitis. Arthritis Rheum. 2005;52(8):2461

Giavina-Bianchi P, Giavina-Bianchi M, Agondi R, Kalil J. Three months' administration of anti-IgE to a patient with Churg-Strauss syndrome. J Allergy Clin Immunol. 2007;119(5):1279

Gross WL. Churg-Strauss syndrome: update on recent developments. Curr Opin Rheumatol. 2002 Jan;14(1):11-4.

Guida G, Vallario A, Stella S, Boita M, Circosta P, Mariani S, Prato G, Heffler E, Bergia R, Sottile A, Rolla G, Cignetti A. Clonal CD8+ TCR-Vbeta expanded populations with effector memory phenotype in Churg Strauss syndrome. Clin Immunol. 2008 Jul;128(1):94-102. Epub 2008 May 23.

Guillevin L, Cohen P, Gayraud M, Lhote F, Jarrouse B, Cassaus P, Churg-Strauss syndrome: clinical study and long-term follow-up of 96 patients, Medicine (Baltimore), Volume: 78, (1999), pp. 26—37

Guillevin L, Pagnoux C, Seror R, Mahr A, Mouthon L, Le Toumelin P; French Vasculitis Study Group (FVSG). The Five-Factor Score revisited: assessment of prognoses of systemic necrotizing vasculitides based on the French Vasculitis Study Group (FVSG) cohort. Medicine (Baltimore). 2011 Jan;90(1):19-27.

Guillevin L, Vignaux O. Cardiac magnetic resonance imaging in Churg-Strauss-syndrome. Impact of immunosuppressants on outcome assessed in a prospective study on 8 patients. Clin Exp Rheumatol. 2010

Guilpain P, Auclair JF, Tamby MC, et al. Serum eosinophil cationic protein: a marker of disease activity in Churg–Strauss syndrome. Ann N Y Acad Sci; 1107:392–399. 2007

Hellmich B, Csernok E, Gross WL. Proinflammatory cytokines and autoimmunity in Churg-Strauss syndrome. Ann N Y Acad Sci. 2005 Jun;1051:121-31.

J.Fraser, V.Arcus, P.Kong, E.Baker, and T.Proft, Superantigens - powerful modifiers of the immune system, Mol.Med.Today 6 125-132 .2000

Jakiela B, Sanak M, Szczeklik W, Sokolowska B, Plutecka H, Mastalerz L, Musial J, Szczeklik A. Both Th2 and Th17 responses are involved in the pathogenesis of Churg-Strauss syndrome. Clin Exp Rheumatol. 2011

Jennette JC, Falk RJ, Andrassy K, et al. Nomenclature of systemic vasculitides: proposal of an international consensus conference. Arthritis Rheum 1994; 37: 187–92.

Jennette, J. C., H. Xiao, and R. J. Falk. Pathogenesis of vascular inflammation by anti-neutrophil cytoplasmic antibodies. J. Am. Soc. Nephrol. 17: 1235-1242. 2006.

Jones RB, Ferraro AJ, Chaudhry AN, Brogan P, Salama AD, Smith KG, Savage CO, Jayne DR. A multicenter survey of rituximab therapy for refractory antineutrophil cytoplasmic antibody-associated vasculitis. Arthritis Rheum. 2009;60(7):2156.

Kararizou E, Davaki P, Spengos K, Karandreas N, Dimitracopoulos A, Vassilopoulos Katzenstein AL. Diagnostic features and differential diagnosis of Churg-Strauss syndrome in the lung: a review. Am J Clin Pathol 2000;114:767–772

Kiene M, Csernok E, Mueller A. Elevated interleukin-4 and interleukin-13 production by T cell lines from patients with Churg-Strauss syndrome. Arthritis Rheum. 44: 469–473. 2001.

Kim S, Marigowda G, Oren E, Israel E, Wechsler ME. Mepolizumab as a steroid-sparing treatment option in patients with Churg-Strauss syndrome. J Allergy Clin Immunol. 2010;125(6):1336.

Krischer JP, Luqmani R, Mahr AD, Matteson EL, Specks U, Stone JH; Vasculitis

Lanham JG, Elkon KB, Pusey CD, et al. Systemic vasculitis with asthma and eosinophilia: a clinical approach to the Churg-Strauss syndrome. Medicine (Baltimore) 1984; 63: 65–81.

Lurati-Ruiz F, Spertini F. Predictive value of antineutrophil cytoplasmic antibodies in small-vessel vasculitis. J Rheumatol; 32:2167–2172. 2005

Manger BJ, Krapf FE, Gramatzki M, et al. IgE-containing circulating immune complexes inChurg–Strauss vasculitis.Scand J Immunol; 21:369–373. 1985

Marmursztejn J, Cohen P, Duboc D, Pagnoux C, Mouthon L, Guilpain P, Legmann P, Masi AT, Hunder GG, Lie JT, et al. The American College of Rheumatology 1990 criteria for the classification of Churg-Strauss syndrome (allergic granulomatosis and angiitis). Arthritis Rheum 1990; 33: 1094–100.

Merkel PA, Cuthbertson DD, Hellmich B, Hoffman GS, Jayne DR, Kallenberg CG,

Metzler C, Csernok E, Gross WL, Hellmich B. Interferon-alpha for maintenance of remission in Churg-Strauss syndrome: a long-term observational study. Clin Exp Rheumatol. 2010 Jan-Feb;28(1 Suppl 57):24-30

Metzler C, Schnabel A, Gross WL, Hellmich B. A phase II study of interferon-alpha for the treatment of refractory Churg-Strauss syndrome. Clin Exp Rheumatol. 2008 May-Jun;26(3 Suppl 49):S35-40.

Morice WG, Kimlinger T, Katzmann JA, Lust JA, Heimgartner PJ, K.C. Halling, Hanson CA, Flow cytometric assessment of TCR-Vbeta expression in the evaluation of peripheral blood involvement by T-cell lymphoproliferative disorders: a comparisonwith conventional T-cell immunophenotyping and molecular genetic techniques, Am. J. Clin. Pathol. 121 (2004) 373—383.

Muschen M, Warskulat U, Perniok A, Involvement of soluble CD95 in Churg-Strauss syndrome. Am. J. Pathol. 155: 915-925.1999 Hattori N, Ichimura M, Nagamatsu M, Li M, Yamamoto K, Kumazawa K, Mitsuma T, Sobue G, Clinicopathological features of Churg–Strauss syndrome-associated neuropathy, Brain 122 (Pt 3)(1999) 427—439.

Neumann T, Manger B, Schmid M, Kroegel C, Hansch A, Kaiser WA, Reinhardt D, Wolf G, Hein G, Mall G, Schett G, Zwerina J. Cardiac involvement in Churg-Strauss syndrome: impact of endomyocarditis. Medicine (Baltimore). 2009 Jul;88(4):236-43.

Oka N, Kawasaki T, Matsui M, Shigematsu K, Unuma T, Sugiyama H. Two subtypes of Churg-Strauss syndrome with neuropathy: the roles of eosinophils and ANCA. Mod Rheumatol. 2010 Dec 29.

Orriols, R, Muñoz, X, Ferrer, J, et al. Cocaine-induced Churg-Strauss vasculitis. Eur Respir J 1996; 9:175.

Pabst S, Tiyerili V, Grohé C. Apparent response to anti-IgE therapy in two patients with refractory "forme fruste" of Churg-Strauss syndrome. Thorax. 2008;63(8):747.

Polzer K, Karonitsch T, Neumann T, et al. Eotaxin-3 is involved in Churg- Strauss syndrome: a serum marker closely correlating with disease activity. Rheumatology (Oxford); 47:804–808. 2008

Ribi C, Cohen P, Pagnoux C, Mahr A, Arène JP, Lauque D, Puéchal X, Letellier P, Delaval P, Cordier JF, Guillevin L, French Vasculitis Study Group.Treatment of Churg-Strauss syndrome without poor-prognosis factors: a multicenter, prospective, randomized, open-label study of seventy-two patients. Arthritis Rheum. 2008;58(2):586

Roufosse FE, Goldman M, Cogan E. Hypereosinophilic syndromes. Orphanet J Rare Dis. 2007 Sep 11;2:37.

Rolla G, Tartaglia N, Motta M, Ferrero N, Bergia R, Guida G, Heffler E. Warning nonrespiratory symptoms in asthma: catastrophic abdominal involvement in a case of Churg-Strauss syndrome. Ann Allergy Asthma Immunol. 2007;98:595-7.

Sable-Fourtassou R, Cohen P, Mahr A, et al. Antineutrophil cytoplasmic antibodies and the Churg–Strauss syndrome. Ann Intern Med; 143: 632–638.2005

Saito H, Tsurikisawa N, Tsuburai T, Oshikata C, Akiyama K. Cytokine production profile of CD4+ T cells from patients with active Churg-Strauss syndrome tends toward Th17. Int Arch Allergy Immunol. 2009;149 Suppl 1:61-5. Epub 2009 Jun 3.

Sallusto F, Lenig D, Forster R, Lipp M, Lanzavecchia A, Two subsets of memory T lymphocytes with distinct homing potentialsand effector functions, Nature 401 (1999) 708–712.

Sanders JS, Huitema MG, Kallenberg CGM, Stegeman CA. Prediction of relapses in PR3-ANCA associated vasculitis by assessing responses of ANCA titres to treatment. Rheumatology; 45:724–729. 2006

Schmitt WH, Csernok E, Kobayashi S, Klinkenborg A, Reinhold-Keller E, Gross WL. Churg-Strauss syndrome: serum markers of lymphocyte activation and endothelial damage. Arthritis Rheum. 1998 Mar;41(3):445-52.

Silva CI, Müller NL, Fujimoto K, Johkoh T, Ajzen SA, Churg AChurg-Strauss syndrome: high resolution CT and pathologic findings. J Thorac Imaging 2005;20(2):74–80.

Sinico RA, Bottero P. Churg-Strauss angiitis. Best Pract Res Clin Rheumatol 23(3):355-66, 2009.

Sinico RA, Di Toma L, Maggiore U, Tosoni C, Bottero P, Sabadini E, Giammarresi G, Tumiati B, Gregorini G, Pesci A, Monti S, Balestrieri G, Garini G, Vecchio F, Buzio C. Renal involvement in Churg-Strauss syndrome. Am J Kidney Dis. 2006;47(5):770-9.

Sinico, R. A., L. Di Toma, U. Maggiore, P. Bottero, A. Radice, C. Tosoni, C. Grasselli, L. Pavone, G. Gregorini, S. Monti, M. Frassi, F. Vecchio, C. Corace, E. Venegoni, and C. Buzio.. Prevalence and clinical significance of antineutrophil cytoplasmic antibodies in Churg-Strauss syndrome. Arthritis Rheum. 52: 2926-2935. 2005

Srouji I, Lund V, Andrews P, Edwards C. Rhinologic symptoms and quality-of-life in patients with Churg-Strauss syndrome vasculitis. Am J Rhinol. 2008 Jul-Aug;22(4):406-9.
Steinman L. A brief history of T(H)17, the first major revision in the T(H)1/T(H)2 hypothesis of T cell-mediated tissue damage. Nat Med. 2007 Feb;13(2):139-45.
Szczeklik W, Sokołowska BM, Zuk J, Mastalerz L, Szczeklik A, Musiał J. The course of asthma in Churg-Strauss syndrome. J Asthma. 2011 Mar;48(2):183-7.
Tougan T, Onda H, Okuzaki D, Kobayashi S, Hashimoto H, Nojima H. Focusedmicroarray analysis of peripheral mononuclear blood cells from Churg-Strauss syndrome patients. DNA Res. Apr 30;15(2):103-14.2008
Tsukadaira A, Okubo Y, Kitano K, et al. Eosinophil active cytokines andsurface analysis of eosinophils in Churg–Strauss syndrome. Allergy Asthma Proc; 20:39–44. 1999
Tsurikisawa N, Saito H, Tsuburai T, et al. Differences in regulatory T cells between Churg–Strauss syndrome and chronic eosinophilic pneumonia with asthma. J Allergy Clin Immunol 122:610–616. 2008.
Vaglio A, Martorana D, Maggiore U, Grasselli C, Zanetti A, Pesci A, Garini G, Manganelli P, Bottero P, Tumiati B, Sinico RA, Savi M, Buzio C, Neri TM; HLA-DRB4 as a genetic risk factor for Churg-Strauss syndrome. .arthritis and Rheumatism, 56(9):3159-66 .2007.
Watts RA, Lane SE, Bentham G, Scott DG. Epidemiology of systemic vasculitis: a ten-year study in the United Kingdom. Arthritis Rheum 2000; 43: 414–19
Wechsler ME, Wong DA, Miller MK, Lawrence-Miyasaki L. Churg-strauss syndrome in patients treated with omalizumab. Chest. 2009 Aug;136(2):507-18
Wei, S., P. Charmley, M. A. Robinson, and P. Concannon. The extent of the human germline T-cell receptor V beta gene segment repertoire. 1994 Immunogenetics 40: 27-36.
Wieczorek S, Holle JU, Epplen JT. Recent progress in the genetics of Wegener's granulomatosis and Churg-Strauss syndrome. Curr Opin Rheumatol. Jan;22(1):8-14. 2010
Worthy SA, Müller NL, Hansell DM, et al.Churg-Strauss syndrome: the spectrum of pulmonary CT findings in 17 patients. AJR Am J Roentgenol 1998;170:297–300
Zhang W, Zhou G, Shi Q, Zhang X, Zeng XF, Zhang FC. Clinical analysis of nervous system involvement in ANCA-associated systemic vasculitides. Clin Exp Rheumatol. 2009 Jan-Feb;27(1 Suppl 52):S65-9.

14

Diagnosis and Treatment of Giant Cell Arteritis (Temporal Arteritis) – Past, Current and Future Aspects

Jan Tore Gran
Department of Rheumatology Oslo University Hospital, Rikshospitalet Oslo, Norway

1. Introduction

Giant cell (temporal) arteritis (GCA) is characterized by a granulomatous inflammatory reaction that penetrates all layers of the wall of medium- to large-sized arteries (1). The transmural vasculitis is particularly prone to involve cranial arteries such as the superficial temporal artery (TA), but not infrequently the disease extends to involve large muscular arteries including the subclavian and axillary arteries and the aorta.

The earliest recorded description of GCA dates to the 10th century when Ali Ibn Isa of Baghdad in his memorandum book remarked on the relationship between inflamed arteries and visual symptoms (2). An even earlier case of GCA is disclosed in a photograph of carving of a blind harpist with swollen eyelids and prominent temporal arteries from a Egyptian tomb of Pa-Aton-Em-Heb dating back to 1350 BC (3). Moreover, the painting by the Flemish painter Jan van Eyck (1436) "The holy Virgin with Canon van der Paele" may also represent an early case of GCA (4). The canon had prominent temporal arteries and diffuse swelling of the hand (5), the latter possibly indicating coexistent PMR. The tortous and inflamed artery seen in the portrait of Lorenzo Gambietti by Piero di Cosimo in 1502 is also suggestive of GCA (5). Thus, although GCA may have existed for several centuries there are rather few definite historical documentations of its existence. As GCA preferentially affects persons aged 50 years and more, one possible explanation is the low average life expectancy in ancient times, exposing few individuals to the risk of contracting GCA.

The first clinical description of GCA was given by Jonathan Hutchinson in 1890 (St. Bartholomew`s Hospital, London) who was asked to examine Mr. Rumbold, an 80 year old father of a porter at the London Hospital who had "red streaks on his head" which were so painful that they prevented him from wearing a hat (6). Forty-two years later (1932), the first histopathological evidence of a granulomatous vasculitis in the temporal arteries was reported by Horton, Magath and Brown at a Mayo Clinic staff meeting in 1932 (7). In 1937, Horton and Magath added to their former report the prominence of headache, the difficulty chewing food, and transient diplopia (8). Blindness as a complication of GCA was, however, first recognized by Jennings in 1938 (9). In 1941, Gilmoure (10) suggested the presence of giant cells as characteristic for the disease which he called "giant cell chronic arteritis".

During the 1930ies, the term "Temporal arteritis" was gradually introduced, whilst the designation "Cranial arteritis" was coined by Kilbourne and Wolff in 1946 (11) to point out that the temporal artery is not the only scalp artery affected in GCA.
The most frequent complaints of GCA are head-ache and malaise. However, GCA may also present as a systemic inflammatory syndrome characterized by non-specific constitutional symptoms related to systemic inflammation in the absence of focal ischemic symptoms. This is often referred to as "silent or masked GCA" (12). On the other hand, the disease may also present with minimal or absent systemic manifestations, but with organ dysfunction such as visual loss or peripheral neuropathy. The term "Occult GCA", coined by Simmons and Cogan in 1962 (13) is often used to denote such a disease variant (14). GCA rather frequently coexists with polymyalgia rheumatica (15), affects most often persons of Nordic origin (15) and almost exclusively involves individuals 50 years or older (15, 16).
The annual incidence of GCA among persons 50 year or older has been estimated to 29/100000 (15), but autopsy studies have indicated a substantially higher incidence (17). It is possible that physician awareness is responsible for the progressive increase in the incidence that has been observed over the past two to five decades in different parts of the world (18, 19), conceivably remaining stable in the recent years (20). Mortality in GCA appears similar to that of the general population (21, 22). The cornerstone of treatment is represented by oral glucocorticosteroids (CS), but new therapeutic options which better control disease activity, exhibiting lower incidences of side effects and reducing disease complications are highly warranted.

2. Age and sex

In GCA, there is a typical female excess across all age groups (15, 16, 20, 23, 24, 25). Although GCA is almost invariably seen in individuals 50 years and older, arteritis of the temporal arteries is occasionally diagnosed in persons younger than 50 years (26). Temporal arteritis in the young may be separated into three groups. First, a localized eosinophilic arteritis confined to the temporal arteries (27), often without evidence of granulomatous inflammation (28). Systemic manifestations may be absent or minimal and the disease generally follows a benign clinical course without ischemic complications (28). Excision of the involved section of the temporal artery is often curative and CS are not required (28). Second, temporal arteritis may accompany other systemic connective diseases such as polyarteritis nodosa, Churg Strauss vasculitis, thrombangitis obliterans, or HIV infection (29). Third, a clinical and histological picture indistinguishable from that seen in adults may be observed. Although well documented, GCA among younger persons is exceptionally rare.

3. Common clinical manifestations

Head-ache At diagnosis, head-ache is reported by the vast majority of patients. In one study (25), it was present at onset in 54.1% and at diagnosis in 84.6%. The head-pain is classically located to the temporal regions, but occipital, frontal, or general headache is often encountered (25, 30, 31). In one case series, 17% of patients with biopsy-proven GCA had an initial presentation of occipital pain (31). Some patients report pain behind the ears which may be associated with vertigo and deafness (32).

4. Constitutional and musculoskeletal manifestations

Constitutional symptoms very often accompany local ischemic manifestations. Asthenia, malaise, low-grade fever, night sweats, loss of appetite and weight loss are reported by more than one third of patients (2, 25, 33, 34). Fever is usually low-grade, but occasionally it is high and associated with night sweats (2). In some cases, fever is the presenting manifestation or the only feature of GCA (35). Patients may report joint pain, but contrary to Polymyalgia rheumatica, frank arthritis appears to be very rare (25, 34).

5. Jaw claudication

Jaw claudication manifests as jaw-pain which is noted particularly when the patient chews solid food or talks at length (2). It is seen in up to 50 % of patients with a full-blown clinical picture of GCA (2, 25, 30, 33), but may in many cases be absent at the very onset of disease (2, 25). Jaw claudication usually develops shortly after some minutes of chewing and is promptly relieved by resting the muscles of mastication (2, 33). It is due to masseter ischemia caused by vasculitis and occlusive stenosis of the maxillary artery, a branch of the external carotid artery. As jaw claudication is explicitly rare in other diseases, it is a high predictor of GCA, although not pathognomonic (30).

6. Ophthalmologic manifestations

The most feared complication of CGA is visual disturbances. The incidence of ophthalmologic manifestations varies from 14-70%, depending on the selection of patients and methods of ophthalmological examinations (25, 36, 37, 38, 39, 40). Consequently, incidences of visual impairment estimated in population surveys range from 1-21%, in hospital-based studies from 0-30% and from 48-65% among patients selected from departments of eye diseases (25). There is no unanimous consensus regarding suggestions of a progressive decline in the proportion of patients with visual manifestations during the last 2 to 3 decades (39, 40, 41).

The most common ophthalmologic manifestation is visual loss (97.7%) followed by diplopia (6-21%). The visual loss is most often unilateral (38), and it may be either transient or permanent (42). Other visual disturbances are bitemporal visual field defects due to vasculitic damage to the arteries that supply that optic chiasm (42), homonymous visual field defects due to vascular involvement of the retrochiasmal visual sensory pathway (42), papillary disturbances and acute ocular hypotony (42). Visual hallucinations may occur, and in most cases these occur after the patient is bilaterally blind (42). Several cases of Charles Bonnet syndrome have been reported (43, 44).

Visual manifestations usually present early in the disease course, and are rarely seen after 2-3 years of disease (25, 45, 46, 47). In one study (25) visual impairment occurred at onset in only 2.7% as opposed to 17.9% at the time of diagnosis. Loss of vision after the first two weeks of CS therapy seems to be exceptionally rare (48). In one study (36), the probability of additional visual loss due to GCA was 13 % at 5 years in patients who presented with visual loss. The probability of visual loss due to GCA was 1 % at 5 years in patients with intact vision when oral CC treatment was started (36). If bilateral visual loss develops, the interval between the first and second eye is usually only a few days (49, 50).

Visual loss is related to anterior ischemic optic neuropathy (AION)(51), which is most commonly caused by narrowing or occlusion of the posterior ciliary arteries (32). These arteries provide blood flow to the optic disc and the choroid (42). Consequently, the early fundoscopic appearance noted in AION consists of slight pallor and oedema of the optic disc with scattered cotton-wool patches and small hemorrhages. Later optic atrophy occurs. Such patients often report a feeling of a shade covering one eye (42). It occurs abruptly or it may be preceded by episodes of transient monocular loss of vision (42). Of all patients with AION, only 5 % have concomitant GCA (42).

Central retinal artery occlusion is the second most common cause of visual loss, affecting 10-13% of patients with visual disturbances (42, 38, 51). However, it should be noted that only 5-10 % of patients with central retinal artery occlusion have GCA (42). Usually, it develops rather abruptly and permanently (42). Posterior ischemic optic neuropathy is much less common (42). A rather rare cause of visual loss in GCA is occipital lobe infarction (52, 53).

Importantly, of patients with visual manifestations, transient visual loss is reported by 5-54 % (47, 54, 55, 56). Transient monoocular blindness (ameurosis fugax) results from insufficient perfusion of the optic nerve, retina or choroid and precedes the development of permanent visual loss by an average of 8.5 days (33, 40, 42, 57). Ameurosis fugax should thus be regarded an ominous sign of impending blindness. In rare cases, transient visual disturbances preceding permanent visual loss may alternate between the two eyes (42).

The risk of developing visual disturbances has been associated with low disease activity (37, 58, 59), high disease activity (37, 45, 60), anemia (61), older age (37, 38), disc swelling (37), and a history of hypertension (62). In some studies, the best predictors for the development of severe cranial ischemic events included the absence of high CRP and ESR levels at diagnosis, absence of systemic manifestations such as fever and weight loss, and a past history of ischemic heart disease (58, 62). On the other hand, one study (60) showed an increased frequency of visual ischemic events in patients with ESR values ranging between 70 and 100 mm/h at the time of disease diagnosis. Similarly, another survey (63), found no increased risk of visual loss or other cranial ischemic events in patients with low ESR (< 40 mm/h). Histologically, the presence of giant cell cells has been associated with increased risk of visual loss (64), but this finding needs to be confirmed. A recent retrospective study showed a frequency of permanent visual loss as high as 70% among patients lacking headache at diagnosis (65). Clearly, further research is needed to define predictors of visual manifestations that can be favorably used in everyday clinical practice.7.

Large vessel vasculitis Involvement of large vessels may be seen in 14-25% of cases with GCA (66, 67, 68, 69). Both aortic aneurysm formation and peripheral large vessel vasculitis of the extremities may be observed (66, 70, 71, 72, 73, 74). In rare cases, arteritis involving the mesenteric vessels may develop both as an initial manifestation of GCA and antedating its diagnosis (75). About 1/3 of such patients die.

In large-vessel arteritis involving the upper extremity, the subclavian and axillary arteries are most often affected (76). In about 1/5 of cases with large vessel vasculitis of the upper extremities, the brachial arteries are involved (68). The clinical picture is characterized by claudication of the arms, bruits over the carotid, subclavian, axillary and brachial arteries and absent or decreased pulses in the neck or arms. Paleness of hands upon use of upper extremity may also be observed (77). Unilateral manifestations are more frequent than bilateral manifestations (68).

In rare instances, lower extremity vasculitis develops in which involvement of the superficial femoral arteries is most frequently seen (68, 71). Other lower extremity vasculitis includes the internal iliac artery, the common femoral artery, the deep femoral artery and the popliteal and anterior tibial arteries (68). Occasionally, GCA may present as a rapidly progressing lower extremity claudication with elevated inflammatory markers whereas cranial symptoms may be absent (71, 78).

In general, TAB may be normal in 50 % of patients with large vessel vasculitis (76). Thus, in many cases the differentiation between GCA and Takayasu arteritis may be difficult, although the latter often occurs at a younger age than the former. Both upper and lower extremity vasculitis in GCA may precede other manifestations of the disease (71), or it may be identified in association with GCA diagnosis and even develop after the onset of GCA (68). According to one study, the outcome of upper and lower extremity vasculitis in GCA seems rather good (68). Approximately 3 years after diagnosis, 80-90% of cases will either experience disappearance or improvement of clinical manifestations (68). Slightly more than 10% will have a deterioration of clinical manifestations (68). However, in another study (71) adressing lower extremity vasculitis exclusively, significant morbidity was observed as several patients were subjected to revascularization surgery and limb amputation. It is thus possible that the outcome differs between patients presenting with rapidly progressing lower limb claudication and those with less predominant clinical manifestations of lower limb vasculitis.

GCA involving the aorta was first described by Sproul and Hawthorne in 1937 (80) and is increasingly recognized conceivably due to improved imaging techniques. Case-series employing PET for diagnosis have found evidence of aortitis in over half the cases (81). Of such cases, both the thoracic and abdominal aorta may be affected (73). A study from the Mayo clinic in 1995 showed that 14 of 96 (15%) patients with GCA had an aortic aneurysm (9 thoracic and 5 abdominal)(69). Thus, patients with GCA were found to be 17.3 times more likely to have a thoracic aortic aneurysm and 2.4 times more likely to develop abdominal aortic aneurysm than age-related controls. Some have suggested it to be more common in men than females (74). Aortic dissection may be the first manifestation of GCA (82), but in the majority of cases, development of aortic disease occurs after the diagnosis of GCA (71). In many cases, aortic aneurysms occur late, years after the onset of the disease and even years after the completion of CS therapy, so that patients will often have left their rheumatologist (69, 76, 83). Moreover, most cases are asymptomatic unless dissection and rupture develop (66, 69, 72, 84). As no absolute correlation between high disease activity and evolvement of aortic disease seem to exist, diagnosis of aortic GCA disease is highly dependent on screening procedures for such events.

Involvement of the aorta may be diagnoses by ultrasonography, CT or MRI (72, 73, 85). Vasculitis of the aorta and peripheral vessels may also be visualized by increased vascular uptake on 18FDG-PET (86, 87, 88, 89), but it is not clear if this is specific to vasculitis or simply a marker of any type of wall injury and tissue repair (76). Its specificity and sensitivity for diagnosing large vessel vasculitis have therefore been questioned (90). Although the recent advent of combined functional and anatomic imaging with PET-CT scanners allows anatomic correlation and exact localization of pathological lesions, PET scanning is associated with high costs and not available in all hospitals. Thus, at present it should not be recommended as a routine screening procedure in GCA. As most aneurysms develop in the ascending aorta, a yearly transthoracic echo and two-view chest radiograph could be considered as a reasonable screening approach (76). A yearly ultrasound screening in GCA for abdominal aneurysms is also likely to be cost effective (76).

In one report (69), 44% of patients with thoracic aortic aneurysm, died suddenly of dissection and 33% developed aortic regurgitation. However, subsequent investigations have concluded with a rather favorable outcome of aortic disease in GCA except for those patients that proceed to develop dissection or rupture (89, 91). In one study, follow-up at 6 months showed complete disappearance in 8.8%, improvement in 47.1%, unchanged in 41.2% and deterioration in 2.9% (72). A French study using CT scans to diagnose aortitis, also disclosed a more favorable prognosis as 10 of 11 patients achieved complete resolution or improvement at follow-up (92).

Risk factors for development of large vessel vasculitis in GCA have been insufficiently investigated. It has, however, been suggested that an aortic insufficiency murmur at the time of GCA diagnosis, hyperlipidemia, coronary artery disease at any time and high ESR in combination with polymyalgic symptoms, and hypertension are factors associated with aortic aneurysm or dissection (76, 83, 93). It should be noted, however, that less than 10 % of patients with noninfectious aortitis have GCA (94).

7. Neurologic manifestations

GCA presenting with neurological manifestations is exceptionally rare, occurring in only four of 260 cases (1.5 %) in one report (34). Neurological manifestations of GCA most probably result from arteritis of the vasa vasorum of peripheral nerves and consist of neuropathies, including mononeuropathies and peripheral polyneuropathies of the upper and lower extremities (95). On the other hand, vasculitis of the central nervous system is extremely rare and inflammatory lesions are very rarely found beyond 5 mm after the artery`s penetration of the dura. Bley et al. (96) studied the thin walled intradural arteries of the circle of Willisi by MRI and did not find any signs on MRI suggestive of mural inflammation. Some rare neurological manifestations are summarized in Table 1.

According to most reports, cerebrovascular ischemic events are found in 3-15% (65, 97, 98) of GCA, but are due to involvement of the extradural segment of the vertebral and carotid arteries. In one study, eight of 287 patients (2.8%) had strokes between the onset of GCA and 4 weeks after the onset of CS (97). Lesions due to involvement of the vertebrobasilar territory were seen more often than those caused by involvement of the carotids (97, 99). Patients with strokes had more commonly permanent visual loss and were more frequently smokers (97). In another study (99), the same incidence (2.8%) of strokes was observed, but the internal carotid arteries were involved in 4 patients and the vertebrobasilar arteries in 3. Interestingly, CT and MRI revealed small cerebral and cerebellar infarction, but at necropsy generalized GCA involving medium and cerebral vessels was found in one case (99). Multiple ischemic strokes despite escalating immmunosuppressive therapy may also develop (100, 101), in which both anterior and posterior circulations are involved bilaterally in a characteristic location where the arteries penetrate the dura (100). Thus, strokes occur in a few patients with GCA and are in the overwhelming majority of cases due to thromboembolic disease localized to the carotid and vertebrobasilar supplied areas of the brain. However, strokes due to atherosclerosis and iatrogenic effects of CS should not be overlooked (101). Finally, in some cases the cause of progressive stroke may be due to CC rather than the disease itself (102), suggesting that replacing GC with anticoagulants should be considered.

8. Scalp necrosis

Scalp necrosis in GCA was first described by Cooke and coworkers in 1946 (103), and remains an explicitly rare disease manifestation of GCA. It is most often localized to the frontal and parietal parts and is often bilateral (Picture 1). As the scalp has an excellent blood supply, development of scalp necrosis signalizes severe vasculitis, involving most superficial arteries of the scalp. Consequently, it is often associated with severe GCA frequently including both cerebral and coronary artery occlusions (41%) and irreversible visual loss (67%)(104). Somewhat surprising, scalp necrosis usually heals completely after a few weeks (105), although sequela in the form of scarring may be seen (106). According to a review of 78 cases reported in the literature, scalp necrosis never developed after onset of therapy with corticosteroids (107). However, a case was recently reported in whom scalp necrosis antedated the initiation of therapeutic corticosteroids (108).

9. Tongue necrosis

The tongue has an excellent blood supply and is usually minimally affected in GCA (109). However, in rare cases, necrosis and gangrene of the anterior portion of the tongue may develop (110). Bilateral lingual necrosis has also been reported (109). It has been suggested that tongue necrosis most often develop during initial tapering of corticosteroid dosage (111). Tongue necrosis is caused by lingual arteritis (109). Occasionally, patients suffering from GCA report loss of taste (112) which may be related to facial artery giant cell arteritis.

Neurological

- Dementia (111)
- Psychosis (33)
- Coma (114)
- Seizures (115)
- Spinal cord infarction (116, 117)
- Subarachnoidal hemorrhage (33)
- Neuropathies (95)
- Mononeuritis multiplex (118)
- Trigeminal neuralgia (119)
- Bilateral peroneal nerve palsy (120)
- Cerebral vein thrombosis (121)
- Occipital infarction (118, 122)
- Transient ischemic attacks (123, 124)

Oral manifestations (125)

- Trismus (125)
- Throat pain (126)
- Hoarsness (126)
- Dysarthria (125, 127, 128)
- Chin numbness (125)
- Glossitis (129, 130)
- Macroglossia (125, 131)
- Lip or tongue necrosis (125)

- Odontogenic pain (33)
- Dysphagia (125)
- A submandibular mass (125)
- Head, neck and facial swelling (132, 133)

Audiovestibular manifestations (134)

- Hearing loss (33, 134)
- Tinnitus (134)
- Vertigo(134)
- Dizziness (134)
- Spontaneous nystagmus (134)
- Earache? (125)

Orbital manifestations

- Ptosis (135)
- Eye pain (125)
- Chemosis (134)
- Ophthalmoplegia (135, 136)
- - Complete abducens nerve palsy (136, 137)- Third nerve palsy (135, 136)
- Lid edema (135)
- Episcleritis (135)
- Proptosis (135, 137)

Other manifestations

- Bowel infarction (138, 139, 140, 141)
- Arteritis of the myometrium,ovaries, paraovarian tissue and fallopian tubes (142, 143, 144)
- Pericardial and pleural effusions (145, 146, 147, 148, 149)
- Pleural thickening, nodules of variable size and reticular lesions (149)
- Cough, sore throat and hoarseness (149)
- Myocardial infarction (150, 151, 152, 153, 154)
- Breast involvement (155, 156)
- Syndrome of inappropriate antidiuretic secretion (157)
- Raynaud`s phenomenon (158)
- Microangiopathic hemolytic anemia (159)
- Carotidynia (160, Cid AR 1998 ref 79)
- Membraneous glomerulopathy and nephrotic syndrome (161)

Table 1. Less commonly reported clinical manifestations in GCA

10. Concomitant polymyalgia rheumatica

Polymyalgia rheumatica (PMR) and GCA frequently coexist (25, 162, 163), an association noted by Porsman as early as in 1951 (164). PMR may precede GCA or develop after GCA diagnosis. Whether or not PMR and GCA represent two separate disease entities which frequently overlap or are one common disease with different clinical expressions remains a controversial issue. The frequent concomitant occurrence of PMR and GCA suggests a common disease denominator whereas the discrepant clinical picture of TA and PMR may indicate two separate disease entities. The occurrence of articular and periarticular inflammation seen almost exclusively in PMR suggests separate disease entities (165). On the other hand, positron emission tomography (PET) scan findings of increased uptake of fluorodeoxyglucose in the thoracic vessels in many patients with PMR suggest a common vasculitic disorder (166, 167). Finally, the reported incidence of biopsy-proven TA among patients with pure PMR varies considerably, from 4 to 70% which makes it difficult to reach an overall conclusion regarding the relationship between TA and PMR (25, 168, 169, 170). Patients presenting with both PMR and GCA often run a severe disease course, and maintenance doses of oral CS are on average often higher compared to patients presenting pure PMR or isolated GCA (171, 172).

11. Clinical examinations

In patients suspected of suffering from GCA rather few clinical examinations are mandatory. As GCA affects individuals older than 50 years who rather frequently suffer from other diseases, a general medical examination is compulsory. Examination of aorta and large arteries of the upper and lower extremities to reveal bruits and diminished pulses is strongly recommended.

Physical examination of the frontal and parietal branches of the temporal arteries may reveal tenderness on palpation, absent or reduced pulsation and thickening of the vessel. General scalp tenderness is rather frequently present and may be worsened by brushing or combing the hair.

A thorough examination for ophthalmological symptoms is strongly recommended. Symptoms indicating coexistent PMR should not be missed. Patients with uncomplicated GCA should be informed about the risk of ischemic complications and asked to report back immediately if such events develop.

12. Laboratory investigations

Acute phase reactants are increased in the overwhelming majority of GCA (25). An ESR of 40 mm/hour or more has been noted in more than 90 % of patients (61, 63). Less than 1-2% have normal levels of both ESR and CRP (25, 173, 174). GCA with normal ESR has, however, been reported (175, 176, 177), even in patients with visual disturbances (176, 178) and devastating central nervous system complications (179). Interestingly, when patients with GCA and normal ESR were followed-up, these patients were never able to mount a high ESR during subsequent episodes of inflammation caused by infection which may imply a genetically determined blunted cytokine response to inflammation (63). ESR and CRP are relatively lower in patients with occult GCA according to some observations (14). These patients often have a longer diagnostic delay (180). Both leucocytosis (61), thrombocytosis (61, 181, 182), and normocytic normochromic anemia (61) may be encountered. Liver function tests are frequently abnormal, particularly elevations of serum alkaline phosphatase (62, 183).

Recent research has explored the potential utility of other biomarkers for disease activity in GCA. A promising cytokine for monitoring disease activity in GCA is IL-6 as it is found in inflamed arterial walls and shows highly elevated serum levels in active GCA (184, 185). In one study, 89% of flares were associated with an elevated level of IL-6 while ESR elevations accompanied 58% of flares (186). However, analyses of IL-6 are not readily available at most centers, and thus not suitable for routine measurements. Finally, more research is needed to explore whether or not serial assessments of circulating TNFα can aid in the monitoring of possible relapses in GCA (187).

13. Imaging

13.1 Ultrasound

Color duplex ultrasonography of the temporal artery has been introduced as a means of improving the diagnosis of GCA. Besides revealing stenosis and vessel occlusions, ultrasound may also detect wall inflammation.

Schmidt and coworkers described in 1997 the presence of a hypoechoic thickening around the lumen of the temporal artery, termed a "halo-sign" which represents edema of the vessel wall (188). The "halo-sign" may also be seen in subclavian, external carotid, occipital, axillary, facial, brachial, ulnar, common carotid, vertebral, radial and popliteal arteries (189). The frequent involvement of the occipital arteries in GCA may also be detected by ultrasonography (190). Thus, an ultrasonographic finding of a hypoechoic halo around the lumen of the temporal arteries has been advocated as a method of making the diagnosis of GCA rendering temporal artery biopsy (TAB) superflous. However, several studies have questioned the sensitivty of the "halo-sign" for the diagnosis of GCA. According to various reports, its sensitivity varies from 10-100% (191, 192, 193). In a meta-analysis of 23 studies, the "halo-sign" had a pooled sensitivity of 69% and a specificity of 82% compared with TAB (194). However, a bilateral "halo-sign" appears almost pathognomonic of GCA (193). In another report, Arida and coworkers (195) conducted an extensive metaanalysis of ultrasonograophy which disclosed a sensitivity of 68% and a specificity of 91% for the unilateral "halo- sign", as well as 43% and 100%, respectively for the bilateral "halo-sign" for GCA diagnosis.

The reasons for apparent discrepancies regarding sensitivity of ultrasound to detect the halo to diagnose GCA may have several explanations. First, sensitivity and specificity are highly dependent on the examiner as the method requires experience and expertice. Second, the quality of the sonographs employed in the different studies may vary. Third, the appearance of vessel wall abnormalities may also vary with the duration of the disease.

A negative ultrasonographic finding at the onset of disease may be due to absence of early adventitial inflammation which is necessary to produce the oedema that causes the halo effect. It should also be noted that the halo disappears after commencement of steroid therapy, usually within 2-4 weeks (188, 189, 193). Finally, in some cases it is difficult to differentiate between inflammatory and noninflammatory temporal artery disease by ultrasonography (196).

At present, ultrasonography should not replace temporal artery biopsy (TAB), but it can serve as a means for identifying sites suitable for surgical biopsies (197). Moreover, ultrasonography appears a promising method for diagnosing GCA in patients who decline surgical biopsies. In such cases, cautious interpretation of the test results based on clinical presentation and pretest probability of the disease is imperative (194). Clinicians responsible for the care of patients with GCA should be encouraged to use ultrasonography to detect large vessel vasculitis in GCA.

14. Magnetic resonance imaging

MRI can detect inflammatory vessel wall changes (198) with a sensitivity of 80.6% and a specificity of 97% compared against a diagnosis of GCA based on the ACR criteria (199). According to other findings, the specificity and positive likelihood ratio of high resolution MRI are sufficiently high that a positive MRI combined with other clinical and laboratory data consistent with GCA may be useful in diagnosing GCA (200). It should be noted, however, that given the relatively low sensitivity of the test, a negative MRI would not be sufficient to rule out the diagnosis of GCA (201).
Moreover, no definite concordance between MRI and acute phase assessed by CRP has been established (86). Finally, to few studies have specifically addressed the suitability of MRI diagnosing arteritis in the temporal arteries (202). Although disputed (201) , MRI appears as a favorable means to detect large vessel vasculitis, in any case when abnormalities such as vessel narrowing or obliteration have developed.

15. ^{18}Fluorodeoxyglucose-positrone emission tomography – 18FDG- pet-scanning)

Similar to MRI, 18FDG-PET may be useful to detect large vessel arteritis but is associated with restricted availability and high costs. However, PET scanning may in the absence of reliable biomarkers for disease activity, represent the only method of disclosing active vessel wall inflammation. Preliminary results indicate that 18F-FDG PET could be a method exhibiting high sensitivity and specificity for GCA-related large-vessel inflammation (203, 204, 205, 206).
Others have found PET as a useful diagnostic tool in early stages of large vessel vasculitis and a powerful instrument to follow the treatment responses (88). However, increased vascular up-take on PET should be interpreted cautiously as it is still unsettled whether or not such uptake represents inflammation requiring anti-inflammatory therapy or indicates inflammation associated with a healing process. One study found only a low, but non-significant correlation of PET with CRP (201). At present, more investigation is needed before PET scan eventually can be included in the routine work-up and monitoring of GCA. The availability of the modality is, however, restricted, and the costs are of great concern.

16. Temporal artery biopsy

According to the British Society for rheumatology guidelines, TAB should be considered whenever a diagnosis of GCA is suspected (207). The EULAR recommendations, however, advocate that a TAB should be performed when GCA is suspected (208). Although a diagnosis of GCA according to the ACR criteria (199) can be made without histological confirmation, these criteria were constructed for use in research. For clinical work, the benefit of a pathological confirmation of the diagnosis should not be underestimated. Both at the start of disease and during disease course, a histological proof of GCA appears reassuring for both patients and clinicians. When patients develop serious adverse-effects due to long-term CS treatment, histopathological proof of the diagnosis helps to buttress the case for continued therapy (209). Moreover, GC therapy may cause serious side effects which may result in a medicolegal case. Morphological evidence of the disease will then provide proof that both diagnosis and treatment were appropriate. Finally, although scalp necrosis, brow droop, chronic skin ulceration and stroke have been described, TAB is associated with low-morbidity (210). As emphazised earlier, an ultrasound should be performed to identify the most suitable location fo biopsy.

Typical histopathological findings in GCA include infiltration of T lymphocytes, dendritic celles and macrophages in all layers of the arterial wall. Moreover, disruption of the internal elastic lamina, chronic granulomatous inflammation, multinucleated giant cells accumulated along the fragmented internal elastic lamina, thickening of the intima and luminal occlusion are frequently observed. In some cases, involvement is in seen exclusively in the small vessels external to the temporal artery adventitia (211). PMR very often accompany GCA in such cases (211).

The minimum length of the biopsy required for a definite diagnosis of GCA has been discussed in several reports. The basis for the discussion is the uneven distribution of arteritic lesions (212). Skip lesions have been described in 8.5-28.3% of positive biopsies (213, 214, 215). Although lengths of biopsies shorter than 10mm are suggested to be sufficient for a diagnosis of GCA (216, 217), most authors recommend a minimum length of at least 1.5-2 cm (218, 219, 220). Such a length would allow for tissue shrinking during fixation which is estimated to approximately 10 %.

If the biopsy yields normal findings, a contralateral biopsy may be considered. However, the diagnostic yield of a second biopsy if the first one is negative is rather small. The percentage of patients with a negative biopsy on one side and a positive biopsy on the other has been reported from 3 to 12.7 % (221, 222, 223). Given the low increase in sensitivity obtained by performing bilateral biopsies, careful diagnostic considerations should be undertaken before requesting a second biopsy. Moreover, a unilateral biopsy preserves an artery in the event that a diagnosis of GCA is considered in the future, and minimizes costs and physician time (224). In any way, commencement of therapy should not be delayed if clinical suspicion of GCA is high in spite of a first negative biopsy.

The administration of immunosuppressive therapy such as CS may have little impact on the possibilities of detecting histological vasculitis during the initial phases of therapy. Specimens might show arteritis after 2-4 weeks of CS therapy (225, 226, 227, 228), although the frequency of positive biopsies is slightly reduced for each week of treatment (227, 229). Active vasculitis observed in TAB has been demonstrated after as long as 9 years after initiation of CS (230). Thus, TAB should be performed in all patients suspected of having GCA, but negative results on biopsy in patients treated for weeks should be interpreted with caution.

In long-term CS treated patients, a histopathological picture of socalled healed-arteritic pattern has been observed. The three most reliable histopathological parameters of CS treated GCA were a complete or incomplete mantle of lymphocytes and epitheloid histiocytes located between the outer muscular layer and the adventitia, large circumferential defects in the elastic lamina and absent or few multinucleated giant cells (231). Patients exhibiting such histopathological features seemed to be at no risk of reactivation, early death, permanent blindness and cerebrovascular accidents (232).

Of major concern is the low number of positive biopsies analyzed by pathological departments. Studies during the years 1976 to 2007 have reported findings of GCA in 13 - 43.7 % of TABs (19, 226, 233, 234, 235). Consequently, predictive markers for a positive biopsy have long been searched for. In one study of TAB performed among patients suspected of having GCA, excluding patients with no evidence of temporal artery abnormalities, scalp tenderness, or jaw claudication, only 48% of the 125 biopsies would have been performed (236). Fiftynine negative biopsies would have been prevented, but six positive biopsies would have been missed (236). The findings jaw claudication, weight loss, pathological temporal artery enlargement, recent head-ache, and scalp tenderness have all been found to predict a positive biopsy (226, 233, 236, 237). It is tentative to suggest that patients exhibiting none of these clinical features combined with a negative ultrasound should not be subjected to TAB before all other causes of current inflammatory manifestations are ruled out. Finally, the frequencies of positive TAB reported in PMR have varied from 4-40% (25, 238), the results depending on the definition of "pure" PMR. At present, it is generally agreed upon that TAB is not indicated in patients with PMR in the absence of cranial manifestations (pure PMR), unless a high inflammatory response is present.

17. Diagnostic and classification criteria

17.1 Clinical suspicion

A diagnosis of GCA should be considered in all patients 50 years or older with unexplained head-ache, a significant inflammatory response that is not explained by infection, other autoimmune diseases or malignancy, visual disturbances or signs of peripheral vasculopathy. The British society for rheumatology (207) recommends that clinical suspicion of GCA should be raised in a patient older than 50 years presenting with either abrupt-onset headache, scalp tenderness, jaw and tongue claudication, visual symptoms, constitutional symptoms, polymyalgic symptoms or limb claudication.

18. Diagnosis

For scientific purpose, the ACR criteria are widely used (199). These criteria attempt to differentiate GCA from other vasculitides and include five items (Table 2). Presence of three or more of these five criteria is associated with a sensitivity of 93.5% and a specificity of 91.2%. It is noteworthy that according to these criteria, a diagnosis of CGA can be made in the absence of histopathological evidence. In a number of studies, patients with biopsy-proven GCA have been studied exclusively, hence hampering comparison with investigations based on the ACR criteria which include both biopsy positive and negative patients. Consequently, results should be presented separately for biopsy positive and negative cases allowing valuable comparison. It should also be noted that occult GCA and patients presenting large vessel vasculitis exclusively may not have been accurately represented in the ACR criteria. Furthermore, as the ACR criteria are not useful for making the diagnosis in individual patients (239), other diagnostic guidelines should be followed.

1. Age 50 years or older
2. New onset of localized headache
3. Temporal artery tenderness or decreased temporal artery pulse,
4. Elevated ESR 50 mm/hour or higher
5. Biopsy sample including an artery, showing necroitizing arteritis, characterized by a predominantly of mononuclear cell infiltrates or a granulomatous process with multinucleated giant cells.

Table 2. The ACR 1990 criteria for giant cell arteritis (199)

A diagnosis of Cranial arteritis requires the histological demonstration of localized vasculitis combined with associated clinical manifestations such as either head-ache and/or jaw claudication, visual loss and constitutional symptoms. Thus, a definite diagnosis of GCA classified as Cranial arteritis rests on the demonstration of inflammatory changes found on biopsy of the temporal arteries. In cases of normal histopathological findings at vessel biopsy, a diagnosis of cranial arteritis should only be made after a thorough exclusion of other causes for the aforementioned clinical manifestations. In such cases, evidence of an elevated acute phase response should be regarded compulsory and detection of a halo by ultrasonography would strongly support the diagnosis of GCA.

In patients with non-specific constitutional symptoms related to systemic inflammation in the absence of focal ischemic symptoms, but with histopathological proof of GCA, the term "Silent or masked GCA" or "systemic inflammatory syndrome" should be preferred. As emphasized by Rahman & Rahman (32), the ACR criteria are likely to result in some false-negative diagnoses of GCA, putting vision at risk. In silent or occult GCA, the risk of ischemic complications resulting in loss of vision is highly significant, requiring a high index of suspicion in order to diagnose GCA in patients with an atypical presentation.

Some patients may show evidence of large vessel vasculitis in the absence of histopathological evidence of GCA, and without significant inflammatory symptoms. Such cases may be indistinguishable from Takayasu arteritis, and should thus be labelled Large vessel vasculitis, or if histopathological proof of granulomatous vasculitis is observed, the term Large vessel giant cell arteritis may be preferred.

19. Differential diagnoses, malignancy and cardiovascular disease

A TAB remains the gold standard test in the diagnosis of GCA, and few diseases can be mistaken for what turns out to be biopsy-proven GCA. Vasculitis of the temporal arteries has been reported in polyarteritis nodosa, Churg Strauss vasculitis, microscopic polyangiitis, Wegener`s granulomatosis, hepatitis B virus-related polyarteritis nodosa, hepatitis C virus-related cryoglobulinemic vasculitis and rheumatoid vasculitis (29, 240, 241, 242), but the clinical features of these diseases distinguish them from TA. Primary systemic amyloidosis may present with a clinical picture of either PMR or GCA or both (243).

Malignancy and Cardiovascular disease in Giant cell arteritis. Although suggested by some (244, 245), the majority of studies have been unable to find an increased risk of malignancy in GCA (246, 247, 248, 249, 250, 251). However, as GCA affects persons 50 years and older, particular attention should be paid to the development of concurrent neoplastic disease which is not uncommon in these age groups. There are several case reports of GCA developing simultaneously with malignant disease such as leukemia (252), lymphoma (253) and lung cancer (254). Previous suggestions of an increased risk of concomitant cancer in patients not responding to treatment with subsequent decline in acute phase reactants have not been subjected to further investigations.

Although an increased incidence of cardiovascular disease in GCA has been suggested (255, 256, 257, 258). these findings have not been corroborated by population surveys (21, 259). Thus, there exists no convincing evidence of an increased risk for development of clinically important cardiovascular disease in GCA, except possibly for the oldest patients with GCA (260). Of note, cardiovascular diseases are in general prevalent in this age group and should not be ignored.

20. Initial treatment

After the first trial of CS therapy for the disease was reported by Schick et al in 1950 (261), CS have remained the mainstay of therapy in GCA. However, much is still unknown regarding their mechanisms of action, the optimal initial dose, speed of taper, and duration of CS therapy.

21. Uncomplicated GCA

In the absence of large vessel vasculitis, severe organ involvement or visual disturbances (uncomplicated GCA), low doses of CS are as effective as low doses (262, 263). Moreover, those patients commencing treatment with low doses of CS do not have more visual or neurological complications than patients treated with higher doses (264). Starting doses of 30-40 mg of prednisolone daily are thus recommended. Both cumulative doses of CS and higher doses are associated with increased toxicity (265, 266, 267).

Side effects may occur in at least one third of patients, and in two thirds if weight gain is included (264). Treatment with alternate-day CS administration is associated with a higher rate of treatment failure than is daily administration (268) and is not recommended.

If a significant response of 30-40 mg prednisolone per day is not obtained within 6-72 hours, an initial dose of oral prednisolone of 60 mg should be administered. There are, however, no studies that clearly show that a higher dose of oral CS yields a higher response rate than lower doses. If response to 60 mg of prednisolone fails to occur, diagnoses other than GCA should be considered. Similarly, in patients whose symptoms persist without elevated acute phase reactants, alternative or concurrent explanations should be sought. Also those patients whose symptoms resolve but the acute phase reactants remain elevated should be subjected to further diagnostic evaluations before continuing GC treatment.

The initial dose of CS is usually given for 2-4 weeks until all reversible signs and symptoms have resolved and acute phase reactants are back to normal. Then, the dose can be gradually reduced (269) each week or every two weeks by a maximum of 10% of the total daily dose with careful follow-up of systemic symptoms and acute phase reactants.

22. Treatment of GCA presenting with visual disturbances and blindness

Historically, experience clearly suggests a protective effect of CS against development of visual complications. Prior to the steroid era, a higher incidence of such ischemic events as compared to recent reports has been observed (17, 36, 270, 271, 272, 273). However, there are no randomized controlled studies proving such a preventive effect. Moreover, a substantial proportion of patients may loose vision in spite of daily treatment with high doses of CS (274, 275, 276). Finally, there is no convincing evidence to suggest that administration of GC results in improvement of established visual loss. Nevertheless, in patients presenting with visual disturbances, administration of CS should be initiated immediately, and not delayed until results of TAB are available. Studies have shown that if therapy is instituted within 24 hours, the chance of visual improvement is much greater than if treatment is delayed (49). Usually, 60 mg of oral prednisolone per day is given (207, 208), with gradual tapering of the dose to 40 mg in 1-2 weeks providing a clinical response appear. Thereafter, the steroid dose is gradually tapered to reach a maintenance dose of 10 mg by 6-9 months, and 5-7.5 mg within 1 year. In one report, the median time to reach the lowest maintenance dose of prednisone at which the ESR and CRP stayed low and stable was 48.7 months (277). However, as pointed out by Hayreh and Zimmerman (277), no generalization is possible for tapering down of CS, and there is no formula because of the infinite variation between individuals.

Patients with loss of vision represent a challenge to the physician. Visual loss from GCA is typically profound and permanent (42, 278). Although still debated (47, 279), most workers recommend administration of 500-1000 mg methylprednisolon i.v. for three days before oral treatment is given (207, 208, 280, 281, 282, 283, 284). The main purpose of this treatment is to protect the contralateral eye (285). If the second eye is to be affected, this most often happens during the first 2 to 14 days (286, 287. Loss of vision after cessation of GC is very rare (36). Alternate day GC is not recommended (268).

23. Treatment of patients with other extratemporal manifestations

Treatment of patients exhibiting large vessel vasculitis involving arteries of the extremities or aorta in addition to temporal arteritis, patients with scalp or tongue necrosis or other serious extratemporal arteritis should be treated vigorously with the same recommendations as for those with visual impairment. For patients with large vessel vasculitis without involvement of the temporal arteries, a low dose regimen of CS may be sufficient (77). For patients developing aortic aneurysms requiering cardiac surgery, medical therapy should be continued at the established dose (93).

23.1 Alternative treatment strategies

In addition to CS-resistance, there are several other compelling reasons to search for alternatives to CS. High initial and cumulative doses of CS often resulting in important side effects, visual impairment despite adequate administration of GC, the development of aortic aneurysm, dilation and dissection in a significant number of patients and the frequent relapses and heterogeneous responses to therapy all are of major concern. Thus, alternate or additive therapy to reduce the CS doses, to better prevent disease complications and to improve therapeutic responses has been the subject of repetitive studies during the recent years.

Trials of methotrexate (MTX) have yielded conflicting results (288, 289, 290). A meta-analysis of three randomized studies (291) showed that treatment with MTX lowers the risk of relapse and reduces exposure to CS. The authors suggested that MTX should be considered as a therapeutic option in addition to standard-of-care treatment with CS for patients with GCA (291). However, most patients are favorably treated with CS monotherapy and may manage with low or modest doses. Consequently, MTX as an adjunctive therapy in GCA should be considered in patients requiring high doses of CS, particularly those having both GCA, PMR and large vessel arteritis (292). MTX may also be added to steroids in patients with peripheral arthritis unresponsive to local CS injections.

Azathioprine and other traditional DMARDs have not been shown to exert any favorable effects in GCA (293, 294, 295), although some steroid sparing effect of azathioprine was found in one double-blind study (293). Similarly, statin therapy does not seem to offer any protection against development of visual complications, large vessel vasculitis, jaw claudication, ischemic heart disease, or cerebrovascular accidents (296).

TNFα has been demonstrated in up to 60% of the cells in all areas of inflamed arteries (297), and inhibition of this cytokine may be an attractive therapeutic option in GCA. Early case reports (298, 299, 300, 301, 302, 303, 304, 305) of favorable response to TNFα inhibitors indicated that biological therapy could be an alternative to CS or at least be used in patients failing to respond to CS. However, suggestions of efficacy of TNFα inhibitors have not withstood further drug trials. In a randomized trial, Hoffman and coworkers (306) found that infliximab therapy did not increase the proportion of patients without relapse at week 22 compared with placebo nor did it increase the proportion of patients whose CS dosages were tapered to 10 mg/d without relapse. The results of drug trials of etanercept are, however, perhaps more promising (299, 300). In a study of etanercept versus placebo, Martinez-Taboada and coworkers showed that among GCA patients with side effects due to CS, etanercept treated patients more often than controls were able to control the disease without CS therapy (299). Clearly, the role of etanercept in CS resistant GCA awaits final clarification.

Much research during the last decade has focused on the role of cytokines in GCA. Cytokines are small proteins that serve as chemical messengers between cells, regulating cell growth and differentiation, tissue repair and remodeling, and many aspects of the immune response (184). In GCA, the different vessel layers produce different cytokines. Interferon-γ secreting T-cells are almost exclusively found in the adventitial layer of the inflamed arteries (184), and appear to be critically involved in modulating the process of intimal hyperplasia, the most destructive consequence of vasculitis. Interferon-Y thus emerges as a prime target for novel therapeutic approaches (184), but no randomized controlled studies have yet emerged. Interestingly, the histological and immunological profile in silent or masked GCA appears different from that of cranial arteritis. The latter is characterized by intimal hyperplasia and production of Interferon-Y, IL-1β and Platelet derived growth factor (PDGF) while in silent GCA there is no intimal hyperplasia and prominent production of IL-2 (33). Whether or not this discrepancy implies different therapeutic approaches and diverging outcome is yet to be shown.

Macrophages in the adventitia produce the proinflammatory cytokines IL-1 and IL-6 (184, 185, 186), and levels of IL-6 has been shown to be potentially helpful in predicting disease severity and may allow for a tailoring of immunosuppressive therapy (186). Thus, preliminary case reports have emerged which may indicate a beneficial effect of the anti IL-6 monoclonal antibody tocilizumab in both polymyalgia rheumatica and GCA (307, 308). Favorable effects of anti-IL-1 receptor antagonists are yet to be documented by randomized controlled trials. Abatacept, a recombinant fusion protein that modulates CD28-mediated T-cell costimulation is another tantalizing therapeutic option in GCA awaiting controlled trials.

In a small series of patients with steroid-resistant Takayasu arteritis, another giant cell vasculitis, treatment with mycophenolate mofetil (MMF) resulted in clinical remission as well as improvement in inflammatory markers (309). However, experience with MMF in GCA is still lacking. Platelet derived growth factor (PDGF) appears to be a critical growth factor in arteries with luminal occlusion (184). Thus, the production of PDGF by multinucleated giant cells and macrophages may be inhibited by tyrosine kinase inhibitors, and preliminary in vitro observations may indicate that imatinib mesylate may have a role in the therapy of GCA (310). Endothelin-1 (ET-1) is one of the most powerful vasoconstrictors identified, and ET-1 concentrations has been found increased at the protein level in temporal artery samples from GCA patients (311). Moreover, plasma ET-1 concentrations appeared higher in patient with ischemic complications (311). However, no study yet has been undertaken to test potential beneficial effects of antagonizing ET-1 in GCA. Finally, the anti-CD20 monoclonal antibody rituximab has not been subjected to

controlled studies, but a case report found improvement of B lymphocyte depletion in a patient requiring unacceptable high doses of CS (312).
At present, no alternatives to daily CS therapy have emerged, but the role of new agents will hopefully be clarified in future drug trials. It is hoped that these new agents will result in better control of markers of inflammation which may translate into lower rates of late atherosclerosis and aortic aneurysms even years after the clinically active phase of the disease has resolved (313). Except for a potential role in patients with visual disturbances, treatment with intravenous methylprednisolone does not appear to offer any long-term CS sparing effect. Moreover, in our experience, intramuscular methylprednisolon has no role in the drug treatment of GCA.

23.2 Additive treatment

Patients with GCA do not seem to be at increased risk of contracting cardiovascular disease (314), but physicians responsible for the treatment of patients with GCA should nevertheless be encouraged to search for cardiovascular risk factors as they are common in this age. Although suggested to be of possible use in other inflammatory rheumatic diseases (315), there are, however, no data to support the use of statins in patients with GCA if they do not have cardiovascular risk factors.
There is an ongoing discussion regarding the use of acetylsalicylic acid in patients with GCA. Some have suggested that treatment with low-dose aspirin may exhibit some protection against cranial ischemic complications (316, 317). However, more recent studies have been unable to detect any definite effects of aspirin in GCA (318). On the other hand, it cannot be excluded that the inflammatory process may have impact on the age-related long-term risk of cardiovascular disease in these patients. In addition to its well-established antiplatelet effect, aspirin may also be beneficial in GCA by virtue of its inhibitory effect on interferon-γ mRNA production, essential for the development of the inflammatory infiltrate of the vessel wall. Thus, low dose aspirin may prevent complications of atherosclerotic cardiovascular disease, not just through its antiplatelet effect, but also by its anti-inflammatory effects during atherogenesis and by increasing plaque stability (313). Finally, the interferon-γ production by the adventitial T lymphocytes in GCA appears relatively resistant to standard CS therapy, but susceptible to aspirin (313). Thus, this may further strengthen the indication for adding aspirin to CS in the standard therapeutic regimen of GCA. However, a prospective study is clearly warranted to define the role of aspirin in GCA. Until then, a low dose regimen of aspirin can be recommended in the absence of specific contraindications as an adjunctive drug in this disease.
Steroid-related side effects are frequently recorded in GCA (264, 265, 266). Among these, the detrimental effects of GC is well known. Although the incidence of CS induced osteoporosis appears rather low in GCA (319, 320), the risk of contracting such complications should not be ignored. Most workers recommend addition of calcium and vitamin-D to female patients with GCA, at least for those patients prone to receive long-term CS therapy and requiring large doses. In the presence of other risk factors for osteoporosis, treatment with bisphonates should be considered.

24. Follow-up and monitoring

24.1 Maintenance therapy (dose and duration)

High doses of oral prednisolone (40-60 mg per day) are maintained for at least 4-6 weeks until systemic symptoms have subsided and markers of disease activity have normalized

(207, 208). Then, the dose is reduced by 10 mg every 2 weeks to 20 mg. Thereafter, the dose is reduced by 2.5 mg every 2-4 weeks to 10 mg. Providing no relapse or development of extracranial complications, CS are further reduced by 1 mg every 1-2 months. In one study (263), mean daily maintenance dose during the first and second year was 6.6 and 4.1 mg, respectively. In another report, the median duration required to reach 7.5 mg/day was 6.5 months (321).

Patients should be monitored closely for relapse, control of disease activity, alleviation of complaints, development of extracranial complications and CS-induced side effects. Which patients that will require higher doses to control the disease are difficult to predict. It has, however, been suggested that a strong systemic inflammatory response is associated with higher CS requirements and a longer duration of therapy (217). Both ESR and CRP should be assessed regularly, but some data indicate that blood concentrations of interleukin 6 are the most sensitive indicators of disease activity and course (185, 186). However, assessment of IL-6 levels is not done in routine laboratories. Thus, both traditional acute phase parameters such as ESR and CRP and clinical evaluation of disease activity and progression represent the basis for deciding the therapeutic dose of CS.

As outlined previously, one approach recommends a minimum of abdominal ultrasound, chest radiographs and transthoracic echocardiogram annually to search for development of aneurysmatic disease. As the incidence of malignant disease in GCA is most likely similar to that of the general population, no recommendations can be given for screening processes to exclude malignancy. The age-group affected by GCA implies, however, attention to coincident development of neoplasia.

25. Cessation of treatment and relapses

Typically, relapses are most commonly occur within the first 18 months (322), but may be observed as late as after 8 years of treatment (321). One or more relapses of GCA occur in 27-62% (323, 324, 325, 326, 327). In patients with visual disturbances, further deterioration of vision usually takes place in the first 5-6 days of steroid initiation (46). Recurrences of visual loss most often occur between 3 and 36 months after the initial visual loss (45). Relapses are most commonly accompanied by increased acute phase parameters. However, both clinical features and acute phase reactants should be considered when diagnosing relapse, as neither CRP nor ESR alone can be depended on to diagnose clinical exacerbations. A rise in ESR/CRP may also spark vigilance that concurrent opportunistic infection is present which should not be overlooked. It is recommended that the initial dose regimen is repeated if relapse develops.

The total duration of GCA treatment is difficult to predict with accuracy on clinical and laboratory grounds. It has been suggested that the slope of prednisolon dose-tapering may identify at an early stage those patients who are at risk of undertaking a long period of treatment (328). Moreover, patients with coexisting AT and PMR appear to demand longer treatment (263, 329). It is still debated whether GCA patients exhibiting visual disturbances require longer periods of GC than those without. In one study (321), the median time to steroid discontinuation was 21.6 months while in another study all patients has discontinued GC within 24 months (329). On the other hands, our experience (263) and also others (330) have demonstrated that after 2 years, 80-90% of patients are still on CS. In the study of Hayreh and Zimmerman (277), 92.5 % of those with visual loss and 86.1 % of those without were still on GC five years after commencement of therapy. Clearly, the duration of

CS treatment is highly variable and careful monitoring of patients cessating treatment is strongly recommended.

26. Concluding remarks

There are still major delays in the recognition and treatment of GCA (65) which partly result in a rather high incidence of irreversible ischemic complications. Patients exibiting less classical clinical manifestations appear to represent a subclass in which diagnosis is particularly problematic. Thus, an important challenge in the care of of patients with GCA is to improve the skill and competence of general practioners as they are the first to meet these patients. Finally, research during the latest years has clearly shown the complexity of the immune pathology in GCA, including both Th1 and Th17 responses (331). Although GC remain the mainstay of therapy in GCA, cocktails of therapies will probably be needed for appropriate disease control (331).

27. References

[1] Gran JT. Some thoughts about the etiopathogenesis of temporal arteritis - a review. Scand J Rheumatol 2002; 31: 1-5.
[2] Hamilton CR, Shelley WM, Tumulty PA. Giant cell arteritis: including temporal arteritis and polymyalgia rheumatica. Medicine 1971; 50: 1-27.
[3] Appelboom T, van Eigem A. How ancient is temporal arteritis? J Rheumatol 1990; 17: 929-31.
[4] Dequeker JV. Polymyalgia rheumatica with temporal arteritis, as painted by Jan van Eyck in 1436. Can Med Assoc J 1981; 124: 1597-8.
[5] Portioli I. The history of polymyalgia rheumatica/giant cell arteritis. Clin Exp Rheum 2000; 18 (4 suppl. 20); S1-S3.
[6] Hutchinson J. Diseases of the arteries. On a peculiar form of thrombotic arteritis of the aged which is sometimes productive of gangrene. Arch Surg 1890; 1 :323-9.
[7] Horton BT, Magath TB, Brown GE. An undescribed form of arteritis of the temporal vessels. May Clin Proc 1932; 7: 700-1.
[8] Horton BT, Magath TB. Arteritis of the temporal vessels; report of seven cases. Staff Meeting Mayo Clinic 1937; 12: 548-53.
[9] Jennings GH. Arteritis of temporal arteries. Lancet 1938; 1: 424-8.
[10] Gilmour JR. Giant cell chronic arteritis. J Pathol Bacteriol 1941;53: 263-77.
[11] Kilbourne ED, Wolff HG. Cranial arteritis: a critical evaluation of the syndrome of temporal arteritis with report of a case. Ann Intern Med 1946; 24: 1- 10.
[12] Liozon E, Boutros-Toni F, Ly K, Loustaud-Ratti V, Soria P, Vidal E. Silent or masked giant cell arteritis is associated with a strong inflammatory response and a benign short term course. J Rheumatol 2003; 30: 1272-6.
[13] Simmons RJ, Cogan DG. Occult temporal arteritis. Arch Ophthalmol 1962; 68: 38-48.
[14] Hayreh SS, Podhajsky PA, Zimmerman B. Occult giant cell arteritis: ocular manifestations. Am J Opthalmol 1998; 125: 521-6.
[15] Gran JT, Myklebust G. The incidence of polymyalgia rheu-matica and temporal arteritis in the county of Aust Agder, South Norway, 1987 - 1994. J Rheumatol 1997; 24: 1739-43.

[16] Smeeth L, Cook C, Hall AJ. Incidence of diagnosed polymyalgia rheumatica and temporal arteritis in the United Kingdom, 1990-2001. Ann Rheum Dis 2006; 65: 1093-8. 17. Østberg G. Temporal arteritis in a large necropsy series. Ann Rheum Dis 1971; 30: 224-35.
[17] Gonzalez-Gay MA, Martinez-Dubois C, Agudo M, Pompei O, Blanco R, Llorca J. Giant cell arteritis: epidemiology, diagnosis and management. Curr Rheum Rep 2010; 12: 436-42.
[18] Nordborg C, Johansson H, Petursdottir V, Nordborg E. The epidemiology of biopsy-proven giant cell arteritis: special reference to changes in the age of the population. Rheumatology 2003; 42: 549-52.
[19] Salvarani C, Crowson CS, O`Fallon M, Hunder GG, Gabriel SE. Reappraisel of the epidemiology of giant cell arteritis in Olmsted County, Minnesota, over a fifty-year period. Arthr Care Res 2004; 51: 264-8.
[20] Gran JT, Myklebust G, Wilsgaard T, Jacobsen BK. Survival in polymyalgia rheumatica and temporal arteritis: a study of 398 cases and matched population controls. Rheumatology 2001; 40: 1238-42.
[21] Matteson EL, Gold KN, Bloch DA, Hunder GG. Long-term survival of patients with giant cell arteritis in the American College of Rheumatology giant cell arteritis classification criteria cohort. Am J Med 1996; 100: 193-6.
[22] Bengtsson BA, Malmwall BE. The epidemiology of giant cell arteritis including temporal arteritis and polymyalgia rheumatica. Incidences of clinical presentations and eye complications. Arthritis Rheum 1981; 24: 899-904.
[23] Salvarani C, Macchioni P, Zizzi F, Mantovani W, Rossi F, Castri C, Capozzoli N, Baricchi R, Boiardi L, Chiaravalloti F. Epidemiologic and immunogenetic aspects of polymyalgia rheumatica and giant cell arteritis. Arthritis Rheum 1991; 34: 351-6.
[24] Myklebust G, Gran JT. A prospective study of 287 patientswith polymyalgia rheumatica and temporal arteritis: clinical and laboratory manifestations at onset of disease and at the time of diagnosis. Br J Rheumatol 1996 ;35: 1161-8.
[25] Pipinos II, Hopp R, Edwards WD, Radio SJ. Giant cell arteritis in a 17 year old male. J Vasc Surg 2006; 43: 1053-5.
[26] Nesher G, Oren S, Lijovetzky G, Nesher R. Vasculitis of the temporal arteritis in the young. Semin Arthritis Rheum 2009; 39: 96-107.
[27] Durant C, Connault J, Graveleau J, Toquet C, Brisseau JM, Hamidou M. Juvenile temporal vasculitis : a rare case in a middle-aged woman. Ann Vasc Surg 2011;25:384: e5-7.
[28] Dinesh KP, Owolabi A, Dwyer-Joyce L, Cronin PM, Schimmer BM, Mo GP. Temporal artery vasculitis in young: a report of two cases. Rheumatol Int 2010; 30: 1393-6.
[29] Gonzalez-Gay MA, Garcia-Porrua C, Amor-Dorado JC, Llorca J. fever in biopsy proven GCA: clinical implications in a defined population. Arthritis Rheum 2004; 51: 652-55.
[30] Jundt J, Mock D. Temporal arteritis with normal erythrocyte sedimentation rate presenting as occipital neuralgia. Arthritis Rheum 1991; 34: 217-9.
[31] Rahman W, Rahman FZ. Giant cell (temporal)arteritis: an overview and update. Surv Ophthalmol 2005; 50: 415-28.
[32] Kawasaki A, Purvin V. Giant cell arteritis: an updated review. Acta Ophthalmol Scand 2009; 87: 13-32.

[33] Becourt-Verlomme C, Barouky R, Alexandre C, Gonthier R, Laurent H, Vital Durand D, Rousset H. Symptomes inauguraux de la maladie de Horton sur une serie de 260 patients. Rev Med Interne 2001; 22: 631-7.
[34] Calamia KT, Hunder GG. GCA (TA) presenting as fever of undetermined origin. Arthritis Rheum 1981; 24: 1414-18.
[35] Aiello PD, Trautmann JC, McPhee TJ, Kunselman AR, Hunder GG. Visual prognosis in giant cell arteritis. Ophthalmology 1993; 100: 550-5.
[36] Loddenkemper T, Sharma P, Katzan I, Plant GT. Risk factors for early visual deterioration in temporal arteritis. J Neurol Neurosurg Psychiatry 2007; 78: 1255-9.
[37] Salvarani C, Cimino L, Macchioni P, Consonni D, Cantini F, Bajocchi G, Pipitone N, Catanoso MG, Biordi L. Risk factors for visual loss in an Italian population-based cohort of patients with giant cell arteritis. Arthritis Rheum 2005; 53: 293-7.
[38] Gonzalez-Gay MA, Miranda-Filloy JA, Lopez-Diaz MJ, Perez-Alvarez R, Gonzalez-Juanatey C, Sanchez-Andrade A, Marin J, Llorca J. Giant cell arteritis in Northwestern Spain. Medicine 2007; 86: 61-8.
[39] Gonzalez-Gay MA, Garcia-Porrua C, Llorca J, Hajeer AH, Branas F, Dababneh A, Gonzalez-Louzao C, Rodriguez-Gil E, Rodrig P, Ollier W. Visual manifestations of giant cell arteritis: trends and clinical spectrum in patients. Medicine 2000; 79: 283-92.
[40] Bas-Lando M, Breuer GS, Berkun Y, Mates M, Sonnenblick M, Nesher G. The incidence of giant cell arteritis in Jerusalem over a 25-year period: annual and seasonal fluctuations. Clin Exp Rheum 2007; 25 (suppl. 44): S15-S17.
[41] Miller NR. Visual manifestations of temporal arteritis. Rheum Dis Clin North Amer 2001; 27: 781-97.
[42] Sonnenblick M, Nesher R, Rozenman Y, Nesher G. Charles Bonnet syndrome in temporal arteritis. J Rheumatol 1995; 22: 1596-7.
[43] Razavi M, Jones RD, Manzel K, Fatal D, Rizzo M. Steroid-responsive Charles-Bonnet syndrome in temporal arthritis. J Neuropsychiatry Clin Neurosci 2004; 16: 505-8.
[44] Chan CCK, Paine M, 0`Day J. Predictors of recurrent ischemic optic neuropathy in giant cell arteritis. J Neuro-Ophthalmol 2005; 25: 14-7.
[45] Danesch-Meyer H, Savino PJ, Gamble GG. Poor prognosis of visual outcome after visual loss from giant cell arteritis. Ophthalmology 2005; 112: 1098-1103.
[46] Hayreh SS, Zimmerman B. Management of giant cell arteritis. Ophthalmologica 2003; 217: 239-59.
[47] Andersson R, Malmwall BE, Bengtsson BÅ. Long-term corticosteroid treatment in giant cell arteritis. Acta Med Scand 1986; 220: 465-9.
[48] Gonzalez-Gay MA, Blanco R, Rodriguez-Valverde V, Martinez-Taboada WM, Delgado-Rodriguez M, Figueroa M, Uriarte E. Permanent visual loss and cerebrovascular accidents in giant cell arteritis. Arthritis Rheum 1998; 41: 1497-1504.
[49] Egge K, Mitbo A, Westby R. Arteritis temporalis. Acta Ophthalmologica 1966; 44: 49-56.
[50] Hayreh SS, Zimmerman B, Kardon RH. Visual improvement with corticosteroid therapy in giant cell arteritis. Report of a large study and review of literature. Acta Ophthalmol Scand 2002: 80: 353-67.

[51] Jallon P, Loron P, Borg M, Viallet F, Jan P, Force L. Cortical blindness from Horton`s disease. Rev Neurol (Paris). 1980; 136: 769-76.
[52] Chisholm IH. Cortical blindness in cranial arteritis. Br J Ophthalmol 1975; 59: 332-3.
[53] Hayreh SS, Podhajsky PA, Zimmerman B. Ocular manifestations of giant cell arteritis. Am J Ophthalmol 1998; 125: 509-20.
[54] Glutz von Blotzheim S, Bourrat FX. Neuro-ophthalmic complications of biopsy proven giant cell arteritis. Eur J Ophthalmol 1997; 7: 375-82.
[55] Wagener HP, Hollenhorst RW. The ocular lesions of temporal arteritis. Am J Ophthalmol 1958; 45: 617-30.
[56] Font C, Cid MC, Coll-Vinent B, Lopez-Soto A, Grau JM. Clinical features in patients with permanent visual loss due to biopsy-proven giant cell arteritis. Br J Rheumatol 1997; 36: 251-4.
[57] Cid MC, Oristrell J, de la Sierra A, Coll-Vinent B, Lopez-Soto A, Vilaseca J, Urbano-Marquez A, Grau JM. Association between strong inflammatory response and low risk of developing visual loss and other cranial ischemic complications in giant cell (temporal) arteritis. Arthritis Rheum 1998; 41: 26-32.
[58] Liozon E, Herrmann F, Ly K, Robert PY, Loustaud V, Soria P. Risk factors for visual loss in giant cell (temporal) arteritis: a prospective study of 174 patients. Am J Med 2001; 111: 211-7.
[59] Lopez-Diaz MJ, Llorca J, Gonzalez-Juanatey C, Pena-Sagredo JL, Martin J, Gonzalez-Gay MA. The erythrocyte sedimentation rate is associated with the development of visual complications in biopsy-proven giant cell arteritis. Semin Arthritis Rheum 2008; 38: 116-23.
[60] Gonzalez-Gay MA, Lopez-Diaz MJ, Barros S, Garcia-Porrua C, Sanchez-Andrade A, Paz-Carreira J, Martin J, Llorca J. Giant cell arteritis. Laboratory tests at the time of diagnosis in a series of 240 patients. Medicine 2005; 84: 277-90.
[61] Salvarani C, Bella CD, Cimino L, Macchioni P, Formisano D, Bajocchi G, Pipitone N, Catasano MG, Restuccia G, Ghinoi A, Boiardi L. Risk factors for severe cranial ischemic events in an Italian population-based cohort of patients with giant cell arteritis. Rheumatology 2009; 48: 250-3.
[62] Salvarani C, Hunder GG. Giant cell arteritis with low erythrocyte sedimentation rate: frequency of occurrence in a population-based study. Arthritis Care Res 2001; 45: 140-5.
[63] Chatelain D, Duhaut P, Schmidt J, Loire R, Bosshard S, Guernou M et al. Pathological features of temporal arteries in patients with giant cell arteritis presenting with permanent visual loss. Ann Rheum Dis 2009; 68: 84-8.
[64] Ezeonyeji AN, Borg FA, Dasgupta B. Delays in recognition and management of giant cell arteritis: result from a retrospective audit. Clin Rheumatol 2011; 30: 259-62.
[65] Nuenninghoff DM, Hunder GG, Christianson TJH, McClelland RL, Matteson EL. Incidence and predictors of large-artery complication (aortic aneurysm, aortic dissection, and/or large-artery stenosis) in patients with giant cell arteritis. Arthritis Rheum 2003; 48: 3522-31.
[66] Klein RG, Hunder GG, Stanson AW, Sheps SG. Large artery involvement in giant cell arteritis. Ann Intern Med 1975; 83: 806-12.

[67] Assie C, Janvresse A, Plissonnier D, Levesque H, Marie I. Long-term follow-up of upper and lower extremity vasculitis related to giant cell arteritis. Medicine 2011; 90: 40-51.
[68] Evans JM, O`Fallon M, Hunder GG. Increased incidence of aortic aneurysm and dissection in giant cell (temporal) arteritis: a population-based study. Ann Intern Med 1995; 122: 502-7.
[69] Schmidt WA, Moll A, Seifert A, Schicke B, Gromnica-Ihle E, Krause A. Prognosis of large-vessel giant cell arteritis. Rheumatology 2008; 47: 1406-8.
[70] Kermani TA, Matteson EL, Hunder GG, Warrington KJ. Symptomatic lower extremity vasculitis in giant cell arteritis: a case series. J Rheumatol 2009; 36: 2277-83.
[71] Marie I, Proux A, Duhaut P, Primard E, Lahaxe L, Girszyn N, Louvet JP, Levesque H. Long-term follow-up of aortic involvement in giant cell arteritis: a series of 48 patients. Medicine 2009; 88: 182-92.
[72] Agard C, Barrier JH, Dupas B, Ponge T, Mahr A, Fradet G, Chevalet P et al. Aortic involvement in recent-onset giant cell (temporal) arteritis: a case-control prospective study using helical aortic computed tomodensitometric scan. Arthritis Care Res 2008; 59: 670-6.
[73] Garcia-Martinez A, Hernandez-Rodriguez J, Arguis P, Paredes P, Segarra M, Lozano E. Development of aortic aneurysm/dilatation during the follow-up of patients with giant cell arteritis: a cross-sectional screening of fifty-four prospectively followed patients. Arthritis Care Res 2008; 59: 422-30.
[74] Sujobert P, Fardet L, Marie I, Duhaut P, Cohen P, Grange C, Gaultier JB, Arrive L, Cabane J. Mesenteric ischemia in giant cell arteritis : 6 cases and systematic review. J Rheumatol 2007; 34: 1727-32.
[75] Bongartz T, Matteson EL. large-vessel involvement in giant cell arteritis. Curr Opin Rheum 2006; 18: 10-17
[76] Brack A, Martinez-Taboada V, Stanson A, Goronzy JJ, Weyand CM. Disease pattern in cranial and large-vessel giant cell arteritis. Arthritis Rheum 1999; 42: 311-7.
[77] Le Hello C, Levesque H, Jeanton M, Cailleux N, Galateau F, Peillon C, Veyssier P, Watelet J, Letellier P, Courtois H, Maiza D. Lower limb giant cell arteritis and temporal arteritis ; Follow-up of 8 cases. J Rheumatol 2001;28: 1407-12.
[78] Schmidt WA, Moll A, Seifert A, Schicke B, Gromnica-Ihle E, Krause A. Prognosis of large-vessel giant cell arteritis. Rheumatology 2008; 47: 1406-8.
[79] Sproul EE, Hawthorne JJ. Chronic diffuse mesaortitis; report of 2 cases of unusual type. Am J Pathol 1937; 13: 311-23.
[80] Bossert M, Prati C, Balblanc JC, Lohse A, Wendling D. Aortic involvement in giant cell arteritis: current data. Joint Bone Spine 2011 e.pub.
[81] Agard C, Ponge T, Fradet G, Baron O, Sagan C, Masseau A, barrier JH, Hamidou M. Giant cell arteritis presenting with aortic dissection: two cases and review of the literature. Scand J Rheumatol 2006; 35: 233-6.
[82] Gonzalez-Gay MA, Garcia-Porrua C, Pineiro A, Pego-Reigosa R, Llorca J, Hunder GG. Aortic aneurysm and dissection in patients with biopsy-proven GCA from northwestern Spain: a population-based study. Medicine 2004; 83: 335-41.
[83] Evans J, Hunder GG. The implications of recognizing large-vessel involvement in elderly patients with giant cell arteritis. Curr Opin Rheum 1997; 9: 37-40.

[84] Narvaez J, Narvaez JA, Nolla JM, Sirvent E, Reina D, Valverde J. Giant cell arteritis and polymyalgia rheumatica: usefulness of vascular magnetic resonance imaging studies in the diagnosis of aortitis. Rheumatology 2005; 44: 479-83.
[85] Both M, Ahmadi-Simab K, Reuter M, Dourvos O, Fritzer E, Ullrich S, Gross WL, Heller M, Bahre M. MRI and FDG-PET in the assessment of inflammatory aortic arch syndrome in complicated courses of giant cell arteritis. Ann Rheum Dis 2008; 67: 1030-3.
[86] Hautzel H, Sander O, Heinzel A, Schneider M, Muller HW. Assessment of large-vessel involvement in giant cell arteritis with 18F-FDG PET: introducing an ROC-analysis-based cutoff ration. J Nucl Med 2008; 49: 1107-13.
[87] Bruschi M, de Leonardis F, Govoni M, Roncali M, Prandini N, La Corte R, Feggi L, Trotta F. 18 FDG-PET and large vessel vasculitis: preliminary data on 25 patients. Reumatismo 2008; 60: 212-6.
[88] Blockmans D, de Ceuninck L, Vanderschueren S, Knockaert D, Mortelmans L, Bobbaers H. Repetitive 18F-Fluorodeaxyglucose positron emission tomography in giant cell arteritis: a prospective study of 35 cases. Arthritis Rheum 2006; 55: 131-7.
[89] Lehman P, Buchtala S, Achajew N, Haerle P, Ehrenstein B, Lighvani H, Fleck M, Marienhagen J. 18F-FDG PET as a diagnostic procedure in large vessel vasculitis - a controlled, blinded re-examination of routine PET scans. Clin Rheum 2011; 30: 37-42.
[90] Neunninghoff DM, Hunder GG, Christianson TJH, McClelland RL, Matteson EL. Mortality of large-artery complications (aortic aneurysm, aortic dissection and/or large-artery stenosis) in patients with giant cell arteritis. Arthritis Rheum 2003;48: 3532-7.
[91] Herve F, Choussy V, Janvresse A, Cailleux N, Levesque H, Marie I. Aortite inflammatoire et maladie de Horton. A propos du suivi evolutif scanographique prospectif d`une serie de 11 patients. Rev Med Interne 2006; 27: 196-202.
[92] Butler N, Mundy J, Shah P. Aortic complications of giant cell arteritis: a diagnostic and management dilemma. J Card Surg 2010; 25: 572-81.
[93] Burke AP, Tavora F, Narula N, Tomaszewski JE, Virmani R. Aortitis and ascending aortic aneurysm: description of 52 cases and proposal of a histologic classification. Hum Pathol 2008; 39: 514-26.
[94] Caselli R, Hunder GG, Whisnant JP. Neurolog disease in biopsy-proven giant cell (temporal) arteritis. Neurology 1988; 38: 352-9.
[95] Bley TA, Geiger J, Jacobsen S, Wieben O, Markl M, Vaith P, Grist T, Langer M, Uhl M. High resolution MRI for assessment of middle artery involvement in giant cell arteritis. Ann Rheum Dis 2009; 68: 1369-70.
[96] Gonzalez-Gay MA, Vasquez-Rodriguez TR, Gomez-Acebo I, Pego-Reigosa R, Lopez-Diaz MJ, Vasquez-Trinanes MC. Strokes at the time of disease diagnosis in a series of 287 patients with biopsy-proven giant cell arteritis. Medicine 2009; 88: 227-35.
[97] Pego-Reigosa R, Garcia-Porrua C, Pineiro A, Dierssen T, Llorca J, Gonzalez-Gay MA. Predictors of cerebrovascular accidents in giant cell arteritis in a defined population. Clin Exp Rheum 2004; 22 (suppl. 36): S13-S17.
[98] Solans-Laque R, Bosch-Gil JA, Molina-Catenario CA, Ortega-Aznar A, Alvarez-Sabin J, Vilardel-Tarres M. Stroke and multi-infarct dementia as presenting symptoms of

giant cell arteritis: report of 7 cases and review of the literature. Medicine 2008; 87: 335-44.

[99] Lu-Emerson C, Walker M, Huber BR, Ghodke B, Longstreth WT Jr, Khot SP. Lethal giant cell arteritis with multiple ischemic strokes despite aggressive immunosuppressive therapy. J Neurol Sci 2010; 295; 120-4.

[100] Fitzgerald AJ, Ironside JW, Summers DM, Dennis MS, McRorie ER. Two cases of recurrent stroke in treated giant cell arteritis: diagnostic and therapeutic dilemmas. J Clin Rheumatol 2010; 16: 225-8.

[101] Staunton H, Stafford F, Leader M, O`Riordan D. Deterioration of giant cell arteritis with corticosteroid therapy. Arch Neurol 2000; 57: 581-4.

[102] Cooke WT, Cloake PCP, Govan ADT. Temporal arteritis: a generalised vascular disease. Q J med 1946; 15: 47-75.

[103] Campbell FA, Clark C, Holmes S. Scalp necrosis in temporal arteritis. Clin Exp Derm 2003; 28: 488-90.

[104] Simon RW, fritz T, Anmann-Vesti BR. An unusual presentation of giant cell arteritis. Vasa 2005; 34: 128-30.

[105] Currey J. Scalp necrosis in giant cell arteritis and review of the literature. Br J Rheumatol 1997; 36: 814-6.

[106] Tsianakas A, Ehrchen JM, Presser D, Fischer T, Kruse-Loesler B, Luger TA, Sunderkoetter C. Scalp necrosis in giant cell arteritis: case report and review of this cutaneous sign og large-vessel vasculitis. J Am Acad Dermatol 2009; 61: 701-6.

[107] Brick KE, Cook-Norris RH, Wetter DA, Warrington KJ. Scalp necrosis in giant cell arteritis after initiation of therapeutic corticosteroids. J Am Acad Dermatol 2010; 63: 343-4.

[108] Rockey JG, Anand R. Tongue necrosis secondary to temporal arteritis: a case report and literature review. Oral Surg Oral Med Oral Pathol Oral Radiol Endo 2002; 94: 471-3.

[109] Davis AE, Davis TP. Gangrene of the tongue caused by temporal arteritis. Med J Aust 1966; 2: 459-60.

[110] Goicochea M, Correale J, Bonamico L, Dominguez R, Bagg E, famulari A, Ameriso S, Sevlever G. Tongue necrosis in temporal arteritis. Headache 2007; 47: 1213-5.

[111] Mathew SD, Bristow K, Higgs J. Giant cell arteritis presenting as ageusia and lower extremity claudication. J Clin Rheumatol 2010; 16: 343-4.

[112] Alisky JM. Giant cell arteritis dementia and other steroid-responsive dementia syndromes are a unique opportunity for clinicialns and researchers. Singapore Med J 2008; 49: 268-70.

[113] Tomer Y, Neufeld MY, Shoenfeld Y. Coma with triphasic pattern in EEG as a complication of temporal arteritis. Neurology 1992; 42: 429-40.

[114] Silbert PL, Stewart-Wynne EG. Seizures and giant cell temporal arteritis: what is the relationship? Aust N Z J Med 1992; 22: 307.

[115] Fruchter O, Ben-Ami H, Schapira D, Gallimidi Z, Gaitini D, Goldsher D. Giant cell arteritis complicated by spinal cord infarction: a therapeutic dilemma. J Rheumatol 2002; 29: 1556-8.

[116] Galetta SL, Balcer LJ, Lieberman AP, Syed NA, Lee JM, Oberholtzer JC. Refractory giant cell arteritis with spinal cord infarction. Neurology 1997; 49: 1720-3.

[117] McAlindon TE, Ferguson IT. Mononeuritis multiplex and occipital infarction complicating giant cell arteritis. Br J Rheumatol 1989; 28: 257-8.
[118] Kawaguchi Y, Ebina M, Sato T, Ishiguro Y, Yagihashi S, Hirota K. A case of trigeminal neuralgia complicated by ipsilateral temporal arteritis. J Anest 2010; 24: 139-42.
[119] Edvardsson B, Eriksson B. Giant cell arteritis and bilateral nerve palsy. Scand J Rheumatol 2010; 39: 269-70.
[120] Donadini M, Dentali F, Squizzato A, Ageno W. An unusual case of cerebral vein thrombosis in a patient with giant cell arteritis. Thromb Haemost 2008; 100: 513-4.
[121] Chisholm IH. Cortical blindness in cranial arteritis. Br J Ophthalmol 1975; 59: 332-3.
[122] Guly CM, Olson JA. Transient ischemic attacks. Giant cell arteritis and transient visual loss. Br Med J 2009; 338:b1809.
[123] Morris OC, Lockie P. Giant cell arteritis presenting as stroke, transient ischemic attacks and dementia. Aust Fam Physician 2005; 34: 653-5.
[124] Paraskevas KI, Boumpas DT, Vrentzos GE, Mikhailidis DP. Oral and ocular/orbital manifestations of temporal arteritis : a disease with deceptive clinical symptoms and devastating consequences. Clin Rheumatol 2007; 26: 1044-8.
[125] Larson TS, Hall S, Hepper NG, Hunder GG. Respiratory tract symptoms as a clue to GCA. Ann Intern Med 1984; 101:594-7.
[126] Lee CC, Su WW, Hunder GG. Dysarthria associated with GCA. J Rheumatol 1999; 26:931-2.
[127] Ramos R, Vila R, Penin R, Cairols MA. Giant cell arteritis presenting as dysarthria and mediastinal mass. Interact Cardiovasc Thor Surg 2010; 11: 337-9.
[128] Levine SM, Hellmann DB. Giant cell arteritis. Curr Opin Rheum 2002; 14: 3-10.
[129] Kinmont PDC, MacCallum DI. The aetiology, pathology and course of giant-cell arteritis. The possible role of light-sensitivity. Br J Derm 1965; 77: 193-202.
[130] Helfrich DJ, Mulhern LM, Luparello FJ, Smith W Jr. Giant cell arteritis of the tongue presenting as macroglossia. J Rheumatol 1988; 15: 1026-8.
[131] Liozon E, Ouattara B, Portal MF, Soria P, Loustaud-Ratti V, Vidal E. Head-and-neck swelling: an under-recognized feature of giant cell arteritis: a report of 37 patients. Clin Exp Rheum 2006; 24 (suppl.41):S20-S25.
[132] Ricketti AJ, Cleri DJ, Godyn JJ, Shenk SH, Vernaleo JR. Giant cell arteritis presenting as facial swelling. Allergy Asthma Proc 2008; 29: 538-50.
[133] Amor-Dorado JC, Llorca J, Garcia-Porrua C, Costa C, Perez-Fernandez N, Gonzalez-Gay MA. Audiovestibular manifestations in giant cell arteritis. A prospective study. Medicine 2003; 82: 13- 26.
[134] Lee AG, Tang RA, Schiffman JS, Feldon SE, Rao N, Pless M, Rubin RM. Orbital presentation of giant cell arteritis. Graefe`s Arch Clin Exp Ophthalmol 2001; 239: 509-13.
[135] Arai M, Katsumata R. Temporal arteritis presenting with headache and abducens palsy. Report of a case. Rhinso Shinkeigaku 2007; 47: 444-6.
[136] Liou LM, Khor TK, Lan SH, Lai CL. Giant cell arteritis with multiple cranial nerve palsy and reversible proptosis: a case report. Headache 2007; 47: 1451-3.
[137] Scola CJ, L C, Upchurch KS. Mesenteric involvement in giant cell arteritis. An unrecognized complication? Medicine 2008; 87: 45-51.
[138] Azeez MA, Browne P, O`Connel P, Roysten D. Giant cell arteritis involving the mesenteric arteries. J Rheumatol 2009; 36:2314-5.

[139] Annamalai A, Francis ML, Ranatunga SK, Resch DS. Giant cell arteritis presenting as small bowel infarction. J Gen Intern Med 2007; 22: 140-4.
[140] Srigley JR, Gardiner GW. Giant cell arteritis with small bowel infarction. A case report and review of the literature. Am J Gastroenterol 1980; 73: 157-61.
[141] Bajocchi G, Zamorani G, Cavazza A. GCA of the female genital tract associated with occult arteritis and FDG-PET evidence of large vessel vasculitis. Clin Exp Rheum 2007;25 (suppl 44):S36-39.
[142] Onuma K, Chu CT, Dabbs DJ. Asymptomatic giant-cell (temporal) arteritis involving the bilateral adnexa: case report and literature review. Int J Gynecol Pathol 2007;26: 352-5.
[143] Hernandez-Rodriguez J, Tan CD, Rodriguez R, Hoffman GS. Gynecologic vasculitis. Medicine 2009; 88: 169-81.
[144] Valstar MH, Terpstra WF, de Jong RS. Pericardial and pleural effusions in GCA. Am J Med 2003; 114: 708-9.
[145] Graffin B, Carli P. Respiratory manifestations of giant cell arteritis : 8 cases and review of the literature. Presse Med 2010; 39: e188-96.
[146] Moulis G, Sailler L, Astudillo L, Vernet J, Couret B, Arlet P. Pericarditis as the presenting manifestation of giant cell arteritis. Rev Med Interne 2010; 31: 46-8.
[147] Kechaou M, Frigui M, Marzouk S, Jallouli M, Frikha F, Kaddour N, Boudawara T, Bahloul Z. Pleural effusion revealing Horton`s disease. Rev Med Liege 2008; 63: 650-3.
[148] Carassou P, Aletti M, Cinquetti G, Banal F, Landais C, Graffin B, Carli P. Respiratory manifestations of giant cell arteritis : 8 cases and review of the literature. Presse Med 2010; 39: e188-96.
[149] Lie JT, Failoni DD, Davies DC Jr. Temporal arteritis with giant cell aortitis, coronary arteritis, and myocardial infarction. Arch Pathol Lab Med 1986; 110:857-60.
[150] Lander H, Bonnin JM. Giant cell arteritis. Report of a case with autopsy. J Path Bacteriol 1956;71:369-73.
[151] Eberhardt RT, Dhadly M. Giant cell arteritis: diagnosis, management and cardiovascular implications. Cardiol Rev 2007; 15: 55-61.
[152] Morris CR, , Scheib JS. Fatal myocardial infarction resulting from coronary arteritis in a patient with polumyalgia rheumatica and biopsy-proved temporal arteritis. A case report and review of the literature. Arch Int Med 1994; 154: 1158-60.
[153] Jithpratuck W, Wason WW, Elsenawy Y. Acute bilateral ischemia of fingers: an unusual complication of temporal arteritis. South Med J 2010; 103: 1178-80.
[154] Kadotani Y, Enoki Y, Itoi N, Kojima F, Kato G, Lee CJ. Giant cell arteritis of the breast: a case report with a review of literures. Breast Cancer 2010; 17: 225-32.
[155] Kariv R, Sidi Y, Gur H. Systemic vasculitis presenting as a tumorlike lesion. Four case reports and an analysis of 79 reported cases. Medicine 2000; 79: 349-59.
[156] Luzar MJ, Whisler RL, Hunder GG. Syndrome of inappropriate secretion of antidiuretic hormone in association with temporal arteritis. J Rheumatol 1982; 9: 957-60.
[157] Mallia C, Coleiro B, Crockford M, Ellul B. Raynaud`s phenomenon caused by giant cell arteritis. A case report. Adv Exp Med Biol 1999; 455: 517-20.

[158] Zauber NP, Echikson AB. Giant cell arteritis and microangiopathic hemaolytic anemia. Am J Med 1982; 73: 928-30.
[159] Chambers BR, Donnan GA, Riddel RJ, Bladin PF. Carotidynia: aetiology, diagnosis and treatment. Clin Exp Neurol 1981; 17: 113-23.
[160] Truong L, Kopelman RG, Williams GS, Pirani CL. Temporal arteritis and renal disease. Case report and review of the literature. Am J Med 1985;78: 171-5.
[161] Salvarani C, gabriel SE, O`Fallon WM, Hunder GG. The incidence of GCA in Olmstead County, Minnesota: apparent fluctuation in a cyclic pattern. Ann Intern med 1995; 123: 192-4.
[162] ranzen P, Sutinen S, von Knorring J. GCA and PMR in a region of Finland: an epidemiologic, clinical and pathologic study. J Rheumatol 1992; 19: 273-80.
[163] Porsman VA. Arthritis in old age. Proc II Congr Europ Rheum (Barcelona). 1951:481-97.
[164] Gran JT, Myklebust G. Incidence and clinical characteristics of peripheral arthritis in polymyalgia rheumatica and temporal arteritis. Rheumatology 2000; 39: 283-7.
[165] Moosig F, Czech N, Mehi C, Henze E, Zenner RA, Kneba M, Schrøder JO. Correlation between 18-fluorodeoxyglucose accumulation in large vessels and serological markers of inflammation in polymyalgia rheumatica: a quantitative PET study. Ann Rheum Dis 2004; 63: 870-3.
[166] Blockmans D, Maes A, Stroobants S, Nuyts J, Bormans G, Knockaert D, Bobbaers H, Mortelmans L. New arguments for a vasculitic nature of polymyalgia rheumatica using positron emission tomography. Rheumatology 1999, 38: 444-7.
[167] Alestig K, Barr J. Giant cell arteritis: a biopsy study of polymyalgia rheumatica, including one case of Takayasu`s disease. Lancet 1963; 1: 1228-30.
[168] Hamrin B, Jonsson N, Landberg T. Arteritis in "polymyalgia rheumatica". Lancet 1964; 1: 397-401.
[169] Nordborg E, Nordborg C. The influence of sectional interval on the reliability of temporal artery biopsies in polymyalgia rheumatica. Clin Rheumatol 1995; 14: 330-4.
[170] Myklebust G, Gran JT. Prednisolone maintenance dose in relation to starting dose in the treatment of polymyalgia rheumatica and temporal arteritis. Scand J Rheumatol 2001; 30: 260-7.
[171] Kyle V, Hazleman BL. The clinical and laboratory course of polymyalgia rheumatica/giant cell arteritis after the first two months of treatment. Ann Rheum Dis 1993; 52:847-50.
[172] Parikh M, Miller NR, Lee AG, Savino PJ, Vacarezza MN, Cornblath W, Eggenberger E, Antonio-Santos A, Golnik K, Kardon R, Wall M. Prevalence of a normal C-reactive protein with an elevated erythrocyte sedimentation rate in biopsy-proven giant cell arteritis. Ophthalmology 2006; 113: 1842-5.
[173] Wise CM, Agudelo CA, Chmelewski WL, McKnight KM. Temporal arteritis with low erythrocyte sedimentation rate: a review of five cases. Arthritis Rheum 1991; 34: 1571-4.
[174] Kansu T, Corbett JJ, Savino P, Schatz NJ. Giant-cell arteritis with normal erythrocyte sedimentation rate. Arch Neurol 1977; 34: 624-5.
[175] Ellis ME, Ralston S. The ESR in the diagnosis and management of polymyalgia rheumatica/giant cell arteritis syndrome. Ann Rheum Dis 1983; 42: 168-70.

[176] Grodum E, Petersen HA. Temporal arteritis with normal erythrocyte sedimentation rate. J Intern Med 1990; 227: 279-80.
[177] Ciccarelli M, Jeanmonod D, Jeanmonod R. Giant cell arteritis with a normal erythrocyte sedimentation rate: report of a case. Am J Emerg Med 2009; 255: e1-3.
[178] Nesh PR, Sergent JS. Giant cell arteritis: a case with unusual neurologic manifestations and a normal sedimentation rate. Arch Intern Med 1991; 151: 378-80.
[179] Desmet GD, Knockaert DC, Bobbaers HJ. Temporal arteritis: the silent presentation and delay in diagnosis. J Int Med 1990; 227: 237-40.
[180] Foroozan R, Danesch-Meyer H, Savino PJ, Gamble G, Mekari-Sabbagh ON, Sergott RC. Thrombocytosis in patients with biopsy-proven giant cell arteritis. Ophthalomology 2002; 109: 1267-71.
[181] Hayreh SS, Podhajsky PA, Raman R, Zimmerman B: GCA: validity and reliability of various diagnostic tests. Am J Ophthalmol 1997; 123: 285-96.
[182] Kyle V. Laboratory investigations including liver in polymyalgia rheumatica/giant cell arteritis. Bailliere`s Clin Rheum 1991; 5: 475-84.
[183] Goronzy JJ, Weyand CM. Cytokines in giant-cell arteritis. Clev Clin J Med 2002; 69: suppl II: 91-4.
[184] Dasgupta B, Panayi GS. Interleukin 6 in serum of patients with polymyalgia rheumatica and giant cell arteritis. Br J Rheum 1990; 29:456-8.
[185] Weyand CM, Fulbright JW, Hunder GG, Evans JM, Goronzy JJ. Treatment of giant cell arteritis: interleukin-6 as a biologic marker of disease activity. Arthritis Rheum 2000; 43: 1041-8.
[186] Garcia-Martinez A, Hernadez-Rodriguez J, Espigol-Frigole G, Prieto-Gonzalez S, Butjosa M, Segarra M, Lozano E, Cid MC. Clinical relevance of peristently elevated circulating cytokines (tumor necrosis factor-α and interleukin-6) in the long-term followup of patients with giant cell arteritis. Arthritis Care Res 2010; 62: 835-41.
[187] Schmidt WA, Kraft HE, Vorpahl, Volker L, Gromnica-Ihle EJ. Color duplex ultrasonography in the diagnosis of temporal arteritis. N Engl J Med 1997;337:1336-42.
[188] Schmidt WA, Natusch A, Moller DE, Vorpahl K, Grominca-Ihle E. Involvement of peripheral arteries in giant celle arteritis: a color doppler sonography study. Clin Exp Rheum 2002; 20: 309-18.
[189] Pfadenhauer K, Weber H. Giant cell arteritis of the occipital arteries - a prospective color-coded duplex sonography study in 78 cases. J Neurol 2003; 250: 844-9.
[190] Houtman PM, Doorenbos BM, Dol J, Bruyn GAW. Doppler ultrasonography to diagnose temporal arteritis in the setting of a large community hospital. Scand J Rheumatol :2008; 37: 316-8.
[191] Maldini C, Depinay-Dhellemmes C, Tra TTS, Chauveau M, Allanore Y, Gossec L et al. Limited value of temporal artery ultrasonography examinations for diagnosis of giant cell arteritis: analysis of 77 subjects. J Rheumatol 2010; 37: 2326-30.
[192] Karahaliou M, Vaiopoulos G, Papaspyrou S, Kanakis MA, Revenas K, Sfikakis PP. Colour duplex sonography of temporal arteries before decision for biopsy: a prospective study in 55 patients with suspected giant cell arteritis. Arthr Res Ther 2006; 8: R116.
[193] Karassa FB, Matsagas MI, Schmidt WA, Ioannidis JPA. Meta-analysis: test performance of ultrasonography for giant cell arteritis. Ann Intern Med 2005; 142: 359-69.

[194] Arida A, Kyprianou M, Kanakis M, Sfikakis PP. The diagnostic value of ultrasonography-derived edema of the temporal artery wall in giant cell arteritis: a second meta-analysis. BMC Musculoskeletal Disorders 2010; 11: 44-51.
[195] Murgatroyd H, Nimmo M, Evans A, MacEwen C. The use of ultrasound as an aid in the diagnosis of giant cell arteritis: a pilot study comparing histological features with ultrasound findings. Eye 2003; 17: 415-9.
[196] Ponge T, Barrier JH, Grolleau JY, Ponge A, Vlasak AM, Cottin S. The efficacy of selective unilateral temporal artery biopsy versus bilateral biopsies for diagnosis of giant cell arteritis. J Rheumatol 1988; 15: 997-1000.
[197] Bley TA, Uhl M, Carew J, Markl M, Schmidt D, Peter HH, Langer M, Wieben O. Diagnostic value of high-resolution MR imaging in giant cell arteritis. Am J Neuroradiol 2007; 28: 1722-7.
[198] Hunder GG, Bloch DA, Michel BA, Stevens MB, Arend WP, American College of Rheumatology 1990 criteria for the classification of giant cell arteritis. Arthritis Rheum 1990; 33: 1122-8.
[199] Khoury K, Hoxworth JM, Mazlumzadeh M, Wellik KE, Wingerchuk DM, demaerschalk BM. The clinical utility of high resolution magnetic resonance imaging in the diagnosis of giant cell arteritis: a critically appraised topic. Neurologist 2008; 14: 330-5.
[200] Both M, Ahmadi-Simab K, Reuter M, Dourvos O, Fritzer E, Ullrich S, Gross Wl, Heller M, Bahre M. MRI and FDG-PET in the assessment of inflammatory aortic arch syndrome in complicated courses of giant cell arteritis. Ann Rheum Dis 2008; 67: 1030-3.
[201] Bley TA, Wieben O, Uhl M, Thiel J, Schmidt D, Langer M. High-resolution MRI in giant cell arteritis: imaging of the wall of the superficial temporal artery. Am J Radiol 2005; 184: 283-7.
[202] Turlakow A, Yeung HWD, Pui J et al. Fluorodeoxyglucose positron emission tomography in the diagnosis of giant cell arteritis. Arch Intern Med 2001; 161: 1003-7.
[203] Meller J, Strutz F, Siefker U et al. Early diagnosis and follow-up of aortitis with (18F) fluorodeoxyglucose PET and MRI. Eur J Nucl Med Mol Imaging 2003; 30: 730-6.
[204] Walter MA, Melzer RA, Schindler C, Muller-Brand J, Tyndall A, Nitzsche EU. The value of (18F) FDG-PET in the diagnosis of large-vessel vasculitis and the assessment of activity and extent of disease. Eur J Nucl Med Mol Imaging 2005; 32: 674-81.
[205] De Leeuw, Bijl M, Jager PL. Additional value of positron emisson tomography in diagnosis and follow-up of patients with large vessel vasculitides. Clin Exp Rheum 2004; 22 (suppl. 36): S21-S26.
[206] Dasgupta B, Borg FA, Hassan N, Alexander L, Barraclough K, Bourke B, Fulcher J. BSR and BHPR guidelines for the management of giant cell arteritis. Rheumatology 2010; 49: 1594-7.
[207] Mukhtyar C, Guillevin L, Cid MC, de Groot K, Gross W, Hauser T et al. EULAR recommendations for the management of large vessel vasculitis. Ann Rheum Dis 2009; 68: 318-23.
[208] Lessel S. Bilateral temporal artery biopsy in giant cell arteritis. J Neuroophthalmol 2000; 20: 220-1.

[209] Carroll SC, Gaskin BJ, Danesh-Meyer H. Giant cell arteritis. Clin Exp Ophthalmol 2006; 34: 159-73.
[210] Belilos E, Maddox J, Kowalewski RM, Kowalewska J, Turi GK, Nochomovitz LE, Khan Y, Carsons SE. Temporal small-vessel inflammation in patients with giant cell arteritis: clinical course and preliminary immunohistopathologic characterization. J Rheumatol 2011: 38: 331-8.
[211] Klein RG, Campbell RJ, Hunder GG, Carney JA. Skip lesions in temporal arteritis. Mayo Clin Proceed 1976; 51: 504-10.
[212] Poller D, van Wyk Q, Jeffrey M. The importance of skip lesions in temporal arteritis. J Clin Pathol 2000; 53: 137-9.
[213] Kawasaki A, Michel P, Maeder P, Borruat FX. Visualizing the skip lesions of giant cell arteritis with CT angiography. Eur Neurol 2009; 61: 374-7.
[214] Albert DM, Ruchman MC, Keitner JL. Skip lesions in temporal arteritis. Arch Ophthalmol 1976; 94: 2072-7.
[215] Mahr A, Saba M, Kambouchner M, Polivka M, Baudrimont M, Brocheriou I, Coste J, Guillevin L. Temporal artery biopsy for diagnosing giant cell arteritis: the longer, the better? Ann Rheum Dis 2006; 65: 826-8.
[216] Arashvand K. The value of temporal artery biopsy specimen length in the diagnosis of giant cell arteritis.
[217] Rheumatol 2007; 34: 1945.
[218] Taylor-Gjevre R, Vo M, Shukla D, Resch L. Temporal biopsy for giant cell arteritis. J Rheumatol 2005;32:1279-82.
[219] Breuer GS, Nesher R, Nesher G. Effect of biopsy length on the rate of positive temporal artery biopsies. Clin Exp Rheum 2009; 27 (suppl 52):S10-S13.
[220] Sharma NS, Ooi JL, Mcgarity BH, Vollmer-Conna U, McCluskey P. The length of superficial temporal artery biopsies. ANZ J Surg 2007; 77: 437-9.
[221] Pless M, Rizzo JF, Lamkin JC, Lessell S. Concordance of bilateral temporal artery biopsy in giant cell arteritis. J Neuro-Ophthlmol 2000; 20: 216-8.
[222] Breuer GS, Nesher G, Nesher R. Rate of discordant findings in bilateral temporal artery biopsy to diagnose giant cell arteritis. J Rheumatol 2009; 36: 794-6.
[223] Boyev LR, Miller NR, Green WR. Efficacy of unilateral versus bilateral temporal artery biopsies for the diagnosis of giant cell arteritis. Am J Ophthalmol 1999; 128: 211-5.
[224] Hall JK, Balcer LJ. Giant cell arteritis. Curr Treatment Options Neurol 2004; 6: 45-53.
[225] arvaez J, Bernad B, Roig-Vilaseca D, Garcia-Gomez C, Gomez-Vaquero C, Juanola X, Rodriguez-Moreno J, Nolla JM, Valverde J. Influence of previous corticosteroid therapy on temporal artery biopsy yield in giant cell arteritis. Semin Arthritis Rheum 2007; 37: 13-19.
[226] Rieck KL, Kermani TA, Thomsen KM, Harmsen WS, Karban MJ, Warrington KJ. Evaluation for clinical predictors of positive temporal artery biopsy in giant cell arteritis. J Oral Maxillofac Surg 2011; 69: 36-40.
[227] Ackar AA, Lie JT, Hunder GG, O`Fallon WM, Gabriel SE. How does previous corticosteroid treatment affect the biopsy findings in giant cell (temporal) arteritis? Ann Intern Med 1994; 120: 987-92.
[228] Ray-Chaudhuri K, Kine DA, Tijani SO, Parums DV, Cartlidge N, Strong NP, Dayan MR. Effects of prior steroid treatment on temporal artery biopsy findings in giant cell arteritis. Br J Ophthalmol 2002; 86: 530-2.

[229] Allison MC, Gallagher PJ. Temporal artery biopsy and corticosteroid treatment. Ann Rheum Dis 1984; 43: 416-17.
[230] Blumberg S, Giansiracusa DF, Docken WP, Kantrowitz FG. Recurrence of temporal arteritis: clinical recurrence nine years after initial illness. JAMA 1980; 244: 1713-4.
[231] Font RL, Venkatesh C, Prabhakaran C. Histological parameters hepful in recognising steroid-treated temporal arteritis: ananalysis of 35 cases. Br J Ophthalmol 2007; 91: 204-9.
[232] ter Borg EJ, Haanen HCM, Seldenrijk CA. Relationship between histological subtypes and clinical characteristics at presentation and outcome in biopsy-proven giant cell arteritis. Clin Rheumatol 2006; 26: 529-32.
[233] Villaseca J, Gonzalez A, Cid MC, Lopez-Viancos J, Ortega A. Clinical usefulness of temporal artery biopsy. Ann Rheum Dis 1987; 46: 282-5.
[234] Fernandez-Herlihy L. Temporal arteritis: clinical aids to diagnosis. J Rheumatol 1988; 15: 1797-1801.
[235] Mari B, Monteagudo M, Bustamante E, Perez J, Casanovas A, Jordana R, Tolosa C, Oristrell J. Analysis of temporal artery biopsies in an 18-year period at a community hospital. Eur J Intern Med 2009; 20: 533-6.
[236] Rodriguez-Pla A, Rossello-Urgell J, Bosch-Gil JA, Huguet-redecilla P, Vilardell-Tarres M. Proposal to decrease the number of negative temporal artery biopsies. Scand J Rheumatol 2007; 36: 111-8.
[237] Younge BR, Cook BE, Bartley GB, Hodge DO, Hunder GG. Initiation of glucocorticoid therapy: before or after temporal artery biopsy. Mayo Clin Proc 2004; 79: 483-91.
[238] Nordborg E, Nordborg C. The influence of sectional interval on the reliability of temporal arterial biopsies in polymyalgia rheumatica. Clin Rheumatol 1995; 14: 330-4.
[239] Rao JK, Allen NB, Pincus T. Limitations of the 1990 American College of Rheumatology classification criteria in the diagnosis of vasculitis. Ann Intern Med 1998; 129: 345-52.
[240] Fraya RA, Abu-Haidar F. Polyarteritis nodosa masquerading as temporal arteritis. J Rheumatol 1979; 6: 76-9.
[241] Nishino H, de Remee RA, Rubino FA. Wegener`s granulomatosis associated with vasculitis of the temporal arteries. Report of five cases. May Clin Proceed 1993; 68: 115-21.
[242] Genereau T, Lortholary O, Pottier MA, Michon-Pasturel U, Ponge T, de Wazieres B, Liozon E, Pinede E, Hachulla E, Roblot P, barrier JH, Herson S, Guillevin L. Temporal artery biopsy: a diagnostic tool for systemic necrotizing vasculitis. French vasculitis study group. Arthritis Rheum 1999; 42: 2674-81.
[243] Salvarani C, Gabriel SE, Gertz MA, Bjørnsson J, Li CY, Hunder GG. Primary systemic amyloidosis presenting as GCA and PMR. Arthritis Rheum 1994;37:1621-6.
[244] Jianguang J, Liu X, Sundquist K, Sundquist J, Hemminki K. Cancer risk in patients hospitalized with polymyalgia rheumatica and giant cell arteritis: a follow-up study in Sweden. Rheumatology 2010; 49: 1158-63.
[245] Haga HJ, Eide GE, Brun J, Johansen A, Langmark F. Cancer in association with polymyalgia rheumatica and temporal arteritis. J Rheumatol 1993; 20: 1335-9.

[246] Kermani TA, Schafer VS, Crowson CS, Hunder GG, Gabriel SE, Ytterberg SR, Matteson EL, Warrington KJ. Malignancy risk in patients with giant cell arteritis: a population-based cohort study. Arthritis Care Res 2010; 62: 149-54.
[247] Kermani TA, Schafer VS, Crowson CS, Hunder GG, Ytterberg SR, Matteson EL, Gabriel SE, Warrington KJ. Cancer preceding giant cell arteritis: a case-control study. Arthritis Rheum 2010; 62: 1763-9.
[248] Hill CL, Cole A, Rischmueller M, Dodd T, Coleman M, Tucker G, Roberts-Thomson P. Risk of cancer in patients with biopsy-proven giant cell arteritis. Rheumatology 2010; 49: 756-9.
[249] von Knorring J, Somer T. Malignancy in association with polymyalgia rheumatica and giant cell arteritis. Scand J Rheumatol 1974; 3: 129-35.
[250] Myklebust G, Wilsgaard T, Koster Jacobsen B, Gran JT. No increased frequency of malignant neoplasms in polymyalgia rheumatic a and temporal arteritis . A prospective longitudinal study of 398 cases and matched population controls. J Rheumatol 2002; 29: 2143-7.
[251] Andersson R, Malmwall BE, Bengtsson BÅ. Long-term survival in giant cell arteritis including temporal arteritis and polymyalgia rheumatica. Acta Med Scand 1986; 220: 361-4.
[252] Shimamoto Y, Matsunaga C, Suga K, Fukushima N, Nomura K, Yamaguchi M. A human T-cell lymphotropic virus type I carrier with temporal arteritis terminating in acute myelogenous leukemia. Scand J Rheumatol 1994; 23: 151-3.
[253] Caldwell DS, McCallum RM. Rheumatological manifestations of cancer. Med Clin North Amer 1986; 70: 385-417.
[254] Lie JT. Simultaneous clinical manifestations of malignancy and giant cell arteritis in a young woman. J Rheumatol 1995; 22: 367-9.
[255] Nordborg E, Bengtsson BÅ. Death rates and causes of deaths in 284 consecutive patients with giant cell arteritis confirmed by biopsy. Br Med J 1989; 299: 549-550.
[256] Bisgård C, Sloth H, Keliding N, Juel K. Excess mortality in giant cell arteritis. J Intern Med 1991; 230: 119-23.
[257] Le Page, Duhaut P, Seydoux D, Bosshard S, Ecochard R, Abbas F et al. Incidence of cardiovascular events in giant cell arteritis: preliminary results of a prospective double cohort study (GRACG). Rev Med Interne 2006; 27: 98-105.
[258] Uddhammar A, Eriksson AL, Nystrøm L, Stenling R, Rantapaa-Dahlquist S. Increased mortality due to cardiovascular disease in patients with giant cell arteritis in Northern Sweden. J Rheumatol 2002; 29: 737-42.
[259] Gonzalez-Gay MA, Rubiera G, Pineiro A, Garcia-Porrua C, Pego-Reigosa R, Gonzalez-Juanatey C, Sanchez-Andrade A, Llorca J. Ischemic heart disease in patients from Northwest Spain with biopsy proven giant cell arteritis. A population based study. J Rheumatol 2005; 32: 502-6.
[260] Ray JG, Mamdani MM, Geerts WH. Giant cell arteritis and cardiovascular disease in older adults. Heart 2005; 91: 324-8.
[261] Schick RM, Baggenstoss AH, Paulley HF. Effects of cortisone and ACTH on periarteritis nodosa and cranial arteritis. Proceed Staff Meeting Mayo Clin 1950; 25: 492-4.
[262] Kyle V, Hazleman BL. Treatment of polymyalgia rheumatica and giant cell arteritis. I. Steroids regimens in the first two months. Ann Rheum Dis 1989; 48: 658-61.

[263] Myklebust G, Gran JT. Prednisolone maintenance dose in relation to starting dose in the treatment of polymyalgia rheumatica and temporal arteritis. Scand J Rheumatol 2001; 30: 260-7.

[264] Delecoeuillerie G, Joly P, de Lara Cohen A, Paolaggi JB. Polymyalgia rheumatica and temporal arteritis : a retrospective analysis of prognostic features and different corticosteroid regimens (11 year survey of 210 patiens). Ann Rheum dis 1988; 47: 733-9.

[265] Nesher G, Rubinow A, Sonnenblick M. Efficacy and adverse effects of different corticosteroid dose regimens in temporal arteritis: a retrospective study. Clin Exp Rheumatol 1997; 15: 303-306.

[266] Nesher G, Sonnenblick M, Friedlander Y. Analysis of steroid related complications and mortality in temporal arteritis: a 15 - year study of 43 patients. J Rheumatol 1994; 21: 1283-6.

[267] Kyle V, Hazleman BL. Treatment of polymyalgia rheumatica and giant cell arteritis. II. Relation between steroid dose and steroid side effects. Ann Rheum Dis 1989;48: 662-6.

[268] Hunder GG, Sheps SG, Allen GL, Joyce JW. Daily and alternate-day corticosteroid regimens in treatment of GCA: comparison in a prospective study. Ann Intern med 1975; 82: 613-8.

[269] Carroll SC, Gaskin BJ, Danesh-Meyer H. Giant cell arteritis. Clin Exp Ophthalmol 2006; 34: 159-73.

[270] Andersen T. Arteritis temporalis (Horton): a symptom of a generalized vascular disease. Acta Med Scand 1947: 128: 151-78.

[271] Wilke WS, Hoffman GS. Treatment of corticosteroid-resistant giant cell arteritis. Rheum Dis Clin North Amer 1995; 21: 59-71.

[272] Hunder GG. Giant cell (temporal) arteritis. Rheum Dis Clin North Amer 1990; 16: 399-409.

[273] Gordon LK, Levin LA. Visual loss in giant cell arteritis. JAMA 1998; 280: 385-6.

[274] Meadows SP. Temporal or giant cell arteritis - ophthalmic aspects. In: Lawton-Smith JL, ed. Neuro-ophthalmology St.Louis; Mosby. 1968:148-57.

[275] Slavin ML, Margolis AJ. Progressive anterior ischemic optic neuropathy due to giant cell arteritis despite high-dose intravenous corticosteroids. Arch Ophthalmol 1988; 106: 1167.

[276] Myles AB, Perera T, Ridley MG. Prevention of blindness in giant cell arteritis by corticosteroid treatment. Br J Rheumatol 1992; 31: 103-5.

[277] Hayreh SS, Zimmerman B. Management of giant cell arteritis. Ophthalmologica 2003; 217: 239-59.

[278] Hayreh SS, Zimmerman B, Kardon RH. Visual improvement with corticosteroid therapy in giant cell arteritis. Report of a large study and review of the literature. Acta Ophthalmol Scand 2002; 80: 355-67.

[279] Chevalet P, Barrier JH, Pottier P, Magadur-Joly G, Pottier MA, Hamidou M. A randomized, multicenter, controlled trial using intravenous pulses of methylprednisolone in the initial treatment of simple forms of giant cell arteritis: a one year followup study of 164 patients. J Rheumatol 2000; 27: 1484-91.

[280] Chan CCK, O`Day J. Oral and intravenous steroids in giant cell arteritis. Clin Exp Ophthalmol 2003; 31: 179-82.

[281] Rosenfeld SI, Kosmorsky GS, Klingele TG, Burde RM, Cohn EM. Treatement of temporal arteritis with ocular involvement. Am J Med 1986; 80: 143-5.
[282] Model DG. Reversal of blindness in temporal arteritis with methylprednisolone. Lancet 1978; feb11: 340.
[283] Diamond JP. Treatable blindness in temporal arteritis. Br J Ophthalmol 1991; 75: 432.
[284] Matzkin DC, Slamovits TL, Sachs R, Burde RM. Visual recovery in two patients after intravenous methylprednisolone treatement of central retinal occlusion secondary to giant-cell arteritis. Ophthalmology 1992; 99: 68-71.
[285] Liu GT, Glaser JS, Schatz NJ, Smith JL. Visual morbidity in giant cell arteritis. Clinical characteristics and prognosis for vision. Ophthalmology 1994; 101: 1779-85.
[286] Salvarani C, Cantini F, Hunder GG. Polymyalgia rheumatica and giant-cell arteritis. Lancet 2008; 372: 234-45.
[287] Cullen JP, Coliro JA. Ophthalmologic complications in giant cell arteritis. Surv Ophthalmol 1976; 20: 247-60.
[288] Hoffman GS, Cid MC, Heiklmann DB et al. A multicenter randomized double blind placebo-controlled trial of adjuvant methotrexate tretament for giant cell arteritis. Arthritis Rheum 2002; 46: 1309-18.
[289] Jover JA, Hernandez-Garcia C, Morado IC, Vargas E, Banares A, Fernandez-Gutierrez B. Combined treatment of giant-cell arteritis with methotrexate and prednisone. Ann Intern Med 2001; 134: 106-114.
[290] Spiera RF, Mitnik HJ, Kupersmith M, Richmond M, Spiera H, Peterson MG. A prospective double-blind, randomized placebo controlled trial of methotrexate in the treatment of giant cell arteritis. Clin Exp Rheum 2001; 19: 495-501.
[291] Mahr AD, Jover JA, Spiera RF, Hernandez-Garcia C, Fernandez-Gutierrez B, La Valley MP, Merkel PA. Adjunctive methotrexate for treatment of giant cell arteritis: an individual patient data meta-analysis. Arthritis Rheum 2007; 56: 2789-97.
[292] Camellino D, Morbelli S, Sambuceti G, Cimmino MA. Methotrexate treatment of polymyalgia rheumatica/giant cell arteritis-associated large vessel vasculitis. Clin Exp Rheum 2010; 28: 288-9.
[293] De Silva M, Hazleman BL. Azathioprine in GCA/PMR: a double-blind study. Ann Rheum Dis 1986; 45: 136-8.
[294] Schauffelberger C, Andersson R, Nordborg E. No additive effect of Cyclosporin A compared with glucocorticoid treatment alone in giant cell arteritis: Results of an open, controlled randomized study. Br J Rheumatol 1998; 37; 464-5.
[295] Wilke WS, Hoffman GS. Treatment of corticosteroid-resistant giant cell arteritis. Rheum Dis Clin North Amer 2995; 21: 59-71.
[296] Narvaez J, Berad B, Nolla JM, Valverde J. Statin therapy does not seem to benefit giant cell arteritis. Semin Arthritis Rheum 2007; 36: 322-7. Commented on in Semin Arthritis Rheum 2008; 38: 63-4.
[297] Field M, Cook A, Gallagher G. Immuno-localization of tumor necrosis factor and its receptors in temporal arteritis. Rheum Int 1997; 17: 113-8.
[298] Ahmed MM, Mubashir E, Hayat S, Fowler M, Berney SM. Treatment of refractory temporal arteritis with adalimumab. Clin Rheumatol 2007; 26: 1353-5.
[299] Martinez-Taboada VM, Rodriguez-Valverde V, Carreno L, Lopez-Longo J, Figueroa M, Belzunegui J, Mola EM, Bonilla G. A double-blind placebo controlled trial of

etanercept in patients with giant cell arteritis and corticosteroid side effects. Ann Rheum Dis 2007; 67: 625-30.

[300] Benucci M, Manfredi M, Puce F, Zuccarini S. Improvement in visual acuity in a patient with ischemic optic neuropathy (Horton arteritis) undergoing therapy with infliximab: a case report. Recenti Prog Med 2007; 98: 624-6.

[301] Airo P, Antonioli CM, Vianelli M, Toniati P. Anti-tumor necrosis factor treatment with infliximab in a case of giant cell arteritis resistant to steroid and immunosuppressive drugs. Rheumatology 2002; 41: 347-9.

[302] Andonopoulos AP, Meimaris N, Daoussis D, Bounas A, Giannopoulos G. Experience with infliximab (anti-TNFα monoclonal antibody) as monotherapy for giant cell arteritis. Ann Rheum Dis 2003; 62: 1116.

[303] Uthman I, Kanj N, Atweh S. Infliximab as monotherapy in giant cell arteritis. Clin Rheumatol 2005; 25: 109-10.

[304] Cantini F, Niccoli L, Salvarani C, Padula A, Olivieri I. Treatment of longstanding active giant cell arteritis with infliximab: report of four cases. Arthritis Rheum 2001; 44: 2933-5.

[305] Tan AL, Holdsworth J, Pease C, Emery P, McGonagle D. Successful treatment of resistant giant cell arteritis with etanercept. Ann Rheum Dis 2003; 62: 373-4.

[306] Hoffman GS, Cid MC, Rendt-Zagar KE, Merkel PA, Weyand CM, Stone JH et al. Infliximab for maintenance of glucocorticosteroid-induced remission of giant cell arteritis: a randomized trial. Ann Intern Med 2007; 146: 621-30.

[307] Hagihara K, Kaware I, Tanaka T, Kishimoto T. Tocilizumab ameliorates clinical symptoms in polymyalgia rheumatica. J Rheumatol 2010; 37: 1075-6.

[308] Seitz M, Reichenbach S, Borel HM, Adler S, Wermelinger F, Villiger PM. Rapid induction of remission in large vessel vasculitis by IL-6 blockade. Swiss Med Wkly 2011; 141: E1-E4.

[309] Shinjo SK, Pereira RMR, Tizziani VAP. Mycophenolate mofetil reduces disease activity and steroid dosage in Takayasu arteritis. Clin Rheumatol 2007; 26: 1871-5.

[310] Lozano E, Segarra M, Garcia-Martinez A, Hernandez-Rodriguez J, Cid MC. Imatinib mesylate inhibits in vitro and ex vivo biological responses related to vascular occlusion in giant cell arteritis. Ann Rheum Dis 2008; 67: 1581-8.

[311] Lozano E, Segarra M, Corbera-Bellalta M, Garcia-Martinez A, Espigol-Frigole G, Pla-Campo A, Hernandez-Rodriguez J, Cid MC. Increased expression of the endothelin system in arterial lesions from patients with giant cell arteritis: association between elevated plasma endothelin levels and the development of ischaemic events. Ann Rheum Dis 2010; 69: 434-42.

[312] Bhatia A, Ell PJ, Edwards JCW. Anti-CD20 monoclonal antibody (rituximab) as an adjunct in the treatment of giant cell arteritis. Ann Rheum Dis 2005; 64: 1099-1100.

[313] Spiera RF, Spiera H. Therapy for giant cell arteritis: can we do better? Arthritis Rheum 2006; 54: 3071-4

[314] Gonzalez-Juanatey C, Lopez-Diaz MJ, Martin J, Llorca J, Gonzalez-Gay MA. Atherosclerosis in patients with biopsy-proven giant cell arteritis. Arthritis Rheum 2007; 57: 1481-6.

[315] Abud-Medoza C, de la Fuente H, Cuevas-Orta E, Baranda L, Cruz-Rizo J, Gonzalez-Amaro R. Therapy with statins in patients with refractory rheumatic diseases: a preliminary study. Lupus 2003; 12: 607-11.

[316] Nesher G, Brkun Y, Mates M, Baras M, Rubinow A, Sonnenblick M. Low-dose aspirin and prevention of cranial ischemic complications in giant cell arteritis. Arthritis Rheum 2004; 50: 1332-7.

[317] Lee MS, Smith SD, Galor A, Hoffman GS. Antiplatelet and anticoagulant therapy in patients with giant cell arteritis. Arthritis Rheum 2006; 54: 3306-9.

[318] Berger CT, Wolbers M, Meyer P, Daikeler T, Hess C. High incidence of severe ischemic complications in patients with giant cell arteritis irrespective of platelet count and size, and platelet inhibition. Rheumatology 2009; 48: 258-61.

[319] Haugeberg G, Myklebust G, Dovland H, Mikkelsen B, Gran JT. No permanent reduction in bone mineral density during treatment of polymyalgia rheumatica and temporal arteritis using low dose corticosteroids. Scand J Rheumatol 2000; 29: 163-9.

[320] Andersson R, Rundgren Å, Rosengren K, Bengtsson BÅ, malmwall BE, mellstrøm D. Osteoporosis after long-term corticosteroid treatment of giant cell arteritis. J Int med 1990; 227: 391-5.

[321] Prøven A, Gabriel SE, Orces C, O`Fallon WM, Hunder GG. Glucocorticoid therapy in giant cell arteritis: duration and adverse outcomes. Arthritis Care Res 2003; 49: 703-8.

[322] Andersson R, Malmwall BE, Bengtsson BÅ. Long-term corticosteroid treatment in giant cell arteritis. Acta Med Scand 1986; 220: 465-9.

[323] auchald P, Rygvold O, Øystese B. Temporal arteritis and polymyalgia rheumatica. Clinical and biopsy findings. Ann Intern Med 1972; 77: 845-52.

[324] Kyle V, Cawston TE, Hazleman BL. Erythrocyte sedimentation rate and C reactive protein in the assessment of polymyalgia rheumatica/giant cell arteritis on presentation and during follow-up. Ann Rheum Dis 1989; 48: 667-71.

[325] von Knorring J. Treatment and prognosis of polymyalgia rheumatica and temporal arteritis: a ten-year survey of 53 patients. Acta Med Scand 1979; 205: 429-35.

[326] Graham E, Holland A, Avery A, Russell RWR. Prognosis in giant-cell arteritis. Br Med J 1981; 282: 269-71.

[327] Hachulla E, Boivin V, Pasturel-Michon U, Fauchais AL, Bouroz-Joly J, Perez-Cousin M, Hatron PY, Devulder B. Prognostic factors and long-term evolution in a cohort of 133 patients with giant cell arteritis. Clin Exp Rheumatol 2001; 19: 171-6.

[328] Liozon E, Gondran G, Ly K, Loustad V, Vidal E. Duration of treatment after eye involvement in giant cell arteritis. J Rheumatol 2008; 35: 1220.

[329] Lundberg I, Hedfors E. Restricted dose and duration of corticosteroid treatment in patients with polymyalgia rheumatica and temporal arteritis. J Rheumatol 1990; 17: 1340-5

[330] Andersson R, Malmwall BE, Bengtsson BÅ. Long-term corticosteroid treatment in giant cell arteritis. Acta Med Scand 1986; 220: 465-9.

[331] Weyand CM, Younge BR, Goronzy JJ. INF-Y and IL-17: the two faces of T-cell pathology in giant cell arteritis. Curr Opin Rheum 2011; 23: 43-9.

15

"Extra-Cranial" Manifestations of Giant Cell Arteritis

Aurélie Daumas, Fanny Bernard, Pascal Rossi and Brigitte Granel
Assistance Publique des Hôpitaux de Marseille
France

1. Introduction

Giant cell arteritis (GCA) is a primitive systemic vasculitis related to a sub-acute inflammatory panarteritis, histologically characterized by segmentary and plurifocal damage, with giant cells and destruction of the internal elastic lamina. GCA involves large and medium sized vessels in subjects over 50, particularly between 75 and 85, and is more common in women (7:3sex-ratio). This arteritis preferentially affects the external carotid and its branches, and more specifically the superficial temporal artery, which explains the usual clinical signs of the disease which are headaches, tenderness and sensitivity of the scalp, painful thickening of the temporal arteries associated with absence of pulsation, and jaw claudication. However, this description of GCA was enriched in 1938 by the first observations of « extra-cranial » manifestations.

A diagnosis of GCA is usually suspected in the elderly subject on the association of focal signs of arteritis prevailing in the head, with a more or less febrile alteration of the general health condition and an inflammatory syndrome. The classification criteria of GCA most used are those of the American College of Rheumatology and which date back to 1990.

Nevertheless, GCA, because of the potential ubiquity of the pathological process, can occur in atypical forms, which renders the etiological approach more complex. The risk is therefore a delay in diagnosis which can jeopardize the prognosis of this disease.

In this chapter, we will approach different atypical aspects of GCA, which can all be inaugural of the disease, whose prognosis will depend on their early recognition. They include aorta and its main branches involvement except arteritis of the branches of the external carotid artery, heart, lung, neurologic, genital and musculoskeletal manifestations.

2. Aortitis and limb arteritis in giant cell arteritis

The diagnosis of GCA is based on clinical, biological and histological elements described in the classification criteria defined by ACR in 1990. The diagnosis is evident in the case of clinical manifestations relative to the involvement of the external carotid branches. However, temporal arteritis is not systematic, and involvement of the aorta and its main branches may be isolated. In this case, diagnosis is complicated by a clinical presentation which is often poor and non-specific, and by the difficulty of obtaining histological proof; the new methods of imagery that we are going to describe can then be useful in diagnostic.

GCA is one of the three main causes of inflammatory aortitis, besides Takayasu's arteritis and Behçet's disease (Launay & Hachulla, 2003). However, involvement of the large vessels, and specifically the aorta, is often little known. Data from series of autopsies evaluate the frequency of aortic involvement up to 70 % during GCA. In the series of Hervé et al. (2006), the frequency of thoracic and abdominal involvement diagnosed by Computer Tomography (CT) scan were close (73 and 82 % respectively); moreover, concomitant thoracic and abdominal involvement was frequent, since it concerned 55 % of the patients. In the study of Agard et al. (2009), 22 patients and 22 controls were screened by CT scan for aortic involvement. Thickening of the aortic wall was more frequent among patients than controls (45.4% versus 13.6%; P 0.02). Aortic thickening was located on the ascending part of the thoracic aorta in 22.7% of the patients, with no evidence of thickening in the controls (P 0.05). Thickening of the abdominal aortic wall was noted in 27.3% of the patients and none of the controls (P 0.02).

Aortic involvement may be the mode of revelation of the disease. It can also occur during corticosteroid decrease or withdrawal in patients carrying a known GCA. The clinical presentation can be limited to a febrile syndrome, an alteration of the general state of health and an inflammatory syndrome. The existence of inflammatory back pains is not systematic. The clinical diagnosis of aortic lesion is often difficult and late in GCA, due to the long latency of this involvement and the absence of clinical presentation (Bossert, 2010). Aortic lesions represent yet another major cause of morbidity and mortality during GCA. They can actually be complicated by aneurisms, aortic dissections and less frequently stenosis. Increased frequency of aortic aneurisms during GCA is established and they expose the patient to the risk of potentially fatal accidents (embol, dissection). In 1995, Evans et al. showed on a retrospective series of 96 patients suffering from GCA a risk 17.3 times higher of developing a thoracic aneurism and 2.4 times higher of developing an isolated abdominal aneurism, in comparison with the population of the same age and sex. In 2003, out of a cohort of 168 patients with GCA, Nuenninghoff et al. (2003) found 30 cases (18 %) of aortic aneurisms, 18 of them in the chest; nine were complicated by aortic dissection, with seven deaths.

Arterial involvement in GCA is not limited only to the thoracic or abdominal aorta. The GCA may be revealed by a lesion in the upper or lower limbs.

Upper and/or lower limb inflammatory arteritis during GCA is not exceptional occurring in 3 to 16% of patients. It is rarely reported in the literature but is probably under-estimated as it is often low symptomatic (Assie & Marie, 2011).

Hamrin et al. were among the first authors as early as 1965 to draw attention to the possibility of "extra-cranial" arterial involvement through the existence of arterial murmurs on the trajectories of the limb arteries. It must not be neglected by the clinicians managing these patients due to the severe ischemic complications that it can trigger, amputation being necessary in 5.6 to 15.8 % of cases (Assie & Marie, 2011).

In the review of 318 cases published by Assie and Marie (2011), it can be noted that the patients present more often a lesion in the upper (63.1 %) than in the lower limbs (32.2 %); with concomitant involvement of both the upper and lower limbs arteries in 4.7 %. It was also observed that the arterial sites involved are in order of frequency:

- subclavian arteries (53.2 %), axillary arteries (37.3 %), brachial arteries (24 %) ;
- iliac arteries (0.43 %), common femoral arteries (2.6 %), superficial femoral arteries (24.9 %), deep femoral arteries (10.3 %), popliteal arteries (16.3 %), tibio-peroneal trunk (1.3 %), and tibial arteries.

If the upper and/or lower limb arterial involvement can be the mode of revelation of GCA, it can also occur during corticosteroid decrease or withdrawal in patients with a known GCA. In the observation by Skopinski et al. (1997), for four women and one man, aged from 67 to 77, the mode of revelation was intermittent claudication of an upper limb in three cases and bilateral Raynaud's syndrome in one case. The discovery was accidental in one case (the general practitioner was anable to measure blood pressure). In all cases there was an absence of peripheral pulse, and it was impossible to measure blood pressure on the side involved. All the patients had a biological inflammatory syndrome. Arteriography showed that all the patients had long and tight stenosis on the subclavian, axillary and humeral arteries. The biopsy of the temporal artery, carried out in all five cases, was positive in three. A surgical act of revascularisation was only necessary once. Evolution of the clinical symptomatology and the inflammatory syndrome was constantly favourable under prednisone. Furthermore Tazi et al.(1997) reported the case of a woman of 67 with no risk factors for atheroma, hospitalised for lower limbs ischemia relative to bilateral occlusion of the superficial femoral arteries. The femoral artery biopsy did not reveal any thrombosis but showed the inflammatory nature of the lesion confirming the diagnosis of GCA. Upper and/or lower limb arterial involvement occurs more frequently in women; in the literature (Assie & Marie, 2011), 58.8 % of the patients were women with a median age of 67. The clinical manifestations included intermittent claudication of a limb (68.6 %), decrease in pulse or absence of a peripheral, limb ischemia (17.9 %), even gangrene of a limb/toe/finger (6.4 %). However limb arterial involvement does not always have a clinical expression in the early stages. Thus involvement must not be neglected by physicians managing these patients due to the severe ischemic complications it can trigger.

In this context, aortitis appears frequent in patients with an upper and/or lower limb arterial involvement complicating a GCA. Weyand and Goronzy (1999) noted an aortitis in 10 to 15 % of these patients. Likewise, in a recent series, an aortic localization was associated with a limb arterial involvement in up to 68.9 % of the cases (Assie et al.2011). In view of the potential gravity of aortic lesions, it would appear justified to carry out a systematic exploration of the aorta and its branches to look for an aortitis in patients presenting a GCA. Interestingly, in the work of Assie et al.(2011), headaches (25 % vs. 77 %), jaw claudication (11 % vs. 35 %), tenderness and sensitivity of the scalp (8 % vs. 67 %) and a positive temporal artery biopsy (69 % vs. 95 %) were all less frequent in the group carrying an upper and/or lower limb arterial involvement than in that who had none. Likewise, Hervé et al.(2006) found less frequent usual inaugural signs of GCA in cases of aortitis. Brack et al. (1999) mentioned that the group of patients carrying a large vessel involvement, compared with those with a predominant cephalic involvement, were younger (66 vs 72) and had less often the classical signs of GCA (headaches, jaw claudication, visual disorders).

Different complementary non-invasive vascular examinations can be carried out to search for a limb or aortic arterial involvement. Arterial Doppler ultrasound is a simple non-invasive examination for studying large arteries in patients. In GCA, arterial inflammation is determined by a circular thickening of decreased echogenicity of the vascular wall around the arterial light (halo of decreased echogenicity). Moreover, studies have found a correlation between the type and the seat of the arterial lesions revealed by arterial Doppler ultrasound and angiography, which confirm the high sensitivity of this examination in detecting upper and/or lower limb arterial involvement in GCA (Schmidt et al. 2005; Agard et al.2009).

On the other hand, arterial Doppler ultrasound presents a limited interest for following up arterial involvement in the patients treated; the thickening of the vascular wall would appear to persist under corticosteroids, which complicates the correlation between the ultrasound data and GCA activity. Angioscan is useful as an examination to detect aortic involvement and limb arterial involvement, and it has the added advantage of being more available and shorter than the MRI angiography. Therefore, Agard et al.(2009) and Hervé et al. (2006) highlighted the diagnostic interest of the angioscan for the diagnosis of inflammatory aortitis in patients suffering from a GCA, as this examination makes it possible to visualize directly the suggestive anomalies of the aortic wall (circumferential parietal thickening, regular and homogeneous, more than 3 mm thick). In addition to this, we can note the interest of the angioscan for the follow-up of GCA aortitis (Hervé et al. 2006).

Lastly positron emission tomography (PET) with 18 FDG, a noninvasive metabolic imaging modality that is well-suited to the assessment of activity and extent of large vessel vasculitis, also appears to be a promising technique. Contrary to the previous radiological examinations, it can detect vasculitis lesions all over the body and it is more sensitive to show inflammatory vascular wall process (Belhocine et al 2002 ;Liozon et al.2010) (figures 1-3); these data suggest the potential clinical interest of the PET in the vascular disease activity, extension and follow-up of patients with GCA (figure 4).

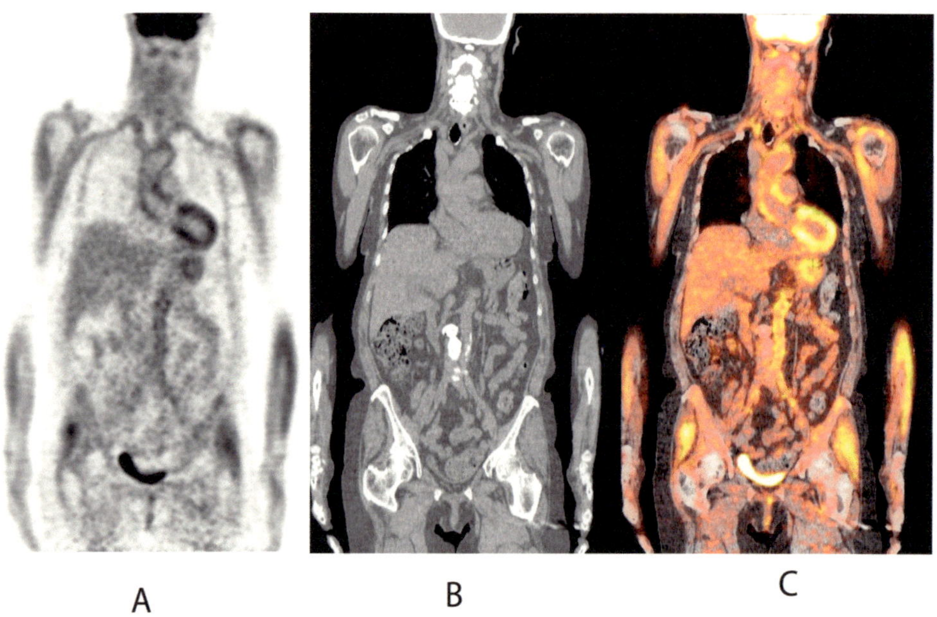

A: PET image.
B: CT-scan image.
C: images fused PET and CT-scan.

Fig. 1. Coronal view of Positron Emission Tomography (PET) showing hyper metabolism of the thoracic and abdominal aorta walls extending to the subclavian arteries indicating aortitis.

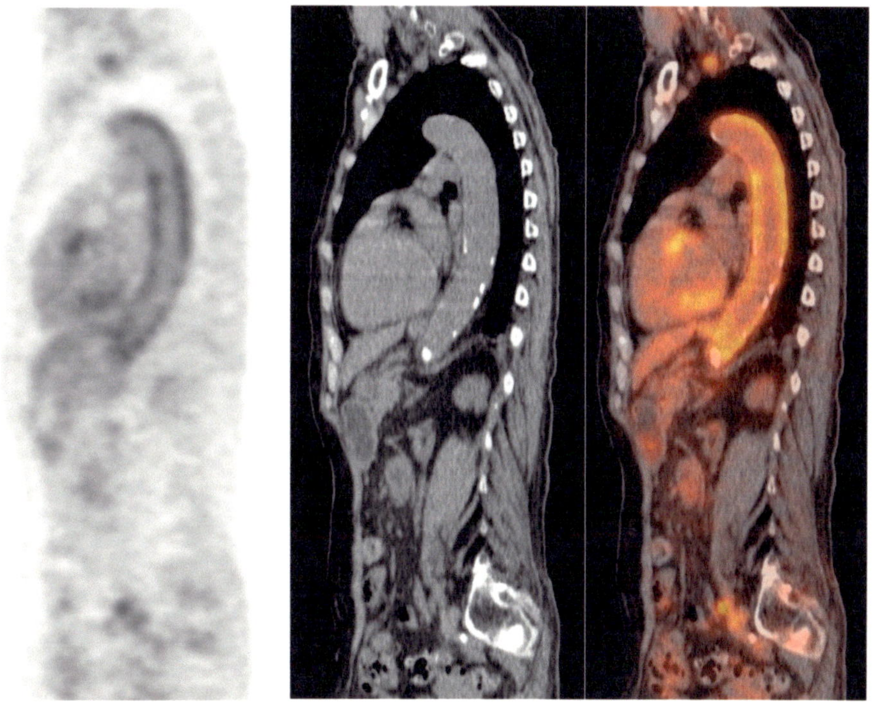

Fig. 2. Sagittal view of inflammation of the descending thoracic aorta (A : PET, B: CT-scan, C: fusion of the PET and CT-scan images).

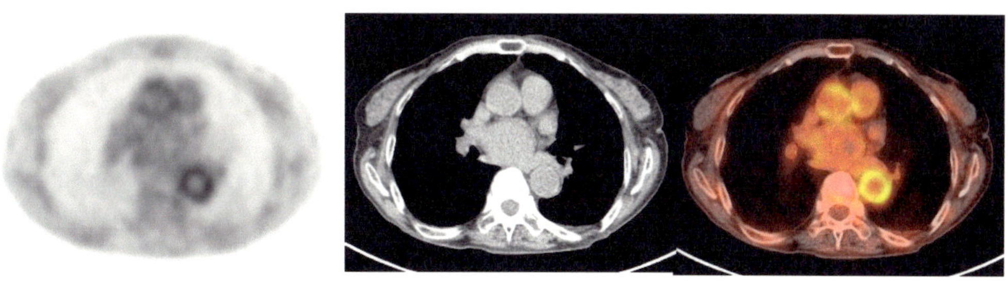

Fig. 3. Axial view showing hyper metabolism of the ascending and descending wall of thoracic aorta, indicating aortitis (A: PET, B: CT scan, C: images fused PET-CT).

One of the limits of PET is its availability and its spatial resolution which does not make it possible to highlight the involvement of arteries with a size of less than 4mm (Loizon et al. 2010).

The treatment of vascular lesions is the same than classical form of GCA relying on corticosteroids. The hypothesis of administration of a higher or longer dose of corticosteroids in the case of aortic and large artery involvement does not reside on any element of proof. The occurrence of thrombotic complications during GCA also leads to discussion on the interest of a treatment by antiplatelet drug or anticoagulants, whose use is not codified. Nesher et al.(2004), in a non-randomized study of 175 GCA patients, reported a reduction of the incidence of neurological ischemic complications in the group of patients treated with aspirin compared with the group which did not receive any (4 % vs. 29 %). In another series, Lee et al. (2006) also mentioned that the risk of occurrence of ischemic complications was three times higher in the group of patients who did not receive an aspirin treatment against the treated group. A few caveats, however, are necessary before one recommends that low-dose aspirin should be added as standard of care in GCA.

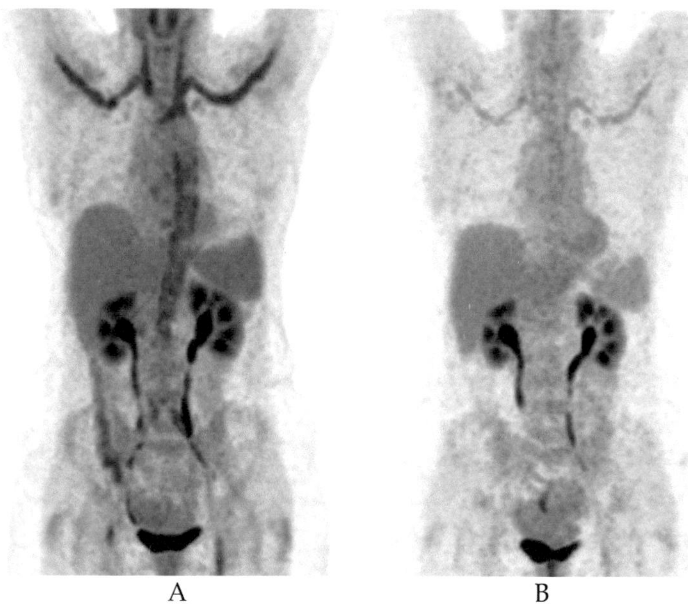

Fig. 4. Maximal Intensity Projection (MIP) of PET showing hyper metabolism of the thoracic and abdominal aorta extending to the subclavian arteries, before (A) and after three months of steroids (B), pointing out the decrease of the inflammation of the arterial walls.

There are very few data, in the form of isolated observations only, relative to the usefulness of anticoagulants in the initial stage of GCA. For some authors, the use of anticoagulants in this indication resides on the following elements: (1) Giant cell arteritis is a granulomatous arterial disease causing sometimes very tight arterial stenosis which can be the seat of an intraluminal thrombosis; (2) the blood rates of the von Willebrand procoagulating factor are increased during GCA. At present, due to the lack of open or randomized studies having analysed the interest of anticoagulants in this context, anticoagulation cannot be recommended systematically for these patients. In practice, in the case of a severe acute ischemic limb involvement, an anticoagulant treatment is usually prescribed.

Immunosuppressive treatments have not been evaluated in these forms. The role of vasodilators remains to be determined. In the series of Benjilali et al. (2009), intravenous prostaglandins had given a good result in a patient with threatening ischemic lesions, in association with corticosteroids and anticoagulants.

To date there is no consensus for the choice of imagery and the rhythm of supervision of aortitis. The follow-up must be regular and on long-term, even after the withdrawal of corticosteroids. As certain authors suggest (Garcia et al.2008), supervision once a year by lung X-ray, transthoracic echocardiography and Doppler ultrasound of the abdominal aorta would seem to be appropriate. Thoracic-abdominal scan with injection and 3D reconstruction is also efficient in this indication (Hervé et al.2006). Lastly, PET would appear to be more interesting than CT scan to evaluate the response of the aortitis to corticosteroids; The vascular metabolic signal disappears, despite the persistence of a perivascular cuff in CT scan (Liozon et al.2010).

3. Mesenteric artery involvement

Described for the first time by Hamrin et al. in 1965, mesenteric inflammatory arteritis is rare in the course of GCA. The majority of articles do not mention GCA among the causes of mesenteric ischemia. From this point of view, analysis of the literature has enabled us to list 33 cases of mesenteric inflammatory arteritis in patients carrying GCA. In the review of the literature (Lorthior et al.2008), diagnosis of mesenteric inflammatory arteritis and GCA was concomitant in 57.6 % of the cases; in the other patients, mesenteric inflammatory arteritis appeared in the development of GCA, usually in the first three months following its diagnosis. The diagnosis of GCA mesenteric arterial lesions is often difficult due to the absence of specific clinical presentation. In all 33 cases, the patients presented: abdominal pains (97%) which were rarely characteristic of mesenteric angina (15.2 %); an occlusive syndrome (42.4 %) or a digestive haemorrhage (6.1 %), and the last patient was asymptomatic from the digestive point of view. These elements suggest that the prevalence of the mesenteric inflammatory arteritis is probably under-estimated during GCA; systematic prospective, vascular imaging studies could make it possible to determine its prevalence along with the incidence in these patients. If the final diagnosis of mesenteric inflammatory arteritis resides, in theory, on the histological examination, arterial biopsies of this kind are an invasive examination, and are not carried out in practice. Colour Doppler ultrasound is an inexpensive and easily available examination, and frequently used at the beginning. At present, the angioscan would appear to be a useful examination to objectivise mesenteric arterial involvement; this examination makes it possible to highlight directly the suggestive anomalies of the mesenteric artery wall: a regular and homogeneous (> 3 mm) thickening, a luminal stenosis and also a periarterial halo and the absence of calcification (Lorthioir et al. 2008). MRI angiography could also be useful for the diagnosis of mesenteric arterial lesion but complementary studies to assess its relevance are necessary. Lastly, PET could also be a useful diagnostic technique in this indication; however, today, it is not possible to analyse small vessels (diameter under 4 mm) with the PET (Liozon et al. 2010). At present, mesenteric arterial lesions are a major cause of morbidity and mortality in GCA. They can be complicated by chronic mesenteric ischemia, mesenteric infarcts, ischemia-related intestinal pseudotumors, or digestive perforations. Some authors (Scola et al. 2008; Sujobert et al. 2008) suggest that the prognosis of patients with only prednisone was better than that of patients who received a medico(prednisone)- surgical treatment; these data seem, partly, to be explained by the fact that the patients treated surgically presented more severe mesenteric arterial complications.

Some patients received, in association with steroids, a complementary treatment with antiplatelet drug. However, the efficiency of these treatments in the reduction of the risk of thrombosis, in patients suffering from a mesenteric giant cell arteritis, remains to be determined.

4. Pericarditis an unusual manifestation

Pericarditis during GCA is rarely reported. In the literature, we were only able to find twelve observations in 20 years (Bablekos et al. 2006; Dupond et al. 1982; Clementz et al. 1989; Garewal et al. 1981; Guillaume et al. 1991; B; Guindon et al. 2007; Preston et al. 1991; Pedro-Botet et al. 1996; Matsue et al. 2011; Moulis et al. 2010; Stanley et al. 1989 & Valstar et al. 2003). In nine of these cases, cardiac symptoms including chest pain, exertional dyspnea or pericardial fremitus were present, but in three of the cases, the pericarditis was silent and was discovered on chest X-ray anomaly (Guindon et al. 2007; Miller 1996; Pedro et al. 1996). In this observations, the classical electrocardiographic anomalies of pericarditis (PR segment depression, repolarization anomalies) are not constant and one case only has been described with signs of ultrasound tamponade which did not however necessitated drainage, the hemodynamics being stable and progression satisfactory with corticosteroids (Valstar et al. 2003).The pericarditis was inaugural of GCA in all the cases, except one incidence of a relapse after one year, following the sudden interruption of the corticosteroids (Valstar et al. 2003). In all the reported cases, the pericarditis was always regressive under corticosteroids. In the review of several cases of pericarditis during GCA carried out by Bablekos et al. (2006), the authors point out that the classical signs of the disease are only present in 2/3 of the cases and highlight the interest of looking for GCA in inflammatory « idiopathic » pericarditis in subjects over 50 (Granel et al. 2001).
The pathogenesis is not known but several hypotheses can be advanced: inflammatory cytokine storm, deposit of complex immunes, and vasculitis of the pericardial arteries or interstitial inflammatory lesion of the pericardium with or without granulomas. It is at present impossible to know its prevalence, especially as pericarditis is not symptomatic in all cases and not searched for by systematic echocardiography. Only a study to evaluate systematic echocardiography during GCA (on diagnosis or in the case of recurrence) could allow us to appreciate its real prevalence and evaluate prospectively its prognostic value.
The treatment and the progression of pericarditis do not seem to differ from those of GCA: corticosensitivity to usual doses is excellent. Even though the risk of chronicity is difficult to appreciate (monitoring in nearly all the observations published does not exceed six months), no case of progression towards constriction have been reported.
In conclusion, we wish to emphasize that pericarditis needs to be added to the list of the numerous unusual presentations of GCA. We suggest relevance of a temporal artery biopsy in elderly patients with general symptoms associated with so-called "idiopathic pericarditis" even in the absence of typical manifestations of temporal arteritis.

5. Giant cell arteritis and myocarditis

Myocarditis belongs among the other cardiac manifestations described during GCA. Classical clinical presentation of GCA is rarely associated. Temporal artery biopsy is essential in confirming the diagnosis of GCA and proposing a specific therapy, in order to prevent cardiovascular ischemic complications. Etiological research of myocarditis must lead to discuss viral or bacterial diseases in the first instance. Certain auto-immune diseases must also be suspected. GCA myocarditis physiopathology is not known and only 3 cases are reported in the literature: two cases of myopericarditis (with alteration of the left ventricular systolic ejection fraction) were described by Teixera et al. (2003)] in two female patients, respectively aged 78 and 65. It must be noted that in these two observations, at no time were any clinical signs suggestive of GCA found; biopsy of the temporal artery was motivated only by the importance of the alteration of the general health condition in an unexplained inflammatory context. A case was described in a woman of 82 hospitalised for chest pain which had for 3 months an alteration of the general health condition with a weight loss of 4 kg, bitemporal headaches and jaw claudication. Transthoracic echocardiography showed a minimal lamina of pericardial effusion, retained left ventricular systolic ejection fraction with normal coronography (Pugnet et al. 2009). Although rare and certainly under-estimated, myocarditis must be known as an expression of GCA with rapid favourable progression under treatment. The diagnosis of GCA must remain in mind faced to myocarditis of the elderly patients with healthy coronaries.

6. Coronary arteritis and giant cell arteritis

Cases of giant cell arteritis in isolated coronary arteries, resulting in myocardial infarction, are unusual and have been infrequently reported in the literature (Cohle et al 1982; Kumar et al.2002; Long-Wei et al 2007 & Saito et al 1994). It is difficult to formally relate signs of coronary heart disease to GCA. However, histologically documented observations describe a thrombosis which develops as a consequence of the coronaritis with giant cells. In most of these reports, the definite diagnosis was based on postmortem examination or on atherectomy specimen evaluation (Saito et al 1994). In the case of Long-Wei and al. (2007), the histopathological diagnosis was based on evaluation of the native heart after heart transplantation. This is the first such case mentioned in the heart transplant literature in which native heart evaluation was used to confirm this diagnosis.The involvement of the coronary arteries is associated with a very severe prognosis. These cases suggest that coronary artery giant cell arteritis should be added to the list of differential diagnoses for patients suspected of myocardial infarction due to coronary artery disease or dilated cardiomyopathy. Treatment of GCA coronaritis is not codified.

7. Respiratory manifestations

The respiratory manifestations of GCA are rare and little known. They can be associated with more typical signs of the disease, but they can also be inaugural and the cause of a delay in care. Cassarou et al. (2010) reported eight observations in 2010 which illustrate the respiratory involvement of the disease. In two observations, the pleuropulmonary manifestations were concomitant with the clinical signs of GCA. In 5 observations out of 8, the pulmonary signs were inaugural with a time lapse of 10 to 21 days before the appearance of the clinical signs suggesting GCA whereas in one observation, these last were never observed.

Cough is the most frequent respiratory manifestation of GCA; pleural effusions and alveolar-interstitial involvement were rarer. The first form of GCA presenting as a chronic cough was described in 1956 by Valleteau de Mouillac. Cough, whether accompanied by a fever or an inflammatory syndrome, can be the first sign of the disease and precede the other signs by several months. In the study by Becourt-Verlomme et al. (2001) which dealt with the inaugural signs of the disease, out of 260 patients with GCA, cough was present in

8 % of the patients. In the study by Letellier et al. (2003) which analyzed 285 patients with GCA, 57 patients (20 %) presented a dry cough with a prolonged fever and this symptom was inaugural in 22 of them (8 %).The cough is irritative, sleep-depriving, and resists symptomatic treatment. After having eliminated the most frequent causes of chronic cough, the age and the importance of the inflammatory syndrome should suggest GCA among the diagnosis hypotheses. To illustrate this involvement, Kassem et al (2010) report the observation of a woman of 70 hospitalized for a dry cough developing over three months, associated secondarily with fever and loss of weight. She had no other functional signs, the clinical examination showed no particularities and it had been identified as a biological inflammatory syndrome. A lung, sinus or digestive pathology was looked for but the chest abdomen pelvis scan was considered as normal. Bronchial fibroscopy found a congestive bronchial mucous with no endoluminal lesions. Taking age into consideration, the alteration of the general state of health and unexplained inflammatory syndrome, a biopsy of the temporal artery was carried out whose histological analysis was characteristic of GCA. The cause of cough in GCA has not been formally identified: it could be related to a pharyngeal involvement whose vascularisation depends on the internal maxillary artery, it could be secondary to an irritation of the cough-exciting centers located in the airways, the diaphragm or the esophagus from the arterial inflammation and finally cough may also be a sign of inflammatory lung involvement which may affect the pulmonary arteries, lung parenchyma and pleura. The evolution of the cough is parallel to that of the disease, and regresses rapidly under steroids with possibility of relapse during decrease or withdrawal of the treatment.

Cases of pulmonary embolism related to GCA are exceptional in the literature (Andrès et al. 2003; Chassagne et al. 1995; Landrin et al. 1997 & Radhamanohar et al. 1991). Chassagne et al (1995) report the case of a woman of 86 with a biopsy proven GCA with a clinical and biological rapid favorable outcome under steroids. She was later hospitalized for febrile dyspnea with cough which revealed pulmonary lesions resulting in a lung infarction with excavation with partial thrombosis of the left pulmonary artery. The favorable development of the symptoms was rapid and durable with an increase in the dosage of steroids (with no associated anticoagulant treatment) which strengthened the hypothesis of an inflammatory thrombosis of the pulmonary artery. In the case reported by Andrès et al. (2003), thrombophilia tests (antithrombin, proteins C and S, factor V Leiden, antiphospholipids and circulating anticoagulant) were negative as was the search for deep vein thrombosis. The post-mortem histological examination revealed a giant cell arteritis infiltrating the three wall linings of the artery with regards to the thrombus.

In the literature, pleural effusion may be unilateral or bilateral, of mild to moderate abundance, generally well-tolerated and not very symptomatic. It may be isolated or associated with a pericardial effusion and sometimes be inaugural of the disease, and render diagnosis difficult (Valstar et al. 2003). The analysis of the liquid is reported around ten times in the literature; exsudative, sterile and with a cellularity of 600 to 3200 elements/mm^3 with a predominance of either neutrophils or lymphocytes (Colnot 1996.; Deraedt et al. 1994 & Marie et al. 2004). The physiopathology of the pleural involvement is not known. Blind pleural biopsies report a non-specific inflammatory reaction or a hyperplasia of mesothelial cells in inflammatory nodules (Colnot 1996). Examination of the pleura is, particularly in histology, more profitable for eliminating differential infectious and neoplastic diagnosis than for confirming GCA. The corticosensitivity of the pleural involvement is specific to the

disease with rapid regression of the effusions, and sometimes total regression in a few days (Colnot 1996.; Deraedt et al. 1994 & Marie et al. 2004).
Parenchymal pulmonary involvement is rare and described inaugurally for a relapse of the disease after reduction or withdrawal of corticosteroids. It is often accompanied by cough but may also be discovered fortuitously in imagery. In practice, the lesions are probably under-diagnosed and under-reported, the cases described in the literature being old ones. The interstitial involvement is predominant of reticulated or reticulo-micronodular type with predominance of the basal type (Karam & Fulmer 1982). Macronodular involvement (Bradley et al. 1984) can take a single or multiple pseudotumoral aspect, sometimes excavated, and leads to discussion on neoplastic aetiology, rheumatoid nodules, infectious (tuberculosis, nocardiosis) or inflammatory (Wegener) granulomatosis. Bronchial fibroscopy and bronchoalveolar lavage play a major role in the bacteriological investigation and the search for a bronchial neoplasia when there are radiological anomalies. On the other hand, they do not supply any diagnostic specificity: the macroscopic aspect shows an inflammatory bronchitis, the cytology of the bronchoalveolar lavage is polymorphic with macrophage predominance in some observations or a lymphocytic alveolitis. Diagnostic procedure of the biopsies carried out during the bronchial fibroscopy is limited. In the observations of Cassarou et al. (2010), the biopsies revealed a non-specific inflammation. The observations of Cassarou et al. (2010) also illustrate well certain problems in diagnosing the respiratory forms of GCA: when lung involvement precedes, sometimes by a few weeks, the clinical signs of GCA and when the histology of the temporal artery is not typical or when it is negative. The differential diagnosis may be difficult with other small and medium sized vessel vasculitis with a much more frequent pulmonary involvement, especially as overlaps were reported between GCA and Churg-Strauss syndrome (Vidal et al. 1992), microscopic polyangitis, periarteritis nodosa (Godeau et al. 1984) or Wegener's disease (Astudillo et al. 2008). A GCA preceding a Wegener's disease by a few years has also been reported (Garrouste et al. 2008). In the eight observations reported by Cassarou et al. (2010), the clinical and radiological lung involvement is sensitive to corticosteroids with no relapse observed. In the same way, Carli et al. (2001) report 2 cases of scattered multiple pulmonary nodules in a context which was suggestive of GCA and totally reversible under corticosteroids after searches for neoplasia have given a negative result.
The knowledge of these different respiratory manifestations during GCA (persistent cough, nodules, pleural effusion) is useful for the clinician. It helps him in prescribing non invasive investigations or even a presumptive steroids therapy, in an often old and weakened patient.

8. Neurologic manifestations

Cerebral vascular accidents (CVA) were reported in 3 to 6 % of cases (Nesher et al. 2000) but have never revealed GCA. Central nervous system findings in GCA are the result of thrombosis of the carotid or vertebral arteries, rather than of a primary neurogenic process or intracranial arteritis. GCA affects vessels that contain, internal elastic lamina. As intracranial vessels lose their internal elastic lamina 5 mm beyond the point of dural perforation, more distal intracranial arteritis is rare. In fact, clinical and pathologic findings suggest that these ischemic events are due to involvement of extradural vertebral and carotid arteries with high-grade stenosis or occlusion rather than intracranial vasculitis. Salvarani et al. (2006) confirm that obstruction and occlusion of internal carotid and/or vertebral arteries are the most frequent causes of cerebrovascular ischemic events in patients with GCA. Involvement of intracranial/intradural arteries in patients with GCA is a rare event and appears to represent a subset of GCA with a fatal course that fails to respond to corticosteroids.

During GCA, strokes occur mostly in the vertebrobasilar territory (as opposed to atheromatosis-related CVA).

Given the frequency of strokes in elderly people, we must discuss the part concerning arteritis, steroids side effect and that of atheromatosis. A CVA can occur before the treatment begins but also at the beginning of treatment (median of 10 days) (Jouquan et al. 1984). The thrombosis-producing role of steroids in the genesis of these CVA has been reported in several retrospective series. The establishment of a steroid treatment could paradoxically favour the onset of cerebral infarcts in patients with intracerebral arteritis and does not prevent often fatal precocious ischemic relapses (Salvarani et al. 2009). This ischemic risk could be decreased by the association of aspirin at a low dosage (3 % against 13 %, p= 0.02) with steroids (Nesher et al. 2004; Lee et al. 2006; Robert et al.2006). But in the study of Berger et al. (2009) severe ischemic events occurred with high prevalence despite established platelet inhibition. Neither platelet count nor size was strongly associated with the risk of severe ischemic events (Berger et al. 2009).

When evaluating patients with dementia, it is common to check for easily reversible problems. Both clinicians and researchers should give more attention to looking for GCA as a routine part of the standard dementia workup. Mental status changes may be a prominent manifestation of GCA and precede and/or overshadow more classic signs and symptoms. Depression, agitation, confusion, and focal intellectual impairment have all been described (Alisky 2008).

For example, Morris and Lockie reported in 2005 a 76-year-old man with acute right-sided periocular pain and diminished vision. He had a sedimentation rate of 73 mm/hr, cilioretinal artery occlusion and "florid" GCA seen on temporal artery biopsy. He was quite impaired cognitively, but prednisolone 50 mg per day produced rapid normalisation of his mental status, and at that point, his family commented that he had actually had dementia for at least a few years. Further investigation revealed that three years before, he had suffered a right-sided middle cerebral artery stroke that had been accompanied by scalp tenderness and right-sided headache. A diagnosis of GCA had been considered at that time but was not pursued because sedimentation rate was only 4 mm/hr.

Peripheral neurological manifestations can be a mode of revelation of GCA but are considered as rare (Reich et al. 1990, Büschges et al. 1984). However, in the series where neurological involvement was systemically looked for, the frequency of peripheral neuropathies was estimated up to 14 %. In the majority of these cases, it is a sensory-motor polyneuropathy which is usually moderate and chronic, a mononeuritis or multineuritis. Radicular involvement, which essentially affects the cervical region, is much rarer. Isolated plexus brachial syndromes in the scope of multineuritis remain exceptional: no cases in the series of 260 GCA by Becourt-Verlomme et al. (2001); one case in 209 proven GCA in the series by Blaise et al. (2005). A review of the literature found around twenty observations of GCA with histological proof, complicated by a plexus brachial syndrome or low cervical radiculopathies on which we wish to focus (Blaise et al. 2005; Soubrier et al. 2002). The involvement is often inaugural and quite constantly involves root C5. There is a male predominance (54 %) of this complication as opposed to the female predilection for temporal arteritis. The unilateral or bilateral involvement with no predominant side occurs usually at the peak of GCA signs. It sometimes precedes the cephalic signs of GCA by a few weeks. Despite the frequent severity of the motor deficit, recuperation is the rule. The usually sudden character of the involvement suggests an ischemic mechanism and the cervical radiculopathies can be due to a florid giant cell arteritis of the lower radicular arteries. Whether ischemic or inflammatory, however, the mechanism of C5-C6 plexopathy is pure speculation.

9. Ophtalmological manifestations

The incidence of ophthalmological manifestations varies according to studies between 14 % and 70 % of cases. In 1998, Hayreh et al. (1998) reported a series of 85 patients suffering from GCA for whom opthalmological involvement was listed: amaurosis fugax 30.5%, loss of visual acuity 97.6%, diplopia 5.9% and ocular pain 8.2%. Therefore, GCA must be suspected in the case of a sudden loss of visual acuity, whether transitory or not, in a patient over 50. This loss of visual acuity might be linked to an acute anterior ischemic optical neuropathy 81.2% according to Hayreh et al. (1998) or, more rarely, central retinal artery occlusion 14.1%, isolated cilioretinal artery occlusion 14.1% and posterior ischemic optic neuropathy in 7%.
The risk of bilateral ocular involvement is major in the case of GCA. It still occurs in around 1 case in 4, even though it is avoidable in most of these cases. In the series by Maalouly et al. (2010), the average time lapse for a bilateralisation of ocular involvement was 17 days (0 to 210 days). This was a bilateral ischemic optical neuropathy: anterior 21 times and posterior twice, a bilateral retinal central artery occlusion 3 times, an ischemic optical neuropathy associated with transitory monocular blindness in the last case. No studied clinical or biological parameters were associated with bilateral ocular involvement risks. Ocular involvement was inaugural in 5 patients (no general signs). Bilateralisation occurred before any steroid treatment 15 times (56 %), 7 times (26 %) at least 5 days after a high dosage steroid treatment and 6 times in a longer-term steroid treatment at variable doses.
Steroids have resulted in a large reduction of the incidence of its ophthalmological complications, whose frequency however remains high for two main reasons: delay in diagnosis and the existence of ophthalmological complications inaugural of the disease. Thus, physicians must be aware of ophthalmological complications of GCA as the severity of the disease can be improved by an earlier diagnosis and treatment.
Berger et al. (2009) have reported a series of 85 GCA patients (78 histologically proven) and investigated how platelet count and size and platelet inhibition with aspirin relate to ischemic complications. Jaw claudication, amaurosis fugax, blurred vision, ischemic stroke and permanent visual loss were classified as "ischemic events"; ischemic stroke and permanent visual loss were sub-grouped as "severe ischemic events". Of the 85 patients, 62 (73%) presented with ischemic events, 29/85 patients (34%) with severe ischemic events. At the time of diagnosis 22/85 patients (26%) were treated with ASA. In multivariate analysis, neither platelet count nor size or aspirin treatment were significantly associated with ischemic or severe ischemic events.

10. Genital involvement

Genital lesions are exceptional. They can affect the ovaries, the uterus and the tubes. They are often discovered by chance, as female patients do not present painful pelvic symptoms.

Thus, in a review of the literature, Ducroix et al. (1990) report 11 cases of isolated ovarian lesions or associated with a uterine or tube lesion. Clinical signs of rhizomelic pseudopolyarthritis were present in four female patients and headaches in two female patients. The differential diagnosis of ovarian lesions of GCA is classically periarteritis nodosa and Wegener's disease. These two diseases can have a gynaecological tropism but the histological aspect is different.

11. Musculoskeletal symptoms

Rhizomelic pseudopolyarthritis is the most frequent rheumatic manifestation of GCA. The frequency of rhizomelic pseudopolyarthritis in the course of certified GCA is on average 40 % (Masson 2010). Conversely, the sub-group of rhizomelic pseudopolyarthritis which does not have, at the time of diagnosis, signs suggesting the coexistence of a GCA would only appear to have a low risk of developing a GCA later: out of a series of 400 cases of rhizomelic pseudopolyarthritis, only four patients (1 %) developed secondarily a clinical GCA (Spiera 1990).

Another work on 230 patients with rhizomelic pseudopolyarthritis with no clinical signs of GCA showed that these biopsies of temporal arteries carried out on a sample of 68 randomly-selected patients were only positive in three cases (4.4 % of the patients) (Mykelust et al. 2003). This frequency of 4 % confirms that most rhizomelic pseudopolyarthritis with no clinical signs of GCA are actually « pure » rhizomelic pseudopolyarthritis. The other rheumatoid manifestations are less frequent. They may be polyarthritis, oligoarthritis or monoarthritis affecting the large joints, and specifically the knees. The interest of the study by Belcourt-Verlomme et al. (2010) is above all to highlight the existence of monoarthritis or oligoarthritis affecting the large joints preceding GCA (nine observations with arthritis affecting large joints,260 with positive temporal artery biopsy in seven patients , with a time lapse of up to 24 months and reacting well to non-steroid anti-inflammatory treatments. Chronic seronegative polyarthritis with a symptomatology comparable to rhumatoid arthritis was also described. In the study of Navaez et al. (2001), the records of 163 cases of rhizomelic pseudopolyarthritis or GCA diagnosed over a 15 year period in one area of Spain were reviewed for the presence and type of musculo-skeletal manifestations. Of 163 patients, 90 had isolated rhizomelic pseudopolyarthritis and 73 had GCA. Eighteen of the 90 patients (20%) with isolated rhizomelic pseudopolyarthritis developed distal peripheral arthritis either at diagnosis or during the course of the disease. When it occurred, synovitis was asymmetrical, transient, and not destructive. Other distal manifestations observed in these patients were carpal tunnel syndrome and distal extremity swelling with pitting oedema. In all cases these manifestations occurred in conjunction with active rhizomelic pseudopolyarthritis. As expected, rhizomelic pseudopolyarthritis was the most frequent musculoskeletal manifestation in patient with GCA, occurring in 56% of cases. On the contrary, only 11% of patients with GCA developed peripheral arthritis. An important finding was that peripheral arthritis in these patients appears to be linked only temporally to the presence of simultaneous rhizomelic pseudopolyarthritis and it is not observed in its absence. The spectrum of distal musculoskeletal manifestations of rhizomelic pseudopolyarthritis in this study is similar to that reported in other populations. By contrast, distal musculoskeletal symptoms are uncommon in GCA.

When the joint fluid was analyzed, it was not specific. The analyses published in the literature show that it is a moderately inflammatory liquid, with less than 3 000 elements, and no specificity.

12. Conclusion

Giant cell arteritis (GCA) is a primary large-vessel vasculitis predominantly seen in the elderly that preferentially involves the external carotid artery and its branches. However, inflammation of the aorta and its branches, pericarditis, myocarditis, respiratory manifestations, neurologic symptoms including, but not limited to, stroke and blindness, as well as musculoskeletal manifestations occur in a subset of patient at diagnosis or during the course of the disease.

Unfortunately, its uncommon findings are frequently overlooked and too often GCA is considered a disease of the temporal arteries only. Awareness of the basic anatomy and pathophysiology of this disease will enable clinicians to recognize many more obscure presentations and provide treatment to prevent serious sequelae.

Extracranial involvement has probably been underestimated and its incidence may be more frequent than suspected. Systematic evaluation of patients with imaging techniques such positron emission tomography (PET) may reveal that the clinical impact of extracranial involvement by GCA may be more relevant than previously thought. In the setting of GCA an early diagnosis is mandatory in order to perform a treatment capable of avoiding the chronic and acute complications associated with an elevated mortality.

13. References

Agard C, Said L, Ponge T, Connault J, Masseau A, Pistorius MA, Planchon B, Dupas B, Barrier JH,

Alisky JM. Giant cell arteritis Dementia and other steroid responsive dementia syndromes are a unique opportunity for clinicians and researchers. *Singapore Med J* 2008; 49 (3):268.

Andrès E, Kaltenbach G, Marcellin L, Imler M. Artérite pulmonaire à cellules géantes révélée par une embolie pulmonaire aiguë. *Presse Med* 2003;33:1328-9.

Assie C, Marie I, Atteintes artérielles des membres supérieurs et inférieurs au cours de la maladie de Horton. *La Presse Médicale* 2011;40:151-161.

Assie C, Janvresse A, Plissonnier D, Levesque H, Marie I. Long-term follow-up of giant cell arteritis. A series of 36 patients. Medicine (Baltimore) 2011;90:40–51. Astudillo L, Pugnet G, Bidegain F, Delsol M, Fortenfant F, Arlet-Suau E. Une maladie de Wegener avec des signes d'artérite temporale. *Rev Med Int* 2008; 29 : 830-831.

Bablekos GD, Michaelides SA, Karachalios GN, Nicolaou IN, Batistatou AK, Charalabopoulos KA. Pericardial involvement as an atypical manifestation of giant cell arteritis: report of a clinical case and literature review. *Am J Med Sci* 2006;332:198–204.

Becourt-Verlomme C, Barouky R, Alexandre C, Gonthier R, Laurent H, Vital Durant D, et al. Symptômes inauguraux de la maladie de Horton sur une série de 260 patients. *Rev Med Interne* 2001;22:631–7.

Belhocine T, Kaye O, Delanaye P, Corman V, Baghaie M, Deprez M, et al. Maladie de Horton et atteintes extratemporales : utilité de la tomographie par émission de positons au 18FDG. À propos de trois observations et d'une revue de la littérature. *Rev Med Interne* 2002;23:584–91.

Benjilali L, Tazi Mezalek Z, Raffali J, El Imadi H and al. Atteinte des artères des membres et maladie de Horton : à propos de cinq cas. *Rev Med Interne* 2009;30:1004-1010.

Berger CT, Wolbers M, Meyer P, Daikeler T and Hess C. High incidence of severe ischaemic complications in patients with giant cell arteritis irrespective of platelet count and size, and platelet inhibition. *Rheumatology* 2009;48:258–261.

Blaise S, Liozon E, Nadalon S, Vidal E. Maladie de Horton etplexite brachiale C5-C6 : une observation avec revue de la littérature. *Rev Med Interne* 2005;26:578-582.

Bossert M, Prati C, Balblanc JC, Lohse A, Wendling D. Atteinte aortique dans la maladie de Horton : aspects actuels . *Revue du Rhumatisme*, In Press, Corrected Proof 2010.

Brack A, Martinez-Taboada V, Stanson A, Goronzy JJ, Weyand CM. Disease pattern in cranial and large-vessel giant cell arteritis. *Arthritis Rheum* 1999;42:311–7.

Bradley JD, Pinals RS, Blumenfeld HB, Poston WM. Giant cell arteritis with pulmonary nodules. *Am J Med* 1984;77:135-40.

Büschges B, De Coninck P, Di Bernardo C, Bouton Y, Plouvier B. Neuropathies périphériques au cours de la pseudo-polyarthrite rhizomélique et de la maladie de Horton. *Presse Med* 1984;13:1636.

Carassou P, Aletti M, Cinquetti G, Banal F, Landais C, Graffin B, Carli P. Atteinte respiratoire de la maladie de Horton : 8observations et revue de la Littérature. *La Presse Médicale* 2010;39:188-196.

Carli P, Na'ftlho A, Marlier S, Crdmades A, Paris JF, Landais C. «Lâcher de ballons », réversible et maladie de Horton : deux observations. *Rev Med interne* 2001; 22suppl4.

Chassagne P, Gligorov J, Dominique S. Pulmonary artery obstruction and giant cell arteritis. *Ann Med Int* 1995;122:732.

Clementz GL, Gold F, Khaiser N, Zolin WD, Jalovec L. Giant cell arteritis associated with pericarditis and pancreatic insufficiency in a patient with psoriatic arthritis. *J Rheumatol* 1989;1:128–9. Cohle SD, Titus JL, Espinola A, et al. Sudden unexpected death due to coronary giant cell arteritis. *Arch Pathol Lab Med* 1982;106:171–2.

Colnot F. Pleurésie révélatrice d'une maladie de Horton. *Rev Med Interne* 1996;17:430-1.

Deraedt S, Cabane J, Genereau T, Imbert JC. Les manifestations respiratoires spécifiques de la maladie de Horton. *Rev Med Interne* 1994;15:813-20.

Ducroix JP, Sevestre H, Humbert G, Smail A, Cohen G, Hoang-Ngoc Minh, Palliez TM, Baillet J. Genital sites of giant-cell arteritis. *Rev Med Interne* 1990;11(4):285-8.

Dupond JL, Leconte des Floris R. Temporal arteritis manifested as an acute febrile pericarditis. *JAMA* 1982;247:2371–2.

Evans JM, O'Fallon WM, Hunder GG. Increased incidence of aortic aneurysm and dissection in giant cell (temporal) arteritis. A population-based study. Ann Intern Med 1995;122:502–7.

Garrouste C, Sailler L, Astudillo L, Lavayssière L, Cointault O, Borel C et al. Fulminant alveolar hemorrhage: evolution of giant cell arteritis to ANCA-positive vasculitis? *Rev Med Interne* 2008;29:232-5.

Godeau P, Lemaitre MO, Wechsler B, Guillevin L, Herson S. Association d'une maladie de Horton et d'une périartérite noueuse. *À propos de 3 cas. Sem Hop Paris* 1984;60:30-4.

Granel B, Serratrice J, Rey J, Pache X, Swiader L, Habib G. La péricardite idiopathique chronique ou récidivante est-elle une maladie inflammatoire autonome ? *Rev Med Interne* 2001;22:1204–12.

Guindon A, Rossi P, Baneres D, Aissi K, Demoux A-L, Bonin-Guillaume S, et al. La péricardite: une manifestation de la maladie de Horton. Rev Med Interne 2007;28:326–31.

Guillaume M, Vachiery F, Cogan E. Pericarditis: an unusual manifestation of giant cell arteritis. Am J Med 1991;6:662–4.

Hamidou MA. Fréquence de l'atteinte de l'aorte abdominale au diagnostic de la Maladie de Horton : étude de 20 patients par échographie-Doppler et angiotomodensitométrie. La Presse Médicale 2009;38:11-19. Hamrin B, Jonsson N, Landberg T. Involvement of large vessels in polymyalgia arteritica. Lancet 1965;33:1193–6.

Hayreh S.S., Podhajsky P.A., Zimmerman B. Occult giant cell arteritis: Ocular manifestations Am J Ophthalmol 1998 ; 125 : 521-526

Hervé F, Choussy V, Janvresse A, et al. Aortic involvement in giant cell arteritis. A prospective follow-up of 11 patients using computed tomography. *Rev Med Interne* 2006;27:196–202.

Jouquan J, Mottier D, Cleuziou A, Pennec Y, Baccino E, Bergeret G, et al. Accident vasculaire cérébral précoce au cours de maladies de Horton traitées. Responsabilité du traitement par corticoïdes? *Ann Med Interne* 1984;135(7):526–9.

Karam GH, Fulmer JD. Giant cell arteritis presenting as interstitial lung disease. *Chest* 1982;82:781-4.

Kassem H, et al. Toux chronique révélant une maladie de Horton. *Rev Med Interne In Press,* Corrected Proof 2010.

Kumar P, Velossaris T, Sheppard MN, et al. Giant cell arteritis confined to intramural coronary arteries. Unforeseen hazards myocardial protection. *J Cardiovasc Surg (Torino)* 2002;43:647–9.

Landrin I, Chassagne P, Bouaniche M. Thrombose des artères pulmonaires dans la maladie de Horton. À propos d'un nouveau cas et d'une revue de la littérature. *Ann Med Int* 1997;148:315-6.

Launay D, Hachulla E. Les aortites inflammatoires. La Presse Médicale 2003;33:1334-1340.

Lee MS, Smith SD, Galor A, Hoffman GS. Antiplatelet and anticoagulant therapy In patients with giant cell arteritis. *Arthritis Rheum* 2006;54:3306-9.

Letellier P, Zoulim A, Ollivier Y, Bonnel N, Lehobey F, Sado E, et al. Toux et maladie de Horton: étude monocentrique prospective portant sur 285 patients. *Rev Med Interne* 2003;24 (Suppl.4):443.

Liozon E, Monteil J, Ly K.H, Vidal E. Place de la tomography par emission de positrons (TEP) au 18FDG dans l'exploration et la surveillance des vascularites. *Rev Med Interne* 2010;31:417- 427.

García-Martínez A, Hernández-Rodríguez J, Arguis P, et al. Development of aortic aneurysm/dilatation during the follow-up of patients with giant cell arte- ritis: a cross-sectional screening of fifty-four prospectively followed patients. *Arthritis Rheum* 2008;59:422–30.

Long-Wei Lin, Shoei-Shen Wang, Chia-Tung Shun. Myocardial Infarction Due to Giant Cell Arteritis: A Case Report and Literature Review. *The Kaohsiung Journal of Medical Sciences* 2007;23:195-198.

Lorthioir A, Marie I,Tetart F, Bernet J, Lévesque H. Artérite inflammatoire mésentérique au cours de la maladie de Horton :) propos de deux observations et revue de la littérature. *Rev Med Interne* 2008 ; 29: 1007-1012.

Maalouly G, Sedira N, Mantout F, I. Rossignol I, S. Feldman S,Benrabah R, Heron E. Atteinte oculaire bilatérale au cours de la maladie de Horton : une série de 27 cas consécutifs. Communications orales / *La Revue de médecine interne* 31S (2010) S35–S83

Marie I, Heliot P, Muir JF, Roussel F, Levesque H, Courtois H. Pleural effusion revealing giant cell arteritis. *Eur J Intern Med* 2004;15:125-7.

Masson C. Pseudopolyarthrite rhizomélique, maladie de Horton. Critères de diagnostic et de suivi. *Revue du rhumatisme* monographies 77 (2010) 76–81.Matsue Y, Ohno M, Nagahori W, Suzuki M, Matsumura A, Hashimoto Y. A case of giant cell arteritis with massive pericardial effusion. *Heart Vessels* 2011 [epub ahead of print]

Miller JP. Pericardial effusion and giant cell arteritis. *Proc R Soc Med* 1972;65:565.

Morris OC, Lockie P. Giant cell arteritis--presenting as stroke, transient ischaemic attack and dementia. *Aust Fam Physician* 2005; 34:653-5.

Moulis G, Sailler L, Astudillo L, Vernet J, Couret B, Arlet P. Péricardite inaugurale de la maladie de Horton. *Rev Med Interne* 2010;31:46-48. Myklebust G, Wilsgaard T, Jacobsen BK, Gran JT.Causes of death in polymyalgia rheumatic. A prospective longitudinal study of 315 cases and matched population controls. Scand J Rheumatol. 2003;32(1):38-4.

Myklebust G, Wilsgaard T, Jacobsen BK, Gran JT.Causes of death in polymyalgia rheumatic. A prospective longitudinal study of 315 cases and matched population controls. Scand J Rheumatol. 2003;32(1):38-4.Nesher G. low dose aspirin and prevention of cranial ischemic complications in giant cell arteritis.*Arthritis Rheum* 2004;50:1332-7.

Narváez J, Nolla-Solé JM, Narváez JA, Clavaguera MT, Valverde-García J, Roig-Escofet D. Musculoskeletal manifestations in polymyalgia rheumatica and temporal arteritis. *Ann Rheum Dis* 2001;60:1060–1063.

Nesher G. Neurologic manifestations of giant cell arteritis. *Clin Exp Rheumatol* 2000;18 (Suppl 20):S24–6.

Nuenninghoff DM, Hunder GG, Christianson TJ, McClelland RL, Matteson EL. Incidence and predictors of large-artery complication (aortic aneurysm, aortic dissection, and/or large-artery stenosis) in patients with giant cell arteritis: a population-based study over 50 years. *Arthritis Rheum* 2003;48:3522–31.

Pedro-Botet J, Coll J, Lopez MJ, Graut JM. Pericadial effusion and giant cell arteritis. *Br Rheumatol* 1996;35:194–5.

Preston J, Warner M. Pericardial effusion as a manifestation of giant cell arteritis. *Am J Med* 1991;91:439–40.

Pugnet G, Sailler L, Vernet J, Astudillo L, Dumonteil N, Couret B, Arlet P . Myocardite aiguë : une présentation exceptionnelle de maladie de Horton. *Rev Med Interne* 2009.30S :S385-S479

Reich KA, Giansiracusa DF, Strongwater SL, Neurologic manifestations of giant cell arteritis, Am. J. Med 1990;89:67–72.

Robert F. Spiera F,Spiera H.Therapy for Giant Cell Arteritis: Can We Do Better? *Arthritis & Rheumatism* 2006;5:3071–3074.

Radhamanohar M. Multiple pulmonary infarctions caused by giant cell arteritis. *Postgrad Med J* 1991;67:491.

Saito S, Arai H, Kim K, et al. Acute myocardial infarction in a young adult due to solitary giant cell arteritis of the coronary artery diagnosed antemortemly by primary directional coronary atherectomy. *Cathet Cardiovasc Diagn* 1994;33:245–9.

Salvarani C, Della Bella C, Cimino L, Macchioni P, Formisano D, Bajocchi G, Pipitone N, Catanoso MG, Restuccia G, Ghinoi A, Boiardi L. Risk factors for severe cranial ischaemic events in an Italian population-based cohort of patients with giant cell arteritis. Rheumatology (Oxford). 2009 Mar;48(3):250-3. Epub 2008 Dec 24

Salvarani C, Giannini C, Miller DV, Hunder G. Giant Cell Arteritis: Involvement of Intracranial Arteries. *Arthritis & Rheumatism (Arthritis Care & Research)* 2006; 55:985–989.

Schmidt WA, Blockmans D. Use of ultrasonography and positron emission tomography in the diagnosis and assessment of large-vessel vasculitis. *Curr Opin Rheumatol* 2005;17:9-15.

Scola CJ, Li C, Upchurch KS. Mesenteric involvement in giant cell arteritis: an underrecognized complication ? Analysis of a case series with clinicoanatomic correlation. *Medicine (Baltimore)* 2008;87: 45–51.

Skopinski S, Constans J, Le Melayer P, Baste JC, Chenfi H, Conn C. Arteriopathie des membres superieurs revelant une maladie de Horton: cinq cas *Rev Med Interne* 1997;18(Supp15)

Soubrier M, Dubost JJ, Tournadre A, Deffond D, Clavelou P, Ristori JM. Cervical radiculopathy as a manifestation of giant cell arteritis. *Joint Bone Spine* 2002; 69: 316–8.

Spiera H.Giant cell arteritis and polymyalgia rheumatic.Hosp Pract (Off Ed). 1990 Nov 15;25(11):71-4, 77-8, 81-4 passim. Review Stanley D, Henderson D, Harris S. Giant cell arteritis associated with pericarditis and large vessel disease. *Aust N Z J Med* 1991;3:353–5.

Sujobert P, Fardet L, Marie I, Duhaut P, Cohen P, Grange C, et al. Mesenteric ischemia: 6 cases and a systematic review. *J Rheumatol* 2007;34:1727–32.

Tazi Z, Cacoub P , Cheysson D, Godeau P, Piette JC. Maladie de Horton démasquée par une artériopathie spécifique des membres inférieurs.Rev Med Interne 1997 ;18 :638-541.

Teixera A, Capitaine E, Congy F, Herson S, Cherin P. Atteinte myopéricardique au cours de la maladie de Horton. *Rev Med Interne* 2003;24:189–94.

Valstar MH, Terpstra WF, de Jong RS. Pericardial and pleural effusion in giant cell arteritis. *Am J Med* 2003;114:708–9.

Vidal E, Liozon F, Rogues AM, Cransac M, Berdha JF, Liozon E. Concurrent temporal arteritis and Churg-Strauss syndrome. *J Rheumatol* 1992;19:1312-4.

Weyand CM, Goronzy JJ. Arterial wall injury in giant cell arteritis. *Arthritis Rheum* 1999;42:844-53.

16

Large Giant Cell Arteritis with Eye Involvement

Jianu Dragoş Cătălin[1,2], Jianu Silviana Nina[3],
Petrica Ligia[1,4] and Şerpe Mircea[2]
[1]"Victor Babeş" University of Medicine and Pharmacy, Timişoara
[2]County Emergency Hospital, Department of Neurology, Timişoara
[3]Military Emergency Hospital, Department of Ophthalmology, Timişoara
[4]County Emergency Hospital, Department of Internal Medicine, Timişoara
Romania

1. Introduction

Giant cell arteritis (GCA), also called Horton, temporal, or granulomatous arteritis, is a primary vasculitis that affects extracranial medium (especially branches of the external carotid artery) and large-sized arteries (aorta and its major branches) (Levine&Hellmann, 2002). The diagnosis of GCA requires age more than 50 years at disease onset, new headache in the temporal area, temporal artery tenderness, and/or reduced pulse, jaw claudication, systemic symptoms, erythrocyte sedimentation rate (ESR) exceeding 50 mm/ hr, and typical histologic findings (granulomatous involvement) in temporal artery biopsy (Hunder et al., 1990). Approximately 40-50% of these patients have ophthalmologic complications, consisting of visual loss secondary to arteritic anterior ischemic optic neuropathy (AION), or central retinal artery occlusion (CRAO), homonymous hemianopsia or cortical blindness (unilateral or bilateral occipital infarction) (Gonzales-Gay, 2005).

2. Epidemiology

Over the last 25–30 years, GCA has been found to be the most common type of vasculitis in Europe and North America. Incidence of GCA is higher in white individuals than those of other ethnicities. The highest incidence rates are reported in Scandinavian countries and North American populations of the same descent. In these regions, the annual incidence rates are generally higher than 17/100,000 people per population age >50 years (Salvarani et al., 1995). The incidence of GCA is lower than 12/100,000 people per population age >50 years in Southern European and Mediterranean countries.

The incidence increases with age and peaks in the 70–79 years age group: 100,000 people per population age >50 years.

In Northern European countries, women are affected more frequently than men (3:1 to 5:1). A lower ratio of women to men was observed in Southern Europe and Israel (Salvarani et al., 1991).

As the population throughout the world continues to age, an increased prevalence of disease should be expected.

Higher physician awareness was proposed as being responsible for the progressive increase of GCA reported in different parts of the world (Gonzales-Gay et al., 2009).

3. Etiology

3.1 Implication of genetic factors

Familial aggregation of GCA has been observed. Genetic predisposition has been reported with an association to the human leukocyte antigen (HLA)-DRB1 molecule, and tumor necrosis factor microsatellite polymorphisms. Moreover, many other studies have shown the implication of genetic variants in key components of immune and inflammatory pathways in GCA susceptibility, because GCA is a polygenic disease. An increased risk of having visual ischemic complications in biopsy-proven GCA patients was found to be associated with the carriage of HLA-DRB1*04 alleles. Moreover, a functional variant of the vascular endothelial growth factor gene was associated with severe ischemic complications in patients with GCA (Gonzales-Gay, 2001).

3.2 Influence of infectious agents

It has been proposed that infectious agents are a possible influence in the pathogenesis of GCA. Several infectious agents have been investigated as possible triggers in a susceptible host, with inconclusive results. Fluctuations of the incidence of GCA in different regions of Denmark, supporting an association with *Mycoplasma pneumoniae*, parvovirus B19, and *Chlamydia pneumoniae* epidemics, were found. An association of parvovirus B19 with GCA was also suggested by Gabriel et al., 1999. French investigators found an association of GCA with human parainfluenza virus type 1 (Gabriel et al., 1999).

Four different recent studies did not confirm any association between the presence of parvovirus B19, *C pneumoniae*, or human herpesvirus DNA in TAB specimens and the histologic evidence of biopsy-proven GCA (Rodriguez-Pla, 2004).

However, the presence of peaks in the incidence and a cyclic pattern observed in other studies suggests that infectious agents may play a role in the pathogenesis of both diseases. They could be the triggers for the development of these conditions in genetically predisposed individuals (Ghanchi, 1996).

3.3 Influence of traditional cardiovascular risk factors

(Duhaut et al, 1999), in a prospective multicenter case-control study on 207 biopsy-proven GCA patients, described a strong association between smoking and previous atheromatous disease in women and GCA. The presence of atherosclerosis risk factors at the time of diagnosis of the disease may influence the development of severe ischemic complications in patients with this vasculitis.

4. Pathogenesis

GCA is an autoimmune vasculitis. It involves predominantly medium-sized arteries, especially the superficial temporal, ophthalmic, posterior ciliary, and other peripheral arteries. The typically predominant extracranial vascular involvement is explained by the affinity of inflammation to the elastic fibers. As intracranial arteries have less elastic fibers in the media, they are seldomly involved. The severity and extent of the involvement are associated with the quantity of elastic tissue in the media of the artery.

Two different types of inflammatory reactions are found in the temporal arteries in patients with GCA. One is related to foreign-body giant-cell reaction, directed at small calcifications of the internal elastic membrana. The foreign-body type of inflamation is focal, affecting only part of the arterial circumference. The other type of lesion is characterized by diffuse inflammation in which mononuclear inflammatory cells invade the layers of the arterial wall in the whole circumference of the vessel. (Weyand et al., 1997).

GCA is an antigen-driven disease with local T cell and macrophage activation in the vessel wall, and with an important role of proinflammatory cytokines. Inflammation of the arterial wall and vessel occlusion through fast and concentric intimal hyperplasia leads to the severe ischemic complications observed in patients with GCA. Dendritic cells localized at the adventitia–media border of normal medium-sized arteries produce chemokines and recruit and locally activate T cells. Moreover, dendritic cells express a singular surface receptor profile, including a series of Toll-like receptors (TLRs). Ligands of TLR-4 promote activation and differentiation of adventitial dendritic cells into chemokine-producing effector cells with high-level expression of both CD83 and CD86, and mediate T cell recruitment through the release of interleukin-18 (IL-18). Activated T cells experience clonal expansion and are stimulated to produce interferon-gamma (IFN-gamma). This leads to the differentiation and migration of macrophages and the formation of giant cells. In the adventitia, macrophages produce proinflammatory cytokines such as IL-1 and IL-6, whereas in the media and intima they contribute to arterial injury by producing metalloproteinases and nitric oxide.

This destructive mechanism of the arterial wall is associated with a repair mechanism that includes the secretion of growth and angiogenic factors (platelet-derived growth factor and vascular endothelial growth factor) through the infiltration of mononuclear cells and multinucleated giant cells. These changes ultimately lead to the degradation of the internal elastic lamina and to occlusive luminal hyperplasia. In addition to IL-1 and IL-6, IFN-gamma specifically seems to play a pivotal role in the pathogenesis and in the clinical expression of GCA. In this regard, IFN- gamma is expressed in nearly 70% of the temporal artery biopsy (TAB) samples from patients with GCA. High transcription of IFN-gamma messenger RNA (mRNA) was associated with the formation of giant cells and with the evidence of cranial ischemic symptoms in GCA patients. The absence of IFN- gamma expression in TAB samples from patients with isolated PMR suggests that its production may be crucial to the development of GCA. TAB specimens from GCA patients with ocular ischemia expressed high amounts of IFN-gammamRNA, whereas those from GCA patients with fever had less IFN-gamma mRNA. Therefore, clinical correlates suggest a role of IFN-gamma in the process of lumenal obstruction. By regulating giant cell formation, IFN-gamma could indirectly control intimal hyperplasia. IFN-gamma may dictate the functional properties of other cell populations in the vascular infiltrates and, by means of this mechanism, guide the response-to-injury reaction of the artery (Weyand et al., 1997).

5. Diagnosis

A definitive diagnosis is made following the criteria of the American College of Rheumatology which include: age, temporal headache, swollen temporal arteries, jaw claudication, eye involvement, the temporal artery biopsy, and its histologic evaluation. The disease affects elderly patients, with a mean age of 70 years.

Diagnostic criteria of temporal arteritis

Three of the five diagnostic criteria for GCA have to be met (Hunder et al., 1990):

1. Age 50 years or more.
2. New developed headache.
3. Tenderness of the superficial temporal artery.
4. Elevated sedimentation rate (ESR), at least 50 mm/h.
5. Giant cell arteritis in a biopsy specimen from the temporal artery.

Large vessel giant cell arteritis is a subgroup of GCA (temporal arteritis) described in at least 17% of cases. In these patients, inflammation occurs also at the level of the aorta and its branches (especially of the subclavian, the axillary arteries, etc), although symptoms of aortic involvement (aortic aneurysm rupture) may appear years after the initial diagnosis of this vasculitis (Martinez-Valle, 2010).

Interestingly, in some cases, the common carotid arteries (CCA) and the internal carotid arteries (ICA) are also involved.

5.1 Clinical features

The typical neurological symptoms and classic clinical features of GCA are presented by new moderate bitemporal headache, especially common at night, jaw claudication, scalp tenderness (which is first noticed when combing the hair), or abnormal superficial temporal arteries (tender, nodular, swollen, and thickened arteries) on palpation (Gonzales-Gay et al., 2005). **(fig.1)**

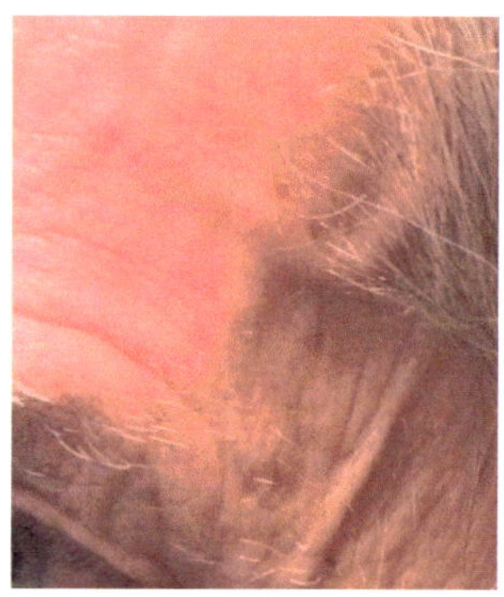

Fig. 1. Patient MM. Dilated and nodular left superficial temporal artery.

Initially, temporal pulsation is present, although the thickened arteries cann't be flattened against the skull. The best location to feel for pulsation is directly in front of the upper pole of the pinna of the ear. Later, the temporal arteries present a decreased pulsatility. Lack of pulsation is very suggestive of GCA because it is most unusual for the superficial temporal arteries to be non-pulsatile in normal elderly individuals. The jaw claudication is the result of ischemia of the masseter muscles, which causes pain on speaking and chewing.

A recent study aiming to establish the best set of clinical features that may predict a positive TAB in a community hospital disclosed that headache, jaw claudication, and abnormal temporal artery on palpation were the best positive predictors of positive TAB in patients on whom a biopsy was performed to diagnose GCA. These authors established clinical differences between biopsy proven GCA and biopsy-negative GCA patients. Moreover, they observed a non-significantly increased frequency of abnormal palpation of the temporal artery on physical examination in biopsy-proven GCA patients (73.3%) compared with biopsy-negative GCA patients (54.2%).

Less common neurologic complications (approximately 4% of patients) include transient ischemic attacks, or stroke, more frequently in the posterior circulation, than in the carotid territory, manifested by homonymous hemianopsia or cortical blindness (unilateral or bilateral occipital infarction), and audiovestibular dysfunction. They occur more commonly at the time of GCA diagnosis or within the first 4 weeks after the onset of corticosteroid therapy. Almost all patients with GCA-associated strokes have a significant acute phase response with elevated ESR and C-reactive protein (CRP). The mortality has been reported to be as high as 75%. The impact of cardiovascular risk factors on the occurrence of cerebral ischemic events has been evaluated in the Reggio Emilia region of Italy in patients with biopsy-proven TA. Both a history of hypertension or ischemic heart disease were associated with a higher risk of stroke (Berger et al., 2009).

Systemic symptoms includ fever, fatigue, malaise, weight loss, and/or polymyalgia rheumatica. Polymyalgia rheumatica (PMR) is a disease characterized by severe bilateral pain and aching involving the neck, shoulder, and pelvic girdles associated with morning stiffness. PMR is more common than GCA, and it may present as an isolated entity, or may be the presenting feature in patients who later develop typical cranial manifestations of GCA (Salvarani et al., 2008). Population-based studies have shown the presence of "silent" biopsy-proven GCA in 9–21% of the patients presenting with PMR features. Also, PMR manifestations are observed in up to 40–50% of patients with biopsy-proven GCA. The nephritic syndrome has been reported in patients with GCA in the setting of focal segmental glomerulonephritis, membranous glomerulonephritis, amyloidosis, and necrotizing glomerulonephritis.

Ocular ischemic complications are the major source of chronic disability among GCA patients. In some cases, the development of blindness may be preceded by episodes of amaurosis fugax. They are generally early manifestations due to the vasculitic involvement of retrobulbar (orbital) vessels deriving from the ophthalmic artery (OA). In unselected patients with biopsy-proven GCA, visual ischemic complications occur in 25% and irreversible visual loss occurs in 10–15% of the patients. There is a significantly increased frequency of severe visual ischemic complications (transient or permanent visual loss) in the group of biopsy-proven GCA patients compared with GCA patients with a negative TAB. These interesting observations are in agreement with two previous population-based studies that disclosed that biopsy-negative patients have less frequency of severe ischemic complications than those with biopsy-proven GCA. Ocular ischemic complications are generally due to arteritic anterior ischemic optic neuropathy (AAION). More rarely, visual loss is caused by central retinal artery occlusion (CRAO), or ischemic retrobulbar neuritis (Gonzales-Gay et al., 2000).

Arteritic anterior ischemic optic neuropathy (AAION) results from short posterior ciliary arteries (SPCA) vasculitis and the consecutive optic nerve head infarction. Human autopsy studies of acute arteritic AION demonstrate optic disc edema with ischemic necrosis of the prelaminar, laminar, and retrolaminar portions of the optic nerve and infiltration of the SPCA by chronic inflammatory cells. In some cases segments of these vessels have been occluded by inflammatory thickening and thrombus (Arnold, 2004).

Patients with an unilateral AAION present the following key features:

a. abrupt, painless, severe loss of vision of the affected eye.
b. anterior segment examination of both eyes is normal.
c. the ophthalmoscopy of the affected eye reveales diffuse pale optic disc edema, but within 1-2 months, the swelling gradualy resolves and the entire optic disc will become atrophic. **(fig.2)**

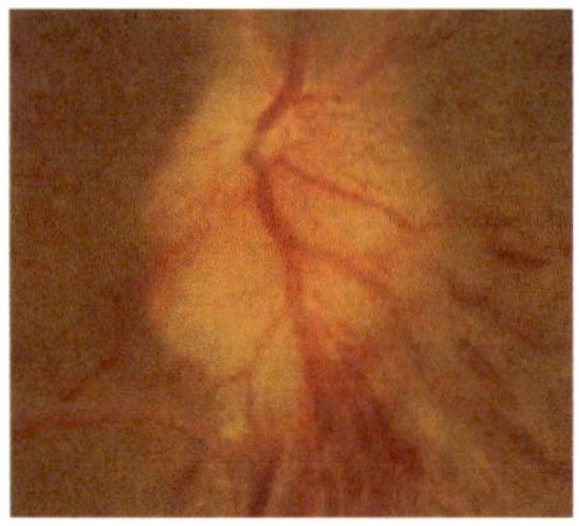

Fig. 2. Pacient TL-Fundus view of the left eye. Arteritic AION. The optic disc demonstrates pale, diffuse edema.

Typically, in AAION the severe visual loss is preceeded by transient visual loss similar to that of carotid artery disease. This symptom is unusual in the nonarteritic form of AION. The ophthalmoscopy indicates that pallor is associated with the edema of the optic disc more frequently in the arteritic than in the non arteritic form of AION. Although simultaneous bilateral involvement is rare in the arteritic form of AION, about 65% of untreated patients become blind in both eyes within a few weeks. The optic disc of the fellow eye is of normal diameter, with a normal physiological cup (absence of „disk at risk", with postulated structural crowding of the axons at the level of the cribriform plate, associating mild disc elevation, and disc margin blurring without overt edema).

Central Retinal Artery Occlusion (CRAO) is the result of an abrupt diminuation of blood flow in CRA, severe enough to cause ischemia of the inner retina. Due to the fact that there are no functional anastomoses between choroidal (posterior ciliary arteries) and retinal circulation (CRA), CRAO determines severe and permanent loss of vision. Therefore, it is very important to identify the cause of CRAO, in order to protect the contralateral eye. Frequently, the site of the blockage is within the optic nerve substance and for this reason, it is generally not visible on the ophthalmoscopy (Ahuja et al., 1999).

Patients with an unilateral CRAO present the following key features:

a. abrupt, painless, severe loss of vision of the affected eye.
b. anterior segment examination is normal in both eyes.
c. the fundus of the affected eye presents: **(fig 3)**
    - ischemic whitening of the retina.
    - cherry-red spot in the center of the retina.
    - the site of obstruction of CRA is not visible on ophthalmoscopy (no embolus is found).

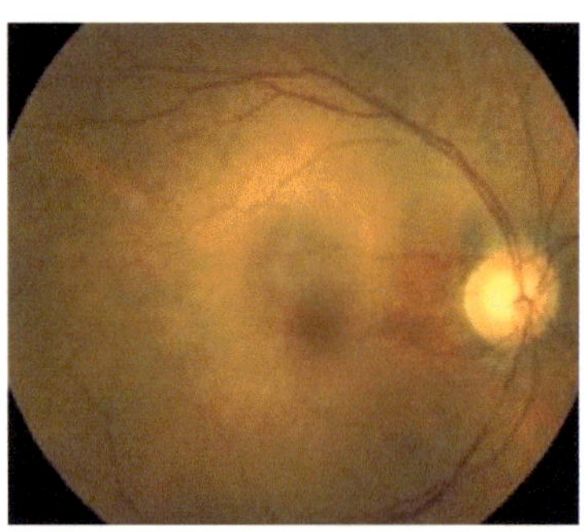

Fig. 3. Patient MM-Fundus view of the left eye. CRAO. A prominent cherry-red spot with cilio-retinal artery sparing in the papillomacular bundle.

In only 20-25% of cases are emboli visible in the CRA or one of its branches, suggesting that an embolic cause is not frequent in CRAO (embolic material from either the heart, the ascending aorta or the ipsilateral ICA). It is currently believed that the majority of CRAO's are caused by thrombus formation due to systemic diseases: haematological disorders, and last but not least, systemic vasculitis (including GCA). For this reason, all patients with CRAO should undergo a systemic evaluation (Duker, 2004).
In CRAO the retina appears white as a result of cloudy swelling. The „cherry-red spot" appearence in the center of the retina is due to the relatively intact choroidal circulation, in contrast to the ischemic retina. (Duker, 2004).

5.2 Laboratory findings

Laboratory findings reveal a raised Erythrocyte sedimentation rate (ESR) and increased values of C-reactive protein (CRP). ESR is often very high in GCA, with levels more than 60 mm/hr. In interpreting the ESR it should be emphasized that the levels of 40 mm/hr may be normal in the elderly and cases of biopsy- proven GCA have been reported in patients with ESR levels lower than 30 mm/hr. Approximately 20% of patients with GCA have a normal ESR. CRP is invariably raised in GCA and may be helpful when the ESR is equivocal (Lopez-Diaz, 2008). This acute phase response is induced by pro-inflammatory cytokines, mainly interleukins (IL) 1, 6 and tumor necrosis factor (TNF) alpha. These are produced by activated macrophages in the vessel wall. The target antigen of the CD4+ T cell immune response in GCA is probably located in the internal elastic layer of the vessel wall which explains that arteries of the anterior intracerebral circulation are infrequently affected because these lack an internal elastic layer (Weyand et al., 2003).
Several imaging modalities may be useful to make a diagnosis of GCA. In this regard, Pipitone et al., 2008performed an elegant review of the role of imaging studies in the diagnosis and follow-up of large vessel vasculitis (Pipitone et. al., 2008).

5.3 Extracranial Duplex sonography

Ultrasonography (US) of the temporal artery has raised great interest in the diagnosis of GCA. Extracranial Duplex sonography investigates almost completely the whole length of the common superficial temporal arteries, including the frontal and parietal branches, and founds that inflammation is segmental (discontinous arterial involvement). The common superficial temporal artery derives from the external carotid artery. It divides into the frontal and parietal ramus in front of the ear. The distal common superficial temporal artery and the rami are localized between the two layers of the temporal fascia, which is like a bright band at ultrasound examination (Schmidt, 2006).

Technical requirements

High-resolution color Doppler US can show the vessel wall and the lumen of the temporal arteries. One should use linear probes with a minimum gray scale frequency of 8 Mhz. Color frequency should be about 10 Mhz (Schmidt, 2006).

Machine adjustments

The pulse repetition frequency (PRF) should be about 2.5khz as maximum systolic velocities are rather high (20-100 cm/s). Steering of the color box and the Doppler beam should be maximal as the rami are paralel to the probe. It is important that the color covers the artery lumen exactly (Schmidt, 2006).

Sonographer training

The sonographer should perform at least 50 Duplex ultrasound of the temporal arteries of subjects without GCA to be sure about the appearance of normal temporal arteries before starting to evaluate patients with GCA (Schmidt, 2006).

Sequence of the Ultrasound examination

The investigation should start at the common superficial temporal artery using a longitudinal scan. The probe should then be moved along the course of the temporal artery to the parietal ramus. On the way back one should deliniate the temporal artery in transverse scans. Using the transverse scan, one can find the frontal ramus, which should then be delineated in both scans (longitudinal and transverse). If the color signals indicates localized aliasing and diastolic flow, one should use the pw-Doppler mode to confirm the presence of stenoses (Schmidt, 2006).

Schmidt et al., 1997 demonstrated that the most specific (almost 100% specificity) and sensitive (73% sensitivity) sign for GCA was a concentric hypoechogenic mural thickening, dubbed halo, which the authors interpreted as vessel wall edema. Other positive findings for GCA are the presence of occlusion and stenosis (Schmidt et al., 1997).

In conclusion, three findings are important for the ultrasound diagnosis of temporal arteritis:

a. *„dark halo" sign* – a typically hypoechoic, circumferential wall thickening around the lumen of an inflamed temporal artery - which represents vessel wall edema and a characteristic finding in temporal arteritis (TA)/GCA (Arida et al., 2010).
b. *stenoses* are documented by blood-flow velocities, which are more than twice the rate recorded in the area of stenosis compared with the area before the stenosis, with wave forms demonstrating turbulence and reduced velocities behind the area of stenosis. **(fig.4.A,B)**.

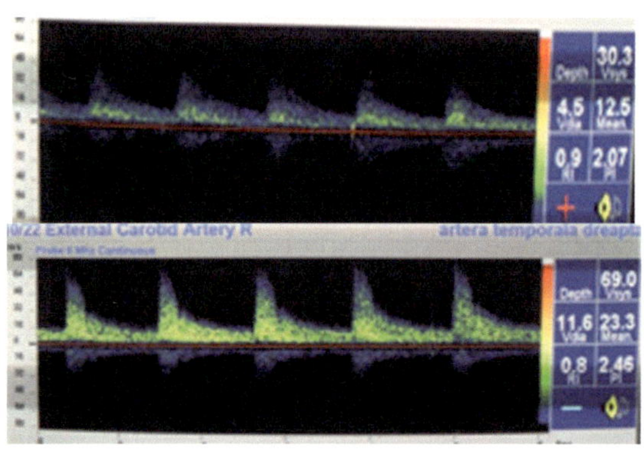

Fig. 4. Patient TL-Spectral analysis CW- 8Mhz -Extracranial Doppler ultrasound of the right temporal artery.

a. Peak flow velocity is 69 cm/s in the area of stenosis, and
b. 30.3 cm/s before the stenosis.
c. *acute occlusions*, in which the ultrasound image is similar to that of acute embolism in other vessels, showing hypoechoic material in the former artery lumen with absence of color signals (Schmidt et al., 1997).

Similar ultrasound patterns can be found in other arteries: the facial, the internal maxilary, the lingual, the distal subclavian, and axilary arteries. **(fig.5A,B.)**

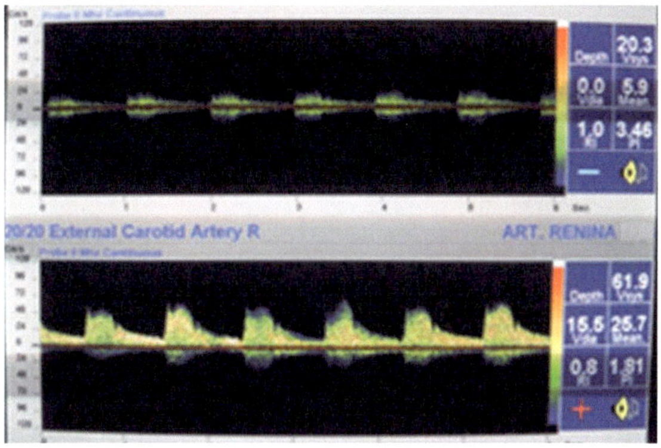

Fig. 5. Patient TL-Spectral analysis CW- 8Mhz -Extracranial Doppler ultrasound of the left lingual artery.

a. Peak flow velocity is 61.9 cm/s in the area of stenosis, and
b. 20.3 cm/s before the stenosis.

Interestingly in some cases the common carotid and the internal carotid arteries (the CCA and the ICA) are also involved (large-vessel giant cell arteritis).(**fig.6, fig.7**).

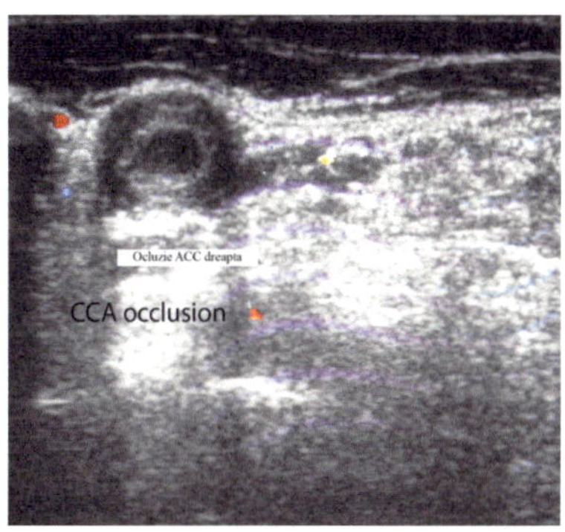

Fig. 6. Patient MM-B mode insonation in large vessel giant cell arteritis. Transverse view of the left CCA. Hypoechoic wall swelling with CCA occlusion.

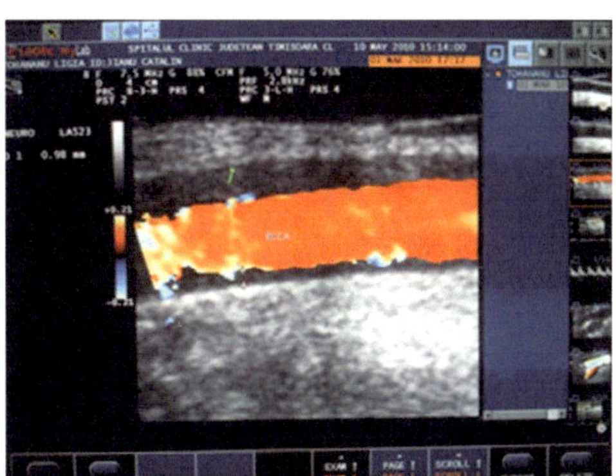

Fig. 7. Patient TL-Color Doppler ultrasound in large vessel giant cell arteritis. *Longitudinal view of the right CCA with hypoechoic wall swelling.*

Ultrasound investigation has to be performed before corticosteroid treatement, or within the first 7 days of treatment, because with corticosteroid therapy the „halo" revealed by temporal arteries ultrasound disappeares within 2-3 weeks. The wall swelling, stenoses, or occlusions of the larger arteries (CCA, ICA) remaines for months, despite the corticosteroid therapy. Nevertheless, diagnostic assessment should not delay the start of therapy. Ultrasound may also detect inflamed temporal arteries in patients with clinically normal temporal arteries. Some patients with the clinical image of polymyalgia rheumatica, but with occult temporal arteritis may be diagnosed by ultrasonography.

Arida et al., 2010 looked for studies that examined the sensitivity and specificity of the „halo" sign demonstrated by temporal artery US for GCA diagnosis versus the American College of Rheumatology (ACR) 1990 criteria for the classification of this vasculitis (used as a reference standard). Only 8 studies involving 575 patients, 204 of whom received the final diagnosis of GCA, fulfilled the technical quality criteria for US. This metaanalysis disclosed a sensitivity of 68% and a specificity of 91% for the unilateral „halo" sign, as well as 43% and 100%, respectively, for the bilateral „halo" sign in temporal artery US for GCA diagnosis when the 1990 ACR criteria are used as the reference standard. The authors confirmed that the halo sign in US is useful in diagnosing GCA (Arida et al., 2010).

Schmidt, 2006 compared the results of temporal artery US examinations with the occurrence of visual ischemic complications in patients with GCA. These US results were compared with the occurrence of AAION, CRAO, branch retinal artery occlusion, diplopia, or amaurosis fugax in 222 consecutive patients with newly diagnosed, active GCA. However, findings of temporal artery US did not correlate with eye complications (Schmidt, 2006).

5.4 Color Doppler Imaging (CDI) of retrobulbar vessels

We used a sonographer with 8-15 MHz linear probe for detecting (by Color Doppler sonography), and measuring (by spectral analysis pulsed Doppler sonography) the blood flow in the orbital vessels: the ophthalmic artery-OA; the central retinal artery-CRA and vein-CRV, posterior ciliary arteries-PCA, and the superior ophthalmic vein-SOV (Tranquart et al., 1997).

The patients with an *unilateral arteritic AAION* present at the Spectral Doppler analysis of the retrobulbar vessels the following aspects:

a. an increased resistance index (RI) in the posterior ciliary arteries (PCA) (the RI is higher on the affected side, than it is on the unaffected side); with severe diminished blood flow velocities (especially end-diastolic velocities) in the PCA. **(fig.8.A, B,C,D)**

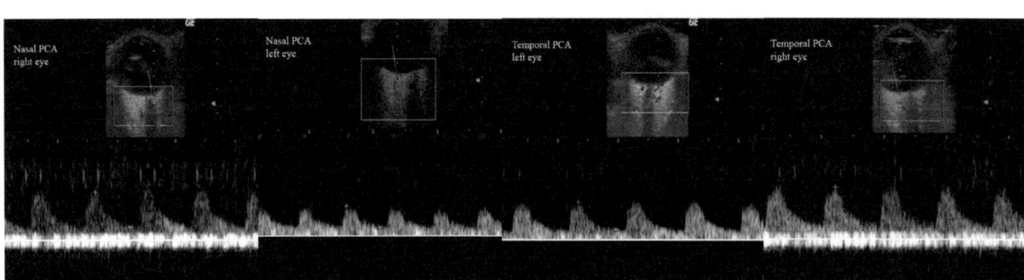

Fig. 8. A,B,C,D. Pacient TL-Spectral Doppler analysis of PCA.

b. less abnormalities are observed in the central retinal arteries (CRA) **(fig.9.A,B)** and in the ophthalmic arteries (OA). **(fig.10.A,B)**

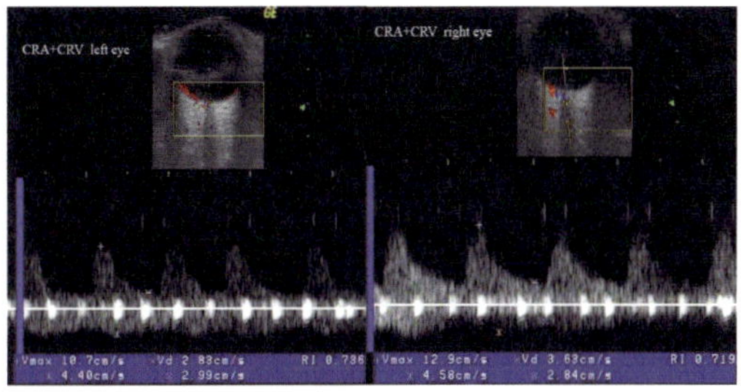

Fig. 9. A,B.Pacient TL-Spectral Doppler analysis of CRA.

In conclusion, the Spectral Doppler Analysis of the orbital vessels in arteritic AION reveales low blood velocities, especially end-diastolic velocities, and high RI in all retrobulbar vessels, in both orbits (with severe diminished blood flow velocities in the PCA, especially on the affected side). In nonarteritic AION blood velocities and RI in PCA are relatively preserved (Jianu D.&Jianu S., 2010).

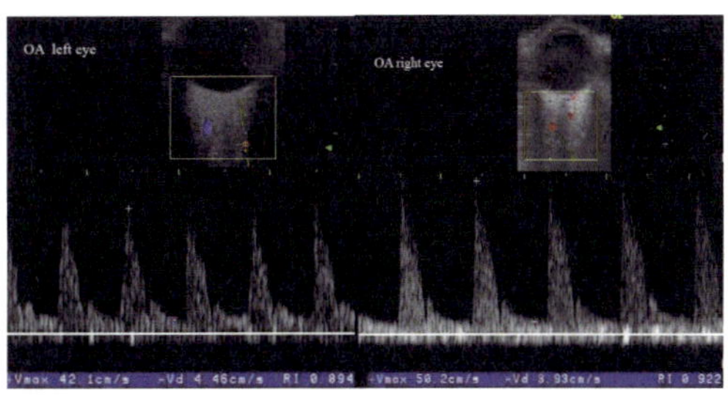

Fig. 10. A,B.Pacient TL-Spectral Doppler analysis of OA.

Fluorescein angiogram and CDI of retrobulbar vessels data support the histopatological evidence of involvement of the entire trunck of the SPCA in the arteritic AION (impaired optic disc and choroidal perfusion in the patients with arteritic AION). In contrast, in the nonarteritic AION, the impaired flow to the optic nerve head is distal to the SPCA themselves, possibly at the level of the paraoptic branches (only 1/3 of the flow of the SPCA) (Collignon-Robe et al., 2004). These branches supply the optic nerve head directly (impaired optic disc perfusion, with relatively conservation of the choroidal perfusion). **(fig.11)**

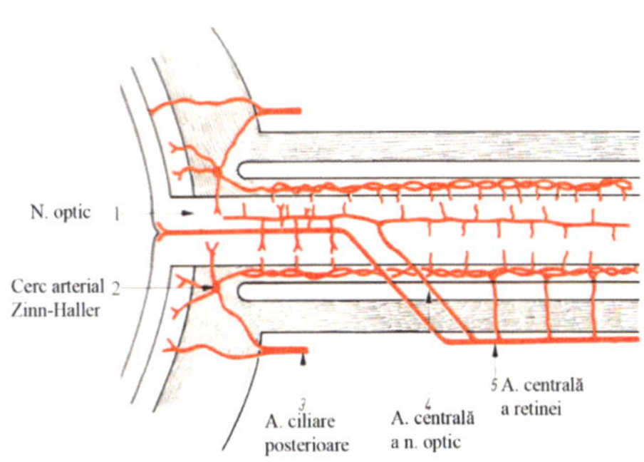

Fig. 11. Arterial vascularisation of the optic nerve.

Extremely delayed or absent filling of the choroid has been depicted as a fluorescein angiogram characteristic of arteritic AION and has been suggested as one useful factor by which arteritic AION can be differentiated from nonarteritic AION.

The patients with an *unilateral CRAO* present at the Spectral Doppler analysis of the retrobulbar vessels the following aspects (Connolly, 2000):

a. an increased resistance index (RI) in the central retinal arteries- CRA (the RI is higher on the affected side, than it is on the unaffected side); with severe diminished blood flow velocities (especially end-diastolic velocities) in the CRA. **(fig.12. A, B)**

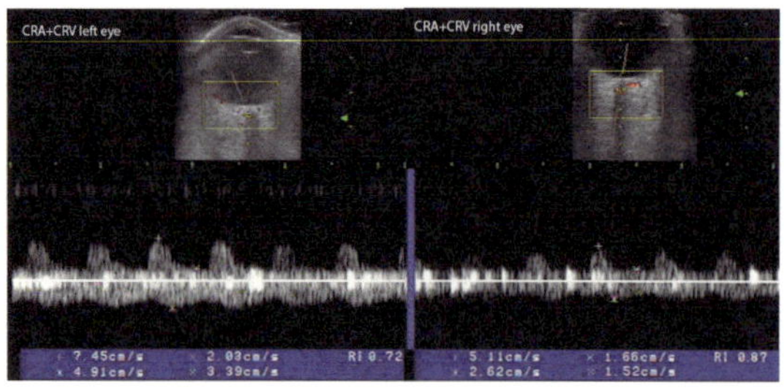

Fig. 12. A,B.Pacient MM-Spectral Doppler analysis of CRA.

b. less abnormalities are observed in the posterior ciliary arteries (PCA), **(fig.13.A,B)** and in the ophthalmic arteries (OA). **(fig.14.A,B)**

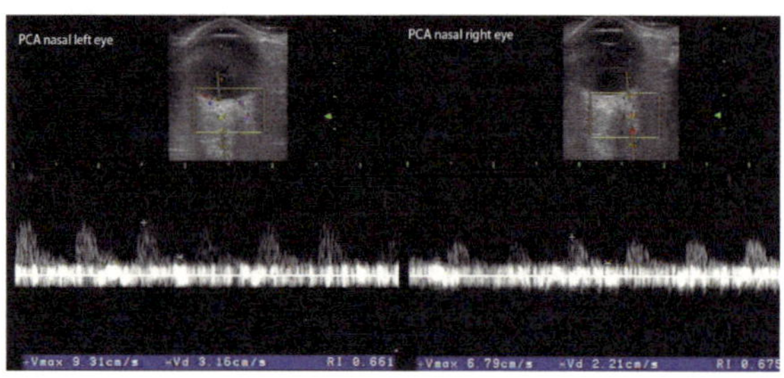

Fig. 13. A,B.Pacient MM-Spectral Doppler analysis of PCA.

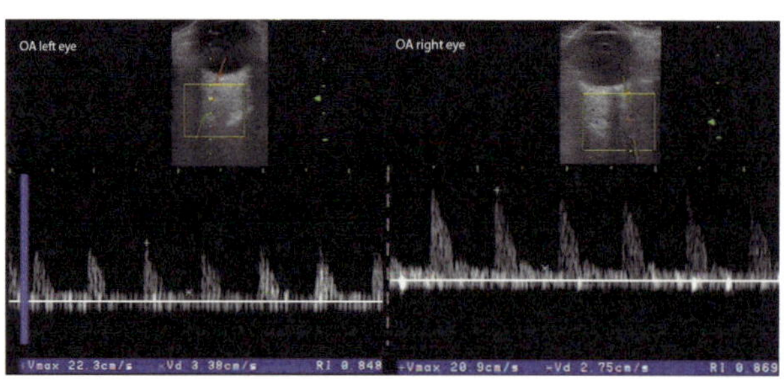

Fig. 14. A,B.Pacient MM-Spectral Doppler analysis of OA.

5.5 Others imaging techniques

Inflammation of the aorta and its branches may occur in a subset of GCA patients, although symptoms of aortic involvement may appear years after the initial diagnosis of this vasculitis (large giant cell arteritis). Therefore, as emphasized by Martinez-Valle et al., 2010 a systematic evaluation of patients with imaging techniques such as magnetic resonance angiography (MRA), computed tomographic angiography (CTA), or positron emission tomography (PET) may reveal that the clinical impact of extracranial involvement by GCA is more relevant than previously thought (Martinez-Valle et al., 2010).

Contrast-enhanced, high-resolution MR imaging allows noninvasive assessment of the mural inflammation. In this regard, Bley et al., 2008 compared the results of high-resolution MRI and color coded duplex US in 59 patients with suspected GCA with the final clinical diagnosis based on the ACR classification criteria for GCA (Bley et al., 2008). Thirty-six of the 59 patients (61%) were ultimately diagnosed as having GCA. Sensitivity of high resolution MRI and color-coded duplex US was 69% and 67%, respectively, while specificity was 91% in both. Temporal artery biopsy findings were positive in 24 of the 41 biopsied patients (59%). Sensitivity of high-resolution MRI and color-coded duplex US compared with temporal artery biopsy was 83% and 79%, respectively, and specificity was 71% and 59%, respectively. Therefore, differences between high-resolution MRI and color-coded duplex US were not significant. According to these observations, the diagnostic power of high-resolution MRI and color-coded duplex US in detecting GCA was comparable. These authors suggest that both noninvasive techniques may be useful in the assessment of patients with suspected GCA.

However, these results are in contrast to those of another study performed in patients with suspected GCA. Ghinoi et al., 2008 performed an interesting study to determine the usefulness of 1 T MRI of the temporal arteries and to compare 1 T MRI with duplex US and physical examination of temporal arteries in the diagnosis of GCA in a series of 20 patients with suspected GCA (Ghinoi et al., 2008). Mural contrast enhancement of the temporal arteries on MRI had a sensitivity of 33.3% and a specificity of 87.5% for the diagnosis of biopsy-proven GCA. Compared with the diagnosis of GCA by the ACR classification criteria, 1 T MRI of the temporal arteries had a sensitivity and specificity of 27.2% and 88.9%, respectively. Temporal artery abnormalities on physical examination and the presence of a hypoechoic halo on US had a higher sensitivity (66.7% and 77.7%, respectively) and a higher specificity. According to these observations, 1 T MRI does not seem useful in the diagnosis of GCA due to its low sensitivity.

Computed tomodensitometric scan allows analysis of the arterial wall and endoluminal part of the aorta and its branches. **(fig.15)**

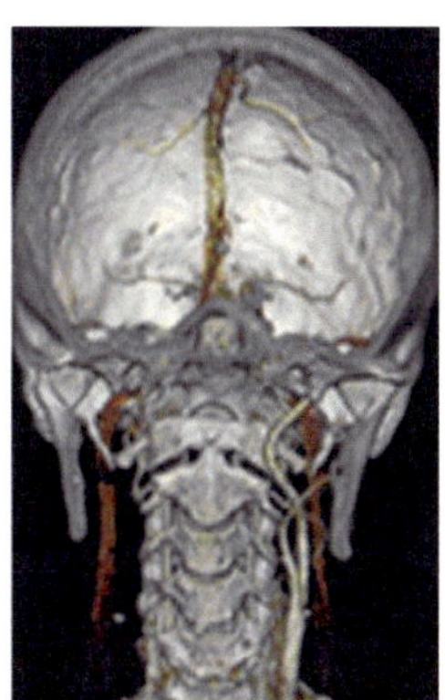

Fig. 15. Patient MM with large giant cell arteritis-CT-Angiography. *Occlusion of the left CCA, ECA, and ICA.*

Because aortitis is a complication of GCA, Agard et al., 2008 conducted a study in a series of 22 patients and 22 controls using computed tomodensitometric scan to assess the presence of aortic abnormalities in patients with recent onset GCA. Thickening of the aortic wall was more frequent among patients with GCA than controls (Agard et al., 2008).

18 Fluorodeoxyglucose (FDG)-PET may be useful to detect large vessel arteritis in the setting of GCA, which can involve the larger thoracic, abdominal, and peripheral arteries. It may be particularly useful in the diagnosis of GCA patients with atypical presentations such as fever of unknown origin or those presenting with asthenia, anorexia, and weight loss without cranial ischemic manifestations. Also, as emphasized by Pipitone et al., 2008 previous reports showed that PET may be more sensitive than MRI in detecting vessel inflammation in the early stage of large giant cell arteritis (Pipitone et al., 2008). However, PET cannot detect inflammation in the temporal arteries; therefore, it is not adequate for the diagnosis of cranial GCA and cannot replace temporal artery biopsy. Moreover, relapses of GCA cannot be predicted by results of previous PET (Henes et al., 2008).

In conclusion, PET/CT seems useful in the diagnosis and re-evaluation of large vessel vasculitis. It allows the evaluation of disease activity and vessel morphology as well as the localization of the inflammatory process in the same session.

5.6 Temporal Artery Biopsy (TAB) and the histopathologic picture

A temporal artery biopsy (TAB) is the gold standard test for the diagnosis of GCA (Duhaut, Pinede, 1999). European League Against Rheumatism recommendations emphasize that TAB should be performed whenever a diagnosis of GCA is suspected. Because corticosteroid therapy is required in most cases for more than 1 year in GCA, the pathologic confirmation of this vasculitis is advisable. However, GCA affects vessels focally and segmentally, yielding areas of inflammatory vasculitic lesions juxtaposed with areas of normal artery. Histologic signs of inflammation may be missed in TABs performed in arteritis-free segments (Foroozan, 2003). Because of segmental (discontinous) involvement of temporal arteries, a biopsy result may be negative in 9-44% of patients with clinical positive signs of temporal arteritis; for this reason the temporal arteries biopsy has to be guided by Doppler Ultrasonography and typical clinical features (tender, swollen portions of temporal arteries). Prior treatment with steroids for more than 7 days may be associated with loss of the histological features of active arteritis. As a consequence, the ultrasound investigations and temporal arteries biopsy has to be performed before corticosteroid treatment. Interestingly, 2 population-based studies have shown that patients with negative biopsy samples have less frequency of severe ischemic complications than those with biopsy-proven GCA (Breuer, 2009).

Taylor-Gjevre et al., 2005 noted that a threshold length of 1.0 cm of postformalin fixed arterial segment was associated with an increased diagnostic yield of GCA (Taylor-Gjevre et al., 2005). They recommended collecting a minimum TAB length of 1.5 cm to allow for tissue shrinkage during fixation that was estimated to be about 10%. More recently, Mahr et al., 2006 reported that a postformalin fixed TAB length of at least 0.5 cm could be sufficient to make a histologic diagnosis of GCA (Mahr et al., 2006). TAB is generally performed on the most symptomatic side. Breuer et al., 2009 performed a study to establish the relationship between TAB length and the diagnostic sensitivity for GCA (Breuer et al., 2009). In this study, the TAB in the subgroup of biopsy-positive GCA patients was significantly longer than in biopsy-negative GCA cases. The rate of positive biopsies was only 19% with TAB length of 5 mm or less but increased to 71-79% with TAB lengths of 6-20 mm, and to 89%

when TAB length was longer than 20 mm. Only 3% of positive biopsies were 5 mm or shorter. These authors concluded that TABs with postfixation length shorter than 5 mm yield an increased biopsy negative rate. As a result, the authors supported the claim that a TAB length longer than 5 mm is required for accurate diagnosis of GCA.

In the presence of unilateral ocular involvement, we took a biopsy from the ipsilateral side representing 2.5 cm of the tender, swollen segments of the affected artery („skip lesions"). Serial sections were examined, as there could be variations in the extent of involvement along the length of the artery (Gonzales-Gay et al., 2001).

However, due to the segmental inflammatory involvement of the temporal artery, a contralateral biopsy may be required in patients with high clinical suspicion of GCA. Breuer et al., 2009 found that performing bilateral TABs increases the diagnostic sensitivity of the procedure by up to 12.7% compared with unilateral biopsies (Breuer et al., 2009).

The definitive diagnosis of GCA requires the pathologic demonstration of a vasculitis with mononucleated cell infiltrates of all mural layers and occurrence of giant cells on a temporal artery biopsy. The degree of intimal hyperplasia on histology findings is associated with neuroophthalmic complications (Makkuni et al., 2008); the presence of giant cells in particular is associated with permanent visual loss (Chatelain et al., 2009).

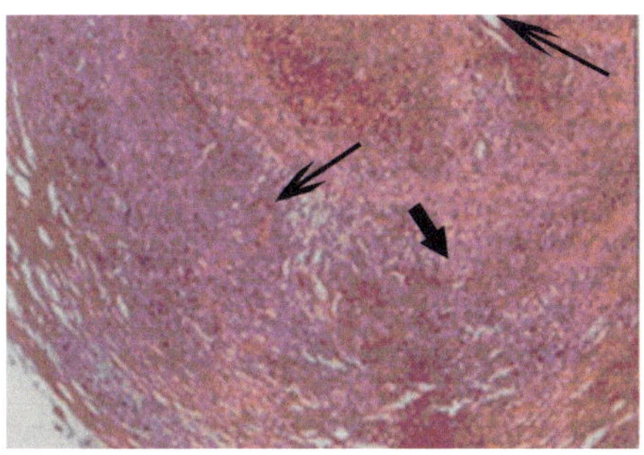

Fig. 16. Typical temporal arteritis **Patient TL.** Higher magnification showing the typical giant cell granulomatous inflammation.

Patient TL. Higher magnification showing the typical giant cell granulomatous inflammation.

In our cases we observed a granulomatous inflammation of the media layer (chronic inflammatory infiltrate with giant cells), with characteristic fragmentation of the internal limiting lamina and intimal thickening. **(fig. 16)**

6. Treatment and evolution

High-dose corticosteroids are the only effective therapy in GCA. Corticosteroid treatment must not be delayed by temporal artery biopsy, because the biopsy is positive even after a few days of steroid treatment. The initial dose of prednisone or its equivalent ranges between 40 and 60 mg/d, as a single or divided dose, for 3-4 weeks .

In our experience, GCA patients without severe ischemic complications have rapid disease improvement with an initial prednisone dose of 40 mg/d. In these patients, the use of corticosteroids has dramatically reduced the frequency of severe visual ischemic complications.

However, in GCA patients who present with visual ischemic manifestations we use higher corticosteroid doses—generally an initial intravenous methyl prednisolone pulse therapy (1 g/d for 3 consecutive days), followed by oral prednisone 60 mg daily for 3-4 weeks.
To assess whether corticosteroid therapy should be given every other day or as a single or divided daily dose, Hunder et al., 1975 carried out a prospective, randomized study to compare oral prednisone treatment in a divided dose t.i.d. (15 mg/ 8 h) with a single daily dose of prednisone (45 mg) and prednisone every other morning (90 mg) (Hunder et al., 1975). After 1 month of treatment, they found a trend toward better disease control in the divided dose group compared with the single daily dose group, but no differences in the side effect profile between the two groups. However, in only 6 of the 20 patients receiving prednisone every other morning was the disease completely suppressed. These results support the need to start treatment with daily prednisone therapy in patients with GCA.
A study compared an initial high-dose pulse of IV methylprednisolone versus classic corticosteroid therapy. The authors performed a double-blind, placebo controlled, randomized, prospective clinical trial: a 3-day course of IV methyl prednisolone pulses (15 mg/kg of ideal body weight/d) in addition to the oral prednisone (n=14) compared with normal IV saline infusions plus oral prednisone (n=13). The initial IV pulse of methylprednisolone therapy yielded more rapid corticosteroid tapering, lower median dose at each visit, and fewer relapses. However, further studies including larger numbers of patients are required to establish the routine use of IV pulse methylprednisolone as the initial corticosteroid therapy for the management of GCA (Mazlumzadeh et al., 2006).
Data show that it is not the absolute dose but rather the time from the onset of symptoms to the first administration of corticosteroids that is predictive of improvement of visual loss. Regrettably, in most cases, once established, the prognosis for significant visual recovery in GCA patients despite corticosteroid therapy is poor. Gonzalez-Gay et al. 2000 assessed the outcome of 29 GCA patients who developed loss of vision shortly before their admission to the hospital (Gonzalez-Gay et al. 2000). Only 8 patients (28%) experienced visual improvement—generally partial—following corticosteroid therapy. The main factor influencing the response to corticosteroids was therapeutic delay. Interestingly, 7 of 12 patients treated within the first 24 h after the onset of visual loss experienced visual improvement. However, when corticosteroid therapy was delayed for more than 1 day, only 1 of the remaining 17 patients experienced some visual recovery. These observations indicate that corticosteroid therapy should not be delayed under any circumstances in GCA patients with suspected visual impairment.
In conclusion the aim of the treatment in patients with GCA with eye involvement is to prevent blindness of the fellow eye, although in a few unfortunate patients with initial unilateral visual loss, the second eye also became blind inspite of prompt steroid administration (Gonzales-Gay et al., 1998). Most GCA symptoms other than blindness (headache, etc) usually begin to improve within 24-72 h after the onset of corticosteroid therapy. Also, normalization of routine laboratory parameters of inflammation (ESR and CRP) occurs within 2-4 weeks after initiation of this therapy. Afterward, the corticosteroid dose can be tapered gradually. However, the duration of corticosteroid therapy is variable, and relapses often occur. Whenever symptoms or acute phase proteins recur during tapering, the last effective dose plus 10 mg should be administered Prednisone is generally reduced by 5 mg every 2-4 weeks down to 25 mg. Then it can be reduced by 2.5 mg every 2-4 weeks until the dose is 10 mg, and later by about 2.5 mg every 2 months. Prednisone tapering is then performed more slowly (Gonzales-Gay et al., 2005).

The duration of treatment (1-2 years) is guided by the patient's symptoms and the levels of the ESR and CRP. In some cases from the literature, symptoms may however recur without a corresponding increase in ESR or CRP or vice versa, requiring indefinite maintenance therapy (Gonzales-Gay et al., 2005).
Up to 80% of patients with GCA experience complications related to steroid therapy. These include diabetes mellitus, osteoporosis with vertebral compression fractures and Cushing syndrome. It is advisable to consider the use of bone protection therapy in patients with GCA (Gonzales-Gay et al., 2005).
In this regard, *alternative corticosteroid-sparing drugs – in particular methotrexate* (MTX) – should be considered in GCA patients with severe corticosteroid-related side effects and/or in patients who require prolonged corticosteroid therapy due to relapses of the disease. With respect to this, to reevaluate the efficacy and safety of adjunctive low-dose MTX in GCA patients, Mahr et al., 2006 performed an individual patient data meta-analysis of three randomized, placebo-controlled trials in patients with newly diagnosed GCA (Mahr et al., 2006). However, the authors found a modest role of MTX (10–15 mg/ wk) in reducing relapse rate and decreasing the cumulative corticosteroid therapy.
In small trials, *anti-tumor necrosis factor-α therapy (infliximab and etanercept)* have been evaluated in patients with GCA and toxicity secondary to steroid therapy. No clear benefit of anti-tumor necrosis factor-α therapy in patients with GCA has been reported. Moreover, the limited number of patients on tumor necrosis factor-α blocker agents included in these studies does not allow us to draw definitive conclusions about tthese drugs (Gonzales-Gay et al., 2005).
It is known that the presence of traditional atherosclerosis risk factors at the time of diagnosis of GCA influences the development of severe ischemic manifestations in patients with this type of vasculitis. Interestingly, two retrospective studies suggested that *antiplatelet and/or anticoagulant therapy* may reduce ischemic complications in patients with GCA (Nesser et al., 2004). Therefore, antiplatelet therapy started before GCA diagnosis may reduce the risk of severe ischemic events in patients with GCA. Thus, aspirin (75–125 mg/d) should be prescribed in patients with GCA. However, no positive impact of antiaggregation therapy on the risk of severe ischemic complications has been confirmed in more recent studies (Lee et al., 2006).

7. Conclusions

GCA is a common disease among older adults from Western countries. Higher physician awareness may have been responsible for the progressive increase in the incidence of these conditions observed in different parts of the world. Diagnostic criteria of GCA are represented by age 50 years or more, new develop headache, tenderness of the superficial temporal artery, elevated ESR, at least 50 mm/h, and giant cell arteritis in a biopsy specimen from the temporal artery. Large vessel giant cell arteritis is a subgroup of GCA occuring also at the level of the aorta and its branches (especially of the subclavian, the axillary arteries, etc.).
The eye involvement in Horton's disease consists in anterior ischemic optic neuropaty or central retinal artery occlusion with abrupt, painless, and severe loss of vision of the involved eye.
The superficial temporal artery biopsy is the gold standard test for the diagnosis of this vasculitis. Several imaging modalities, particularly US, are useful in making a diagnosis of

GCA („dark halo" sign). However, findings of temporal artery US did not correlate with eye complications. For this reason, Color Doppler Imaging of the retrobulbar vessels may be helpful to detect the blood flow in the orbital vessels, especially in cases of opacity of the medium, or when the clinical appearance of ophthalmologic complications in temporal arteritis is athypical. The Spectral Doppler Analysis of the orbital vessels in GCA reveales low blood velocities, especially end-diastolic velocities, and high resistance index in all retrobulbar vessels, in both orbits, for all patients (especially on the affected side).
Corticosteroids are the cornerstone of treatment in GCA. Alternative corticosteroid- sparing drugs, in particular MTX, should be considered in GCA patients with severe corticosteroid-related side effects and/or in patients who require prolonged corticosteroid therapy due to relapses of the disease.
Key words: Giant cell arteritis, temporal headache, superficial temporal artery biopsy, "dark halo" sign, central retinal artery obstruction, arteritic anterior ischaemic optic neuropathy.

8. References

Agard C, Barrier JH, Dupas B, et al. (2008): Aortic involvement in recent-onset giant cell (temporal) arteritis: a case-control prospective study using helical aortic computed tomodensitometric scan. *Arthritis Rheum* 2008, 59:670–676.

Ahuja R.M., Chaturvedi S., Elliot A., et al. (1999) – Mechanism of retinal arterial occlusive disease in African, American and Caucasian patients, *Stroke* 1999 Aug; 30(8): 479-84.

Arida A, Kyprianou M, Kanakis M, Sfikakis PP (2010): The diagnostic value of ultrasonography-derived edema of the temporal artery wall in giant cell arteritis: a second meta-analysis. *BMC Musculoskelet Disord* 2010, 11:44.

Arnold A.C. (2004) - Chapter 191 - Ischemic optic neuropathy, in *Ianoff M., Duker J.S.*, ed., Ophtalmology, second edition, Mosby, 2004:1268-1272.

Berger CT, Wolbers M, Meyer P, et al.(2009): High incidence of severe ischaemic complications in patients with giant cell arteritis irrespective of platelet count and size, and platelet inhibition. *Rheumatology* (Oxford) 2009, 48:258–261.

Bley TA, Reinhard M, Hauenstein C, et al.(2008): Comparison of duplex sonography and high-resolution magnetic resonance imaging in the diagnosis of giant cell (temporal) arteritis. *Arthritis Rheum* 2008, 58:2574–2578.

Breuer GS, Nesher R, Nesher G (2009): Effect of biopsy length on the rate of positive temporal artery biopsies. *Clin Exp Rheumatol* 2009, 27(Suppl 52):S10–S13.

Collignon-Robe N.J., Feke G.T., Rizzo J.F. (2004) - Optic nerve head circulation in nonarteritic anterior ischemic optic neuropathy and optic neuritis, *Ophthalmol.* 2004; 111: 1663-72.

Connolly B.P., Krishnan A., Shah G.K., Whelan J., Brown G.C., Eagle R.C. Jr., Shakin E.P. (2000) – Characteristics of patients presenting with central retinal artery occlusion with and without giant cell arteritis, *Can. J. Ophthalmol.* 2000 Dec; 35(7):379-84.

Duhaut P, Bosshard S, Calvet A, Pinede L, Demolombe-Rague S, Dumontet C, et al (1999), for the Groupe de Recherche sur l'Arterite a` Cellules Geantes. Giant cell arteritis, polymyalgia rheumatica, and viral hypotheses: a multicenter, prospective case-control study. *J Rheumatol* 1999;26:361–9.

Duhaut P, Pinède L, Bornet H, et al.(1999): Biopsy proven and biopsy negative temporal arteritis: differences in clinical spectrum at the onset of the disease. Groupe de Recherche sur l'Artérite à Cellules Géantes. *Ann Rheum Dis* 1999, 58:335–341.

Duker J.S.(2004), - Chapter 114 - Retinal arterial obstruction, in Yanoff M., Duker J.S., ed., *Ophtalmology*, second edition, Mosby, 2004:856-63.

Foroozan R, Deramo VA, Buono LM, et al.(2003): Recovery of visual function in patients with biopsy-proven giant cell arteritis. *Ophthalmology* 2003, 110:539–542.

Gabriel SE, Espy M, Erdman DD, Bjornsson J, Smith TF, Hunder GG (1999). The role of parvovirus B19 in the pathogenesis of giant cell arteritis: a preliminary evaluation. *Arthritis Rheum* 1999;42:1255–8.

Ghanchi F.D., Williamson T.H., Lim C.S., Butt Z., Baxter G.M., McKillop G., O`Brien C.(1996) - Color Doppler imaging in giant cell (temporal) arteritis: serial examination and comparison with non-arteritic anterior ischaemic optic neuropathy, *Eye* 1996; 10(4):459-64.

Ghinoi A, Zuccoli G, Nicolini A, et al.(2008): 1 T magnetic resonance imaging in the diagnosis of giant cell arteritis: comparison with ultrasonography and physical examination of temporal arteries. *Clin Exp Rheumatol* 2008, 26(Suppl 49):S76–S80.

Gonzalez-Gay MA.(2001) Genetic epidemiology: giant cell arteritis and polymyalgia rheumatica. *Arthritis Res* 2001;3:154–7.

Gonzalez-Gay M.(2005) The diagnosis and management of patients with giant cell arteritis. *J Rheumatol* 2005;32:1186–8.

Gonzalez-Gay MA, Barros S, Lopez-Diaz MJ, Garcia-Porrua C, Sanchez-Andrade A, Llorca J. (2005) Giant cell arteritis: disease patterns of clinical presentation in a series of 240 patients. *Medicine* (Baltimore) 2005;84:269–76.

Gonzalez-Gay MA, Blanco R, Rodriguez-Valverde V, et al.(1998): Permanent visual loss and cerebrovascular accidents in giant cell arteritis: predictors and response to treatment. *Arthritis Rheum* 1998, 41:1497–1504.

Gonzalez-Gay MA, Garcia-Porrua C, Llorca J, et al.(2001): Biopsynegative giant cell arteritis: clinical spectrum and predictive factors for positive temporal artery biopsy. *Semin Arthritis Rheum* 2001, 30:249–256.

Gonzalez-Gay MA, Garcia-Porrua C, Llorca J, Gonzalez-Louzao C, Rodriguez-Ledo P. (2001) Biopsy-negative giant cell arteritis: clinical spectrum and predictive factors for positive temporal artery biopsy. *Semin Arthritis Rheum* 2001;30:249–56.

Gonzalez-Gay MA, Garcia-Porrua C, Llorca J, Hajeer AH, Branas F, Dababneh A, et al.(2000) Visual manifestations of giant cell arteritis: trends and clinical spectrum in 161 patients. *Medicine* (Baltimore) 2000;79:283–92

Gonzalez-Gay MA, Vazquez-Rodriguez TR, Lopez-Diaz MJ, et al.(2009): Epidemiology of giant cell arteritis and polymyalgia rheumatica *Arthritis Rheum* 2009, 61:1454–1461.

Henes JC, Müller M, Krieger J, et al.(2008): [18F] FDG-PET/CT as a new and sensitive imaging method for the diagnosis of large vessel vasculitis. *Clin Exp Rheumatol* 2008, 26(Suppl 49):S47–S52.

Hunder G.G., et al.(1990) - The American College of Reumatology 1990 criteria for the classification of giant cell arteritis, *Arteritis Rheum*. 1990; 33:1122-28.

Hunder GG, Sheps SG, Allen GL, Joyce JW (1975): Daily and alternate day corticosteroid regimens in treatment of giant cell arteritis: comparison in a prospective study. *Ann Intern Med* 1975, 82:613–618.

Jianu D.C., Jianu S.N.(2010) - Chapter 8 - Aportul CDI in studiul neuropatiilor optice, in Jianu D.C., Jianu S.N., ed., *Ecografia Doppler Color. Interferente oftalmo-neurologice*, Mirton, 2010:154-74

Lee MS, Smith SD, Galor A, Hoffman GS (2006): Antiplatelet and anticoagulant therapy in patients with giant cell arteritis. *Arthritis Rheum* 2006, 54:3306–3309.

Levine SM, Hellmann DB. (2002) Giant cell arteritis. *Curr Opin Rheumatol* 2002;14:3–10.

Lopez-Diaz MJ, Llorca J, Gonzalez-Juanatey C, et al.(2008): The erythrocyte sedimentation rate is associated with the development of visual complications in biopsy-proven giant cell arteritis. *Semin Arthritis Rheum* 2008, 38:116–123.

Mahr AD, Jover JA, Spiera RF, et al.(2007): Adjunctive methotrexate for treatment of giant cell arteritis: an individual patient data metaanalysis. *Arthritis Rheum* 2007, 56:2789–2797.

Mahr A, Saba M, Kambouchner M, et al.(2006): Temporal artery biopsy for diagnosing giant cell arteritis: the longer, the better? *Ann Rheum Dis* 2006, 65:826–828.

Martínez-Valle F, Solans-Laqué R, Bosch-Gil J, et al.(2010): Aortic involvement in giant cell arteritis. *Autoimmun Rev* 2010, 9:521–524.

Mazlumzadeh M, Hunder GG, Easley KA, et al.(2006): Treatment of giant cell arteritis using induction therapy with high-dose glucocorticoids: a double-blind, placebo-controlled, randomized prospective clinical trial. *Arthritis Rheum* 2006, 54:3310–3318.

Nesher G, Berkun Y, Mates M, et al.(2004): Low-dose aspirin and prevention of cranial ischemic complications in giant cell arteritis. *Arthritis Rheum* 2004, 50:1332–1337.

Pipitone N, Versari A, Salvarani C (2008): Role of imaging studies in the diagnosis and follow-up of large-vessel vasculitis: an update. *Rheumatology* (Oxford) 2008, 47:403–408.

Rodriguez-Pla A, Bosch-Gil JA, Echevarria-Mayo JE, Rossello-Urgell J, Solans-Laque R, Huguet-Redecilla P, et al. (2004) No detection of parvovirus B19 or herpesvirus DNA in giant cell arteritis. *J Clin Virol* 2004;31:11–5.

Salvarani C, Cantini F, Hunder GG (2008): Polymyalgia rheumatica and giant-cell arteritis. *Lancet* 2008, 372:234–245.

Salvarani C, Gabriel SE, O'Fallon WM, Hunder GG. (1995) The incidence of giant cell arteritis in Olmsted County, Minnesota: apparent fluctuations in a cyclic pattern. *Ann Intern Med* 1995;123:192–4.

Salvarani C, Macchioni P, Zizzi F, Mantovani W, Rossi F, Castri C, et al. (1991) Epidemiologic and immunogenetic aspects of polymyalgia rheumatica and giant cell arteritis in northern Italy. *Arthritis Rheum* 1991;34:351–6.

Schmidt W.A. (2006) Takayasu and temporal arteritis, in Baumgartner R.W. (ed.): Handbook on Neurovascular Ultrasound. *Front.Neurol.Neurosci.*Basel, Karger, 2006, 21:96-104.

Schmidt WA, Kraft HE, Vorpahl K, et al.(1997): Color duplex ultrasonography in the diagnosis of temporal arteritis. *N Engl J Med* 1997, 337:1336–1342.

Taylor-Gjevre R, Vo M, Shukla D, Resch L (2005): Temporal artery biopsy for giant cell arteritis. *J Rheumatol* 2005, 32:1279–1282.

Tranquart F., Aubert-Urena A.S., Arsene S., Audrierie C., Rossazza C., Pourcelot L. (1997) - Echo-Doppler couleur des arteres ciliaires posterieures dans la neuropathie optique ischemique anterieure aigue, *J.E.MU.* 1997; 18(1):6871.

Weyand CM, Goronzy JJ. (2003) Giant-cell arteritis and polymyalgia rheumatica. *Ann Intern Med* 2003;139:505–15.

Weyand CM, Tetzlaff N, Bjornsson J, Brack A, Younge B, Goronzy JJ. (1997) Disease patterns and tissue cytokine profiles in giant cell arteritis. *Arthritis Rheum* 1997;40:19–26.

17

Kawasaki Disease in a Tertiary Pediatric Referral Center in Athens, Greece and Review of the Literature

Chrysanthi L. Skevaki[1,2], Elpida Charalampaki[1], Georgia Pinna[1], Michail Pararas[2], Athanassios Tsakris[2] and Dimitrios A. Kafetzis[1]
[1]*P & A Kyriakou" Children's Hospital, Second Department of Pediatrics, University of Athens,*
[2]*Department of Microbiology, School of Medicine, University of Athens, Athens, Greece*

1. Introduction

Kawasaki disease (KD), an acute febrile mucotaneous lymph node syndrome, was initially described as a distinct clinical entity in 1967 by the Japanese physician, Dr Tomisaku Kawasaki (Kawasaki et al., 1974). Today the disease is recognized as an acute self - limited vasculitis of unknown etiology that predominantly affects young children of all racial and ethnic groups (Shulman et al., 1987). It is characterised by prolonged fever unresponsive to antibiotics, a polymorphous skin rash, erythema of the oral mucosa, lips and tongue, erythema of the palms and soles, bilateral conjunctival injection and cervical lymphadenopathy. This disease has become the leading cause of acquired heart disease among children in the developed world, with coronary artery aneurysms occurring in up to 25% of untreated cases (Newburger & Fulton, 2004).

2. Epidemiology

Approximately 85% of children with KD are aged less than five years, with a relatively higher incidence reported for boys (Chang, 2002). Patients either younger than three months or older than five years are scarcely encountered and are regarded to be at a higher cardiovascular risk (Burns et al.,1986; Stockheim et al., 2000). Occurrence beyond late childhood is extremely rare. Less than 100 cases of adult KD have actually been reported in the world literature since the recognition of this illness, according to a 2010 case series and review of the disease in adults (Gomard - Mennesson et al., 2010; Wolff et al., 2007). In fact, many of the reported cases in adults have been misdiagnosed as KD, while the correct diagnosis was toxic shock syndrome (Meissner & Leung 1995; Shulman et al., 1995).
The epidemiology of KD is best documented in Japan, where regular nationwide epidemiological surveys are being conducted every two years since 1970. Based on the recent 20th survey, the number of patients with KD are continuously increasing, with an average annual incidence rate in 2007 and 2008 that reached 217/ 100.000 children younger

than five years of age, while the same value was 184.6/100.000 for the years 2005 and 2006 (Nakamura et al., 2010, 2008).Over the past years, incidence figures have also been reported based on surveys upon hospital admission from Korea, Taiwan, the United States of America and the United Kingdom, enabling comparisons to be made. The highest incidence rate of KD per 100.000 children less than five years of age is recorded in Japan. Korea and Taiwan hold the second and third place respectively (Huang et al., 2009; Park et al., 2011). The United Kingdom and the United States are credited with a significantly lower annual incidence, which however, shows an increasing tendency over the past years (Harnden et al., 2002; Holman et al., 2010).

A study performed from 1996 through 2001, showed that the annual incidence rate for KD among children younger than five years of age was 45.2 in Hawaii, the highest figure in the United States (Holman et al., 2005). Interestingly, the study showed that Japanese children in Hawaii were more likely to develop Kawasaki disease than children of other races in the same state or even children living in Japan. It is thus suggested that the incidence rate is higher in children either living in East Asia or being of Asian ancestry and living in other parts of the world. The overall prevalence in the United States is the highest among Asian and Pacific Islanders, intermediate in non-Hispanic African-Americans and the lowest for Caucasians (Holman et al., 2010a, 2010b).

Other than the racial variations in the different geographical areas, a seasonal parameter in the distribution of KD cases also seems to exist. In most countries that hold records of KD occurrence, the greatest frequency is noted during winter months. In Japan, the disease shows a bimodal seasonality, that peaks once in January and secondly in June and July (Burns et al., 2005). Moreover, a bimodal pattern of occurrence is reported in Korea (Park et al., 2011). In Taiwan, recent studies have shown that KD is noted most frequently in the summer and least frequently in the winter (Huang et al., 2009). It is therefore noticed that although the period may not always be the same, seasonal clustering of the disease does take place. Such seasonality and temporal occurrence suggest that infectious agents or other environmental factors that are yet unknown, might trigger the onset of the disease.

The standardized mortality ratio associated with KD is 1,14 (Nakamura et al., 2008). There is a slightly increased mortality ratio in boys with the disease, which is mainly recorded during the acute phase and returns to baseline thereafter. This likely reflects the fact that cardiac and coronary artery abnormalities occur more frequently in boys than in girls and that most deaths related to KD are due to acute phase coronary disease or cardiac complications. In a study conducted in Japan, researchers have concluded that the mortality rate among males with cardiac lesions due to KD appeared to be higher than in the general population. Meanwhile, the mortality for girls with cardiac sequelae and for both male and female patients without sequelae, was not elevated (Nakamura et al., 2008).

In a retrospective study we conducted in "P & A Kyriakou" Children's Hospital, a tertiary pediatric referral center in Athens, Greece, we retrieved thirty-four cases of KD within a period of 16 years (1989-2005). The age upon diagnosis was between 2 months to 11 years (average: 2.9 years) and there was no significant gender preference (18 girls versus 16 boys). The duration of hospitalization varied from 5 to 29 days depending on the severity of associated symptoms. Thirty two children were Greek and 2 were of Albanian origin. In regards to seasonality, 58.8% of the cases occurred between November and March of any given year as depicted in figure 1.

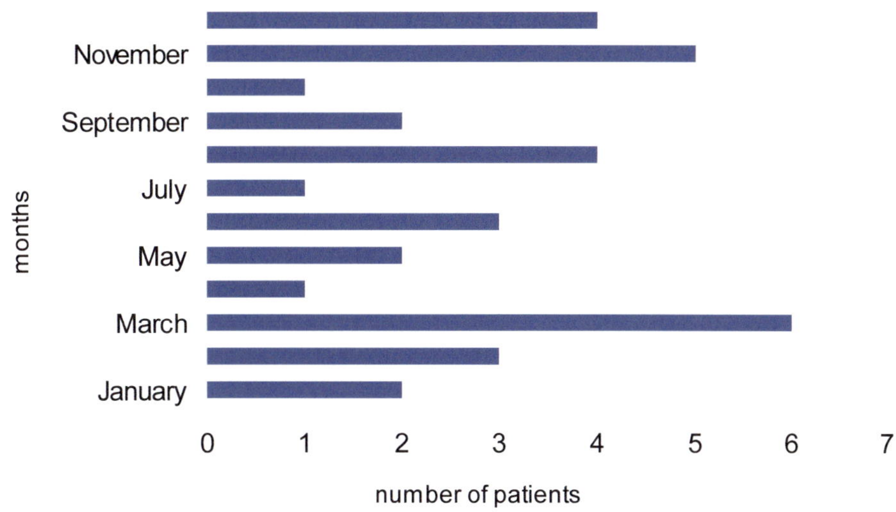

Fig. 1. Monthly distribution of the 34 cases hospitalized for Kawasaki disease in "P & A Kyriakou" Children's Hospital in Athens, Greece between the years 1989 and 2005

3. Aetiology

The cause of KD remains unknown. Most investigators suspect the existence of an infectious agent or the response to one or more pathogens to be responsible for the development of the disease. Evidence supporting this hypothesis includes the following:

a. Seasonal clustering of KD during the winter months in most geographical areas (Burns et al, 2005).
b. Geographical distribution of recorded periodic epidemics (Kao et al., 2008; Yanagawa et al., 1999).
c. The fact that the disease occurs most often among toddlers, with only rare cases of infants younger than three years of age, which suggests the involvement of transplacental antibodies. Maternal immunoglobulin G may offer some protection to young infants and this protection diminishes as levels of maternal antibodies decrease (Burns & Glode, 2004).
d. The 3-5 % of recurrency among cases in Japan, that may suggest either an aberrant immune response in this particular group of patients or the existence of more than one infectious agents responsible for the disease (Hirata et al., 2001).
e. The clinical presentation of the disease with fever, cervical lymphadenitis, exanthema and conjunctivitis that resembles other infectious diseases such as scarlet fever and toxic shock syndrome (TSS).

While the infectious agent hypothesis remains plausible, research on associating KD with a specific pathogen has been yet fruitless. A wide variety of microbiological and molecular methods have been employed in order to isolate pathogens from body fluidsand/or detect agent – specific nucleic acids retrospectively, however with,limited results (Kawasaki et al., 1974; Melish et al., 1976; Rowley et al., 1994). Although there have been numerous reports suggesting the involvement of infectious agents such as Parvovirus B19, Bocavirus, Cytomegalovirus or other viruses, *Propionibacterium acnes*, Rickettciae, and Yersiniae, none of these agents have been seen consistently isolated in children with KD (Catalano-Pons et al., 2007; Esper et al., 2005; Wang et al., 2004). Among the 34 cases of children hospitalized with KD in our study, some were examined for a variety of infectious agents as presented in table 1. Most of the children were tested negative for recent exposure to the tested infectious agents. Nevertheless, the small number of subjects tested and the lack of a control population precludes any definitive conclusions.

	Children tested	% IgM (+)	% IgM (-)	% IgG (+)	% IgG (-)
EBV	16	-	100	12,5	87,5
Parvo B19	10	-	100	30	70
CMV	14	-	100	21,4	78,6
Coxsackie - Virus	10	10	90	10	90
	1	-	100	10	90
	1	10	90	-	100
ECHO - Virus	13	23	77	-	-

Table 1. Microbiological findings among the 34 cases of Kawasaki disease identified in "P & A Kyriakou" Children's Hospital, Second Department of Pediatrics, University of Athens, Greece during the period 1989-2005

Due to the aforementioned clinical resemblance of KD with scarlet fever and TSS, it was suggested that superantigens, especially toxic shock syndrome toxin – 1 (TSST–1) and group A streptococcal exotoxins A, B and C (SPEA, SPEB, SPEC) may be involved in the pathogenesis of the disease (Table 2). This was strongly supported by a study that reported associated increase of IgM antibodies against TSST–1, streptococcal pyogenic exotoxin A and staphylococcal enterotoxin A (Matsubara & Fukaya, 2007). However, an earlier multicentre, prospective study detected no difference in the isolation of superantigen-producing bacteria between patients with the disease and febrile controls, thus complicating the matter further (Leung et al., 2002). On the other hand, bacterial toxins'-induced clonal expansion of T–cell receptors Vβ2 and Vβ8 is found among a subset of patients at the early stages of disease. This expansion seems to withdraw during the convalescent phase and may be responsible for the non specific T–cell activation that can lead to massive cytokine release and the development of KD (Abe et al.,1992; Brogan et al., 2008).

Another hypothesis for the etiology of KD involves the implication of an environmental cause, such as pesticides, chemicals, heavy metals, toxins and pollutants. However, poisoning with environmental agents does not usually manifest acutely and is the result of chronic exposure. Nonetheless, some studies correlate KD to recent exposure to freshly shampooed carpets, habitation near a body of stagnant water and the use of a humidifier (Rauch et al., 1991; Treadwell et al., 2002).

	Kawasaki disease	Scarlet fever	Toxic shock syndrome
Age at onset	<5 years of age	>4 years of age	90% girls reaching the menstrual age
Epidemic	+	+	-
Cause	unknown	A streptococcal pyrogenic exotoxin (SPE- A, B,C)	Staphylococcus enterotoxin (TSST-1)
Features of rash	Polymorphous rash	Diffuse erythema	Diffuse erythema
Conjunctival injection	+	_	+
Labial and oral hyperemia	Whole area	Localized to pharynx, soft palate	Whole area
Cervical lymphadenopathy	+	+	-
Strawberry tongue	+	+	+
Erythema of the palms and soles	+	+	+
Palmar desquamation	+	+	+
Recurrence	3 – 4 %	rare	30,00%
Shock or hypotension	_	_	+
Coronary arteriitis	+	_	_

Table 2. Comparison of clinical features of Kawasaki disease, Scarlet fever, and Toxic shock syndrome

Other researchers have found evidence of an oligoclonal antibody response, suggesting that the disease is elicited by a conventional antigen rather than a superantigen (Rowley et al., 2001).

The predilection of the disease for children either living in Asia or being of Asian ancestry as well as the relatively higher recurrence within families point towards a genetic predisposition for developing KD (Caquard et al., 2006; Uehara et al., 2003). In Japan, the relative risk of developing the disease among siblings is 10, and it reaches to 13 when referring to twins (Harada et al., 1986). Several studies have been conducted, trying to link susceptibility to KD or disease outcome to genetic polymorphisms (Ahn et al., 2003; Burns et al., 2005; Furuno et al., 2004; Sato et al., 2009). However, most of these studies have been carried out on single small cohorts of KD patients and findings were reported without validation in additional case-control studies. Other limitations include the small scale number of alleles examined, control and sample populations heterogeneity that complicates comparison and the existence of silent undiagnosed cases within the control group. As opposed to candidate gene studies, genome-wide studies, which search for disease causing mutations within the whole genome, seem very promising. One such recent study, has identified inositol 1,4,5-trisphosphate 3-kinase C (ITPK-C) gene as a susceptibility gene for KD (Onouchi et al., 2008). A functional single nucleotide polymorphism was recognized and associated with disease development but also with increased risk for the formation of coronary artery lesions. This polymorphism is shown to reduce splicing efficiency of ITPK-C mRNA. While ITPK-C is shown to act as a negative regulator of T-cell activation through the Ca^{2+}/nuclear factor of activated T-cells signal pathway, the reduced splicing efficiency may contribute to immune hyperreactivity and thus the pathogenesis of KD (Onouchi, 2010). Further research on the biological significance of ITPK-C in other immune or non-immune cells may lead to better understanding of the disease pathogenesis.

4. Pathology

The histological findings of KD are consistent with those of a systemic vasculitis affecting medium sized arteries and veins to a lesser extent, with inflammatory lesions in virtually every organ. With the exception of arterial lesions, inflammatory lesions heal without residual changes (Amano et al., 1980; Masuda et al., 1986). Our understanding of the histopathological findings in KD is restricted due to the scarcity of study material for reasons such as the low mortality rate and the difficulties encountered upon sampling medium sized arteries, especially coronary arteries.

After the encounter of a genetically predisposed individual with the unknown trigger, an activation of mononuclear cells and platelets occurs (Jennette, 2002). The two latter cell populations interact with the endothelium that expresses surface adhesion molecules leading to margination of circulating cells, especially large mononuclear cells, lymphocytes and IgA plasma cells (Brown et al., 2001;Rowley et al., 2001). Activated endothelial cells also secrete monocyte chemoattractant protein 1 (MCP-1), which further attracts monocytes and vascular endothelial cell growth factor (VEGF), which increases vessel permeability (Asano & Ogawa, 2000; Maeno et al., 1998; Yasukawa et al., 2002) . Afterwards, platelets adhere to the vascular wall, while inflammatory cells cross the endothelium, gather in the intima, and liberate proinflammatory molecules such as interleukins, tumor necrosis factor α (TNFα), and matrix metalloproteinases (MMP) (Eberhard et al., 1995; Gavin et al., 2003; Lin et al., 1992). Neutrophils release neutrophil elastase which destroys the internal elastic lamina and contributes to disruption of the extracellular matrix. Active inflammation is succeeded by progressive fibrosis and finally scar formation.

In the heart, perivasculitis and endarteritis of the three major coronary arteries are seen during the acute phase, followed by panvasculitis in the consequent two weeks period. Aneurysms, phlebitis, formation of intraluminal thrombi and potential pancarditis with lesions of the conduction system are also present during this phase of the disease. As the disease progresses, inflammation is replaced by granulation in the form of scarring, stenosis of major coronary arteries, fibrosis of the myocardium, coagulation necrosis, and endocardial fibroelastosis (Fujiwara & Hamashima, 1978).

Inflammatory changes of the lungs, spleen, lymph nodes and salivary glands remain for more than 61 days from the onset of the disease, while in other organs these changes resolve much earlier. A predilection of KD for duct systems such as the prostate, pancreas, bile ducts and salivary glands has also been documented. However, in contrast to the irreversible changes that may occur in the cardiovascular system, histological changes on other parts of the body seem to fully recover after the convalescent phase of the disease (Amano et al., 1980).

The histological findings in KD strongly resemble polyarteriitis nodosa, and even though fine differences between the two illnesses do exist, differential diagnosis can only be made clinically. Most importantly, KD manifests with lymphadenopathy, which is usually absent in patients with polyarteritis nodosa (Jennette, 2002).

5. Diagnosis & clinical features

Signs and symptoms of KD develop over the first ten days of the illness and then gradually disappear spontaneously in most patients. In 20–25 % of the cases the disease is complicated by coronary artery lesions that may remain silent and diagnosed only years later, after the occurrence of a myocardial infarction episode or sudden death (Burns et al., 1996; Kato et al., 1992). The disease may be separated in three phases according to its clinical presentation. The acute phase, which may last 7-14 days, the sub-acute phase from the 10th to the 24th day of the disease, and finally the convalescent phase, typically lasting 6-8 weeks. Diagnosis of the disease during the acute phase is of utmost significance, as treatment with high dose of intravenous immunoglobulin within the first 10 days of onset reduces the risk of coronary artery lesions (Newburger et al.,1986, 1991). However, diagnosis of the disease is quite challenging, first because it remains clinically silent for some time, and secondly because there is no specific diagnostic test available. Aside from key elements of the history and physical examination, as well as indications based on laboratory markers of inflammation, the disease is presently diagnosed by the use of a case definition created for epidemiological surveys in Japan. The diagnostic criteria for complete and incomplete KD are presented in Table 3 and Table 4 respectively.

a.	Fever lasting for at least 5 days
b.	Presence of 4 of the following 5 conditions: 1. Bilateral conjunctival injection 2. Changes of the mucous membranes of the upper respiratory tract: injected pharynx, injected or/and dry fissured lips, strawberry tongue 3. Polymorphous rash, primarily truncal. 4. Changes of the extremities such as peripheral edema, peripheral erythema, and periungual desquamation. 5. Cervical lymphadenopathy.
c.	Absence of any other reasonable explanation for the illness.

Table 3. Diagnostic criteria for complete Kawasaki disease

a.	Fever lasting for at least 5 days.
b.	At least 2 of the 5 clinical criteria for Kawasaki disease (Table 3: $B_{1\text{-}5}$).
c.	Absence of any other sensible explanation for the illness.
d.	Laboratory findings, consistent with severe systemic inflammation.

Table 4. Diagnostic criteria for incomplete/ atypical Kawasaki disease

Although according to the criteria diagnosis requires a minimum of 5 days of fever, many experts prefer to treat classic KD earlier than the 5th day. The reason is that the case definition of KD is of questionable value as a clinical tool (Stapp & Marshall, 2002; Witt et al.,1999). A broader definition of the disease would ensure identification of all patients who could benefit from intravenous immunoglobulin treatment. It is very common that the criteria for diagnosis of KD are not all present at the same time during the course of the illness (Newburger & Fulton, 2004). Patients with an inflammatory disorder that did not meet all the clinical criteria but with echocardiographic abnormalities of the coronary arteries have been identified. It should also been noted that 5 of the patients in Kawasaki' s original report of 50 patients did not fulfill the current criteria for the diagnosis of the disease (Burns, 2002).

The lack of a specific and sensitive diagnostic test remains a great obstacle in the identification of all patients with KD. Besides the possibility that the illness may be underdiagnosed, there is an almost equally high chance that the disease is overdiagnosed since clinicians use non specific laboratory markers of inflammation to support their diagnosis. Thus, differential diagnosis among diseases that require different treatment remains a challenge (Table 5).

- Scarlet fever
- Toxic shock syndrome (TSS)
- Staphylococcal scalded skin syndrome (SSSS)
- Measles and other febrile viral exanthems
- Drug reactions
- Steven - Johnson' s syndrome
- Juvenile rheumatoid arthritis

Table 5. Selected differential diagnosis of Kawasaki disease

Acknowledgement of the protective role that early administration of intravenous immunoglobulin may play in the disease has placed a significant burden on clinicians to consider diagnosis in patients with unexplained fever with rash. Certain features of KD that may potentially deceive physicians include sterile pyuria misdiagnosed as urinary tract infection, cerebrospinal fluid (CSF) pleiocytosis misdiagnosed as aseptic meningitis, rash that may resemble a viral or drug side-effect sign, and cervical lymphadenopathy that is often confused with bacterial adenitis (Dengler et al., 1998; Wu et al, 2005).

The clinical symptoms upon presentation of the disease for the 34 hospitalized cases identified in our hospital between the years 1989 and 2005, are shown in Table 6. The predominant symptom was -as expected - fever with an average duration of 7,8 days. Other symptoms in decreasing order of frequency were rash, desquamation, conjunctivitis, lymphadenitis, fissured lips, glossitis, edema of the extremities, gastrointestinal abnormalities and arthritis. Aneurysms were identified in only 5 cases, and while tachycardia was absent in all cases, a 1st degree AV block was noted in 1 child.

Laboratory indices at the time of entrance were suggestive of a generalized activation of the inflammatory system. Average white blood cell (WBC) count was 16.193 cells/μl, average erythrocyte sedimentation rate (ESR) was 74.7 mm, average level of C-reactive protein (CRP) was 120,2 mg/l and average platelet count was 45.700/μl. Liver transaminases (aspartate aminotransferase, AST and alanine aminotransferase, ALT) were elevated in only 3 of the children. Urine analysis revealed the existence of aseptic pyuria in a 76,5% of the patients. An immune workup was performed for 10 of the children and is shown in Table 7. Finally, level of a1 - antithrypsin was tested in 3 cases and was found to be elevated in all three of them.

Clinical symptoms	Number of patients	% of patients
1. fever	34	100
2. rash	33	97,1
3. desquamation	27	79,4
4. conjunctivitis	26	76,5
5. lymphadenitis	26	76,5
6. fissured lips	26	76,5
7. glossitis	14	41,2
8. edema of the extremities	11	32,4
9. aneurysms	5	14,7
10. gastrointestinal abnormalities	5	14,7
11. arrhythmia	1	2,9
12. arthritis	1	2,9

Table 6. Clinical presentation upon admission of the 34 cases of patients hospitalized for Kawasaki disease in "P & A Kyriakou" Children's Hospital in Athens, Greece between the years 1989 and 2005

	Number of patients with **normal titer**	Number of patients with **elevated titer**	Number of patients with **decreased titer**
IgG	3	3	4
IgM	3	7	-
IgA	6	4	-

Table 7. Immune workup of the ten patients that underwent the examination in "P & A Kyriakou" Children's Hospital in Athens, Greece between the years 1989 and 2005.

Even if the underlying cause remains unknown, there is an ever increasing need for the development of a unique diagnostic test that can help in identification of the disease. Although non specific markers of inflammation such as serum procalcitonin, interleukin-18 (IL-18), WBC count, ESR, and CRP are all found elevated in KD, no association to the severity of the illness has yet been established (Mitani et al., 2005; Nomura et al., 2004; Okada et al., 2004). Unfortunately, the diagnosis of the disease currently depends largely on increased clinical awareness.

6. Cardiovascular complications

Kawasaki disease has become the leading cause of acquired heart disease among children in the developed world, even surpassing the impact of rheumatic fever in this respect. Twenty to 25% of untreated patients with KD develop coronary artery aneurysms and myocardial infarction with an associated considerable morbidity and mortality (Taubert et al., 1994) . Other cardiovascular complications related with the disease include coronary artery stenosis, myocarditis, pericarditis with effusion and mitral valvulitis (Akagi et al.,1990; Dajani et al., 1993). Cardiac imaging is hence very important in the evaluation of patients with suspected KD. Echocardiography is both a sensitive and specific method to recognize coronary artery aneurysms in the acute and subacute phase of the disease (Yoshikawa et al., 1979). Serial ultrasound studies can provide evidence of aneurysm formation, they may help evaluate left ventricular function as well as detect possible existence of pericardial effusion (McMorrow Tuohy et al.,2001; Scott et al., 1999). Doppler echocardiography can assist in the identification of mitral valve regurgitation and is also advisable in the presence of a pansystolic murmur upon auscultation. Morphological assessment of coronary arteries is of high significance, as the prognosis of aneurysms in patients with KD depends on the size and shape of the aneurysm. These features are best evaluated with three-dimensional echocardiography (Miyashita et al., 2007). Coronary artery aneurysms are characterized as small if less than 5 mm in internal diameter, medium if 5-8 mm, or giant if larger than 8 mm (Dayani et al., 1993, 1994). Fusiform aneurysms with a diameter of less than 8 mm have the best outcome, while giant aneurysms more than 8 mm have the worst. The latter is attributed to the fact that giant coronary aneurysms are highly probable to cause ischemic heart disease (Kamiya et al., 1995; Tatara & Kusakawa, 1987). On the contrary, small and medium diameter aneurysms have been reported to regress in approximately 50% of the cases and progress to stenosis in another 20% of patients (Kato et al., 1996). However, the value of echocardiographic detection of thrombi and coronary artery stenosis is questionable. In a selection of patients with KD, a series of other tests are recommended, aiming at better visualization of the coronary arteries. These include angiography, intravascular ultrasound, transesophageal echocardiography, magnetic resonance imaging, magnetic resonance angiography and ultrafast computed tomography (Greil et al., 2002; Naiser et al., 2008; Newburger et al., 2004; Suzuki et al., 1996). Interestingly, coronary artery lesions following KD may remain silent until the patient becomes 30 or even 40 years old. Especially patients without pathological findings in their echocardiogram during the acute and subacute phases of the disease usually remain clinically asymptomatic for at least a decade. To this end, a pediatric history of illness resembling KD should be sought in young adults presenting with myocardial infarction or sudden death (Burns et al., 1996; Kato et al., 1992).

Suggested risk factors for coronary artery formation include fever that endures even after intravenous immunogobulin administration, elevated CRP, low hemoglobin, thrombocytopenia, hypoalbuminemia, hyponatremia, male sex and age under one year (Honkanen et al., 2003; Koren et al., 1986; Mori et al., 2002). A proposed stratification of patients according to the relative risk for developing myocardial ischemia is presented, in table 9 (Newburger et al.2004).

7. Treatment

7.1 Initial treatment

Coronary artery aneurysms develop in 20 - 25% of patients left untreated. During the acute phase, the primary objective is to ascertain the diagnosis of the disease, provide supportive

Risk level	Pharmacological therapy	Follow - up & diagnostic tests	Invasive tests
1 (no coronary artery changes at any stage of illness)	None beyond first 6–8 weeks	Cardiovascular risk assessment, counseling every 5 years	-
2 (transient coronary artery ectasia disappears within first 6–8 weeks)	None beyond first 6–8 weeks	Cardiovascular risk assessment, counseling every 3-5 years	-
3 (1 small-to-medium coronary artery aneurysm/ major coronary artery)	Low-dose aspirin (3–5 mg/kg aspirin/day), at least until aneurysm regression is documented	ECHO+ECG, cardiovascular risk assesment, counseling annually. Stress test/ evaluation of myocardial perfusion scan every 2 years	Angiography, if noninvasive test suggests ischemia
4 (1 large or giant coronary artery aneurysm, or multiple or complex aneurysms in the same coronary artery, without obstruction)	Long-term antiplatelet therapy and warfarin (target INR 2.0–2.5) or low-molecular-weight heparin (target: antifactor Xa level 0.5–1.0 U/ml) should be combined in giant aneurysms.	ECHO+ECG twice annually. Stress test /evaluation of myocardial perfusion annually.	First angiography at 6–12 months or sooner if clinically indicated; repeated angiography if noninvasive test, clinical, or laboratory findings suggest ischemia; elective repeat angiography under some circumstances
5 (coronary artery obstruction)	Long-term low-dose aspirin. Warfarin or low-molecular-weight heparin if giant aneurysm persists. Use of beta blockers to reduce myocardial O_2 consumption should also be considered	ECHO+ECG twice annually. Stress test /evaluation of myocardial perfusion annually.	Angiography recommended to address therapeutic options

Table 9. Risk stratification for Kawasaki disease (ECHO: echocardiography, EKG electrocardiogram, INR: International normalized ratio)

care whenever needed (fluid and electrolytes), aim to attenuate the inflammatory process and prevent the formation of coronary artery aneurysms. Echocardiographic identification of coronary artery aneurysms not only redirects primary treatment plan, but also contributes to establishing the diagnosis of KD when there is absence of symptoms other than fever. It is thus suggested to consider echocardiography in a child with high fever of unknown etiology lasting more than 5 days and concurrent signs of generalized inflammation.

Intravenous immunoglobulin G is the cornerstone of treatment for KD during the acute phase. Several studies have shown that intravenous immunoglobulin G administration early in the course of the disease (before the 10th day from fever onset) reduces total duration of clinical symptoms as well as the incidence of coronary artery aneurysms (Durongpisitkul et al., 1995; Furusho et al., 1984). It has been demonstrated that a single dose of 2 g/kg intravenous immunoglobulin G infused over 10–12 hours is more effective than multiple doses, and together with aspirin (Kato et al., 1996) now comprise the standard therapy in the USA, UK, Europe, Australia and many parts of Asia (Brogan et al., 2002). Although treatment should be instituted within the first ten days of illness, intravenous immunoglobulin G administration to children beyond the tenth day of illness is also recommended if they have either persistent fever without other explanation or aneurysms and ongoing systemic inflammation (Marasini et al., 1991; Newburger et al., 2004) . The molecular basis for the anti-inflammatory action of intravenous immunoglobulin G is a field of extended research. Several mechanisms have been proposed including induction of immune inhibitory receptors such as FcγIII on macrophages (Samuelsson et al., 2001), blocked interaction between endothelial and natural killer (NK) cells, necrosis-like changes in morphologic features of neutrophils (Sugita et al., 2005), accelerated apoptosis of circulating neutrophils (Tsujimoto et al, 2002) and down-regulation of genes expressed mainly by monocytes (Abe et al., 2005; Popper et al., 2007). Gamma globulin is a biological product manufactured from pooled donor plasma and adverse effects vary according to the product infused. Generally, adverse effects are considered mild, comprising of headache, myalgia, fever, chills, backache, chest pain, nausea, vomiting, as well as increased plasma viscosity. These effects are usually self-limited, rarely demanding cessation of therapy, although slowing down of the infusion may be required (Rosenfeld et al., 1995) Live virus vaccines should not be administered to patients for at least eleven months following treatment, due to reduced immunogenicity related to passive antibodies in the infused product.

Aspirin may also be administered in the acute phase of the disease in order to enhance the efficacy of intravenous immunoglobulin G. Currently, 80–100 mg/kg (divided in four doses) are administered in the acute inflammatory stage of the disease, while a single dose of 3–5 mg/kg is given when patients have been afebrile for 3-7 days. Aspirin may be continued indefinitely in children that have already developed coronary artery abnormalities,. Despite the fact that aspirin has an important anti-inflammatory effect at high doses and an anti-platelet action at low doses, it does not shorten the frequency of coronary artery aneurysm complications (Terai & Shulman, 1997). The latter, along with aspirin's adverse effects and the risk for developing Reye's syndrome raise an important question regarding the value of exposing children with KD to high doses of aspirin.

Corticosteroids are the golden standard in the treatment of other forms of vasculitis. Nevertheless, their use in children with KD is limited (Shulman, 2003) even though they are found to suppress markers of inflammation and decrease total fever duration (Nonaka et al., 1995; Okada et al., 2003).

If initial therapy during the acute stage is successful, the primary objective at the subacute phase is to diminish platelet adhesion (usually by means of low dose aspirin administration), provision of supportive care when needed and monitoring patients in case of cardiovascular involvement. In both the subacute and convalescent phase, management plans are adjusted to coronary artery involvement and risk level, individualized for each patient (Newburger et al., 2004).

For the 34 cases included in our study, treatment comprised primarily of intravenous immunoglobulin G and aspirin as shown on Table 10. Aspirin was administered to 31 patients (91,2 %) during an average treatment duration of 5,7 days. Among children treated with aspirin, 23 continued with an antiplatelet dose (74,2%) after fever regression and only 1 patient had to discontinue aspirin treatment due to related hepatotoxicity. Twenty eight patients were treated with γ-globulin (82,4%) with an average treatment duration of 1,9 days. Additional therapy consisted of penicillin in 2 children, carbamazepine that was later replaced by sorvitole in 1 child, clindamycin in 1 and finally a combination of ampicillin and netilmycin in another 1 of the children. In terms of patients' management, there was also a case admitted to the intensive care unit of the hospital due to sepsis and multiple organ failure.

Treatment with various doses of aspirin		
dosage	Number of patients treated with aspirin	% of patients treated with aspirin
5 mg/ kg	3	9,6
60 mg/ kg	3	9,6
80 mg/ kg	13	41,9
85 mg/ kg	1	3,2
100 mg/kg	11	35,5
Treatment with intravenous immunoglobulin G		
dosage	Number of patients treated with IVIG	% of patients treated with IVIG
1 g/ kg	2	3,6
2 g/ kg	19	67,9
400 mg/ kg/ 24 h	7	25

Table 10. Treatment of the patients hospitalized for Kawasaki disease in "P & A Kyriakou" Children's Hospital in Athens, Greece between the years 1989 and 2005

7.2 Treatment of persistent or recrudescent fever

About 10–15% of children with KD that are treated with high dose aspirin and 2 g/kg intravenous immunoglobulin G will not become afebrile (Burns et al., 1998). Fever that is not reduced 36 hours after the completion of the initial intravenous immunoglobulin G infusion is defined as persistent or recrudescent fever. This subgroup, consisting of unresponsive to intravenous immunoglobulin G patients, is proved to be at a higher risk for developing coronary artery aneurysms (Newburger, 2000). Unfortunately, no studies have yet proven the efficacy of a specific secondary treatment. Clinicians should first re-evaluate initial diagnosis and then move to selection of an appropriate secondary treatment. Most experts recommend re-treatment with intravenous immunoglobulin G, while plasmapheresis and treatment with corticosteroids, cyclophosphamide, methotrexate and monoclonal antibodies against TNF- α have also been suggested (Ahn &Kim, 2005; Al Mayouf, 2004; Mori et al., 1995; Weiss et al., 2004).

7.3 Treatment of cardiovascular complications

Treatment of coronary disease in patients with KD depends on the severity and extent of coronary involvement. Prevention of thrombosis and myointimal proliferation that leads to stenosis are the main objectives when managing patients with coronary aneurysms. Early coronary thrombosis occurs almost exclusively among patients with giant aneurysms (Takahashi, 1996). Unfortunately, no prospective data exist to guide clinicians towards the ideal plan; therefore, treatment of this subgroup of patients is still based on experts' recommendations. Prevention of thrombosis is accomplished by the administration of an antiplatelet or an anticoagulant agent, or most frequently by a combination of both.

Antiplatelet agents play a significant role in managing patients at every stage of the disease, since platelet activation is a fundamental component of thrombosis development in KD (Burns et al., 1984, Kuramochi et al., 2000). Therefore, low dose aspirin (3–5 mg/kg daily) is the backbone of therapy for asymptomatic patients with mild and stable disease. Use of other antiplatelet agents (such as clopidogrel or dipyridamole) alone or combined with aspirin, may be more effective in suppressing platelet activation with more advanced coronary abnormalities (O'Brien et al., 2000). Randomized trials are needed to establish the role of low molecular heparin, monoclonal antibodies against IIB/IIIA receptor and warfarin in the long term management of patients with giant aneurysms (Brogan et al., 2002; Williams et al., 2002).

In contrast to adult patients with aneurysms, the thrombus burden in children with KD is not related to the form of plaque instability and rupture (Kuramochi et al., 2000). Hence, randomized controlled trials involving children with coronary thrombosis are needed to set up the role of thrombolytic medication (traditionally used in adults) such as streptokinase, urokinase and tisue plasminogen activator.

Mechanical restoration of coronary blood flow is the other option in this group of patients that develop thrombosis. Coronary bypass grafting is the recommended surgical therapy upon evidence of reversible ischemia in stress imaging, if viable myocardium is present in the area of distribution of the affected vessel and when there is absence of coronary disease distal to the planned graft site (Kitamura et al., 1994). (Yoshikawa et al., 2000). Initially, the saphenous vein was used as the graft for this procedure; however, early failures in younger children led to the introduction of internal mammary arterial grafts (Kitamura et al., 1994). It was later found that patency rates of arterial grafts were higher as opposed to venal grafts. However, despite the encouraging results during the first decade after coronary artery bypass surgery, the arterial graft patency in later adult life is still unknown (Tsuda & Kitamura, 2004).

Catheter intervention (such as balloon angioplasty, stent implantation, rotational ablation and transluminal coronary revascularization) is indicated in the presence of ischemic symptoms, reversible ischemia on stress testing and at least 75% stenosis of the left anterior descending coronary artery. Although the use of percutaneous coronary rotational ablation is still limited, this procedure may be the most appropriate catheter intervention for patients with KD. The advantage is the high success rate even among patients with calcified coronary artery stenoses (Ishii et al., 2002; Sugimura et al., 1997), which renders this method a potential therapeutic option also for postponing coronary artery bypass surgery (Lee et al., 2005). Contraindications to catheter intervention include vessels with multiple, ostial, or long-segment lesions (Akagi, 2011; Ishii et al., 2001).

8. Conclusion

Kawasaki disease is a systemic vasculitis of early childhood and comprises one of the leading causes of acquired heart disease in the western world. Although great efforts have been made in order to improve our understanding of the cause, pathogenesis and natural history of the disease, many of these aspects remain vague. Physical examination, laboratory markers of inflammation, and a case definition created for epidemiological surveys in Japan are the main tools currently available for the diagnosis of KD. Treatment with intravenous immunoglobulin in association with aspirin early in the course of the disease shortens the duration of symptoms and decreases the frequency of coronary artery abnormalities.

During the period 1989–2005, 34 children with KD were admitted in our hospital. Analysis of different clinical manifestations and laboratory indices showed similar results to other studies. All children presented with fever, while the other most common symptoms were conjunctivitis, lymphadenitis, fissured lips and desquamation. Laboratory analyses were suggestive of non-specific inflammation. Patients responded well to treatment with aspirin and γ - globulin, and with the exception of one patient that was admitted to the intensive care unit, all other children did not develop any severe complications.

Therapy of intravenous immunoglobulin-resistant KD remains obscure. What is the main concern, is the extent to which it is going to influence adult cardiovascular disease. Long term management of patients with KD is therefore very important and evidence-based approaches are required in order to define the best medical practice. Further research is also essential in elucidating the cause of the disease and developing high sensitivity and specificity diagnostic tests.

9. References

Abe J, Jibiki T, Noma S, et al. Gene expression profiling of the effect of highdose intravenous Ig in patients with Kawasaki disease. *J Immunol* 2005; 174:5837–5845

Abe, J., Kotzin, B.L., Jujo, K. *et al.*: Selective expansion of T cells expressing T-cell receptor variable region V 2 and V 8 in Kawasaki disease. Proc Natl Acad Sci USA 1992; 89: 4066–4070.

Ahn SY, Jang GC, Shin JS, Shin KM, Kim DS. Tumor necrosis factor-alpha levels and promoter polymorphism in patients with Kawasaki disease in Korea. *Yonsei Med J.* 2003 Dec 30;44(6):1021-6.

Ahn SY, Kim DS. Treatment of intravenous immunoglobulin-resistant Kawasaki disease with methotrexate. *Scand J Rheumatol* 2005; 34:136–139.

Akagi T. Catheter interventions for kawasaki disease: current concepts and future directions. *Korean Circ J.* 2011 Feb;41(2):53-7. Epub 2011 Feb 28.

Akagi T, Kato H, Inoue O, Sato N, Imamura K. Valvular heart disease in Kawasaki syndrome: incidence and natural history. *Am Heart J* 1990; 120: 366–72

Al Mayouf SM. The use of corticosteroid therapy in refractory Kawasaki patients. *Clin Rheumatol* 2004; 23:11–13.

Amano S, Hazama F, Kubagawa H, Tasaka K, Haebara H, Hamashima Y. General pathology of Kawasaki disease. On the morphological alterations corresponding to the clinical manifestations. *Acta Pathol Jpn.* 1980 Sep;30(5):681-94.

Asano T, Ogawa S. Expression of monocyte chemoattractant protein-1 in Kawasaki disease: the anti-inflammatory effect of gamma globulin therapy. *Scand J Immunol.* 2000;51:98–103.

Burns JC. Translation of Dr Tomisaku Kawasaki's original report of fifty patients in 1967. Pediatr Infect Dis J 2002; 21: 993–95.

Burns JC, Capparelli EV, Brown JA, Newburger JW, Glode MP, Multicenter KD Study Group. Intravenous gamma globulin treatment and retreatment in Kawasaki disease. *Pediatr Infect Dis J* 1998; 17: 1144–48.

Burns JC, Cayan DR, Tong G, Bainto EV, Turner CL, Shike H, Kawasaki T, Nakamura Y, Yashiro M, Yanagawa H. Seasonality and temporal clustering of Kawasaki syndrome. *Epidemiology.* 2005 Mar;16(2):220-5.

Burns JC, Glode MP. Kawasaki syndrome. *Lancet* 2004; 364:533–544.

Burns JC, Glode MP, Clarke SH, Wiggins J Jr, Hathaway WE Coagulopathy and platelet activation in Kawasaki syndrome: identification of patients at high risk for development of coronary artery aneurysms. *J Pediatr* 1984; 105:206-211

Burns JC, Shike H, Gordon JB, Malhotra A, Schoenwetter M, Kawasaki T. Sequelae of Kawasaki disease in adolescents and young adults. *J Am Coll Cardiol* 1996; 28: 253–57.

Burns JC, Shimizu C, Gonzalez E, et al. Genetic variations in the receptorligand pair CCR5 and CCL3L1 are important determinants of susceptibility to Kawasaki Disease. *J Infect Dis* 2005; 192:344-349.

Burns JC, Wiggins JW, Toews WH, et al. The clinical spectrum of Kawasaki syndrome in infants less than six months of age. *J Pediatr* 1986; 109: 759–63.

Brogan PA, Bose A, Burgner D, et al. Kawasaki disease: an evidence based approach to diagnosis, treatment, and proposals for future research. *Arch Dis Child* 2002; 86:286–290.

Brogan PA, Shah V, Clarke LA, Dillon MJ, Klein N. T cell activation profiles in Kawasaki syndrome. Clin Exp Immunol. 2008 Feb;151(2):267-74. Epub 2007 Dec 6.

Brown TJ, Crawford SE, Cornwall ML, Garcia F, Shulman ST, Rowley AH. CD8 T lymphocytes and macrophages infiltrate coronary artery aneurysms in acute Kawasaki disease. *J Infect Dis.* 2001;184:940–943.

Caquard M, ParlierG, Siret D. Family observation of Kawasaki disease: 2 cases in sister and brother. *Arch Pediatr* 2006; 13:453–455.

Catalano-Pons C, Giraud C, Rozenberg F, Meritet JF, Lebon P, Gendrel D. Detection of human bocavirus in children with Kawasaki disease. *Clin Microbiol Infect.* 2007 Dec;13(12):1220-2. Epub 2007 Sep 10.

Chang RK. Hospitalizations for Kawasaki disease among children in the United States, 1988-1997. *Pediatrics.* 2002 Jun;109(6):e87.

Dajani AS, Taubert KA, Gerber MA, Shulman ST, Ferrieri P, Freed M, Takahashi M, Bierman FZ, Karchmer AW, Wilson W, et al.Diagnosis and therapy of Kawasaki disease in children. *Circulation.* 1993 May;87(5):1776-80

Dajani AS, Taubert KA, Takahashi M, Bierman FZ, Freed MD, Ferrieri P, Gerber M, Shulman St, Karchmer AW, Wilson W, et al. Guidelines for long-term management of patients with Kawasaki disease. Report from the Committee on Rheumatic Fever, Endocarditis, and Kawasaki Disease, Council on Cardiovascular Disease in the Young, American Heart Association. *Circulation.* 1994;89:916–922.

Dengler LD, Capparelli EV, Bastian JF, Bradley DJ, Glode MP, Santa S, Newburger JW, Baker AL, Matsubara T, Burns JC. Cerebrospinal fluid profile in patients with acute Kawasaki disease. *Pediatr Infect Dis J.* 1998 Jun;17(6):478-81.

Durongpisitkul K, Gururaj VJ, Park JM, Martin CF. The prevention of coronary artery aneurysm in Kawasaki disease: A meta-analysis on the efficacy of aspirin and immunoglobulin treatment. *Pediatrics.* 1995;96:1057–1061.

Eberhard BA, Andersson U, Laxer RM, Rose V, Silverman ED. Evaluation of the cytokine response in Kawasaki disease. *Pediatr Infect Dis J.* 1995; 14:199–203.

Esper F, Shapiro ED, Weibel C, et al. Association between a novel human coronavirus and Kawasaki disease. *J Infect Dis.* 2005; 191:499–502

Fujiwara H, Hamashima Y. Pathology of the heart in Kawasaki disease. Pediatrics. 1978 Jan;61(1):100-7

Furuno K, Yuge T, Kusuhara K, et al. CD25ώ CD4ώ regulatory T cells in patients with Kawasaki disease. *J Pediatr* 2004; 145:385–390.

Furusho K, Kamiya T, Nakano H, et al. High-dose intravenous gamma globulin for Kawasaki disease. *Lancet* 1984; 2: 1055–58

Gavin PJ, Crawford SE, Shulman ST, Garcia FL, Rowley AH. Systemic arterial expression of matrix metalloproteinases 2 and 9 in acute Kawasaki disease. *Arterioscler Thromb Vasc Biol.* 2003;23:576–581.

Gomard-Mennesson E, Landron C, Dauphin C, Epaulard O, Petit C, Green L, Roblot P, Lusson JR, Broussolle C, Sève P. Kawasaki disease in adults: report of 10 cases. Medicine (Baltimore). 2010;89(3):149.

Greil GF, Stuber M, Botnar RM, et al. Coronary magnetic resonance angiography in adolescents and young adults with Kawasaki disease. *Circulation* 2002; 105: 908–11.

Harada F, Sada M, Kamiya T, et al. Genetic analysis of Kawasaki syndrome. *Am J Hum Genet* 1986; 39:537–539.

Harnden A, Alves B, Sheikh A. Rising incidence of Kawasaki disease in England: analysis of hospital admission data. *BMJ.* 2002 Jun 15;324(7351):1424-5.

Hirata S, Nakamura Y, Yanagawa H. Incidence of recurrent Kawasaki disease and related risk factors: for the results of nationwide surveys of Kawasaki disease in Japan. *Acta Pediatr* 2001; 90: 40–44.

Holman RC, Belay ED, Christensen KY, Folkema AM, Steiner CA, Schonberger LB. Hospitalizations for Kawasaki syndrome among children in the United States, 1997-2007. *Pediatr Infect Dis J.* 2010 Jun;29(6):483-8.

Holman RC, Christensen KY, Belay ED, Steiner CA, Effler PV, Miyamura J, Forbes S, Schonberger LB, Melish M. Racial/ethnic differences in the incidence of Kawasaki syndrome among children in Hawaii. *Hawaii Med J.* 2010 Aug;69(8):194-7.

Holman RC, Curns AT, Belay ED, Steiner CA, Effler PV, Yorita KL, Miyamura J,Forbes S, Schonberger LB, Melish M. Kawasaki syndrome in Hawaii. *Pediatr Infect Dis J*. 2005 May;24(5):429-33.

Honkanen E, McCrindle BW, Laxer RM, Feldman BM, Schneider R, Silverman ED. Clinical relevance of the risk factors for coronary artery inflammation in Kawasaki disease. *Pediatr Cardiol* 2003; 24: 122–26.

Huang WC, Huang LM, Chang IS, Chang LY, Chiang BL, Chen PJ, Wu MH, Lue HC, Lee CY; Kawasaki Disease Research Group. Epidemiologic features of Kawasaki disease in Taiwan, 2003-2006. *Pediatrics*. 2009 Mar;123(3):e401-5. Epub 2009 Feb 23.

Ishii M, Ueno T, Akagi T, et al. Guidelines for catheter intervention in coronary artery lesion in Kawasaki disease. *Pediatr Int* 2001; 43:558–562.

Ishii M, Ueno T, Ikeda H, et al. Sequential follow-up results of catheter intervention for coronary artery lesions after Kawasaki disease: quantitative coronary artery angiography and intravascular ultrasound imaging study. *Circulation*. 2002;105:3004–3010

Jennette JC. Implications for pathogenesis of patterns of injury in small- and medium-sized-vessel vasculitis. *Cleve Clin J Med*. 2002;69 Suppl 2:SII33-8.

Kamiya T, Suzuki A, Ono Y, Arakaki Y, Tsuda E, Fujiwara M et al. Angiographic follow-up study of coronary artery lesion in the cases with a history of Kawasaki disease—with a focus on the follow-up more than ten years after the onset of the disease. In: Kato H, ed. *Kawasaki Disease. Proceedings of the 5th International Kawasaki Disease Symposium, Fukuoka, Japan, 22–25 May 1995. New York, NY*: Elsevier Science; 1995:569–573.

Kao AS, Getis A, Brodine S, Burns JC. Spatial and temporal clustering of Kawasaki syndrome cases. Pediatr Infect Dis J. 2008 Nov;27(11):981-5.

Kato H, Inoue O, Kawasaki T , Fujiwara H, Watanabe T, Toshima H. Adult coronary artery disease probably due to childhood Kawasaki disease. *Lancet* 1992; 340: 1127–29

Kato H, Sugimura T, Akagi T, et al. Long-term consequences of Kawasaki disease: 10–21-year follow-up study of 594 patients. *Circulation* 1996; 94: 1379–85.

Kawasaki T, Kosaki F, Okawa S, Shigematsu I, Yanagawa H. A new infantile acute febrile mucocutaneous lymph node syndrome (MLNS) prevailing in Japan. *Pediatrics* 1974;54:271- 6.

Kitamura S, Kameda Y, Seki T, et al. Long-term outcome of myocardial revascularization in patients with Kawasaki coronary artery disease. *J Thorac Cardiovasc Surg* 1994; 107:663–674.

Koren G, Lavi S, Rose V, Rowe R. Kawasaki disease: review of risk factors for coronary aneurysms. *J Pediatr* 1986; 108: 388–92.

Kuramochi Y, Ohkubo T, Takechi N, Fukumi D, Uchikoba Y, Ogawa S. Hemodynamic factors of thrombus formation in coronary aneurysms associated with Kawasaki disease. *Pediatr Int*. 2000;42:470–475.

Lee JY, Song JY, Kim SJ, et al. Coronary rotational ablation for calcific coronary artery stenosis in a young child. *Int J Cardiol* 2005; 99:349- 350.

Leung DY, Meissner HC, Shulman ST, et al. Prevalence of superantigensecreting bacteria in patients with Kawasaki Disease. *J Pediatr* 2002; 140: 742–746.

Lin CY, Lin CC, Hwang B, Chiang B. Serial changes of serum interleukin-6, interleukin-8, and tumor necrosis factor alpha among patients with Kawasaki disease. *J Pediatr.* 1992;121:924–926

Maeno N, Takei S, Masuda K, Akaike H, Matsuo K, Kitajima I, Maruyama I, Miyata I. Increased serum levels of vascular endothelial growth factor in Kawasaki disease. *Pediatr Res.* 1998;44:596–599.

Marasini M, Pongiglione G, Gazzolo D, Campelli A, Ribaldone D, Caponnetto S. Late intravenous gamma globulin treatment in infants and children with Kawasaki disease and coronary artery abnormalities. *Am J Cardiol.* 1991;68:796–797.

Masuda H, Shozawa T, Naoe S, Tanaka N. The intercostal artery in Kawasaki disease. A pathologic study of 17 autopsy cases. *Arch Pathol Lab Med.* 1986 Dec;110(12):1136-42.

Matsubara K, Fukaya T. The role of superantigens of group A Streptococcus and Staphylococcus aureus in Kawasaki disease. *Curr Opin Infect Dis* 2007; 20:298–303.

McMorrow Tuohy AM, Tani LY, Cetta F, Lewin MB, Eidem BW, Van Buren P, Williams RV, Shaddy RE, Tuohy RP, Minich LL. How many echocardiograms are necessary for follow-up evaluation of patients with Kawasaki disease? *Am J Cardiol.* 2001;88:328–330.

Meissner HC, Leung DY. Kawasaki syndrome. Curr Opin Rheumatol. 1995 Sep;7(5):455-8.

Melish ME, Hicks RM, Larson EJ. Mucocutaneous lymph node syndrome in the United States. *Am J Dis Child* 1976; 130: 599–607.

Miyashita M, Karasawa K, Taniguchi K, et al. Usefulness of real-time 3-dimensional echocardiography for the evaluation of coronary artery morphology in patients with Kawasaki disease. *J Am Soc Echocardiogr* 2007; 20:930–933 .

Mitani Y, Sawada H, Hayakawa H, et al. Elevated levels of high-sensitivity C-reactive protein and serum amyloid-A late after Kawasaki disease: association between inflammation and late coronary sequelae in Kawasaki disease. *Circulation* 2005; 111:38–43.

Mori M, Imagawa T, Yasui K, Kanaya A, Yokota S. Predictors of coronary artery lesions after intravenous gamma globulin treatment in Kawasaki disease *J Pediatr* 2000; 137: 177–80.

Mori M, Tomono N, Yokota S. Coronary arteritis of Kawasaki disease unresponsive to high-dose intravenous gammaglobulin successfully treated with plasmapheresis. Nihon Rinsho Meneki Gakkai Kaishi 1995; 18:282–288.

Naiser JA, Schaller FA, Bannout R, Tak T. Kawasaki disease causing giant saccular aneurysms of the coronary arteries: echocardiographic and 64-slice computed tomographic angiographic findings.*Tex Heart Inst J.* 2008;35(3):369-70.

Nakamura Y, Aso E, Yashiro M, Uehara R, Watanabe M, Oki I, Yanagawa H. Mortality among persons with a history of kawasaki disease in Japan: mortality among males with cardiac sequelae is significantly higher than that of the general population. *Circ J.* 2008 Jan;72(1):134-8.

Nakamura Y, Yashiro M, Uehara R, Oki I, Watanabe M, Yanagawa H. Epidemiologic features of Kawasaki disease in Japan: results from the nationwide survey in 2005-2006. *J Epidemiol.* 2008;18(4):167-72. Epub 2008 Jul 18.

Nakamura Y, Yashiro M, Uehara R, Sadakane A, Chihara I, Aoyama Y, Kotani K, Yanagawa H. Epidemiologic features of Kawasaki disease in Japan: results of the 2007-2008 nationwide survey. *J Epidemiol.* 2010;20(4):302-7. Epub 2010 Jun 5.

Newburger JW. Kawasaki disease: who is at risk? *J Pediatr* 2000; 137: 149–52.

Newburger JW, Fulton DR. Kawasaki disease. *Curr Opin Pediatr* 2004; 16:508–514.

Newburger JW, Takahashi M, Beiser AS, et al. Single infusion of intravenous gamma globulin compared to four daily doses in the treatment of acute Kawasaki syndrome. *N Engl J Med* 1991; 324: 1633–39.

Newburger JW, Takahashi M, Gerber MA, Gewitz MH, Tani LY, Burns JC, et al. Diagnosis, treatment, and long-term management of Kawasaki disease: a statement for health professionals from the Committee on Rheumatic Fever, Endocarditis and Kawasaki Disease, Council on Cardiovascular Disease in the Young, American Heart Association. *Circulation* 2004;110(17):2747–71

Newburger JW, Takahashi M, Burns JC, et al. Treatment of Kawasaki syndrome with intravenous gamma globulin. *N Engl J Med* 1986; 315: 341–47.

Nomura Y, Masuda K, Maeno N, et al. Serum levels of interleukin-18 are elevated in the subacute phase of Kawasaki syndrome. *Int Arch Allergy Immunol* 2004; 135:161–165.

Nonaka Z, Maekawa K, Okabe T, Eto Y, Kubo M. Randomized controlled study of intravenous prednisolone and gamma globulin treatment in 100 cases with Kawasaki disease. In: Kato H, ed. *Kawasaki Disease. Proceedings of the 5th International Kawasaki Disease Symposium, Fukuoka,Japan, 22–25 May 1995*. New York, NY: Elsevier Science; 1995:328–331

Park YW, Han JW, Hong YM, Ma JS, Cha SH, Kwon TC, Lee SB, Kim CH, Lee JS, Kim CH. Epidemiological features of Kawasaki disease in Korea, 2006-2008. *Pediatr Int*. 2011 Feb;53(1):36-9. doi: 10.1111/j.1442-200X.2010.03178.x

O'Brien M, Parness IA, Neufeld EJ, Baker AL, Sundel RP, Newburger JW.Ticlopidine plus aspirin for coronary thrombosis in Kawasaki disease. *Pediatrics*. 2000 May;105(5):E64.

Okada Y, Minakami H, Tomomasa T, et al. Serum procalcitonin concentrationin patients with Kawasaki disease. *J Infect* 2004; 48:199–205.

Okada Y, Shinohara M, Kobayashi T, Inoue Y, Tomomasa T, Kobayashi T, Morikawa A, Gunma Kawasaki Disease Study Group. Effect of corticosteroids in addition to intravenous gamma globulin therapy on serum cytokine levels in the acute phase of Kawasaki disease in children. *J Pediatr*. 2003; 143:363–367.

Onouchi Y. Identification of susceptibility genes for Kawasaki disease. Nihon Rinsho Meneki Gakkai Kaishi. 2010;33(2):73-80.

Onouchi Y, Gunji T, Burns JC, Shimizu C, Newburger JW, Yashiro M, Nakamura Y, Yanagawa H, Wakui K, Fukushima Y, Kishi F, Hamamoto K, Terai M, Sato Y, Ouchi K, Saji T, Nariai A, Kaburagi Y, Yoshikawa T, Suzuki K, Tanaka T, Nagai T, Cho H, Fujino A, Sekine A, Nakamichi R, Tsunoda T, Kawasaki T, Nakamura Y, Hata A. ITPKC functional polymorphism associated with Kawasaki disease susceptibility and formation of coronary artery aneurysms. *Nat Genet*. 2008 Jan;40(1):35-42. Epub 2007 Dec 16.

Popper SJ, Shimizu C, Shike H, Kanegaye JT, Newburger JW, Sundel RP, Brown PO, Burns JC, Relman DA.Gene-expression patterns reveal underlying biological processes in Kawasaki disease. *Genome Biol*. 2007;8(12):R261.

Rauch AM, Glode MP, Wiggins JW Jr, Rodriguez JG, Hopkins RS, Hurwitz ES, Schonberger LB. Outbreak of Kawasaki syndrome in Denver, Colorado: association with rug and carpet cleaning. *Pediatrics*. 1991 May;87(5):663-9.

Rosenfeld EA, Shulman ST, Corydon KE, Mason W, Takahashi M, Kuroda C. Comparative safety and efficacy of two immune globulin products in Kawasaki disease. *J Pediatr.* 1995;126:1000-1003.

Rowley AH, Shulman ST, Spike BT, et al. Oligoclonal IgA response in the vascular wall in acute Kawasaki Disease. *J Immunol* 2001; 166:1334–1343

Rowley AH, Wolinsky SM, Relman DA, Sambol SP, Sullivan J, Terai M, Shulman ST. Search for highly conserved viral and bacterial nucleic acid sequences corresponding to an etiologic agent of Kawasaki disease. Pediatr Res.1994 Nov;36(5):567-71.

Samuelsson A, Towers TL, Ravetch JV. Anti-inflammatory activity of IVIG mediated through the inhibitory Fc receptor. *Science* 2001;291: 484–86.

Sato S, Kawashima H, Kashiwagi Y, Fujioka T, Takekuma K, Hoshika A. Association of mannose-binding lectin gene polymorphisms with Kawasaki disease in the Japanese. Int J Rheum Dis. 2009 Dec;12(4):307-10.

Scott JS, Ettedgui JA, Neches WH. Cost-effective use of echocardiography in children with Kawasaki disease. *Pediatrics.* 1999;104:e57 .

Shulman ST. Is there a role for corticosteroids in Kawasaki disease?*J Pediatr.* 2003;142:601-603.

Shulman ST, De Inocencio J, Hirsch R. Kawasaki disease. Pediatr Clin North Am. 1995 Oct;42(5):1205-22.

Shulman ST, McAuley JB, Pachman LM, Miller ML, Ruschhaupt DG1. Risk of coronary abnormalities due to Kawasaki disease in urban area with small Asian population. *Am J Dis Child.*1987 Apr;141(4):420-5.

Stapp J, Marshall GS. Fulfillment of diagnostic criteria in Kawasaki disease. *South Med J* 2000; 93: 44–47.

Stockheim JA, Innocentini N, Shulman ST. Kawasaki disease in older children and adolescents. *J Pediatr* 2000; 137: 250–52.

Sugimura T, Yokoi H, Sato N, et al. Interventional treatment for children with severe coronary artery stenosis with calcification after long-term Kawasaki disease. *Circulation.* 1997;96:3928–3933.

Sugita K, Hirao J, Arisaka O, Eguchi M. Gamma-globulin-induced modulation with necrotic-like morphology of peripheral blood neutrophils. *Eur J Pharmacol* 2005; 513:141–144.

Suzuki M, Yamagishi M, Kimura K, et al. Functional behavior and morphology of the coronary artery wall in patients with Kawasaki disease assessed by intravascular ultrasound. *J Am Coll Cardiol* 1996; 27: 291–96.

Takahashi M. Management of giant coronary artery aneurysms due to Kawasaki disease. *ACC Curr J* Rev. 1996:74-76

Tatara K, Kusakawa S. Long-term prognosis of giant coronary aneurysm in Kawasaki disease: an angiographic study. *J Pediatr.* 1987;111:705–710.

Taubert KA, Rowley AH, Shulman ST. Seven-year national survey of Kawasaki disease and acute rheumatic fever.*Pediatr Infect Dis J.* 1994 Aug;13(8):704-8.

Terai M, Shulman ST. Prevalence of coronary artery abnormalities in Kawasaki disease is highly dependent on gamma globulin dose but independent of salicylate dose. *J Pediatr.* 1997;131: 888–893.

Treadwell TA, Maddox RA, Holman RC, Belay ED, Shahriari A, Anderson MS, Burns J, Glodé MP, Hoffman RE, Schonberger LB. Investigation of Kawasaki syndrome risk factors in Colorado. *Pediatr Infect Dis J*. 2002 Oct;21(10):976-8.

Tsuda E, Kitamura S; Cooperative Study Group of Japan. National survey of coronary artery bypass grafting for coronary stenosis caused by Kawasaki disease in Japan. *Circulation*. 2004;110:II61–II66.

Tsujimoto H, Takeshita S, Nakatani K, Kawamura Y, Tokutomi T, Sekine I. Intravenous immunoglobulin therapy induces neutrophil apoptosis in Kawasaki disease. *Clin Immunol*. 2002 May;103(2):161-8.

Uehara R, Yashiro M, Nakamura Y, Yanagawa H. Kawasaki disease in parents and children. *Acta Paediatr*. 2003 Jun;92(6):694-7.

Wang X, Zhang G, Liu F, et al. Prevalence of human parvovirus B19 DNA in cardiac tissues of patients with congenital heart diseases indicated by nested PCR and in situ hybridization. *J Clin Virol*. 2004; 31:20–24.

Weiss JE, Eberhard BA, Chowdhury D, Gottlieb BS. Infliximab as a novel therapy for refractory Kawasaki disease. *J Rheumatol*. 2004;31:808–810.

WilliamsRV, Wilke VM, Tani LY, Minich LL.Does abciximab enhance regression of coronary aneurysms resulting from Kawasaki disease? *Pediatrics* 2002; 109:e4.

Witt MT, Minich LL, Bohnsack JF, Young PC. Kawasaki disease: more patients are being diagnosed who do not meet American Heart Association criteria.*Pediatrics*. 1999 Jul;104(1):e10.

Wolff AE, Hansen KE, Zakowski L. Acute Kawasaki disease: not just for kids. *J Gen Intern Med*. 2007 May;22(5):681-4.

Wu CY, Hsieh KS, Chiou YH, et al. Prolonged fever and pyuria: a urinary tract infection presentation of incomplete Kawasaki disease. *Acta Paediatr* 2005; 94:375–377.

Yanagawa H, Nakamura Y, Ojima T, Yashiro M, Tanihara S, Oki I. Changes in epidemic patterns of Kawasaki disease in Japan. *Pediatr Infect Dis J*. 1999 Jan;18(1):64-6.

Yasukawa K, Terai M, Shulman ST, Toyozaki T, Yajima S, Kohno Y, Rowley AH. Systemic production of vascular endothelial growth factor and fms-like tyrosine kinase-1 receptor in acute Kawasaki disease. *Circulation*. 2002;105:766–769.

Yoshikawa Y, Yagihara T, Kameda Y, Taniguchi S, Tsuda E, Kawahira Y, Uemura H, Kitamura S. Result of surgical treatments in patients with coronary-arterial obstructive disease after Kawasaki disease. *Eur J Cardiothorac Surg*. 2000;17:515–519.

Yoshikawa J, Yanagihara K, Owaki T, et al. Cross-sectional echocardiographic diagnosis of coronary artery aneurysms in patients with mucocutaneous lymph node syndrome. *Circulation* 1979; 59: 133–39.

18

Neurological Manifestations in Behcet Disease

E. Ait Ben Haddou, A. Benomar, W. Regragui and M. Yahyaoui
Departement of Neurology B and Neurogenetic, Hopital des Spécialités, Rabat, Mohammed V Souissi University, Faculty of Medicine of Rabat, Morocoo

1. Introduction

Behçet disease is a multisystem disease of unknown cause in which an inflammatory perivasculitis can arise in almost any tissue (Sakane et *al.*, 1999). Neurologic involvement in Behçet disease was first reported by Knapp in 1941. It represented between 4-49% of manifestations of BD (Haghighi et *al.*, 2005). There is one of the most serious causes of long term morbidity and mortality in Behçet's Disease. As well as, involvement of the central nervous system occurs late in the course of the disease (10–25%) (Ildan et *al.*, 1996; Nakasu et *al.*, 2001). It is caused by primary neural parenchymal lesions or is secondary to major vascular involvement (Adnan et al, 2009).
Treatment of the most cases of NB should be given as infusion of intravenous methyl prednisolone followed by a slowly tapering course of oral steroids. (Adnan et *al.*, 2000,). Immunopressives agents should be used in its severity forms of NB such as meningoencephalitis, deep veins thrombosis and myelopathy. In this Review, we summarise and describe the clinicals manifestations of neurobehcet disease.

2. Epidemiology

Epidemiological, Clinical characterization and pattern of neurological involvement of Behcet's disease have been reported in different series (Hentati et al., 1993; bohlega et al., 1993; nakamura et al., 1994; Farah et al,1998; Kidd et al.,1999; Akman et al.,1999; Al fahad et al.,1999).
Retrospective and prospective studies found that the prevalence of Neurobehcet disease (NBD) is very variable. Neurologic involovement were occured in 2-49% of cases, other authors estimated their prevalence of 3-50% of cases (Borhani et al., 2009). The age of onset of NBD is usually 20–40 years with an average age of 39 years. In two the last decade, Neurological complications have also been described in children. (Adnan et al., 2005 ; Araji et al., 2009).
The highest incidence is in the Middle East, the Mediterranean basin, and the Far East regions, but it is rare in Europe and North America. The frequency was 13% in men and 5 • 6% in women. Neurological manifestations commonly develop a few years after the onset of the other systemic features of BD; The mean duration between onset of BD and development of NBD ranged from 3 to 6 years. (Siva et al., 2001). However, neurological syndrome might coincide or come in advance (~6% of patients) with other systemic

symptoms features of BD, in that case diagnosis can be difficult and causes ambiguity with other systemic diseases (Akman et *al.,* 1999).

3. Classification

There are two categories of neurological involvement in BD that have been generally accepted: parenchymal involvement and non-parenchymal involvement, also called cerebral angio-Behcet's syndrome. The most syndromes often involved in NBD were meningoencephalitis, myelopathy and deep veins thrombosis which presented 80% in retrospective series (Tohme et al., 2008)

4. Neuropathology

NBD is considered as an inflamatory perivasculitis disease, in an acute meningoencephalitis the most common neuropathologic findings are Severe and acute inflammation consisting mainly of lymphocytic, eosinophils, macrophages, and neutrophilic infiltrations of the perivascular spaces and parenchyma. These lesions can lead to necrotizing and disseminated encephalitis involving the basal ganglia, brainstem, cerebellum and diencephalon.

In the progressive phase, authors found the inflammatory infiltration of lymphocytes and cytokines remains and cuts down. (Hirohata et al., 2008; Heo et al., 2008; Hadfi et al., 1996; Arai et al., 2006; Scardamaglia et al., 2001).

5. Clinical characteristics

In order to the accumulated data, it's now obvious that it is necessary to handle parenchymal CNS involvement and non parenchymal CNS involvement in Behçet'sdisease separately.

5.1 Parenchymal CNS involvement

About 70 à 80% CNS involvement

First of all, Subacute meningoencephalitis accounts for 75% of cases in parenchymal NBD, which performs adverse symptoms, depending on the topography of lesions.

It's and often associated with exacerbation of the systemic features of BD, including fever, malaise, orogenital ulcers, skin lesions, or uveitis (Akman et *al.,* 2003; Joseph et *al.,* 2007).

The onset of signs is in the most cases acute or subacute. More rarely, the onset is chronic (Akman *et al.,* 1999). Onset is usually with an attack of headache, hemiparesis and / or gradual behavioural changes. The symptoms and signs are taking a few days to attempt Summit and during several weeks, rely on depending on the extent of the lesion and on how rapidly treatment is initiated. However, spontaneous remissions of symptoms could be taken before initiation of therapy as it has been reported (Hirohata et *al.,* 2007).

Different syndromes might be encountered during the course of parenchymal NBD.

The patient may frequently show brainstem signs, including pyramidal bilateral and cebellar syndromes, ophthalmoparesis and cranial neuropathy. Moreover, there is evidence for additional cerebral or spinal cord involvement like a day time sleeping with or without hyperphagia and which might be indicative of hypothalamic dysfunction (Wechsler et al., 2002; Houmana et *al.,* 2009)

Second a progressive form of the disease which represents 10% of cases of NBD, including, a worsening subcortical dementia, were usually accompanied by ataxia.
Third, symptoms and signs suggestive of cerebral hemispheric involvement include encephalopathy, hemiparesis, Hemisensory loss, seizures, dysphasia, and mental changes with cognitive dysfunction and psychosis.
Fourth, symptoms and signs of spinal cord involvement include pyramidal signs in the limbs, sensory level dysfunction, and, commonly, sphincter dysfunction.
Finally, asymptomatic (silent) parenchymal NBD is diagnosed if there are no neurological symptoms, but neurological signs on examination (usually pyramidal signs). Recognition of these clinical syndromes might help clinicians dealing with BD to predict the pattern of involvement. They might also help neurologists to remember BD in the differential diagnosis of a patient who presents with one of these neurological syndromes. In addition, other clinical syndromes might arise in BD, and although uncommon, it is important that these syndromes are recognized.

5.1.1 Epilepsy

Neuro-BD-related epileptic disorder has been previously reported in a large series of Behçet disease. Generalized seizures are the predominant type (Aykutlu et *al.*, 2002). Convulsions were observed in 2 - 5% of large series (Al-Fahad et al., 2001).Behcet's syndrome may present with partial seizure and epilepsia partialis continua (Aktekin et *al.*, 2006. Partial seizures were a presenting feature of NBD in one report (Chroni et *al.*, 2008).

5.1.2 Brain tumour

Since the first described case in 1987; Focal necrotic lesions in the cerebral cortex; only a few cases have been published. (Litvan et *al.*, 2005; Matsuo et *al.*, 2005; Appenzeller et *al.*, 2005; Kosters et *al.*, 2006; Bennett et *al.*, 2004; Park et *al.*, 2002).
The regions usually affected are, brainstem, diencephalon, basal ganglia, and internal capsule. The clinical presentation depends on the localizations of brain tumors; usually include intracranial hypertension syndrome and/or impaired of consciousness. These lesions cause a diagnosis problem with the brain tumor and a multiple metastatic tumors.

5.1.3 Movement disorders

Extrapyramidal manifestations whitch are indicating basal ganglion excessive dysfunction, are rare in most series of patients with NBD.

5.1.4 Acute meningeal syndrome

Aseptic meningitis commonly exists with many parenchymal CNS manifestations of BD. The signs and symptoms are relatively common in parenchymal NBD. However, isolated meningitis might only rarely be the presenting feature of NBD (Kidd et al., 1999; Akman et *al.*, 1999; Al-Fahad et *al.*, 1999).

5.1.5 Optic neuropathy

Optic neuropathy is rare in BD, it has been described only in0.4% of the main series of behçet disease. It can be bilateral and can be recurrent over many years. The severity of the visual loss and its recovery can be very variable, even in the same patient (Voros et al., 2006; Tarzi et al., 2005).

5.1.6 Spinal cord involvement

Involvement of the spinal cord as part of the diffuse type of parenchymal NBD pattern is rare , represent 11% as reported by the most studies, thurly the spinal cord is commonly found to be involved in autopsy series of Behcet's disease. More frequently a combination of spinal cord symptoms with other syndromes of parenchymal NBD, However isolated acute transverse myelitis is an exceptional presentation of NBD (Joseph, 2007).

Most commonly patients presented with sensory-motor symptoms, sphincter and/or sexual dysfunction evolving over days. Although spinal cord involvement has a n worse prognosis compared with other types of p-NBD. The myelopathy can have a severe primary progressive course, a secondary progressive course after initial attack(s), or an acute attack with severe residual sequela after attacks (Houman et *al.*, 2007; Moskau et *al.*, 2003).

14% had predominantly spinal cord involvement (10 with isolated spinal cord involvement and 13 with additional brainstem and/or hemispheric involvement. The cervical and/or dorsal areas can be involved (Kocer, 1999; Kizilkilic, 1998; Tunc et *al.*, 2003; Calguneri et *al.*, 2005).

5.2 Non-parenchymal NBD

5.2.1 Cerebrovascular involvement

Also called cerebral angio-Behcet's syndrome, encompassing mainly those instances with dural sinus thrombosis. Cerebrovascular complications include strokes, carotid aneurysm formation and cerebral venous thrombosis (Hadfield et *al*, 1996; Tunc et *al.*, 2004; B'chir-Hamzaoui et *al.*, 2009)

5.2.1.1 Cerebral venous thrombosis

In 1959, with headache and bilateral papilloedema. CVT constituted about 18% of NBD cases in the studies included, it's reported to affect men more often than women and occurs at an earlier age. Clinical onset is acute or subacute in most patients. Chronic onset is less frequent. Patient has an intracranial hypertension. a focal deficits, seizures and /or counsiousness impairement (Yesilot et al., 2006; Bousser et al., 2007; Akman et al., 1999).

The superior sagittal sinus is the most common site of thrombosis, followed by transverse sinuses, deep cerebral veins and cavernous sinuses, respectively (Mossadeq et al., 2004).

Deep cerebral vein thrombosis is a specific clinical pattern of neuroBehçet. The clinical features of Rosenthal or internal cephalic vein thrombosis predominate. The clinical presentation is highly suggestive of diagnosis confirmed by Imaging ; it's a mesencephalic diencephalitis syndroma combining hemiparesis, hémiataxie and / or movement disorders and ophthalmoplegia by damage of III (Mossadeq et al., 2004).

5.2.1.2 Ischemic stroke and cerebral vasculitis

are unusual manifestations during the course of BD, it was reported in1-5% of major series in the literature (1999; Al-Araji et al., 2003; Al-Fahad et al., 1999; Barros et al., 2007; Benamour et al., 2006; Borhani-Haghighi et al., 2006; Houman et al., 2007; Joseph et al., 2007; Monaco et al., 2006; Turker et al., 2008).

5.2.1.3 Aneurysm formation

Aneurysm formation is common in the visceral arteries in BD, but extremely rare in the intracranial.vasculitis may be involved in the etiology of intracranial aneurysms in patients with BD (Kaku et al., 2007).

5.2.2 Intracranial hypertension

Hypertension manifests as an acute or, more commonly, subacute evolution of headache (92%), papilledema (80%), focal neurologic deficits (32%), seizures (20%), sixth-nerve palsy (16%) and/or altered consciousness (8%). Intracranial hypertension with or without cerebral vein thrombosis appears in 11-35% of all patients. Dural sinus thrombosis, more frequently the superior sagittal sinus; is the main cause of raised intracranial pressure.

In the other side, intracranial without sinus thrombosis or MRI abnormalities have been reported in NBD (Pamiret al., 1981; Akman et al., 1996).

5.3 Others

5.3.1 Psychiatric and cognitive disorders

Psychiatric or cognitive symptoms might be the earliest presentation of NBD, patient can have a dementia as a sole presentation of the disease. Patients have usually a special pattern of cognitive decline in with impaired memory, attention, and frontal lobe functions, and poor motivation and personality change, by contrast with relatively preserved linguistic, arithmetic, visuospatial, abstraction, and problem-solving abilities (Akman et al., 1999).

Psychosomatic symptoms, such as anxiety and depression, are the most commonly encountered, in BD. These symptoms are mostly related to the underlying systemic disease, fatigue, functional deterioration, and sociological handicap, but are only rarely due to direct involvement of the CNS (Taner et *al.*, 2007). Behavioural changes were common; where as major psychiatric symptoms were less common in large series (Akman et *al.*, 1999; Al-Fahad et *al.*, 1999; Siva, 2001).

It is possible that psychiatric symptoms could be the first manifestation of the disease. To our knowledge, this is the first case report of Neuro-Behçet 's Syndrome that presents with an acute psychotic attack (Orhan, 2009).

Abnormal cognitive performances were present in 87.8% of the patients, with the most commonly and most severely affected function being long term memory for both verbal and visual modalities, followed by attention, and executive functioning, whereas only 9% of BD patients also showed cognitive deficits in visuospatial functions

(Roberto, 2004) found that the main cognitive domain. Previous papers reporting cognitive dysfunction in BD patients in- cluded participants with neurological involvement (Akman et *al.*, 1999; Oktem et *al.*, 1999).

However the recent studies reported that BD patients without overt neurological involvement are more likely to have cognitive impairment (Al-Arajiet *al.*, 2009; Wechsler et *al.*, 2002; Taner et *al.*, 2007).

5.3.2 Peripheral nervous system involvements

Peripheral nervous system manifestations are relatively rare in BD. Isolated cases of peripheral neuropathy or myopathy have been reported in Behçet's disease, they are essentially a case of multiple neuropathies, sensorimotor peripheral neuropathy, neuropathy autonomic dysfunction a Guillain Barré syndrome and hearing loss (Namer *et al.*, 1987). Causes of

sensorineural hearing loss include central Causes of sensorineural hearing loss include central and peripheral nerve disorders. In particular, sensorineural hearing loss due to peripheral neuropathy was reported to be very rare (AK, 2004). Few series have described the clinical manifestations (Namer et *al.*, 1987; Worthmann et *al.*, 1996; Ben Ghorbel et *al.*, 2005).
Muscle involvement seems to be exceedingly rare in adults but more common in children. Patients present with a myositis, occasionally localised, that can be detected by electromyography. The rarity of these reports should encourage clinicians to investigate extensively for alternatives before accepting BD as the diagnosis.

5.3.3 Headache

The study has revealed a very high prevalence of headache in an unselected population of patients with Behçet's syndrome. The majority of headaches is of neurovascular type and the prevalence of visual or sensory aura is higher than that seen in the general population of migraine sufferers (Kidd et al., 2006). Headache is the most common neurological symptom in patients with BD, and occurs in about 70% of patients. . The frequency of headache in BD was similar to the prevalence of headache
Headache syndromes (e.g., migraine and tension-type headache) affect about 50% of patients with BD, and account for 70% of all causes of headaches in BD. The characteristics of these primary symptoms in BD did not differ when compared with a headache clinic population (Aykutlu et *al.*, 2006).
The features of this headache varied between migraine, migraine like, and tension type (Borhani-Haghighi et *al.*, 2008; Aykutlu et *al.*, 2006; Saip et *al.*, 2005).
The most widely accepted criteria for the diagnosis of BD are the International BD Study Group criteria (panel 1).

Panel 1: International Behçet's Disease Study Group criteria for the diagnosis of Behçet's disease[5]

For diagnosis, patient must have had the following symptoms:
Recurrent oral ulceration—minor aphthous, major aphthous, or herpetiform ulceration observed by physician or patient that recurred at least three times in one 12-month period

Plus two of the following:
Recurrent genital ulceration—aphthous or scarring, observed by physician or patient
Eye lesions—anterior uveitis, posterior uveitis, or cells in vitreous on slit lamp examination; or retinal vasculitis observed by ophthalmologist
Skin lesions—erythema nodosum observed by physician or patient, pseudofoliculitis, papulopustular lesions; or acneiform nodules observed by physician in post-adolescent patients not on corticosteroids
Positive pathergy test—read by physician at 24–48 h

Findings applicable only in the absence of other clinical explanations.

6. Diagnosis

The diagnosis of neurological involvement in BD is done mainly by clinical means; the ancillary investigations noted below help to suggest alternatives, and especially infective complications of treatment, but there is no diagnostic test for NBD (Adnan et *al.*, 2009). No validated criteria for the diagnosis of NBD exist. Blood count and biochemical screening is used to identify the nature and severity of the systemic disorder and to identify signs of a superimposed infective complication. (Yazici et *al.*, 2007).

6.1 Blood test

Blood count and biochemical screening is used to identify the nature and severity of the systemic disorder and to identify signs of a superimposed infective complication (Yazici et *al.*, 2007). Erythrocyte sedimentation rate has been found to be associated with disease activity.

HLA type B51 has been reported to be present in 60–70% of Turkish and Japanese patients, although in only 10–20% of European patients (Borhani et *al.*, 2009). Patients with HLAB51 have a six-time increased risk of BD, and the disease is usually more severe in such patients (Yazici et al., 2007).

In the case of cerebral venous thrombosis (CVT), a thrombophilia screen should be undertaken. Early reports suggested a higher prevalence of antiphospholipid antibodies and factor V Leiden mutations, but these findings have not been confirmed (Adnan et *al.*, 2009).

6.2 Cerebrospinal fluid (CSF)

CSF constituents are altered in around 70–80% of patients with parenchymal complications. CSF protein is modestly raised in most cases, sometimes to over 1 g/dL, and oligoclonal bands are usually absent (Akman et *al.*, 1999). The CSF cell count is often prominently raised. (Borhani et *al.*, 2008; Houman et *al.*, 2007).

In Hamzaoui et al. study, elevated CSF levels of IL-15 were seen in patients with NBD in comparison with the patients with non-inflammatory neurological disease (Hamzaoui et *al.*, 2006).

CSF levels of some major pro-inflammatory (IL-6, 8, TNF-_and interferon) and anti-inflammatory (IL-10) cytokines in patients with different subtypes of NBD, In Niino et al. study, the concentration of macrophage migration inhibitory factor in CSF was significantly elevated in patients with NBD compared with control group and correlated well with CSF cell count (Niino et al. , 2000).

Significance of elevation of interleukin 6 in patients with parenchymal NBD was found (A. Borhani et a.l, 2009).

The level of interleukin-6 dropped when the disease activity subsided.

These changes were in parallel with IgM isotype of anticardiolipin antibodies (Wong et *al.*, 1992).In Hirohata et al. study 11 patients with progressive NBD showed significant elevation of CSF interleukin-6 activities in comparison with patients with active BD without progressive neurological manifestations.

Serum interleukin-6 activities of these groups did not revealed significant difference (Hirohata et *al.*, 1997).

CSF interleukin-6 levels were used as a parameter for investigation of response of six patients with NBD to low dose methotrexate.

After 12 months trial CSF interleukin-6 levels were significantly decreased. However six months after discontinuation of methotrexate, all patients showed significant exacerbation evidenced by a decrease in verbal intelligence quotients along with the marked elevation of CSF interleukin 6(Hirohata et *al.*, 1998).

6.3 MRI

However, there were still limitations in differential diagnosis with tumor, abscess, multiple sclerosis, and other vasculitis (Joseph et *al.*, 2007; Miller et *al.*, 1987.; Litvan et *al.*, 1987; Mnif et al., 2006; Neudorfer et *al.*, 1993; Imoto et *al.*, 2002; Tuzgen et *al.*, 2002; Bennet et al., 2004; A. Tourba et al., 2011).

In Neurobehçet's disease, the most common site was brainstem and the next most common sites were basal ganglia and white matter.

Cerebellar lesion was reported in a few cases (Kocer et *al.*, 1999; Jae-Hyeok et *al.*, 2008).

Patients with a more diffuse meningoencephalitis show hyper intense T2 lesions within the subcortical white matter of the temporal, frontal, and hypothalamic regions, but the scan might also be normal.

Patients with spinal cord involvement show a single lesion, which might look like a demyelinating plaque, but might extend over two or three segments.

Venous sinus thrombosis is readily seen on magnetic resonance venography and brain CT venography. Patients who present with idiopathic intracranial hypertension have normal imaging studies (Ak man et *al.*, 2003; Coban et al., 1999; Siva et *al.*, 2009).

7. Treatment

The severe nature of the neurological involvement in BD obligates the innovation of markers of disease activity or prognosis that can be determined early in the disease course (Guls et *al.*, 2008). There have no controlled or comparative trials of treatment of any aspect of neurological involvement in BD. Based on scattered evidence, corticosteroids and immunosuppressive have proved effective in improving clinical symptoms of NBD. Remission can be defined as complete or nearly complete absence of symptoms.

Corticosteroids should be given as infusions of intravenous methylprednisolone: 1g IV daily for 3 to 5 days followed by prednisone 0.5 to 1 mg/kg/d for acute attacks. Therefore prevention treatment for early relapses consists of prednisone which must be very gradually tapered over 2 to 3 months (Siva et *al.*, 2000), followed by a slowly tapering course of oral steroids (Adnan et *al.*, 2009).

However , there is controversy about the choice of immunosuppressant therapy as an adjuvant to corticosteroids; immunosuppressive agents or tumor necrosis antagonists should be used at the same time or later depends on the nature of the disease, its severity, the response to steroids, and whether the patient has had previous attacks. In the retrospectives series, immunosuppressive therapy not be used until the second attack occurs, or if the disease is aggressive. Similarly, no treatment trial has been undertaken CVT.

For dural sinus thrombosis associated with Behçet disease, concurrent use of corticosteroids and anticoagulants is suggested (Bank et *al.*, 1984). Either intravenous unfractionated heparin or subcutaneous low-molecular-weight heparin can be used (Siva et *al.*, 2001).

Some neurologists do not use anticoagulants at all, choosing instead to give steroids and immunosuppressants alone.

Other neurologists prefer to use anticoagulants, but recent data show that immunosuppressants are underused (Adnan et *al.*, 2009).

In the literature, several immunosuppressive agents were previously reported, such as Azathioprine, Cyclophosphamide, Chlorambucil, thalidomide and Methotrexate. In most series, the most used immusupressant were Azathioprine and methotrexate. Cyclophosphamide (CPM) is only reported in only sporadic cases, and used in second intention (Homan et *al.*, 2008; Hatemi et *al.*, 2008; Kotter et *al.*, 2005).

More recently, some immunomodulators such as interferon, infliximab and thalidomide have been used successfully in treating some cases of Neurobehçet, but their effectiveness has been proven with any controlled study (Siva et *al.*, 2009).

In the study by O'Duffy et *al.*, Chlorambucil with or without corticosteroids was more effective than corticosteroids alone for meningoencephalitis or recurrent meningitis (O'Duffy et *al.*, 1984). In the Hirohata et al study, low-dose methotrexate reduced the CSF interleukin-6 level and seemed to ameliorate the course of neuropsychiatric manifestations (Hirohata, 1998).

For patients with parenchymal Neurobehçet's disease without any poor prognostic factor, Azathioprine or methotrexate and corticosteroids are recommended as the first line treatment. For high risk patients, intravenous Cyclophosphamide and corticosteroids are recommended (Borhani et *al.*, 2009).

8. Prognosis

Neurobehçet's disease has a high mortality rate, up to 25% within the first year after developing neurological manifestations (Wolf et *al.*, 1965).

Most patients who have an acute parenchymal inflammatory episode recover well after steroid treatment. Retrospective series from 10–15 years ago reported a mean of 20–30% of patients with residual neurological impairments, and a high 10-year mortality of 10%.However, non-parenchymal CNS involvement is prominently associated with a better prognosis than parenchymal CNS involvement (Wechsler et *al.*, 1992; Akman-Demir et *al.*, 1996; Siva et *al.*, 1997). It should be noted that certain factors influence the course and prognosis of Neurobehçet cases. I a previous reported the most important of these is the correlation between the acute-stage CSF findings and the clinical cours (Akman-Demir et *al.*, 1996) normal CSF at the acute stage is associated with a better prognosis, stable course and less disability, while high cellular and/or protein content is significantly associated with a worse prognosis (Gu¨lsen Akman-Demir et *al.*, 1999)

9. Conclusion

Neurological involvements are actually classified in two categories; a parenchymal and none parenchymal diseases. Their manifestations come many years after the outset of BD. The diagnosis is based according to the international criteria of a group study of Behçet disease.

Moreover, clinical manifestations are critical and should be diagnosed earlier. The most serious involvements are parenchymal and vascular diseases because they engage vital and functional prognosis.

Therefore intensive therapy based on corticosteroids anticoagulation therapy and immunosuppressive only guarantees of improving their prognosis.

10. References

A.Tohme, S.Koussa, S.Haddad-Zébouni, B.El-Rassi,E.Ghayad (2008). Etude de 22 observations de Neurobehçet dans une série de 170 maladies de Behçet, *Presse médicale*.

Adnan al Araji, kidd P Desmond. (2009). Neuro-Behçet's disease: epidemiology, clinical characteristics, and management. *Lancet Neurol*, 8: 194-204.

AK E, Harputluoglu U, Oghan F, Baykal B. (2004). Behçet's disease and hearing loss. *Auris Nasus Larynx*, 31, 29-33.

Akman Demir G, Bahar S, Baykan-Kurt B, Gurvit IH, Serdaroglu P. (1996). Intracranial hypertension in Behçet's disease. *Eur J Neurol*, 3, 66–70.

Akman-Demir G, Bahar S, Coban O, Tasci B, Serdaroglu P. (2003). Cranial MRI in Behc¸et's disease: 134 examinations of 98 patients. *Neuroradiology*; 45:851–9.

Akman-Demir G, Baykan-Kurt B, Serdaroglu P, Gu¨rvit H, YurdakulS, Yazici H, et al. (1996). Seven-year follow-up of neurologic involvement in Behçet syndrome. *Arch Neurol*, 53: 691–4.

Akman-Demir G, Serdaroglu P, Tasci B. (1999). Clinical patterns of neurological involvement in Behçet's disease: evaluation of 200 patients. The Neuro-Behcet Study Group. *Brain*; 122: 2171–82.

Al-Araji A, Sharquie K, Al-Rawi Z. Prevalence and patterns of neurological involvement in Behçet's disease: a prospective study from Iraq. *J Neurol Neurosurg Psychiatry*, 74, 608–13.

Al-Fahad S, Al-Araji A. Neuro-Behçet's disease in Iraq: a study of 40 patients. (1999). *J Neurol Sci*, 170, 105–11.

Appenzeller S, de Castro R, de Souza Queiroz L, et al. (2005). BrainSchmolck H. Large thalamic mass due to neuro-Behcet disease. Neurology, 65, 436.

Appenzeller S, de Castro R, Queiroz Lde S, Madegan L, Soledade C,Zanardi Vde A, et al. (2006). Brain tumor-like lesion in Behçet disease. *Rheumatol Int*, 26(6): 577–80.

Arai Y, Kohno S, Takahashi Y, Miyajima Y, Tsutusi Y (2006). Autopsy case of neuro-Behcet's disease with multifocal neutrophilic perivascular infl ammation. *Neuropathology*, 26, 579–85.

Aykutlu E, Baykan B, Akman-Demir G, Topcular B, Ertas M. Headache in Behcet's disease (2006). *Cephalalgia*, 26, 180–86.

Aykutlu E, Baykan B, Serdaroglu P, Gokyigit A, Akman-Demir G (2002). Epileptic seizures in Behcet disease. *Epilepsia*, 43, 832–35

B. Pourabbase, M.A. Nazariniaf, Z. Habibagahif, M.J. Fattahig, A. Ghaderig. (2009). CSF levels of cytokines in Neurobehçet's disease. *Clinical Neurology and Neurosurgery*; 111, 507–510.

Bank I, Weart C. (1984). Dural sinus thrombosis in Behçet's disease. *Arthritis Rheum*; 27: 816–818.

Barros R, Santos E, Moreira B, et al. (2007). Clinical characterization and pattern of neurological involvement of Behc¸et's disease in fifteen Portuguese patients. *Clin Exp Rheumatol*, 24(Suppl. 42), S31.

Ben Ghorbel I, Ibnelhadj Z, Zouari M, Nagi S, Khanfir M, Hentati F, et al. (2005). Behçet's disease associated with peripheral neuropathy. *Rev Neurol*, 161, 218–20.
Benamour S, Naji T, Alaoui F-Z, Kabli H, El Aidouni S. (2006). Manifestation neurologiques de la maladie de Behc¸et. *Rev Neurol*, 162, 1084–90.
Bennett DL, McCabe DJ, Stevens JM, Mifsud V, Kitchen ND, Giovannoni G. (2004). Tumefactive Neurobehçet disease. *Neurology* Aug 24; 63(4):709.
Borhani Haghighi A. (2008). Comment on "histopathology of central nervous system lesions in Behçet's disease". *J Neurol Sci*; 270: 211.
Borhani HaghighiA. (2009). Treatment of Neuro-Behçet's disease: an update. *Expert Rev Neurother*. Apr; 9(4):565-74.
Borhani-Haghighi A, Afl aki E, Ketabchi L.(2008). The prevalence and characteristics of different types of headache in patients with Behcet's disease, a case-control study. *Headache*; 48, 424–29.
Borhani-Haghighi A, Samangooie S, Ashjazadeh N, et al. (2006). Neurological manifestations of Behçet's disease. *Saudi Med Journal*, 1542–6.
Bousser MG, Ferro JM. (2007). Cerebral venous thrombosis: an update. *Lancet Neurol*, 6, 162–70.
Calguneri M, Onat AM, Ozturk MA, et al. (2005). Transverse myelitis in a patient with Behçet's disease: favourable outcome with a combination of interferon-alpha. *Clin Rheumatol*, 24, 64–66.
Chroni E, Monastirli A, Polychronopoulos P, Pasmatzi E, Georgiou S, Tsambaos D. (2008). Epileptic seizures as the sole manifestation of Neurobehçet's disease: complete control under interferon-alpha treatment. Seizure; Dec, 17(8): 744-7.
Coban O, Bahar S, Akman-Demir G, Tas¸ci B, Yurdakul S, Yazici H, et al. (1999). Masked assessment of MRI findings: is it possible to differentiate Neurobehçet's disease from other central nervous system diseases? *Neuroradiology*; 41: 255–60.
D. Kidd (2006). The prevalence of headache in Behçet's syndrome. *Rheumatology*, 45, 621–623
Ebru Aykutlu, Betül Baykan, Piraye Serdarolu, Aysen Gökyiit, Gülsen Akman-Demir (2002). Epileptic seizures in Behcet disease. *Epilepsia*, 43, 832–35.
Gu¨lsen Akman-Demir, Piraye Serdaroglu, Banu Tasc and the Neuro-Behc¸et Study Group*. (1999). Clinical patterns of neurological involvement in Behçet's disease: evaluation of 200 patients *Brain*; 122, 2171–218.1
Guak TH, Kim YI, Park SM, Kim JS. (2002). Paroxysmal focal dystonia in neuro-Behçet by a small ipsilateral thalamic lesion. *Eur Neurol*, 47, 183–84.
Guls_en Akman-Demir , Erdem Tuzun , Sema _Icoz , Nilufer Yes_ilot , Sibel P. Yentur , Murat Kurtuncu , Melike Mutlu a, Guher Saruhan-Direskeneli . (2008). Interleukin-6 in neuro-Behcet's disease: Association with disease subsetsand long-term outcome. *Cytokine 44*; 373–376.
Hadfi eld MG, Aydin F, Lippman HR, Kubal WS, Sanders KM. (1996). Neuro-Behcet's disease. *Clin Neuropathol*, 15, 249–55.
Hamzaoui K, Hamzaoui A, Ghorbel I, Khanfir M, Houman H. (2006). Levels of IL-15 in serum and cerebrospinal fluid of patients with Behçet's disease. *Scand J Immunol*; 64(December (6): 655–60.
Hatemi G, Silman A, Bang D, Bodaghi B, Chamberlain AM, et al. (2008). Management of Behçet's disease: a systematic literature review for the EULAR evidence-based recommendationsEULARExpert Committee. *Ann Rheum Dis*; 67:1656-62.

Hirohata S, Isshi K, Oguchi H, Ohse T, Haraoka H, Takeuchi A, et al. (1997). Cerebrospinal fluid interleukin-6 in progressive NeuroBehçet's syndrome. *Clin Immunol Immunopathol;* 82(January (1):12–7.

Hirohata S, Suda H, Hashimoto T. (1998). Low dose weekly methotrexate for progressive neuropsychiatric manifestations in Behçet's disease. *J Neurol Sci;* 159:181–5.

Hirohata S.(2007). Potential new therapeutic options for involvement of central nervous system in Behcet's disease (neuro-Behcet's syndrome). *Curr Rheumatol Rev,* 3, 297–303.

Hirohata S.(2008). Histopathology of central nervous system lesions in Behcet's disease. *J Neurol Sci,* 267, 41–47

Houman MH, Neffati H, Braham A, et al. Behçet's disease in Tunisia.(2007). Demographic, clinical and genetic aspects in 260 patients. *Clin Exp Rheumatol;* 25(Suppl. 45):S58–64.

Houman MH, Smiti-Khanfir M, Hamzaoui K. (2008). Traitements actuels et perspectives thérapeutiques dans la maladie de Behc¸et. *Presse Med;* 37: 25–35

Imoto H, Nishizaki T, Nogami K, Sakamoto K, Nomura S, Akimura T, et al. (2002). Neuro-Behcet's disease manifesting as a neoplasm-like lesion case report. *Neurol Med Chir (Tokyo)* Sep; 42(9):406–9)

Jae-Hyeok Heo, Soon-Tae Lee, Kon Chu, Manho Kim. (2008) Neuro-Behcet's disease mimicking multiple brain tumors: Diffusion-weighted MR study and literature review *Journal of the Neurological Sciences 264;* 177–181

Joseph FG, Scolding NJ. (2007). Neurobehçet's disease in Caucasians: a study of 22 patients. *Eur J Neurol* Feb; 14(2):174–80.

Kaku Y, Hamada JI, Kuroda JI, Kai Y, Morioka M, Kuratsu JI. (2007). Multiple peripheral middle cerebral artery aneurysms associated with Behçet's disease. *Acta Neurochir (Wien),* 149: 823–27.

Kidd D, Steuer A, Denman AM, Rudge P (1999). Neurological complications of Behcet's syndrome. *Brain,* 122: 2183–94.

Kizilkilic O, Albayram S, Adaletli I, Ak H, Islak C, Kocer N. Mascalchi M, Cosottini M, Cellerini M, Paganini M, Arnetoli G.(1998). MRI of spinal cord involvement in Behçet's disease: case report. *Neuroradiology,* 40, 255–57.

Kocer N, Islak C, Siva A, Saip S, Akman C, Kantarci O, et al. (1999). CNS involvement in neuro-Behcet syndrome: an MR study. *AJNR Am JNeuroradiol* Jun–Jul; 20(6):1015–24.

Kosters K, Bos MM, Wesseling P, Smeets SM, van der Ven AJ, Bredie SJ.(2006). An unusual cause of a cerebral tumour in a young patient. Behçet's disease. *Neth J Med,* 64: 152.

Kotter I, Gunaydin I, Batra M, Vonthein R, Stubiger N, Fierlbeck G, et al. (2005). CNS involvement occurs more frequently in patients with Behc¸et's disease under cyclosporin A (CSA) than under other medications-results of a retrospective analysis of 117 cases. *Clin Rheumatol;* 1–5.

Kuriwaka R, Kunishige M, Nakahira H, et al. (2004). Neuro-Behcet's disease with chorea after remission of intestinal Behcet's disease. *Clin Rheumatol,* 23: 364–67.

Lee SH, Yoon PH, Park SJ, Kim DI. (2001). MRI findings in neuro-Behcet's disease. *Clin Radiol,* 56, 485–94.

Litvan I, Roig C, Rovira A, Ruscalleda J. (1987). Behçet's syndrome masquerading as tumor. *Neuroradiology;* 29:103.

Lo Monaco A, La Corte R, Caniatti L, Borrelli M, Trotta F (2006). Neurological involvement in North Italian patients with Behçet disease. *Rheumatol Int*, 26, 1113-9.

M.H. Houmana, R. Salem, T. Ben Salem (2009). Neurological involvement in Behçet disease Les manifestations neurologiques de la maladie de Behçet. *La Revue de médecine interne*.

Matsuo K, Yamada K, Nakajima K, Nakagawa M. (2005). Neuro-Behçet disease mimicking brain tumor. *Am J Neuroradiol*, 26, 650-73.

Miller HD, Ormerod IEC, Gibson A, du Boulay EP, Rudge P,McDonald WI. (1987). MR brain scanning in patients with vasculitis: differentiation from multiple sclerosis. *Neuroradiology*; 29:226-31.

Mnif N, Rajhi H, Mlika N, Kechaou S, BenAbdallah N, Hamza R. (2006). Aspect En IRM du Neurobehçet. *J Neuroradiol*; 33:250-4.

Moskau S, Urbach H, Hartmann A, Schmidt S. Multifocal myelitis in Behcet's disease (2003). *Neurology*, 60: 517.

Mossadeq R, Karouache A, Bouraza A, et al. (2004). Neuro-Behçet's syndrome and thrombosis of Rosenthal's basilar vein: a report of twelve cases. *Rev Neurol*, 160, 935-8.

Namer IJ, Karabudak R, Zileli T, et al. (1987). Peripheral nervous system involvement in Behçet's diseases. Eur Neurol; 26:235-40.

Namer IJ, Karabudak R, Zileli T, Ruacan S, Ku¨c¸u¨kali T, KansuE. (1987). Peripheral nervous system involvement in Behçet's disease. *EurNeurol*, 26, 235-40.

Neudorfer M, Feiler-Ofri V, Geyer O, Reider I. (1993). Behçet's disease presenting as a cerebral tumour. *Neuroradiology; 35:145.*

Niino M, Ogata A, Kikuchi S, Tashiro K, Nishihira J.(2000). Macrophage migration inhibitory factor in the cerebrospinal fluid of patients with conventional and optic-spinal forms of multiple sclerosis and neuro-Behcet's disease. *JNeurol Sci*; 179(October (Suppl. 1-2)):127-31.

O'Duffy JD, Robertson DM, Goldstein NP. (1984). Chlorambucil in the treatment of uveitis and meningoencephalitis of Behc¸et's disease. *Am J Med*; 76:75- 84.

Oktem-Tanor O, Baykan-Kurt B, Gurvit IH, Akman-Demir G, Serdaroglu P.(1999). Neuropsychological follow-up of 12 patients with neuro-Behçet disease. *J Neuro*, 246, 113- 9.

Orhan Deniza, Ali C, aykoylub, Gonul Vural a, Yakup Albayrakb,, S ' adiye Temela. (2009). A case study of Neuro-psycho-Behçet's Syndrome presenting with psychotic attack. *Clinical Neurology and Neurosurgery*; 111 877 - 879

Pamir MN, Kansu T, Erbiengi A, Zileli T. (1981). Papilloedema in Behçet's syndrome. *Arch Neurol*, 38, 643-45.

S. B'chir-Hamzaoui, T. Larbi, M. Abdallah, A. Harmel, M. Ennafaa, K. Bouslama, M. Ben Dridi, S.M'rad (2009). Pour le groupe Behçet Maghreb Behçet's disease in Maghreb: Behçet Maghreb study about 1460 cases *La Revue de médecine interne*, 30S S229-S231

Saip S, Siva A, Altintas A, et al.(2005). Headache in Behcet's syndrome. *Headache*, 45, 911-19.

Scardamaglia L, Desmond PM, Gonzales MF, Bendrups A, Brotdmann A, Kay TWH. (2001). Behcet's disease with cerebral vasculitis. *Int Med J*, 31, 560-61.

Schmolck H. (2005). Large thalamic mass due to Neurobehçet disease. *Neurology* Aug 9; 65(3):436.

Siva A, Fresco I. (2000). Behçet's disease. *Curr Treat Options Neurol*; 2: 435- 448.

Siva A, Kantarci OH, Saip S, et al. (*2001*) Behçet's disease: diagnostic and prognostic aspects of neurological involvement. *J Neurol;* 248: 95–103.

Siva A, Saip S, Kantarci O, Hamuryudan V, Koc¸er N, Islak C, et al. (1997). Neuro-Behc¸et syndrome (NBS): clinical and imaging features. *Neurology;* 48 (3 Suppl): A362.

Siva A, Saip S. (2009). The spectrum of nervous system involvement in Behçet's syndrome and its differential diagnosis. *J Neurol;* 256:513–29.

Siva A. (2001). Vasculitis of the nervous system. *J Neurol.;* 248: 451- 468.

Taner E, Cos¸ar B, Burhano˘glu S, Caliko˘glu E, Onder M, Arikan Z. (2007). Depression and anxiety in patients with Behc¸et's disease compared with that in patients with psoriasis. *Int J Dermatol*, 46, 1118–24.

Tarzi MD, Lightman S, Longhurst HJ. (2005). An exacerbation of Behçet's syndrome presenting with bilateral papillitis. *Rheumatology (Oxford*), 44, 953–54.

Tunc R, Saip S, Siva A, et al. (2004). Cerebral venous thrombosis is associated with major vessel disease in Behcet's syndrome. *Ann Rheum Dis;*63, 1693–4.

Tunc R, Saip S, Siva A, Yazici H. (2003). Cerebral venous thrombosis Moskau S, Urbach H, Hartmann A, Schmidt S. Multifocal myelitis in Behcet's disease. *Neurology*, 60, 517.

Turker H, Terzi M, Bayrak O, Cengiz N, Onar M, Us O.(2008). Visual evoked potentials in differential diagnosis of multiple sclerosis and neuro-behc¸et's disease. Tohoku J Exp Med, 216, 109–16.

Tuzgen S, Kaya AH, Erdincler D, Oguzoglu SA, Ulu O, Saip S. (2003). Two cases of neuro-Behcet's disease mimicking cerebral tumor. *Neurol India* Sep; 51(3):376–8.

Voroos Gm, Sandhu SS, Pandit R.(2006). Acute optic neuropathy in patients with Behcet's disease. Report of two cases. *Ophthalmologica*, 220, 400–05.

Wang CR, Chuang CY, Chen CY. (1992). Anticardiolipin antibodies and interleukin-6 in cerebrospinal fluid and blood of Chinese patients with Neurobehçet's syndrome. *Clin Exp Rheumatol;* 10: 599–602.

Wechsler B, Sbaï A, Du-Boutin LT, Duhaut P, Dormont D, Piette JC. (2002). Manifestations neurologiques de la maladie de Behc¸et. *Rev Neurol*, 158, 926–33.

Wechsler B, VidailhetM, Piette JC, BousserMG, Dell Isola B, Ble´tryO, et al. (1992). Cerebral venous thrombosis in Behçet's disease. *Neurology;* 42: 614–8.

Wolf SM, Schotland DL, Phillips LL. (1965). Involvement of nervous system in Behcet's syndrome. *Arch Neurol;* 12:315–25.

Worthmann F, Bruns J, Turker T, Gosztonyi G. (1996). Muscular involvementin Behc¸et's disease. [Review]. *Neuromuscul Disord*, 6, 247–53.

Yazici H, Fresko I, Yurdakul S. (2007). Behcet's syndrome: disease manifestations, management, and advances in treatment. *Nat Clin Pract Rheumatol;* 3: 148–55.

Yesilot N, Celiktas S, Mutlu M, et al. (2006). Cerebral venous and dural sinus thrombosis associated with Behcet's disease. *Clin Exp Rheumatol*, 24 (suppl 42): S30.

Yesilot N, Mutlu M, Gungor O, Baykal B, Serdaroglu P, Akman-Demir G. (2007). Clinical characteristics and course of spinal cord involvement in Behcet's disease. *Eur J Neurol*, 14, 729–37.